Symptoms and Signs in Pediatric Surgery

Georges L. Kaiser
Author

Symptoms and Signs in Pediatric Surgery

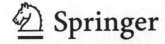 Springer

Author
Prof. em. Georges L. Kaiser
University of Berne
Department of Pediatric Surgery
Inselspital
Berne
Switzerland

Originally published: Georges Kaiser: Leitsymptome in der Kinderchirurgie.
© Verlag Hans Huber, 2005

ISBN 978-3-642-31160-4   ISBN 978-3-642-31161-1   (eBook)
DOI 10.1007/978-3-642-31161-1
Springer Heidelberg New York Dordrecht London

Library of Congress Control Number: 2012950009

Printed on acid-free paper

Springer is part of Springer Science+Business Media (www.springer.com)

Dedicated to my parents Otto and Angela Kaiser and to my wife Regine Kaiser-Schillig

Foreword

Pediatric surgery as a medical specialty is undeniably living a niche existence. This is generally reflected in university curriculums where the transmission of knowledge and skills in pediatric surgery plays only a minor role – understandable, given the immense width and depth of today's medical knowledge. This marginalization of the young in need of surgery presents a problem for doctors' advanced and continuing education and calls for growing a new generation of specialists in this field in order to secure knowledge, care, and scientific advancement. Let us not forget the persons directly concerned: newborns, young children, adolescents, and their parents. Even though pediatric surgery weighs little in medical curriculums, it is crucial for the patients and their kin. Circumstances necessitating a pediatric surgical intervention are often far-reaching and tragic for all family members, and the doctor thus needs to stand by them not only as an expert but as an empathetic human being.

In 2001, Prof. Georges Louis Kaiser, M.D., submitted a proposal to the e-learning development team of the Institute of Medical Education (University of Bern) for the creation of pediatric surgical tutorials over the Internet. His aim was to make available worldwide the abundant material he had accrued over the years in pursuit of his vision: preventing any suffering that can be averted through the dissemination of knowledge. The contents-to-be were processed over a period of 10 years, in order to meet didactic and professional requirements. The quintessence of Prof. Kaiser's work as author of this project is the book at hand, and the "book/Internet" duality renders the question of pluses and cons of one or the other irrelevant because they were made to complement each other.

That said, we invite the readers to broaden and consolidate their knowledge in pediatric surgery and to contribute to its scientific and clinical advancement, for there are many who depend on help from professionals in this medical field.

Bern, Switzerland   Stefan Minder
Bern, Switzerland   Béatrice Boog

Preface

This book is written for physicians who care for children: pediatricians, general practitioners, pediatric surgeons, general surgeons, and specialists whose activity includes also children. This book has been put together based on many years of personal experience, serves as source of specific informations about pediatric surgery for people who need them occasionally or day-to-day, and represents basic and comprehensive knowledge for pediatric surgeons in training and afterward.

The central target of this book concerns the clinical significance and presentation, differential diagnostic delineation, and indication for specific treatment of most disorders of pediatric surgery and of some in related fields. This book intends to lead the reader and specifically the pediatric surgeon of developed and developing countries to a total care of the confided child even if she/he or another physician cannot or will not take over surgery in each field.

The reader wonders how this book should or can be used: (1) If the reader wants a specific information about a known disorder, the index or table of contents leads her or him to the desired chapter and by stereotypically arranged headlines "occurrence, clinical significance or presentation, workups or differential diagnosis, and treatment or prognosis" to the specific informations of the chosen disorder; (2) If the reader starts from a characteristic leading symptom or sign without precise knowledge of the most probable disorder, she or he chooses first the involved body area (they are arranged in the following order "head, neck, chest, abdomen, urogenital system, and back") and finds there the most suitable leading symptom or sign of which totally 35 are available and correspond each to a main chapter. The reader finds at the beginning of each chosen main chapter an introduction to the assessment of the leading symptom or sign and to correlate it with specific disorders of the differential diagnosis; (3) Although the diagrams of this book display essential clinical, radiological, and operative characteristics of some disorders in an abstracted manner, the reader wants realistic pictures; therefore, she or he is referred to the e-learning box at the end of each main chapter that allows her or him to choose from a relatively large number of clinical, radiological, and intraoperative findings the wanted disorder by Internet without any additional expenses; (4) Although the often large list of references is not complete, some case reports enable the reader to participate in the clinical everyday work, some more detailed papers to complete the knowledge in some specific fields, and other publications to perform her or his own literature research; (5) Treatment and prognosis in general and those in specific fields change continually. In the last two decades, minimally invasive surgery has increasingly entered many fields of pediatric surgery. The description of some common open interventions does not deal with technical aspects of minimally invasive surgery although it is basic to it. But its significance, indications and contraindications, and advantages or drawbacks are mentioned in some disorders under the headline "indication for surgery" or in some references. It is possible that the next decades lead to a balance between disorder in which minimally invasive surgery is superior to open surgery and those in which open surgery is still the golden standard if minimally invasive surgery is not only performed because it can be technically done ("l'art pour l'art") but also global aspects of pediatric surgical training, restricted resources, and wear of materials are considered.

This book is based on the experience as author and coauthor of the textbook "Bettex M, Genton N, Stockmann M (1982) *Kinderchirurgie Diagnostik, Indikation, Therapie, Prognose Begründet von M. Grob*.Thieme, Stuttgart," and as author of the booklet "Kaiser G (2005) *Leitsymptome in der Kinderchirurgie*. Hans Huber, Bern."

Many thanks are dedicated to the lector Dr. med. Klaus Reinhardt of Hans Huber Publishers and especially to Gabrielle Schroeder, editorial director of Springer Publishing, and her lector who provided me with possibility to publish in Springer and designed the final, appropriate, and handsome shape, to Joe Arun S.A., Project Manager, and the staff at SPi Global, India, to Stefan Minder and Felix M. Schmitz of the Institute of Medical Education (University of Bern) for development and implementation of their e-learning tool "Blended Learning and Formative Assessments for Specialist Training and Continuing Education in Pediatric Surgery," to Hans Holzherr for his diagrammatic drawings, and to Ursula Güder for her IT support. Finally, I thank the numerous children and their parents for whom I was directly or indirectly the responsible pediatric surgeon, my medical staff and nurses, my medical students and faculty colleges, and all trainees in pediatric surgery or other fields for their trust, challenge, inputs, criticism, and gratitude.

Contents

Tumors, Tumorlike Masses, and Abnormalities of Scalp, Calvaria, and Adjacent Regions

Masses and abnormalities of the scalp and calvaria occur frequently, are caused by a wide variety of possible pathologies, and are often underestimated in their significance by the primary care provider. Table 1.1 gives a surview of the possible lesions and marks them according to their frequency. **Dermoid and epidermoid cysts** belong to the most frequently quoted masses, **atretic cephalocele, ossified cephalhematoma, eosinophilic granuloma, and hemangioma** to the next frequent masses in the pediatric neurosurgical literature and **pilomatricoma** in the dermatological papers. Up to one third of the lesions have an intracranial and almost half of these an intradural extension.

History and physical findings often allow a preliminary differentiation and evaluation of the considered visible and palpable lesions:

- **Time of recognition** by the caregiver or patient, **growth** during the observation time until the first consultation, and **appearance** of local and general **signs and symptoms**. Vascular malformations are present since birth. Hemangiomas (defined as growing vascular tumors) become visible in the second half of the first month of life and grow in the second to third month and thereafter. A visible mass of the scalp, pain, and signs of infection or bleeding are the most frequently observed presenting symptoms.
- At first consultation, **age** (congenital vs. acquired pathologies), **location** (midline vs. lateral site of the lesion; congenital midline lesions have more

Table 1.1 Tumors, tumorlike masses, and abnormalities of the scalp, calvaria, and adjacent regions*

Congenital pathologies
- Dermoid and epidermoid cysts
- o Special forms of dermoid and epidermoid cysts (midline forms)
- o Vascular malformations
- o Atretic cephalocele (abortive encephalocele)
- o Cephalocele (encephalocele)
- o Nasal glioma (glial heterotopia of the nose)
- o Sinus pericranii
- o Congenital scalp and skull defects

Traumatic pathologies
- Cephalhematoma
- o Growing or enlarging skull fracture (leptomeningeal cyst)
- Subperiosteal and subgaleal (subaponeurotic) hematoma

Inflammatory pathologies
- o Infections of the galea and osteomyelitis of the skull

Neoplastic pathologies
- Hemangioma
- o Rare tumors and tumorlike masses of the soft tissue including pilomatrixoma
- o Osteoma
- o Fibrous dysplasia
- Eosinophilic granuloma (histiocytosis X)
- o Rare benign and malignant skull tumors (including neuroblastoma metastasis, melanotic neuroectodermal tumor)

*Some pathologies of the adnexes of eye and nose
- = relatively frequent pathologies
o = relatively rare pathologies, characteristic pathologies are quoted as single pathologies

likely an intracranial extension than lateral ones), and **local findings** are of crucial importance for the differential diagnoses: changes of the overlying skin; presence of a minute opening; tenderness, consistency, and mobility of the mass; volume changes on crying or depending on posture and emptying of the contents.

Essential knowledge of the frequent or typical pathologies and careful clinical examination allows frequently a preliminary diagnosis without or with minimal additional examinations. On the other hand, sophisticated work-ups may be indispensable for specification of a lesion and its possible intracranial expansion, or the final diagnosis can only be achieved by histological examination of the excised mass.

The **possible work-up examinations** include plain skull x-ray, ultrasound (with Doppler), CT (with contrast, 3D reconstruction), MRI (T1-/T2-weighted, dynamic studies with gadolinium [Ga-DTPA]), and scintiscans. CT or MRI combined with angiography may replace invasive angiography.

These methods and/or their modifications help to characterize the different pathologies and their relation to extra- and intracranial structures. They should be applied according to the suspected pathology and their diagnostic power instead of a whole battery of possible examinations. Whenever possible, **complete surgical removal** should be performed. The techniques depend on the expected pathology and should be followed by a histological examination (if needed, combined with specific methods such as immunochemistry) in every case because a precise preoperative diagnosis or differential diagnoses are possible at best in approximately 90 %.

1.1   Congenital Pathologies

1.1.1   Dermoid and Epidermoid Cysts

Occurrence

Dermoid cysts are the most common congenital masses of galea, calvaria, and of the adjacent regions (>50 %). They are remnants of the superficially or deeply sequestrated ectoderm,

develop into elements of the whole skin including its appendages or epidermis, and persist as cysts and/or sinuses. According to the published series with histological work-up, most of them are dermoid # and not epidermoid tumors.

Types

Differentiation between lateral and midline forms is important. They lie under the skin, are located partially or exclusively in the calvaria, and may extend as far as the dura (categories 1–3 ##). At their periphery, the dermoid and epidermoid cysts are connected with the skin, and a visible opening leading to a sinus tract may be present.

Mainly in the midline posterior (occipital including posterior fontanel) and anterior (nasofrontal including nasal tip) forms, an epidural mass or an intradural and intraparenchymatous part can be observed (categories 4 and 5, Fig. 1.1).

Clinical Significance

• Increase in size, perforation, infection, and rare malignant degeneration are inherent risks apart from the parent's concern about cosmesis and malignancy.

History, Clinical Findings

Dermoid and epidermoid cysts are present since birth. Their size may increase with body growth or more rapidly, and the first consultation occurs in developed countries mostly in infancy.

The preferential site is periorbital (up to 50 % of all head and neck dermoid tumors). Pathognomonic is a roundish, usually nontender, and firm *mass of the lateral eyebrow* that is fixed to the periosteum of the orbital rim in the area of the frontozygomatic suture #.

Less frequently is an analogous *mass of the medial eye corner* #. Additional sites are the *galea and/or calvaria lateral to the midline* preferably over the cranial sutures or in the frontoparietal region, sometimes combined with a tuft of hair #. Some of them are recognized by chance on a lateral skull x-ray performed for other reasons. The round or oval bone defect with a sclerotic rim is characteristic for the intraosseous dermoid tumor #.

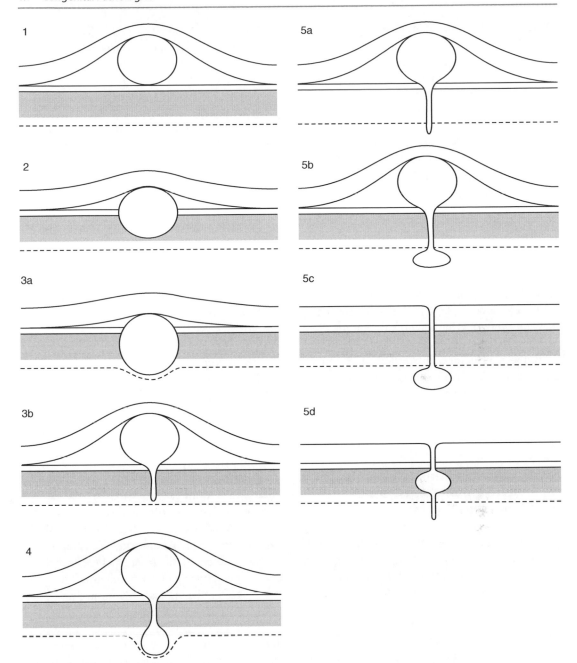

Fig. 1.1 Types and categories of epidermoid and dermoid cysts. *1*: cyst strictly below the skin. *2*: cyst underneath the skin and within the skull. *3a* and *b*: cyst or fistula mainly within the skull. Both variants extend to the dura. *4*: depression of the dura by the cyst that perforates the bone like a sandglass. *5a–d*: variants of the cyst that perforate the dura either without/with a fistula or with/without an orifice at the surface of the skin. The knowledge of these categories is important due to the inherent danger of complication and for total excision. The categories apply also to other types of cysts and masses

Differential Diagnosis, Work-Up Examinations

The frequent dermoid and epidermoid cyst of the lateral eyebrow does not need additional examinations. In case of a dermoid tumor of the frontoparietal region, a lateral skull x-ray demonstrates possible calvarial involvement (categories 2 and 3 are possible). Dermoids of the medial eye corner have several differential diagnoses, and work-up examinations are necessary similar to the frontonasal midline masses.

Therapy, Prognosis

A prompt and complete resection with a spindle of the overlying skin is necessary in every case. At the same time, a possible extension of the dermoid tumor (cyst or sinus tract) to the dura must be carefully considered, and in every case of gross epidural involvement and intradural extension, a pediatric neurosurgeon must be consulted before surgery.

If these principles are followed, permanent cure is achieved on condition that the histological examination confirms the diagnosis and previously no suppuration or spontaneous perforation has occurred.

1.1.2   Special Forms of Dermoid and Epidermoid Cysts (Midline Forms)

Preferred sites are the anterior fontanel and the back of the head and nasal region although dermoid tumors can be observed everywhere along the sagittal and frontal suture. In contrast to the former regions with possible intradural extension, it is unusual in parietal, anterior fontanel, and frontal dermoid cysts.

The **dermoid cyst of the anterior fontanel** # amounts to round 25 % of all calvarial dermoid tumors, and the black component in a population may be important for their frequency. They differ from those of other sites by the rapid growth in some of them and may contain a clear fluid, which is explained by the activity of exocrine sweat glands.

The nontender, broadly sessile mass over or close to the anterior fontanel is round, nonpulsatile,

and does not increase on crying, which allows clinically together with other findings a differentiation from other pathologies such as cephalhematoma, encephalocele, and hemangioma or vascular malformations. Depending on the age at presentation, a roundish skull defect may be present.

Instead of CT or MRI, ultrasound allows a delineation of the dura and the sagittal sinus in early infancy #.

The **surgeon** must consider in a category 3 variety a possibly tight adhesion of the dermoid cyst with the sagittal sinus.

The **frontonasal form** occurs between the glabella and the tip of the nose #. The term **nasal dermal sinus cyst** considers the frequency of an associated sinus in up to 50 % and its clinical implications.

A painless, cystic enlargement at any part of the nose, possibly associated with one or several dimples, a minute opening #, and possibly protruding hair, first or recurrent localized inflammation(s) and pus discharge, nasal airway obstruction, and meningitis or cerebral abscess are the presenting symptoms, signs, or hints in the history.

The extracranial dermoid tumor lies either subcutaneously and/or in the deep nasal structures (in about 80 %) or extends intracranially (in up to 20 %) to the leaves of the falx through the foramen cecum, cribriform plate, or fonticulus nasalis. A combination with widening of the nasal dorsum or hypertelorism is possible.

The differential diagnoses include encephalocele, nasal glioma, and in asymmetric forms, dermoid cyst of the medial eye corner and other pathologies of the eye adnexes.

The work-up examinations are CT for evaluation of frontobasal osseous structures with signs of intranasal and intracranial extension (wide septum, broad frontonasal suture, large foramen cecum, and bifid crista galli) and MRI for differential diagnosis and for the location, structure of the dermoid tumor, and its possible complications. Nasal fiber endoscopy can be a useful adjunct.

The **surgical approach** is transnasal, and in case of intracranial extension, combined with an intracranial access as multidisciplinary procedure (excision of the whole dermoid tumor and sinus tract and repair of the frontobasal hole and dura).

Prognosis depends on the time and type of surgery (prophylactic vs. therapeutic intervention after preceding infection) and its completeness, for example, repeated abscesses after incomplete removal of the intranasal part of the dermoid tumor.

In the **dermoid cyst of the base of the columella,** neither an intranasal nor an intracranial extension is observed.

Dermal sinus and dermoid tumor of the posterior fossa: Its *external orifice is located at the level of the posterior fontanel, inion, and occiput* (including the lateral part such as the lambdoid suture and rarely a supratentorial site). The anomaly has *a sinus tract with/without a subgaleal dermoid tumor which extends mostly either to the subdural space or to the cerebellum* (mostly ending as dermoid tumor and rarely with a blind end) #. The same principles of work-up examinations, therapy, and prognosis as in frontonasal forms are applicable for the dermoid tumor of the back of the head. The **surgery** as outpatient is not appropriate, the adherence of the sinus tract to the torcular Herophili, and the possibility of spilling of the cyst content must be considered (rupture with severe hemorrhage, recurrent cyst, or aseptic meningitis).

1.1.3 Vascular Malformations

Occurrence
Severe genuine vascular malformations are infrequent in comparison to hemangiomas of whom 50 % occur in the region of the head and mainly in the face. In contrast to the well-known venous vascular malformations (the so-called cavernous hemangiomas) of the brain, those of the galea and calvaria are rare #.

Types, Clinical Significance
Depending on the histopathological appearance and the hemodynamics, four major categories can be differentiated: Pure and complex-combined vascular malformations, each of them either as slow- or fast-flow type. To the pure slow-flow types belong **capillary, lymphatic, and venous vascular malformations**, to the fast-flow the **arteriovenous vascular malformations**. To the slow- and fast-flow complex-combined vascular malformations belong known syndromes such as **Sturge-Weber syndrome**. Their clinical significance is as follows:

- Vascular malformations in general and capillary vascular malformations (port wine stain) specifically may be red flags signaling significant pathologies such as atretic cephalocele or Sturge-Weber syndrome.
- Venous and more frequently arteriovenous vascular malformations may lead to pain, bleeding, ulceration, infection, mass effect, recurrent thrombosis, and congestive heart failure.
- Severe bleeding may be observed after head injury or during surgery (vascular connections to the sagittal sinus and/or superficial cerebral veins).

Clinical Presentation
Vascular malformations *are present at birth, albeit not always evident or recognized, and grow proportionately to the child except for possible increases after trauma or during puberty.*

The faint blue spots or soft blue masses are localized or diffuse, compressible, and increase or decrease depending on the posture.

Arteriovenous malformations that consist of arterial feeding vessels, arteriovenous fistulas, and enlarged veins may appear during childhood. They present as *red and warm overlying skin, distinct tumor, and palpable buzz (whirr) or audible (thrill-bruit) noise.*

The term **sinus pericranii** is possibly only a complex of symptoms with different etiologies and not a pathological entity as such. It means an impressive network of dilated veins close to the midline that may be combined with corresponding irregular skull defects.

Differential Diagnosis, Work-Up Examinations
Although vascular malformations and their type can be recognized by history and clinical findings

in more than 90 %, hemangioma, cephalocele, dermoid cyst, and other tumorlike masses that are associated with some characteristics of a vascular malformation must be considered, for example, if they are compressible or display a specific color or shape.

Ultrasound with color Doppler as screening permits a differentiation between slow- and fast-flow vascular malformations. MRI (gadolinium, MR angio-/venography) delineates the size, the relationship to the adjacent structure, hemodynamics, and allows preoperative planning of surgery. Venous vascular malformations exhibit high signal intensity on T2-weighted images, and the pathognomonic phleboliths are recognizable by round signal voids in T1- and T2-weighted pictures. CT (contrast) is useful in case of calvarial involvement.

Therapy, Prognosis
In general, treatment is indicated in venous and arteriovenous vascular malformations to prevent the inherent or already occurring complications and to improve cosmesis.

Therapy includes laser (capillary vascular malformations), sclerotherapy, or superselective arterial embolization combined with resection (venous or arteriovenous vascular malformations) and, whenever possible, closure of the defect with normal galea by different techniques of plastic surgery including expansion of the adjacent skin by subcutaneous silicone bags.

The prognosis concerning permanent cure and cosmesis depends on the complexity and sequels of the vascular anomalies, the possibility to treat the whole malformation, and the availability of sufficient normal galea.

1.1.4 Atretic Cephalocele (Abortive Encephalocele)

Definition, Pathoanatomy
Atretic cephalocele is one of the four types of cephalocele and may be described as a lesion that gives no clue to its nature before modern neuroimaging and/or surgery is performed. The mass is cystic, parenchymatous, or mixed and attached to the dura or the intradural structures by

a solid stalk or a sinus tract through the osseous defect. It contains meninges, glias, neurons, and/or vascular and fibrous tissue.

Clinical Significance
• Discovery of atretic cephalocele is important because the lesion may be combined with other intracranial malformations (hydrocephalus, microencephaly, and structural abnormalities) and mental retardation or a red flag of a syndrome as in overt encephalocele.

Occurrence, Clinical Presentation
The mass is sometimes *present at birth, however, only recognized later in the occipital or parietal midline region and covered by alopecic skin that is thinned out toward its dome and may contain a dimple and/or a vascular abnormality ##. It is combined with a well-defined osseous defect* (which may be palpable). Spontaneous pain or *tenderness* may be present; the mass does not change its shape on crying or postural change and is not pulsatile in every case as in common types of cephalocele.

Differential Diagnosis, Work-Ups
Adopting the described characteristics, atretic cephalocele can be suspected clinically although other pathologies such as *vascular malformations or former hemangiomas and aplasia cutis # or dermoid tumor* are not excluded. CT and MRI confirm the clinical diagnosis.

Treatment, Prognosis
Surgery includes excision of the atrophied skin, removal of the stalk or sinus tract, and possibly dural repair, closure of the osseous defect, and skin plasty. Permanent cure is possible with complete excision.

1.1.5 Cephalocele (Encephalocele)

Occurrence, Pathoanatomy
Present since birth, encephalocele continues to grow postnatally. In Southeast Asia including north of India and to a lesser degree in Africa, the occurrence of anterior (sincipital) cephalocele

is similar to that of occipital encephalocele in the western countries (today <1 in 3–5,000 live births).

Encephalocele is a congenital herniation of cranial contents through a defect in the dura and the skull bone (and vertebrae in the suboccipital subtype). Rarely, they may be combined with lipomas (lipoencephalo- or lipomeningocele). Secondary encephaloceles occur after head injury or craniofacial surgery.

Seventy to eighty percent include **occipital cephaloceles #** (osseous defect somewhere between inion and foramen magnum) or the suboccipital subtype in the western countries. The remainder are **cranial vault cephaloceles** including the subtypes at the pterion or asterion, **anterior (frontoethmoidal or sincipital) types** with three subtypes protruding to the nasal root or the orbit, **basal types of encephalocele** with five subtypes protruding into the anterior or posterior nasal cavity, epipharynx, orbit, or pterygopalatine fossa, and **cranioschisis** (absent neurocranium).

Only 10–20 % of the occipital and cranial vault cephaloceles have no neural tissue (cranial meningocele), and the remaining 80–90 % contain brain tissue (meningoencephalocele).

Clinical Significance
- Cephalocele is the cranial counterpart of spina bifida. Combinations are possible.
- Disfigurement depending on its size.
- Mental and/or motor deficit in occipital and encephalocele of the cranial vault # (parietal encephalocele) except for encephalocele of the pterion (temporal encephalocele) and asterion.
- Combinations with CNS and other malformations such as hydrocephalus, microencephaly, agenesis of corpus callosum, or syndromes (e.g., **Meckel-Gruber syndrome**) occur frequently.
- Risks of complications such as ulceration with CSF leakage or meningitis and epilepsy, respiratory impairment in anterior and basal cephalocele, and progressive endocrinological and visual deficit in the latter.

Clinical Presentation, Types and Subtypes
The visible pedunculated or sessile mass lies mostly in the midline, is totally or partially covered with alopecic skin which is thinned out on its dome, contains hair and possibly a port wine stain at its base, and is cystic or mixed solid-cystic on palpation. The cephalocele sac may be tender, its tension depends on the present ICP, and its size is variable from a fingertip in some basal to a mass as large as the rest of the head in some occipital or parietal encephaloceles #.

A clinical diagnosis is possible referring to the described characteristics including transillumination. In contrast to the size, a sessile base and mixed consistency point to a meningoencephalocele.

In contrast to the **occipital, parietal, and anterior** (sincipital) **cephalocele** *with a visible mass that is uni- or multilobulated on the nasal root # or at the inner eye corner in the latter*, **basal cephalocele** is often recognized much later or by chance (e.g., in cleft palate). *Nasal airway obstruction* (e.g., RDS, apneic episodes, disorder of feeding), *mucous discharge, suspected nasal or epipharyngeal tumor, CSF leakage, hemorrhage, and meningitis* (spontaneously or after erroneous biopsy) belong to the signs and complications. In sincipital and basal cephalocele, there is usually no mental and/or motorial deficit; the former has *telecanthus and a variable degree of hypertelorism*; the latter may be associated with *facial midline anomalies* (e.g., cleft palate), *endocrinological (pituitary dysfunction) and/or visual disorders*. The latter may develop early or late on follow-up due to the involvement of the hypophysis and/or chiasm in the cephalocele sac or primary anomaly.

Differential Diagnosis, Work-Ups
In anterior (sincipital) cephalocele, nasal glioma, midline or eye corner dermoid cyst, pathologies of eye adnexes (e.g., mucocele of the lacrimal duct), and orbital tumors must be considered, and in basal cephalocele, nasal polyp, mucocele, glioma, dermoid cyst, teratoma, vascular malformation, hemangioma, and rhabdomyosarcoma or non-Hodgkin sarcoma.

MRI, CT, and rhinoscopy, as well as complete hormone screening, (in basal subtypes) permit the diagnosis of cephalocele and its site, extension, and contents, as well as possible asso-ciated malformations of the brain and other organs (e.g., optic nerve). 3D CT depicts the skull and its base for planning surgery. Endoscopically, the site of the mass in the nasal cavity allows a prelimi-nary differential diagnosis (e.g., intranasal enceph-alocele close to the septum in contrast to the more lateral site of **mucocele** or **nasal polyp**).

Therapy, Prognosis

Indication for and type of surgery depends on the type of cephalocele.

In many occipital and parietal types, surgery should be withheld after birth in case of severely defective patients with meningoencephalocele combined with considerable malformations as microencephaly and only be performed for care if they survive the neonatal period #. On the other hand, anterior and basal cephalocele should be operated electively as early as possible before the possible complications arise.

In general, **surgery** includes transection of the neck (if needed, resection of dysplastic brain tis-sue), watertight dural repair, autologous bone plasty of skull defect, and skin or mucous mem-brane closure. Except for the already mentioned types of encephalocele, early elective surgery to minimize the lifetime risk and to enable optimal remodeling is indicated in all patients, and depend-ing on the type, by a multidisciplinary team.

In sincipital cephalocele, the correction of the medial orbital wall by orbitomy and, if needed, the reconstruction of the nose must be included in the treatment of cephalocele by the often possible one-stage intra- and extracranial approach. In basal cephalocele, transoral, transpalatinal access is less harmful in posterior subtypes than tran-scranial (avoidance of damage to or resection of pituitary parts). In anterior subtypes, transcranial approach is mandatory.

Prognosis depends on the type of encephalo-cele, its content, and the possible associated mal-formations. In anterior and basal cephalocele, postoperative CSF leakage and possible infection are the main complications; pre- or postoperative transitory CSF diversion may minimize or treat this risk.

1.1.6 Nasal Glioma (Glial Heterotopia of the Nose)

Occurrence

The extranasal variety of nasal glioma and the already described nasal cephalocele (encephalo-cele) are rare lesions, are visible at birth, and occur also as intranasal form.

Clinical Significance, Clinical Presentation

- The extranasal variety of nasal glioma is one of the differential diagnoses of a nasal root mass.
- Possibility of nasal root widening, hypertelor-ism, and space occupying effect on the orbit.
- The intranasal variety leads to nasal airway obstruction.

The sessile or pedunculated round mass lies often asymmetrically over the bridge of the nose or close to the inner canthus, is smooth, firm, and noncompressible on palpation, and *covered by* nearly *normal skin #.*

Differential Diagnosis, Work-Ups

The mass does not enlarge with crying or strain-ing which allows together with other characteris-tics a differentiation from a typical cephalocele. The intranasal form is attached to the lateral wall on rhinoscopy in contrast to the intranasal cepha-locele that lies on the nasal septum.

CT and MRI are necessary for recognition of a possible additional intranasal or intracranial extra-dural site of the nasal glioma and for differentia-tion from cephalocele, dermoid cyst, pathologies of the eye adnexes, or a polyp. In cephalocele, there is a patent intracranial connection.

Therapy and Prognosis

Total removal of the mass together with the adherent skin leads to permanent cure because the mass deals histologically with simple glial tissue and vascularized fibrous tissue that con-tinues to grow. In the presence of a fibrous stalk, an intranasal or intracranial continuation must be considered (rhinotomy or craniotomy needed, possibility of creation of a CSF leak by surgery).

1.1.7   Sinus Pericranii

Sinus pericranii is a rare clinical entity composed of abnormal extracranial vascular tissue that communicates directly with intracranial sinuses via dilated emissary or diploic veins of the skull. It is either congenital or posttraumatic acquired (with or without endothelial lining).

Clinical Significance, Clinical Presentation
- The impressive appearance causes anxiety.
- Massive bleeding, air embolism, and infection are possible complications especially in trauma to the head.

Sinus pericranii is *mostly observed in the first decade of life and consists of gorgeous soft and fluctuant masses near the midline in the frontal and parieto-occipital region which vary in size with positional changes and with Valsalva's experiment #.* They are mostly asymptomatic although headache, localized pain, and other symptoms may occur.

The underlying skull contains often irregular (sometimes palpable) defects that accompany the venous plexuses and their intracranial communications #.

Differential Diagnosis, Work-Ups
Vascular malformations and hemangioma, different types of cephalhematoma and their sequels, cephalocele and leptomeningeal cyst (growing skull fracture) must be considered.

CT (3D CT) and MRI (MR angio-/venography) # not only permit, together with the clinical findings, the diagnosis but also a differentiation of the three types (type 1: circulation in a closed system from and to the sinus; type 2: circulation coming from the sinus and peripheral extracranial passage with possible high flow; type 3: pseudosinus pericranii with arterial participation). Red flags signaling type 2 are prominent scalp veins in addition to the masses and large holes of the skull.

Therapy and Prognosis
Although spontaneous regression is quoted in the literature, surgery is indicated to prevent possible complications and for cosmesis. The excision of the lesion must consider the possibility of massive bleeding especially in presence of large holes containing communicating veins.

Prognosis is good in prophylactic surgery provided precise work-up examinations have been performed and a careful control of the inherent bleedings is carried out including possible blood transfusion.

1.1.8   Congenital Scalp (Aplasia Cutis Congenita) and Skull Defects

Occurrence Pathoanatomy
Aplasia cutis congenita occurs spontaneously, familially, or inherited. It may be combined with CNS and other anomalies, associated with trisomy 13–15, and attributed to the intake of teratogens by the mother. The cause of the focal skin defects that are present at birth is not known.

Clinical Significance
- Disfigurement and/or loss of protection of the skull or brain if large enough.
- If combined with skull defect, risk of meningitis, sinus thrombosis, or hemorrhage.
- Congenital scalp defect is a possible red flag signaling a specific disease, syndrome, or chromosomal aberration.

Clinical Presentation
Aplasia cutis congenita is *in 60 % limited to the scalp with a preferential site on the vertex (80 %) although lateral, multiple, and extracranial localizations may occur. The diameter of the oval defect with irregular edges of atrophic skin varies from a few mm or 1–2 cm to much larger lesions in which the underlying calvarial bone may be involved in 20 % of the cases with a visible sinus and dura #.* Rarely the dura may be also missing. Aplasia cutis occurs in 40 % on the limbs or the trunk either isolated or combined with scalp lesions.

Congenital skull defects are either an integrated part of a congenital pathology, for instance, in cephalocele or aplasia cutis, or an isolated disorder without involvement of skin and meninges. Examples of the latter disorder are

foramina parietalia permagna, midline defects of the vertex (from the bregma to the occiput with sizes of 1–10 cm), or uni- or bilateral defects in the supraorbital region as small to very large frontal forms.

In contrast to the skull defects combined with aplasia cutis with occasional and delayed ossification, spontaneous closure does not occur in all other skull defects. The paired and oval foramina parietalia are localized in the posterior half of the vertex and appear sometimes as single defect early in infancy.

Differential Diagnosis, Work-Ups

Depending on the stage of the natural history of aplasia cutis with gradual spontaneous epithelization of the defect within several weeks after birth, atretic cephalocele, other alopecic lesions, heterotopic scalp tissue, and a so-called **nuchal bleb** must be considered in the differential diagnosis. Posttraumatic or surgical skull defects are also possible differential diagnoses. The term nuchal bleb is used in fetal cystic hygroma and for other disorders of back head and nape.

CT and, depending on the individual history and clinical examination, additional work-ups are necessary (e.g., genetic consultation and chromosomal examinations); the former examination delineates a possible skull defect and CNS malformations. Screening for skeletal, urological, or CNS malformations can be performed by ultrasound.

Therapy, Prognosis

In **aplasia cutis**, **management options** (wound dressing vs. operative skin closure) and timing of interventions (skin and, if needed, osseous closure in the neonatal period vs. staged procedure with early skin closure and later skull closure, if spontaneous ossification does not occur within the first years of life) are controversial.

Depending on the location (midline vs. lateral), the size (primary closure vs. preliminary skin expansion), the depth of the defect (isolated skin vs. dural defect), and the general condition and life expectancy, the appropriate management and schedule must be chosen individually.

Early skin closure by a rotational flap combined with repair of a possible calvarial defect with autologous calvarial bone in the neonatal period is probably the best option. On the other hand, it is possible to wait for spontaneous closure in very large skin defects with appropriate conservative management and make use of the spontaneous skin expansion by the retracting scar which gets much small than the original defect and allows assessment a possible ossification in the first half of infancy #.

In **the other forms of skull defects**, the use of autologous calvarial bone in early infancy is probably superior to postponement of this method and/or of acrylic cranioplasty in the toddler.

The prognosis concerning survival depends on the individual type of aplasia cutis and on the chosen management. It achieves today nearly the same good functional and cosmetic results as that for congenital skull defects.

1.2 Traumatic Pathologies

1.2.1 Cephalhematoma

Occurrence

Cephalhematoma is related to birth and instrumental delivery that add a considerable risk of its development. The reported incidence amounts to 0.2–2.5 % and more and depends on the composition of the investigated group of parturients and neonates.

Clinical Significance

- Cephalhematoma may be combined with severe head injury such as linear, growing, or depressed skull fracture (e.g., celluloid ball fracture), intracranial hematoma, and cerebral contusion.
- Cephalohematoma is a risk of complications such as infection (local or generalized such as osteomyelitis, meningitis, and/or septicemia), anemia and shock, and jaundice and hyperbilirubinemia (due to enclosed hemorrhage).
- Cephalhematoma may lead to disfiguring persistent ossified cephalhematoma still visible after several years (in 1.6–3.2 to 10 %) #.
- Incidence of cephalhematoma may be a quality sign of obstetrical care.

Clinical Presentation

The clinical presentation is dependent on the stage after birth. In the **acute stage**, *an oblong-oval mass becomes visible within 1–4 days after birth. It is confined to one (rarely to two or more) calvarial bone(s)* (in 85–91 % to the parietal, in 10 % to the occipital, and rarely to the frontal or another bone) and it *is soft to tense and fluctuating on palpation*. It may grow in size in the following days.

Although the majority of cephalhematomas are spontaneously resorbed within 1–6 weeks with a median time of 3–4 weeks, several may go through different stages of ossification, and some end up in a permanent ossification with either slow resolution by merging into the general contour of the growing calvaria or with a persistent disfiguring osseous mass #.

Differential Diagnosis, Work-Ups

In the acute stage, the differential diagnosis of cepalhematoma includes **caput succedaneum** (pasty swelling of the soft tissue without limitation to a certain calvarial bone and with poorly defined margins). It disappears within a few days, but it may be superimposed on a cephalhematoma and hide it, or a **subaponeurotic cephalhematoma** # (this rarely observed hematoma extends broadly under the epicranial aponeurosis and is a sign of a massive life-threatening hemorrhage due to birth trauma and/or a congenital or acquired platelets or coagulation disorder). In addition, a dermoid cyst, vascular malformation, cephalocele, growing skull fracture, and congenital neoplasm must be considered although less probable because of their specific characteristics.

In stage 1 or 2 of ongoing ossification (palpable ridge around the edges of or pliable layer over the cephalhematoma like rustling parchment), a depressed skull fracture or bone tumor must be considered, and in permanent ossification with a firm or hard osseous mass, the differential diagnosis includes **plagiocephaly or bone tumor,** especially if the initial diagnosis of cephalhematoma is not known.

CT (including 3D) and MRI allow the differential diagnosis, the definition of suspected head injury combined with acute cephalhematoma, and its stage of ossification after 6 weeks, describes the expansion of the ossified cephalhematoma, and possible depression of the inner table and other sequels of intracranial trauma.

Therapy, Prognosis

Each cephalhematoma needs appropriate follow-ups.

In the **acute stage**, evacuation is indicated in large cephalhematoma (size ≥5 cm diameter or size of a walnut to an apple) by proper punction in time (beyond day 6 after birth) and followed by mild compressive bandage, or in case of suspected infection, delayed resorption or increase in size, erythema of the overlying skin, and/or clinical or hematological signs of system infection.

In **persistent ossification**, removal of the osseous mass is indicated for cosmesis and rarely for repair of sequels of former head injury. Remodeling can be achieved either by excision of the outer table including the residual inner part of cephalhematoma or by removal of the whole cephalhematoma which allows remodeling outside of the patient by correction of the depressed inner table.

Spontaneous resolution of cephalhematoma occurs in up to 90 %. Except for risk of death and diminished quality of life in combined head injury, the outcome is uneventful if an ossified cephalhematoma is avoided by punction of large cephalhematomas or managed by appropriate treatment and if the possible complications in the acute stage are recognized quickly.

1.2.2   Growing or Enlarging Skull Fracture (Leptomeningeal Cyst)

Occurrence, Pathoanatomy

Children of less than ≤3 years are involved in 90 % and infants of ≤12 months in 50 %. They occur following a severe localized trauma to the head (falls and motor vehicle accident) or less frequently after reconstructive surgery.

An unhealed and enlarging skull fracture develops from a linear fracture that is regularly combined with a dural tear. Because of the unrestrained CSF pulse and expansion of the cranial vault to suit to the rapidly growing brain, there is a progressive widening of the fracture that is often filled up within 3–4 months by a leptomeningeal cyst underneath the skin formed after entrapment of the arachnoid membrane.

Clinical Significance
- Enlarging skull fracture is mostly combined with cerebral contusion at the site of the local impact and leads depending on the site to focal neurological signs (such as contralateral hemiparesis in the preferred parietal localization and convulsions).
- Delayed diagnosis leads to a leptomeningeal cyst with secondary damage to the brain that needs a larger surgical procedure.

Clinical Findings
Considering the pathoanatomy, a skull defect is palpable in the early stage that may be pulsating and increasing in fullness on crying and in supine position. A soft, pulsating, and fluctuant mass that becomes larger in supine and smaller in upright position is a late presentation #.

In the absence of a palpable skull defect, radiological diastasis of the fracture of ≥4–5 mm points to an enlarging skull fracture #.

The intrauterine (due to a blow to the mother's belly) or perinatally acquired enlarging skull fracture (after instrumental delivery) needs special consideration due to the rapid development of the local findings. In the former, the palpable defect may be overlooked, and in the latter, the huge mass close to the anterior fontanel and coronal suture may be attributed to a caput succedaneum, cephalhematoma, subaponeurotic cephalhematoma, or encephalocele.

Differential Diagnosis, Work-Ups
The differential diagnosis includes causes of unhealed skull fractures such as rickets, scurvy, hypophosphatemia, osteogenesis imperfecta, and large fractures in teenagers.

In the neonatal period, a stage 2 cephalhematoma may be mixed up with an enlarging skull fracture on palpation, and the former may conceal it from detection.

Initial work-ups include plain skull x-ray, CT, and MRI. In case of initial suspicion of an enlarging skull fracture, serial plain skull x-rays may be unnecessary because the diagnosis is possible by palpation 1 month after the accident and can be confirmed by MRI. CT and MRI delineate the dimension of the fracture and demonstrate the possible intracranial lesions: ipsilateral localized cerebral contusion, atrophy, porencephaly, ventricular dilatation, leptomeningeal cyst, subdural hematoma, and hydrocephalus.

Therapy Prognosis
Surgery is always indicated and should be performed as early as possible. It includes optional decompression of the leptomeningeal cyst, dural repair with periosteum or fascia lata, and cranioplasty. In addition, shunting of the hydrocephalus or the porencephalia may be needed.

Prognosis depends on the possible intracranial lesions and the time of revision.

1.2.3 Subperiosteal and Subgaleal (Subaponeurotic Cephalhematoma) Hematoma

Occurrence, Clinical Significance
Both hematomas are frequent sequels of head injury. In contrast to the common periosteal cephalhematoma of the newborn # that is associated with a linear or ping-pong skull fracture only in 10–20 %, subperiosteal hematomas of older children are mostly combined with an underlying skull fracture. This association occurs less frequently in subgaleal hematoma. The clinical significance is as follows:
- Ignorance or underestimation of a fall or a blow to the head may lead to unexpected recognition of a tumorlike mass while the hair is washed by the mother.
- Large subperiosteal or subgaleal hematoma may lead to anemia and even to shock, especially in the subgaleal hematoma of the newborn.
- Galeal hematomas may be sign of battered child syndrome, even if it is slight #.

Clinical Presentation

In **subperiosteal** hematoma, a fluctuant or firm mass is palpable which is confined to the fracture site. After a while, it feels like a depressed skull fracture due to a peripheral ridge and a central dell (coagulated blood in the periphery and liquefied in the center).

The **subgaleal** hematoma occurs less often, it may be much larger (because its extension is not limited by the sutures), feels like a diffuse or fluctuant swelling, and shifts after change of the head's position. The neonatal subgaleal hematoma is mainly observed after instrumental delivery and may lead to shock and/or death (the total subgaleal space may contain 250 ml; 20–40 % of the circulating blood volume leads in a newborn to shock). Subgaleal hematoma in older children is due to falls, blows to the head, to **vigorous hair combing** and tight braiding, or to hair pulling by the patient or someone else. Minimal scalp edema may progress to a nontender massive edema of the scalp and bilateral periorbital edema over 1–2 weeks with pallor, tachycardia, fever, and slowly spontaneous recovery thereafter.

Differential Diagnosis, Work-Ups

The differential diagnosis is age-dependant: In subgaleal hematoma of the newborn, cephalocele, vascular malformation, and perinatal growing skull fracture must be considered and in older children, depressed skull fracture, leptomeningeal cyst, subgaleal hygroma, hemangioma, eosinophilic granuloma, and other soft tissue tumors.

Work-ups include plain skull x-ray or ultrasound and, depending on the size and general condition, CT, MRI, and hematological examinations including coagulation studies and blood testing.

Therapy, Prognosis

In many cases, close clinical follow-ups with blood counts are needed. Resorption occurs within 1–5 week. In large cephalhematoma and subgaleal hematoma of the newborn, blood transfusions and coagulation products are urgent, and evacuation by puncture and surgical drainage and/or stanching may be necessary.

Prognosis depends on the time of recognition of the pathologies and on the taken measures.

Occasionally, coagulation defects are recognized such as Willebrand disease.

1.3 Inflammatory Pathologies

1.3.1 Infections of the Galea and Osteomyelitis of the Skull

Occurrence

In contrast to the infrequent acute hematogenous osteomyelitis of the skull, infectious pathologies of the galea and skull are mostly related to galeal and calvarial masses (dermoid cyst, hemangioma, cephalhematoma), to head injury # (abrasion, laceration, hematomas, and implanted devices), and to delayed infections in contiguous sites (paranasal sinuses, otitis, dental abscess).

Clinical Significance

- Involvement of skull must be considered in galea infection and intracranial spread or origin (intracranial abscess, ventriculitis) in osteomyelitis.

Clinical Presentation

It includes *discomfort and headache, persistent fever (in spite of treatment of the primary pathology), and inflammatory signs of the overlying soft tissue.*

Differential Diagnosis, Work-Ups

The former includes primary or secondary malignant and benign tumors of the soft tissue and the skull, fibrous dysplasia (teenager), vascular tumors of the bone, and other inflammatory pathologies or complications. The occurrence of **mastoiditis** depends on the nonappropriate antibiotic treatment of acute otitis. Swelling, redness, fluctuation, and pain behind the auricle that is protruding are the clinical signs possibly combined with lowering of the posterior auditory passage on otoscopy and radiological bone destruction of the mastoid.

The work-ups include plain skull x-ray corresponding to the site of the lesion and its possible origin, CT, MRI (skull defect and possible extension, subperiosteal or epidural abscess; characterization of the soft tissue mass and delineation of possible intracranial spread). Nuclear bone scan may be indicated to discover earliest objective abnormalities of the bone in osteomyelitis and to localize tissue site of infection. In addition, inflammatory blood signs and microbiological examinations of swab, punctate, and blood are necessary.

Therapy, Prognosis

Appropriate i.v. antibiotics and abscess evacuation by punction or incision. In addition, excision of the underlying galea or calvarial mass à froid or treatment of the contiguous focus of infection, and resection of the osteomyelitic skull and treatment of the intracranial spread are necessary.

Prognosis depends on the cause of the infected galea and/or skull and its stage. Although permanent cure is possible, restrictions concern a possible recurrence of a galea or calvarial mass and possible sequels in intracerebral abscess of an eloquent area.

1.4 Neoplastic Pathologies

1.4.1 Hemangioma

Occurrence, Clinical Significance

Fifty percent occur in the head region and mainly in the face although also the galea and rarely the skull may be involved. Their clinical significance is as follows:

- Facial hemangiomas are a problem of cosmesis and in some also of function (nose, lip, orbit, and parotid gland hemangioma).
- Hemangiomas are prone to complications such as ulceration with hemorrhage #, infection, obstruction, final cicatrization, and disseminated intravascular coagulation (exclusively in **Kasabach-Merritt syndrome**).
- Ulceration and cicatrization are important in all hemangiomas of the head and obstruction specifically in facial hemangiomas.
- Hemangiomas may be a red flag of an additional pathology.

Forms, Subgroups

More than 85 % are superficial, about 1.5 % involve profound soft tissues, and more than 10 %

are combined forms ##. About 85 % belong to the subgroup of solitary hemangiomas with regular margins.

Clinical Presentation

The proliferative period starts often in the second part of the first month of life which leads to the clinical recognition. After a period of (sometimes excessive) growth, first signs of spontaneous regression may occur in the second half of infancy #; gross involution can be observed either in the second to fifth year of life or at puberty. Complete regression occurs in approximately 70 %; involution is either partially or even missing in the remainder.

Hemangioma is recognizable from the outside as a prominent, light or dark red tumefaction without the characteristics of normal skin depending on the stages of natural history and the form, and/or palpable as a partially compressible soft tissue mass or recognizable as an osseous calvarial mass on x-ray.

Grayish spots on the surface and stabilization or decrease in size of a former growing hemangioma are signs of regression. Finally, a whitish, thin, and pliable skin scar marks the possible end result of involution #.

Differential Diagnosis, Work-Ups

Deep and combined forms may be mixed up initially or after regression of the superficial part with vascular malformations and sinus pericranii, midline and rare lateral encephalocele or atretic encephalocele, soft tissue tumors, and the osseous hemangioma with calvarial masses.

Especially in hemangioma with excessive growth, short-term follow-ups are needed with measurement of the tumor size and photographic documentation. Additional examinations include mainly in combined and deep forms ultrasound with Doppler, MRI (MRI angiography), and possibly CT.

Therapy, Prognosis

Treatment depends on the site, form, subgroup, and evolution of the individual hemangioma. Today, delayed treatment with observation of the natural course of the hemangioma is often not the golden standard. Depending on the size, contact cryotherapy in small (≤1 cm) or pulsed color laser in large superficial hemangiomas are excellent options. In galeal and calvarial hemangiomas with or without complications, primary excision or resection en bloc without or with transposition flaps avoids the need for repeated sessions and a hairless zone and allows histological examinations. In deep and osseous forms, possible intracranial vascular communications must be considered.

In general, 30 % of hemangiomas do not regress spontaneously or only partially, and the mentioned treatment options lead in single hemangiomas to complete cure combined with good aesthetic results.

1.4.2 Rare Tumors and Tumor-like Masses of the Soft Tissue (Galea)

Occurrence, Clinical Significance
Similar to the calvarial masses, many tumors and tumorlike masses of the galea are rare pathologies. Their clinical significance is as follows:
- Some rare tumors of the galea are specific for this site and/or may also include or occur in the skull.
- Some galeal soft tissue tumors may feign sarcoma.

Pathologies, Clinical Presentation
Cranial fasciitis is a benign proliferative scalp lesion of immature fibroblasts within a myxoid matrix which occurs mainly in children less than 3 years including newborns and is similar to the nodular fasciitis of the trunk and extremities of adults (most common **pseudosarcoma** in adults). *It increases rapidly in size within 2–3 months, lies mostly off the midline, and feels firm, tender, and fixed to the bone and not to the skin on palpation. Exceptionally, categories 3–5 and/or primary localization in the skull may be observed.* The correct diagnosis can only be determined by histopathological examination.

Infantile myofibromatosis (congenital generalized fibromatosis) occurs in the different skin layers, skeletal muscle, bone, and visceral organs. It is a proliferation disorder of a mixture of mesenchymal elements, exhibits either a nodular or diffuse growth, and represents in its solitary form as a common and **partly benign** fibrous tumor at birth or in the first 3 months of life.

On the head, *a firm, circumscribed, painless mass of some millimeter diameter is observed*; the occurrence within the skull is less frequently. Although spontaneous regression is possible, it must be resected completely to avoid recurrence (e.g., in those arising from the dura).

The prognosis of the less common generalized form with involvement of skin, bone, and visceral organs is poor with a mortality of 75 % in contrast to the multicentric form without visceral involvement and possible disappearance of the lesions within 1–2 years.

Congenital desmoid tumor is a benign tumor of bundles of fibroblasts mixed with collagen material. It exhibits an aggressive behavior with **invasion of the surrounding structures** and occurs usually in the third to fifth decade in the abdominal wall, mesentery, and other sites (e.g., women of childbearing age). *The scalp mass is firm and partially adherent to the skin and the deep structures.* Complete excision is necessary to prevent recurrence which may occur in up to 70 % of children within the first 3–6 months.

Other pathologies include **lipoma #, histiocytofibroma, neurofibroma #, neurinoma,** primary galeal and/or calvarial **meningioma,** and calcifying epithelioma of Malherbe (**pilomatrixoma**) of whom some may point to congenital pathologies and syndromes, and the latter is mainly observed on the face and occurs also on the chest wall, back, and extremities.

Congenital and differentiated sarcoma and **rhabdomyosarcoma** belong to the **malignant soft tissue tumors**; the latter needs special attention: 50 % of all childhood soft tissue sarcomas belong to this entity which occurs in two thirds in less than 10 years of age and has a median age distribution of 5 years. Although one third occurs in the head and neck region, 50 % are so-called parameningeal and 25 % orbital tumors, and only 25 % concern the galea, the superficial and deep orofacial, and neck region.

The rapidly growing irregular mass of the galea may arrode the underlying calvaria.

Differential Diagnosis, Work-Ups

It includes all already and later mentioned galeal or calvarial tumors, vascular malformations, hemangiomas, dermoid cyst, and encephalocele (particularly the lateral forms), traumatic and spontaneous hematomas, and osteomyelitis.

Work-ups are ultrasound with Doppler, plain skull x-ray, CT, MRI, and in every case, histopathological examination. In malignancies, staging (by surgery, bone scanning, CT of visceral organs, etc.) and biological characterization are necessary for treatment and prognostication.

In cranial fasciitis, plain skull x-ray may show indentation and scalloping of the underlying calvaria or possibly as in infantile myofibromatosis, a lytic defect with partially sclerosed margins. CT and MRI demonstrate an often isodense soft tissue mass and their extension (including the basal and facial skull or the brain in case of possible local extension and invasiveness of the tumor).

Therapy, Prognosis

Considering the demonstrated properties of some of the so-called benign pathologies, complete resection should be performed whenever possible. In obvious malignancies such as rhabdomyosarcoma, the first intervention is usually a surgical biopsy for determination of the type and the biological characterization (60 % of the head and neck rhabdomyosarcoma have an embryonal type).

Although, in such superficial head and neck tumors, primary excision and possibly re-excision that consider conservation of cosmesis and function are often possible, additional radiation and/or chemotherapy must be applied depending in the individual case.

Prognosis depends on the pathology and the completeness of resection, and in rhabdomyosarcoma on its primary site and the presence of metastatic disease; without the latter, 5-year survival is >80 %.

1.4.3   Osteoma

Occurrence, Clinical Significance

Osteoma of the skull is not uncommon in teenagers although its peak age is the third decade of life. Its preferential site is the frontal supraorbital region.

- Disfigurement and/or space-occupying effect on the frontal sinus, anterior fossa, or orbit are possible sequels because of the inward growth.

Clinical Presentation

Osteoma presents as *slowly increasing osseous and painless mass above the supraorbital ridge or somewhere on the skull and/or local signs depending on the site of inward growth. The lesion is hard and fixed on palpation. It may be discovered accidentally on plain skull x-ray.*

Differential Diagnosis, Work-Ups

It includes all tumors of the calvaria especially monostotic fibrous dysplasia, hemangioma, and **meningioma of the skull**.

Plain x-ray of the skull reveals a mass of hyperostotic bone with a partially recognizable sclerotic rim. CT and MRI are work-up examinations to delineate the morphology and extent of the mass similar to the other rare bone tumors of the skull.

Therapy, Prognosis

Complete en bloc resection, if needed, combined with cranioplasty leads to a permanent cure.

1.4.4   Fibrous Dysplasia

Occurrence, Forms, Clinical Significance

In fibrous dysplasia, the normal bone is replaced for unknown causes by fibro-osseous connective tissue (primarily the medullary, later the cortical part). This process of bone de- and reconstruction that is unpredictable in the individual case starts in the first years of life, is active and/or reveals periods of more and less activity at first, gradually becomes inactive and/or ceases to grow with termination of skeletal growth in many of the involved patients but not in all.

In the **monostotic form**, only one bone is involved (>70 % of the patients with craniofacial fibrous dysplasia); in the **polyostotic form**

(<30 %), several long tubular bones are involved frequently on the same body side (>80 % are unilateral); and in other less frequent forms, cutaneous hyperpigmentation on the same side and single or multiple endocrinopathies (e.g., precocious puberty in girls) are combined with the polyostotic form (**McCune-Albright syndrome, <5 %**).

Their clinical significance is as follows:

- In all forms, the skull vault and/or base and face including the orbit may be involved (the frontal, sphenoid, and ethmoid bones are the most frequently affected bones).
- The disorder may lead to visible craniofacial disfigurement, to increased intracranial or intraocular pressure, and to neurological, sensorial, and other functional deficits.
- The clinical behavior of the individual case is variable and unpredictably concerning time and extension.
- A seemingly monostotic form may point to a polyostotic form without or with McCune-Albright syndrome.
- Malignant transformation may occur rarely in adulthood, for example, osteosarcoma.

Clinical Presentation

The most common clinical signs are *craniofacial or calvarial asymmetry, disfigurement (>80 %) due to a painless and irregular osseous mass, and proptosis and other signs of orbital involvement.*

Less frequently, neurological and/or sensorial deficits may be observed such as optic atrophy and visual loss up to blindness (>10 %) due to narrowing of the optic canal (>30 % in orbitocranial fibrous dysplasia), hearing disorders (involvement of the temporal and petrous bone), or epiphora (nasolacrimal duct obstruction).

Differential Diagnosis, Work-Ups

It includes osteoma, eosinophilic granuloma, neuroblastoma, rare benign and malignant tumors and tumorlike masses of the skull, and in cranioorbital asymmetry, neurofibromatosis, and tuberous sclerosis, intracranial or intraorbital tumors such meningioma, unilateral coronal synostosis, chronic temporal fossa hygroma, and facial hemihypertrophy.

Interpretation of radiological imaging may be difficult because it may mimic other **fibro-osseous lesions** or **osteosarcoma**, and fibrous dysplasia may be combined with other pathologies.

They include plain skull x-ray, CT, and MRI (3D reconstruction), neurological, ophthalmological (e.g., fundoscopy), and ENT (e.g., audiometry) examinations, and whenever possible, confirmation of the suspected fibrous dysplasia by a surgical biopsy. Nuclear bone scanning is useful to exclude a polyostotic form and may demonstrate a single focus prior conventional x-ray.

In the long tubular bones, fibrous dysplasia shows a well-defined radiolucent medullary lesion that is irregular, expansive, and displays a hazy opacity. The cortical part is bulging and arroded, and the whole bone is widened due to subperiosteal reossification. These characteristics are less distinct in the craniofacial bone. In addition, irregular bone regrowth and increasing calcification of the mass can be demonstrated, and pagetoid and sclerotic forms exist.

Therapy, Prognosis

Depending on the individual case, some of the work-ups should be performed in addition to the clinical examinations in regular short- or long-term intervals (e.g., visual loss may develop insidiously).

Decompression is absolutely indicated in aggressive lesions with imminent or already present loss of function.

For several reasons (possibility of indefinite regrowth in polyostotic forms including McCune-Albright syndrome beyond the physiological arrest of skeletal growth; recurrences after partial resection and bone contouring in symptomatic and asymptomatic cases; beneficial effect with radical surgery in cases with absolute indication and in slowly progressive and disfiguring cases including prevention of loss of function), **complete resection** and **immediate reconstruction** is today the preferred method in some tertiary centers in monostotic forms independent of age (e.g., fibrous dysplasia of the orbit or the temporal and petrous bone, respectively; follow-up times of >10 years).

In slowly progressive cases without any functional impairment, **simple bone contouring** may be discussed in monostotic cases after arrest of skeletal growth. In polyostotic forms, complete resection and reconstruction of the craniofacial focus is needed for this purpose.

Prognosis depends on the form, the involved site, and the dynamic of the disease process during childhood and adolescence, and the promptness of decompression in symptomatic cases. The outcome of complete resection and immediate reconstruction is superior to partial resection. The results of remodeling surgery depend on the age of intervention and/or the natural history of the individual fibrous dysplasia case.

1.4.5 Eosinophilic Granuloma (Histiocytosis X)

Forms, Occurrence

Eosinophilic granuloma is the localized form of **Langerhans' cell histiocytosis** (histiocytosis X) and the most frequently observed type of it (70 %). **Hand-Schüller-Christian** and **Abt-Letterer-Siwe syndromes** are disseminated or multifocal forms of histiocytosis X, have a chronic or acute clinical course, and occur in small children and infants.

In contrast, eosinophilic granuloma has a peak age of 5–10 years, mostly only one focus or less often several focuses in the same or in different bones, occasionally involvement of the lymph nodes or lungs, and is in some series the third most common tumor in the differential diagnoses of scalp and calvarial masses because the skull is with more than two thirds the most frequently involved bone.

Clinical Significance

- Most of eosinophilic granulomas of the head need surgical treatment and can be cured permanently although occasional spontaneous regression may occur.
- Profound work- and follow-ups are necessary in a tertiary center because a continuous

transition from localized to disseminated forms may be possible clinically (multiple skull focuses are also observed in Hand-Schüller-Christian syndrome together with other organ involvement) or recurrences and manifestations of a disseminated type.

- Eosinophilic granuloma may lead rarely to acute or subacute epidural hematoma due to intratumoral hemorrhage or involvement of a venous sinus.

Clinical Presentation

Local pain and enlarging skull mass are the most frequently observed complaints although an osteolytic focus on a plain skull x-ray may be found occasionally that has been performed due to head injury #.

The tender and fluctuant mass is fixed to the skull on palpation #.

Differential Diagnosis, Work-Ups

Dependent on age, history, and additional findings, an enlarging or depressed skull fracture, a subcutaneous or subperiosteal hematoma, a hemangioma or vascular malformation including sinus pericranii, osteomyelitis, and a primary or secondary malignancy must be considered.

Plain skull x-ray in lateral or in another projection demonstrates one or less frequently several osteolytic focus(es) with irregular map-like margins and beveled edges (partially sclerosed margins are also possible).

CT and MRI (and MR venogram) delineate the skull focus (sequestration is also possible) and a possible epidural and rarely transdural spread with involvement of a venous sinus. Scintiscan excludes skeletal (mostly femur, ribs, mandible, spine, and other long hallow bones) or parenchymatous involvement. Histological (including cyto- and immunochemistry) and ultrastructural examinations permit together with history, clinical findings, and radiology the diagnosis of Langerhans' cell histiocytosis and its form; positive stains for CD1a antigen and protein S-100 and Birbeck granules (intracytoplasmic organelles) are diagnostic for eosinophilic granuloma.

Treatment, Prognosis

In case of typical single focus accessible to surgery, complete resection by curettage or limited craniectomy is indicated. In case of inaccessibility, incomplete resection, or recurrence, localized radiation, and of multifocal involvement, chemotherapy is necessary.

Risk of local or distant recurrence depends on the age (< or >5 years), uni- or multifocal involvement, etc., 20–30 % recurrences in unifocal involvement beyond 5 years of age. Follow-up of 10 years is recommended. Transition to the disseminated type occurs rarely and mostly within 6 months.

1.4.6 Rare Benign and Malignant Skull Tumors

Occurrence

They encompass **all known benign, semimalignant, and malignant neoplasms, and both primary and secondary types** and those already mentioned in the preceding sections. Many of them are extremely rare because their preferential site is not the skull and/or their peak age may concern the third or fourth decade.

Clinical Significance

In spite of their rarity, the individual case needs an appropriate radiological and a final, sometimes sophisticated histological work-up because the history and clinical findings are usually similar, the radiological findings may be characteristic but not specific, and the treatment depends largely on the most probable or final diagnosis.

Clinical Findings

The following are possible as single or combined findings: (1) Enlarging hard and nonmobile tumescence of the skull that may be combined with local pain or discomfort and is tender on palpation. The overlying skin is often inconspicuous albeit the galea may be affected sometimes; (2) Signs of increased intracranial pressure, neurological deficit, and eye signs (proptosis, chemosis, exophthalmos, and cranial nerve deficits) depending on the inward bulge or growth;

(3) Occasionally radiological involvement of the skull is discovered by chance.

Pathologies

The following pathologies may be observed: **benign osteoblastoma**, cavernous hemangioma (of the skull) and intradiploic meningioma, aneurysmatic bone cyst (ABC) and giant cell tumor (GCT), **primary osteosarcoma, Ewing's sarcoma**, and spindle cell sarcomas, **melanotic neuroectodermal tumor**; histiocytic bone lymphoma (non-Hodgkin lymphoma), primary or secondary granulocytic sarcoma in AML (acute myelogenous leukemia); metastases of neuroblastoma, renal and adrenal gland tumors, sarcomas, and melanoma.

The **melanotic neuroectodermal tumor** is an example of a rare benign tumor of infancy below the age of 6 months (the origin of this tumor is melanin-forming leptomeningeal cells trapped on the periosteum during embryonal development). It concerns mostly the maxilla and mandible and the less frequently the neurocranium.

A malignant form is observed in the brain and long bones of infants and young children. In the first years of life and in close vicinity, a **poorly differentiated meningeal tumor** may be observed that amounts to one fourth of all childhood meningeal tumors (the remainder three fourths are meningioma usually recognized beyond 10 years of age). Focal neurological deficits, increased intracranial pressure, and seizures are the presenting signs of these meningeal malignancies which occur also in other sites such as mediastinum or epididymis and are usually diagnosed after a medium time of 7 weeks in an advanced stage.

The benign form of the **melanotic neuroectodermal tumor** of the neurocranium *displays a rapid growth with doubling in size over a 1–2-month(s) period. … The nontender and firm subcutaneous mass that lies mostly on the top of the head and less frequently laterally, is initially freely movable and becomes later fixed to the neurocranium and dura but not to the scalp.*

The location in the bones close to or including the orbit is a classic type of **metastasis in neuroblastoma**. This characteristic manifestation and the age peak (median age of neuroblastoma 2 1/2 years) may point to the diagnosis or aid to differentiate it from calvarial and facial bone metastases of other malignancies #.

Work-Ups, Differential Diagnosis

Plain skull x-rays #, CT (e.g., bone window in high-resolution CT), and MRI are the main work-ups. Depending on the suspected diagnosis, preoperative surgical biopsy and bone scintiscan are examples of additional examinations.

The following radiological findings are characteristic examples of some of the quoted pathologies: (1) **Plain skull x-rays**: Lytic lesion with sclerotic rim in benign osteoblastoma, lytic mass with ballooning of the tables in ABC, hyperostotic ring-like area in GCT, signs of periosteal remodeling with growth of bone matrix and bone destruction in osteosarcoma, soft tissue mass superimposed on the involved bone, and erosion of one of the tables in Ewing's sarcoma. (2) **CT and/or MRI**: Hypo- or hyperdense osteolytic lesion with thinning or destruction of the tables in benign osteoblastoma; enhancing heterogenous multilocular lesions containing fluid levels in ABC; hyperostotic tumor associated with central calcareous deposits in GCT; assessment of soft tissue involvement by CT and definition of tumor anatomy by MRI in osteosarcoma; extradural, hypertense, and lentiform lesion with erosion of the inner skull table on CT or extradural cystic mass with isointensity on T1- and low intensity in its center on T2-weighted MRI with enhancement after gadolinium in examples in Ewing's sarcoma. In the melanotic neuroectodermal skull tumor of the neurocranium, a characteristic sunburst appearance of spicules may be seen radiating in all directions.

The differential diagnosis includes the more frequent bone tumors such as **osteoma, fibrous dysplasia, eosinophilic granuloma (histiocytosis X), and neuroblastoma metastases**, intracranial tumors, and tumorlike masses (e.g., meningioma [may also occur as primary calvarial or galeal types] or posttraumatic intradiploic arachnoid cyst) with outward growth, **osteomyelitis, and ossified cephalhematoma**.

Therapy, Prognosis

In most of the quoted pathologies, a total en bloc resection of the involved skull is indicated although some less invasive procedures may be possible in some lesions. On the other hand, malignant tumors need preoperative surgical biopsy and work-up for staging, chemotherapy, and thereafter resection.

In infants with melanotic neuroectodermal tumor, en bloc resection of periosteum, skull, and dura are necessary (dural involvement is recognizable by black pigmentation).

In most quoted pathologies, permanent cure is possible by surgery. In ABC, the secondary type (combined with fibrous dysplasia, chondroblastoma, GCT, or osteosarcoma) must be considered by a thorough histopathological examination, and recurrences are possible after curettage or incomplete resection; in GCT, initial malignancy, malignant transformation, and recurrences are well known; in osteosarcoma, Ewing's sarcoma, and the other malignant tumors, outcome depends on numerous prognostic factors and the therapeutical progresses and possibly on the calvarial localization.

Webcodes

The following webcodes can be used on www. psurg.net for further images and data.

101 Dermoid cyst	124 MRI, irregular skull defect and
102 Dermoid cyst, category 2	125 Grotesque Venectasia, sinus pericranii
103 Dermoid cyst, category 3	126 Congenital aplasia cutis, skull defect
104 Epidermoid cyst, lateral eye brow	127 Spontaneous epithelization
105 Epidermoid cyst, medial eye corner	128 Ossified cephalhematoma
106 Parietal dermoid cyst	129 Skull x-ray, ossified cephalhematoma
107 Intraosseous dermoid cyst, sclerotic rim	130 Subaponeurotic hematoma
108 Dermoid cyst anterior fontanel	131 Leptomeningeal cyst

Bibliography

Section 1.1.1

Armon N, Sharmay S, Maly A, Margulis A (2010) Occurrence and characteristics of head cysts in children. Eplasty 10:e37

Dutta S, Lorenz HP, Albanese CT (2006) Endoscopic excision of benign forehead masses: a novel approach for pediatric general surgeons. J Pediatr Surg 41:1874–1878

Martinez-Lage JF, Capel A, Costa TR, Perez-Espejo MA, Poza M (1992) The child with a mass on its head: diagnostic and surgical strategies. Childs Nerv Syst 8: 247–252

Ruge JR, Tomita T, Naidich TP, Hahn YS, McLone DG (1988) Scalp and Cal-varial masses of infants and children. Neurosurgery 22:1037–1041

Thaller SR, Bauer BS (1987) Cysts and cyst-like lesions of the skin and subcutaneous tissue. Clin Plast Surg 14:327–339

Willatt JM, Quaghebeur G (2004) Calvarial masses of infants and children. A radio-logical approach. Clin Radiol 59:474–486

Yoon SH, Park SH (2008) A study of 77 cases of surgically excised scalp and skull masses in pediatric patients. Childs Nerv Syst 24:459–465

Section 1.1.2

Bächli H, Zettl AS, Köppl R, Mayr J (2007) Vorsicht vor mittellinigen nasalen Pickeln im Kindesalter! (Midline nasal pimple in infancy: caution!). Schweiz Med Forum 7:862–863

Blake WE, Chow CW, Holmes AD, Meara JG (2006) Nasal dermoid sinus cysts. A retrospective review and discussion of investigation and management. Ann Plast Surg 57:535–540

Caldarelli M, Massimi L, Kondageski C, di Rocco C (2004) Intracranial midline dermoid and epidermoid cysts in children. J Neurosurg 100:473–480

Fermin S, Fernandez-Guerra RA, Lopez-Camacho O, Alvarez R (2001) Congenital dermoid cyst of the anterior fontanel in mestizo-mulatto children. Childs Nerv Syst 17:353–355

Hanikeri M, Waterhouse N, Kirkpatrick N, Peterson D, Macleod I (2005) The management of midline transcranial nasal dermoid sinus cysts. Br J Plast Surg 58:1043–1050

Hedlund G (2006) Congenital frontonasal masses: developmental anatomy, malformations, and MRI imaging. Pediatr Radiol 36:647–662

Martinez-Lage JF, Quinonez MA, Poza M, Puche A, Casas C, Costa TR (1985) Congenital epidermoid cyst of the anterior fontanelle. Childs Nerv Syst 1:319–323

Okuda Y, Oi S (1987) Nasal dermal sinus and dermoid cyst with intrafalcial extension: case report and review of the literature. Childs Nerv Syst 3:40–43

Schijman E, Monges J, Cragnaz R (1986) Congenital dermal sinuses, dermoid and epidermoid cysts of the posterior fossa. Childs Nerv Syst 2:83–89

Stokes RB, Saunders CJ, Thaller SR (1996) Bregmatic epidermoid inclusion cyst eroding both calvarial tables. J Craniofac Surg 7:148–150

Tateshima S, Numoto RT, Abe S, Yasne M, Abe T (2000) Rapidly enlarging dermoid cyst over the anterior fontanel: a case report and review of the literature. Childs Nerv Syst 16:875–878

Vinchon M, Soto-Ares G, Assaker R, Belbachir F, Dhellemmes P (2001) Occipital dermal sinuses: report of nine pediatric cases and review of the literature. Pediatr Neurosurg 34:255–263

Section 1.1.3

Kang GC, Song C (2008) Forty-one cervicofacial vascular anomalies and their surgical treatment – retrospection and review. Ann Acad Med Singapore 37:165–179

Yoshida D, Sugisaki Y, Shimura T, Teramoto A (1999) Cavernous hemangioma of the skull in a neonate. Childs Nerv Syst 15:351–353

Section 1.1.4

Martinez-Lage JF, Sola J, Casa C, Poza M, Almagro MJ, Girona DG (1992) Atretic cephalocele: the tip of the iceberg. J Neurosurg 77:230–235

Yamazaki T, Enomoto T, Iguchi M, Nose T (2001) Atretic cephalocele – report of two cases with special reference to embryology. Childs Nerv Syst 17:674–678

Section 1.1.5

Chen CS, David D, Hanieh A (2004) Morning glory syndrome and basal encephalocele. Childs Nerv Syst 20:87–90

Dehdashti AR, Abonzeid H, Momjian S, Delavelle J, Rilliet B (2004) Occipital extra- and intracranial lipoencephalocele associated with tectocerebellar dysraphia. Childs Nerv Syst 20:225–228

Formica F, Iannelli A, Paludetti G, Di Rocco C (2002) Transsphenoidal meningoencephalocele. Childs Nerv Syst 18:295–298

Mahapatra AK, Tandon PN, Dhawan IK, Khazanchi RK (1994) Anterior encephaloceles: a report of 90 cases. Childs Nerv Syst 10:501–504

Martinez-Lage JF, Gonzalez-Tortosa XY, Poza M (1982) Meningocele of the asterion. Childs Brain 9:53–59

Parizek J, Mericka P, Nemecek S, Nemeckova J, Zemankova M, Sercl M, Häringova M (1996) Allogeneic cartilage used for skull base plasty in children with primary intranasal encephalomeningocele associated with cerebrospinal fluid rhinorrhea. Childs Nerv Syst 12:136–141

Traumer BI, Singh S, Ketch L (1989) An unusual case of temporal encephalocele. Childs Nerv Syst 5:371–373

Section 1.1.6

Choudhury AR, Bandey SA, Haleem A, Sharif H (1996) Glial heterotopias of the nose. A report of two cases. Childs Nerv Syst 12:43–47

Verney Y, Zanolla G, Teixeira R, Oliveira LC (2001) Midline nasal mass in infancy: a nasal glioma case report. Eur J Pediatr Surg 11:324–327

Section 1.1.7

Wen CS, Chang YL, Wang HS, Kno MF, Tu YK (2005) Sinus pericranii: from gross and neuroimaging findings to different pathophysiological changes. Childs Nerv Syst 21:482–488

Section 1.1.8

Bang RL, Ghoneim IE, Gang RK, Al Najjadah I (2003) Treatment dilemma: conservative versus surgery in cutis aplasia congenita. Eur J Pediatr Surg 13:125–129

Chakrabortty S, Oi S, Suzuki H, Izawa I, Yamaguchi M, Tamaki N, Matsumoto S (1993) Congenital frontal bone defect with intact overlying scalp. Childs Nerv Syst 9:485–487

Martinez-Lage JF, Almagro MJ, Lopez-Hernandez F, Poza M (2002) Aplasia cutis congenital of the scalp. Childs Nerv Syst 18:634–637

Steinbock P (2000) Repair of a congenital cranial defect in a newborn with autologous calvarial bone. Childs Nerv Syst 16:47–250

Section 1.2.1

Kaiser GL, Oesch V (2009) Sagittal craniosynostosis combined with ossified cephalhematoma – a tricky and demanding puzzle. Childs Nerv Syst 25:103–110

Section 1.2.2

Djientcheu VD, Rilliet B, Delavelle J, Argyropoulo M, Gudinchet F, de Tribolet N (1996) Leptomeningeal cyst in newborns due to vacuum extraction: report of two cases. Childs Nerv Syst 12:399–403

Johnson DL, Helman T (1995) Enlarging skull fractures in children. Childs Nerv Syst 11:265–286

Papaefthymion G, Oberbauer R, Pendl G (1996) Craniocerebral birth trauma caused by vacuum extraction: a case of growing skull fracture as a perinatal complication. Childs Nerv Syst 12:117–120

Section 1.2.3

Donmouchtsis SK, Arul Kumaran S (2006) Head injuries after instrumental vaginal deliveries. Curr Opin Obstet Gynecol 18:129–134, Lippincott Williams & Wilkins

Fujisawa H, Yonaha H, Oka Y, Uehava M, Nagata Y, Kajiwara K, Fuji M, Kato S, Akimura T, Suzuki M (2005) A marked exophthalmos and corneal ulceration caused by delayed massive expansion of subgaleal hematoma. Childs Nerv Syst 21:489–492

Uhing MR (2005) Management of birth injuries. Clin Perinatol 32:19–38

Section 1.3.1

Prasad A, Madan VS, Suri ML, Buxi TBS (1992) Cryptogenetic osteomyelitis of the skull and intracerebral abscess. Childs Nerv Syst 8:142–143

Section 1.4.1

Brandling-Bennett HA, Metry DW, Baselga E, Lucky AW, Adams DM, Cordisco MR, Frieden IJ (2008) Infantile hemangiomas with unusually prolonged growth phase. Arch Dermatol 144:1632–1637

Mulliken JB, Fishman SJ (1998) Vascular anomalies: hemangiomas and malformations. In: O'Neill JA (ed) Pediatric surgery, vol II, 5th edn. Year Book, Inc, St. Louis

Mulliken JB, Glowacki J (1982) Hemangiomas and vascular malformations in infants and children. A classification based on endothelial characteristics. Plast Reconstr Surg 69:412–420

Section 1.4.2

Im SH, Wang KC, Kim SK, Oh CW, Kim DG, Hong SK, Kim NR, Chi JG, Cho BK (2001) Childhood meningioma: unusual location, atypical radiological findings, and favourable treatment and outcome. Childs Nerv Syst 17:656–662

Lang DA, Neil-Dwyer G, Evans BT, Sarsfield P, Nenji E (1996) Cranial fasciitis of the orbit and maxilla: extensive resection and reconstruction. Childs Nerv Syst 12:218–221

Martinez-Lage JF, Acosta J, Sola J, Poza M (1996) Congenital desmoids tumor of the scalp: a histologically benign lesion with aggressive clinical behaviour. Childs Nerv Syst 12:409–412

Martinez-Lage JF, Torroba A, Lopez F, Manzoms MC, Poza M (1997) Cranial fasciitis of the anterior fontanel. Childs Nerv Syst 13:626–628

Niimura K, Shirane R, Yoshimoto T (1997) Infantile myofibromatosis located in the temporal bone. Childs Nerv Syst 13:629–632

Tsuji M, Inagaki T, Kasai H, Yamanouchi Y, Kawamoto K, Uemura Y (2004) Solitary myofibromatosis of the skull: a case report and review of the literature. Childs Nerv Syst 20:366–369

Wiener ES (1998) Rhabdomyosarcoma. In: O'Neill JA (ed) Pediatric surgery, vol I, 5th edn. Year Book, Inc, St. Louis

Yamada H, Sakata K, Kashiki Y, Okuma A, Takada M (1979) Peculiar congenital parieto-occipital head tumor. Report of 3 cases. Childs Brain 5:426–432

Section 1.4.3

Viswanatha B (2011) Characteristics of osteoma of the temporal bone in young adolescents. Ear Nose Throat J 90:72–79

Section 1.4.4

Ameli NO, Rahmat H, Abbassioun K (1981) Monostotic fibrous dysplasia of the cranial bones: report of fourteen cases. Neurosurg Rev 4:71–77

Kim YH, Song JJ, Choi HG, Lee JH, Oh SH, Chang SO, Koo JW, Kim CS (2009) Role of surgical management in temporal bone fibrous dysplasia. Acta Otolaryngol 5:1–6

Kusano T, Hirabayashi S, Eguchi T, Sugawara Y (2009) Treatment strategies for fibrous dysplasia. J Craniofac Surg 20:768–770

Lädermann A, Stern R, Ceroni D, De Coulon G, Taylor S, Kaelin A (2008) Unusual radiological presentation of monostotic fibrous dysplasia. Orthopedics 31:282

Maher CO, Friedman JA, Meyer FB, Lynch JJ, Unni K, Raffel C (2002) Surgical treatment of fibrous dysplasia of the skull in children. Pediatr Neurosurg 37:87–92

Moore AT, Buncic JR, Munro IR (1985) Fibrous dysplasia of the orbit in childhood. Clinical features and management. Ophthalmology 92:12–20

Posnick JC, Wells MD, Drake JM, Buncic JR, Armstrong D (1993) Childhood fibrous dysplasia presenting as blindness: a skull base approach for resection and immediate reconstruction. Pediatr Neurosurg 19:260–266

Rahman AM, Madge SN, Billing K, Anderson B, Leibovitch I, Selva D, David D (2009) Craniofacial fibrous dysplasia: clinical characteristics and long-term outcomes. Eye (Lond) 23:2175–2181

Valentini V, Cassoni A, Marianetti TM, Terenzi V, Fadda MT, Iannetti G (2009) Craniomaxillofacial fibrous dysplasia: conservative treatment or radical surgery? A retrospective study of 68 patients. Plast Reconstr Surg 123:653–660

Wei YT, Jiang S, Cen Y (2010) Fibrous dysplasia of skull. J Craniofac Surg 21:538–542

Section 1.4.5

Allen CE, McClain KL (2007) Langerhans cell histiocytosis: a review of past, current and future therapies. Drugs Today (Barc) 43:627–643

Mut M, Cataltepe O, Bakar B, Cila A, Akalan N (2004) Eosinophilic granuloma of the skull associated with epidural haematoma: a case report and review of the literature. Childs Nerv Syst 20:765–769

Section 1.4.6

Dammann O, Hagel C, Allers B, Grubel G, Schulte FJ (1995) Malignant melanotic neuroectodermal tumor of infancy. Childs Nerv Syst 11:186–188

Ersalin Y, Mutener S, Demirtas E (2000) Intraosseous neurinoma of the parietal bone. Childs Nerv Syst 16:181–183

Germano A, Caruso G, Caffo M, Galatioto S, Belvedere M, Cardia E (1998) Temporal osteoclastoma: an exceptional lesion in infancy. Childs Nerv Syst 14:213–217

Guida F, Rapana A, Conti C, Cagliari E, Civelli F, Trincia G (2001) Cranial aneurysmal bone cyst: a diagnostic problem with review of the literature. Childs Nerv Syst 17:297–301

Martinez-Lage JF, Garcia S, Torroba A, Sola J, Poza M (1996) Unusual osteolytic midline lesion of the skull: benign osteoblastoma of the parietal bone. Childs Nerv Syst 12:343–345

Martinez-Lage JF, Martinez Perez M, Domingo R, Poza M (1997) Posttraumatic intradiploic arachnoid cyst of the posterior fossa. Childs Nerv Syst 13: 293–296

Otah K, Kondoh T, Yasuo K, Kohsaka Y, Kohmura E (2003) Primary granulocytic sarcoma in the sphenoid bone and orbit. Childs Nerv Syst 19:674–679

Salvati M, Ciappetta P, Capone R, Santoro A, Raguso M, Raco A (1993) Osteosarcoma of the skull in a child: case report and review of the literature. Childs Nerv Syst 9:437–439

van den Berg H, Kroon HM, Slaar A, Hogendoorn P (2008) Incidence of biopsy-proven bone tumors in children: a report based on the Dutch pathology registration "PALGA". J Pediatr Orthop 28:29–35

Walsh JW, Stand RD (1982) Melanotic neuroectodermal tumor of the neurocranium in infancy. Childs Brain 9:329–346

Yasuda T, Inagaki T, Yamanouchi Y, Kawamoto K, Kohdera U, Kawasaki H (2003) A case of primary Ewing's sarcoma of the occipital bone presenting with obstructive hydrocephalus. Childs Nerv Syst 19:792–799

Macrocrania

This presenting sign is easy to recognize if the head is too large in relation to the face or to the remaining body with the naked eye #. More often, measurement of the head circumference demonstrates a value above the normal range, too high in relation to the body length, or that exceeds one percentile after the other on follow-up #.

Because head circumference is measured in the fronto-occipital plane, it may be an indication of a too large skull volume, as the normal values have been obtained from a mean population of different age that show a slightly longitudinal-oval shape.

In children with dolicho- or brachycephaly, the measured values fall often into the upper or lower percentiles for geometric reasons and may therefore simulate a relative macrocrania or microcephalia, for example, in craniosynostoses.

In the individual case or in longitudinal measurements, the head circumference does not at all follow a harmonious way as it is recognizable from the common percentile curves. This must be considered in case of small deviations of head circumference values, for example, in constitutional macrocrania.

A wrong measurement is not always excluded, too. Therefore, the mean value of three head circumference measurements should be calculated. After 1 year of age, 87.5 %, after 5 years, 93.3 % of the final value is attained, and with approximately 13 years (girls) or 15 years (boys), the adult values of 51.5–58 cm are achieved.

In Table 2.1, mainly the surgically relevant pathologies of macrocrania are listed. The significance of some of the pathologies has got smaller in comparison to older similar surveys, in part, due to prenatal ultrasound performed in developed countries for diagnosis of CNS malformations that belong together with the urogenital to the most frequently encountered pathologies.

2.1 Hydrocephalus

Occurrence, Etiology, Forms

Due to prenatal diagnosis and abortion or to a lesser degree due to prevention of spina bifida by preconceptional enrichment of the food with folic acid, congenital hydrocephalus is observed less frequently than peri- or postnatally acquired hydrocephalus, whereas the latter is possibly increased because of increased survival of premature infants with intraventricular hemorrhage (former prevalence 1 isolated hydrocephalus in 1,000 live births).

The percentage of congenital and postnatally acquired hydrocephalus and of the different etiologies depends on the inclusion of children and adults, for example, 41 % congenital and 59 % acquired types if both ages are considered. Nevertheless, 60–90 % of the cases are treated in the first year of life.

There are numerous etiologies and different forms of hydrocephalus. In **congenital and connatal hydrocephalus**, malformative or prenatally acquired causes exist such as aqueductal stenosis, spina bifida (due to aqueductal stenosis and Chiari II malformation), Dandy-Walker malformations

Table 2.1 Differential diagnosis of macrocrania

• Hydrocephalus
Shunt failure, shunt infection, abdominal CSF pseudocyst, slit ventricle syndrome, isolated fourth ventricle hydrocephalus, Chiari II and I malformations
• Constitutional macrocrania (benign familial macrocephaly)
• Intraventricular (periventricular/intraventricular) hemorrhage of the newborn
Transient ventriculomegaly, progressive hydrocephalus
o Catch-up growth of head circumference
o Congenital intracranial cysts
Arachnoid cyst, Dandy-Walker malformation and variant, porencephalic cyst, septum pellucidum cyst, cavum vergae and velum interpositum cyst
o Subacute and chronic subdural hematoma (hygroma)
External (extraventricular) hydrocephalus, subdural collection due to meningitis
o Encephalopathies, metabolic disorders with brain involvement

(e.g., Dandy-Walker cyst), or hydrocephalus after infections transmitted by the pregnant women (e.g., toxoplasmosis) and after intracerebral hemorrhage (e.g., as expanding porencephalic cyst).

About 2 % of the patients with congenital hydrocephalus have an **x-linked hydrocephalus** that occurs only in boys and may be a part of a MASA syndrome.

Among the **peri- or postnatally acquired hydrocephali**, previous infections (such as hydrocephalus after pneumococcal meningitis in the western world and after tuberculous meningitis in the western Cape district of South Africa and other parts of the world with high incidence of tuberculosis, or aqueductal stenosis after mumps encephalomeningitis), intraventricular or subarachnoidal hemorrhage (such as in prematurity, trauma to the head, or spontaneously), and brain tumors (such as axial tumors of the posterior fossa) belong to the most common causes.

Hydrocephalus is a disorder of CFS circulation by blockage at different sites of its pathway with dilatation of the prestenotic parts (e.g., triventricular hydrocephalus in aqueductal stenosis or dilatation of all ventricles in obstruction of the foramina of the fourth ventricle), increased intraventricular pressure, and decreased cerebral blood flow. The former are noncommunicating forms, whereas obstructions outside of the ventricles such as those at the level of the basal cisterns belong to the communicating forms of hydrocephalus.

In light of recent research results, the possibility of other CSF absorptive mechanisms must be considered in addition to the classic concept of CSF circulation such as CSF absorption by lymphatics after clearance of CSF along the sheets of the cranial nerves.

Clinical Significance
- The recognition of ventriculomegaly by prenatal screening is important because it may be combined with cerebral and/or extracerebral malformations and/or chromosomal aberrations, and may be the start of progressive hydrocephalus.
- Pathology, pathophysiology, clinical presentation, and prognosis depend not only on the hydrocephalus but also substantially on its etiology.
- The disorder of the cerebrospinal fluid (CSF) circulation can be treated always effectively in contrast to the etiology.
- Non- or delayed treatment leads to death, mental, and neurological deficit.
- Treated hydrocephalus needs lifelong follow-ups.

Clinical Presentation
Prenatal screening and diagnosis: In general, **ventriculomegaly** is the most frequent issue on ultrasound. In contrast to hydrocephalus that is defined as ventriculomegaly combined with abnormal increase of head circumference, ventriculomegaly means only a lateral ventricle

atrium larger than 10 mm independent of term on ultrasound or MRI (measurements in the coronal and/or axial plane; >15 mm = severe ventriculomegaly). During the second half of gestation, the atriocerebral ratio (ratio between atrial diameter and biparietal brain diameter) decreases normally from 13.6 to 8 %. Ventriculomegaly is caused by CSF accumulation, brain atrophy, or dysgenesis; in one third of the patients, a resolution, and in less than two thirds, stabilization is observed during gestation. The recognition of ventriculomegaly is important because it is often combined with cerebral and/or extracerebral malformations and/or chromosomal aberrations (in up to three fourths and one third, respectively), and can be beginning of progressive hydrocephalus (>10 %). In general, isolated mild ventriculomegaly (10–15 mm) means a postnatal development delay in round 10 %.

A posterior asymmetric enlargement of the ventricles and the parieto-occipital subarachnoid spaces may be a precursor of an external hydrocephalus.

Depending on the age of the child, the type of progression, or stage of hydrocephalus, the clinical presentation is different. The latter include acute, progressive, or chronic, compensated, arrested, or shunted hydrocephalus with overt or insidious blockage or with compensation or arrest.

Newborns and infants: Unspecific symptoms and signs are food refusal, irritability, apathy, and arrest or loss of developmental milestones. On inspection and/or palpation, the following findings are present: *macrocrania pre- or postnatally, or progressive increase of head circumference (HC) afterward with crossing of one percentile after the other with disproportion of the large neurocranium in relation to a small face (normal values of HC are at term ≤37 cm in boys and ≤36 cm in girls). Furthermore, distended scalp veins, widening of the cranial sutures, enlarged, tense, and bulging anterior fontanel (the normal anterior fontanel is soft and sunken in the quiet patients held in upright position), and setting sun sign # are encountered.*

Older children: Depending on the acuteness of development of the disorder of CSF circulation, *more or less distinct signs of increased intracranial pressure (ICP) are prominent such as headache (characteristically also at night and in the morning), vomiting, papilledema on fundoscopy, and split cranial sutures on plain skull x-ray. In addition, abducens nerve palsy, paralysis of upward gaze (Parinaud's syndrome), and other ophthalmological and neurological deficits may be encountered.*

In case of compensation, *the signs of increased ICP may be discreet except for macrocrania. The preserved language (chatterbox) and memory abilities delude the examiner about the deficits of general and school performance, of behavior, and neuropsychological examination. Episodes of spontaneous exacerbation of hydrocephalus, for example, after head injury may lead to aggravation and specification of the clinical presentation.*

Shunt failure: Although shunt failure corresponds often to an acute or subacute hydrocephalus with *possible clouding of consciousness from apathy to coma*, there is often a *dissociation of the common symptoms and signs of increased ICP and findings of neuroradiological imaging*, and uncommon, isolated complaints are possible such as blurred vision, etc.

In shunted patients, shunt failure must always be considered, and the needed work-ups must be carried out timely because severe deficits may develop, for example, visual loss in approximately 2 % that is completely irreversible in at least one third of the involved children. On checking the valve, the only reliable sign of obstruction is a permanently flat chamber after single decompression (#/#).

The **work-up examinations** are the same as quoted under slit ventricle syndrome. Ultrasound of the optic nerve sheath yields somewhat earlier and more reliable pathological findings than fundoscopy (lacking papilledema after optic atrophy). Normal are values of <4 and <4.5 mm in infants and older children, respectively. Nevertheless, variation from the asymptomatic baseline value is the most sensitive variable in determining development of hydrocephalus in the individual case.

Natural History

Without treatment, 45 % of the patients with hydrocephalus are still alive 7 years after the initial diagnosis, and at least two thirds of them have severe mental and neurological deficits, and all are conspicuous in everyday life. To a lesser degree, the same applies to patients with **compensation of hydrocephalus after shunt blockage**. As in native hydrocephalus, acute exacerbation of hydrocephalus with fatal outcome is possible even after several years.

After shunting and long-term observation, several types of shunt dependency are observed with the majority remaining shunt-dependent (Fig. 2.1).

Differential Diagnosis, Work-Ups

The differential diagnosis includes pathologies with apparent or real macrocrania, with clouded consciousness or unconsciousness (acute hydrocephalus, spontaneous exacerbation of hydrocephalus, or in shunt failure) and with signs of increased ICP or other neurological presentations. In addition to the pathologies described in this chapter and those quoted in the chapter on clouded consciousness or unconsciousness, the following disorders must be considered: fourth ventricle hydrocephalus, (Arnold) Chiari II and I malformations, and syringobulbia and -myelia; the latter occurs mostly combined with Chiari I and II malformations.

Isolated fourth ventricle hydrocephalus occurs usually after long-term conventional shunting in children with postmeningitic, posthemorrhagic, and hydrocephalus with former shunt infection or due a congenital malformation; communicating hydrocephalus, aqueductal stenosis, or occlusion of the foramina of the fourth ventricle may be present, for example, in Dandy-Walker cyst. The increased volume of the fourth ventricle with or without a clinical symptomatology is due to an imbalance between the supra- and infratentorial ventricular system with increased IVP of the latter and upward shift of the brain stem on condition that there is an aqueductal stenosis or insufficiency on the one hand and an occlusion of the fourth ventricle foramina on the other hand.

Clinically, there is either a slowly progressive symptomatology with ataxia, apathia, and diplopia over years or an acute life-threatening clinical presentation of a posterior fossa mass with cranial nerve deficits and cerebellar tonsil herniation. Treatment option is either a double shunt (ventricular and fourth ventricle catheter with a common valve and distal catheter) or endoscopic stenting in addition to a conventional shunt. Isolated shunt of the fourth ventricle and, to a lesser degree, a double shunt are prone to complications such as primary or secondary injury of the brain stem parenchyma or of the floor of the fourth ventricle or overdrainage with brain stem tethering with the appearance of cranial nerve deficits.

In Chiari II malformation, there is a hindbrain deformity with a small posterior fossa and

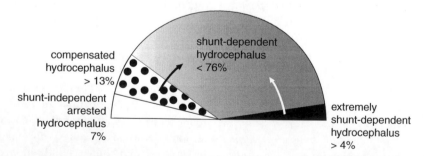

Fig. 2.1 After long-term shunting, several types of shunt dependency arise. The majority remains shunt-dependent. Some become extremely shunt-dependent with slit ventricle syndrome. On the other hand, arrested hydrocephalus occurs in 5–10 % of the patients following gradual loss of shunt function. This group should be differentiated from compensated hydrocephalus in which the shunt does not work anymore without obvious clinical signs. Nevertheless, decompensation of hydrocephalus is possible any time

impaction of the posterior cerebellum through the foramen magnum; the elongated fourth ventricle extends as far as the cervical canal and its foramina are obstructed by parts of the cerebellum and arachnoidal adhesions. Precise individual pathoanatomical and flow characteristics can be determined by CT and MRI. *By compression and/or distortion of the cranial nerves and the brain stem, life-threatening symptoms may occur such as apneic or cyanotic attacks, respiratory distress syndrome, difficulty in swallowing, and vocal cord paresis.* There is no consensus about the most appropriate initial therapy in symptomatic Chiari II malformation. In already shunted children, a throughout evaluation of shunt function is needed because the symptomatology disappears or is lessened by optimal shunt function. In case of life-threatening and persistent severe symptoms, despite a normal shunt function, decompression of the upper cervical canal (occipital decompression is not necessary in large foramen magnum) and dural expansion are indicated. It may lessen the symptoms and those of an associated syringomyelia in at least 75 %; the latter needs only a syrinx shunt to the subarachnoid or peritoneal space in case of failure of decompression. Rarely, decompression must be combined with a double ventriculo- and cisterna magna-peritoneal shunt.

In Chiari I malformation, there is a descent of the cerebellar tonsils into the cervical canal. It is diagnosed by MRI (abnormal position of the cerebellar tonsils below the foramen magnum) during work-ups of skeletal abnormalities of the cervical spine, craniocervical junction, or scoliosis in which associated Chiari I malformation is often encountered or due to neurological deficits in the second decade. *The symptomatology is caused by compression/distortion of the dura, brain stem, lower cranial nerves, cerebellum, or by an associated syringomyelia. It includes occipital or cervical pain that is paroxysmal (triggered by Valsalva maneuver such as coughing) or persistent (analogous presentation in young children by crying and neck hyperextension), weakness and spasticity of extremities, and in*

20 %, sings such as vocal cord paresis, recurrent aspiration, and down beating nystagmus. In addition, weakness of the upper limbs (intrinsic hand muscles) or only absence of superficial abdominal reflexes may be observed. The treatment includes foramen magnum decompression and dural expansion that is not indicated in asymptomatic patients except for those with scoliosis.

Work-ups: Ultrasound, CT, and MRI belong to the main imaging procedures #/#/#. They confirm the clinical diagnosis of hydrocephalus, describe its degree (volume of the lateral or all four ventricles, brain mantle thickness, etc.) and the involved parts (e.g., triventricular hydrocephalus), demonstrate possible additional findings, and allow the differential diagnosis from other pathologies. The involved parts of the CSF compartments and additional findings point to the probable site of obstruction and/or possibly to the etiology.

For follow-ups, it is important to know that changes of ventricular size in ventriculomegaly are only recognizable from 20 % upward by the naked eye.

With the advent of endoscopic surgery, preoperative evaluation of the type of hydrocephalus (e.g., noncommunicating vs. communicating) and postoperative monitoring (determination of stoma patency, changes in ventricular volume) became indispensable; phase-contrast cine flow MRI and air encephalography are examples of such examinations.

Neurological, ophthalmological, neuropsychological, genetic examinations and laboratory blood and CSF tests (e.g., increased CSF levels of IgM and IgG anti-paramyxovirus in aqueductal stenosis after mumps) allow to demonstrate the etiology of hydrocephalus and possible associated pathologies, malformations, and syndromes for prognostic purposes or to describe the hydrocephalus for further follow-ups.

CSF pressure measurement of 24–48 h by an intracranial route allows the differentiation between shunt-dependent compensated and shunt-independent arrested hydrocephalus in apparently asymptomatic patients who have been shunted or not (##).

Therapy

Most commonly used are the ventriculoperitoneal (VP) shunt and endoscopic procedures such as third ventriculostomy (ETV). In contrast to the generally applicable shunting, endoscopic procedures need specific indications because the success rate depends on the age, on the site of CSF blockage, and on the etiology, respectively. Both methods have different advantages and drawbacks.

Fetal surgery by placement of a ventriculo-amniotic shunt has been disappointing so far. Actually, the prerequisites that concern meaningful indications (e.g., type of hydrocephalus in which there will be irreversible damage if left untreated) and suitable surgical methods are not yet established for a renewed trial. The outcome depends specifically on the time of onset of hydrocephalus in general and/or on the stage, type, and clinical category of congenital hydrocephalus (perspective classification of congenital hydrocephalus).

Shunt implants are expensive especially in case of repeated shunt failure. Shunt revisions performed in time are nearly impossible in not accessible parts of the third world.

In contrast to the differential pressure valves that produce an unphysiologically negative ICP pressure in upright position, the newer generation of valves (hydrostatic valves, programmable valves, antisiphon devices, and so-called variable-resistance or flow-regulated valves) overcome or lessen overdrainage but may be combined with the drawbacks of significant risks of shunt insufficiency. Radiological signs of overdrainage are postponed, and occurrence of SVS is possibly decreased.

Shunt surgery (Fig. 2.2): If one lateral ventricle is larger than the other, this side is chosen for shunting. The child is in supine position with the head turned to the contralateral side, and the planned incisions are marked: transverse incision lateral to the umbilicus and hockey stick incision in the parieto-occipital angle or lateral to the anterior fontanel. The skin is covered by a film, and the parts of the shunt never touch the naked skin. After the cranial and abdominal incision, the shunt passer is introduced from one to the other

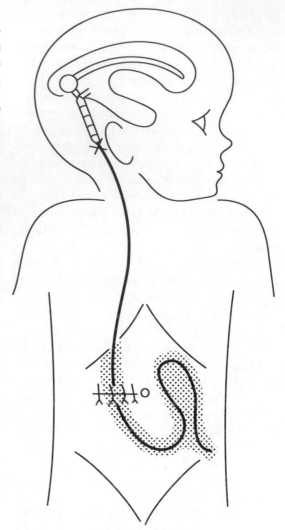

Fig. 2.2 Ventriculoperitoneal shunt. The ventricular catheter is introduced from a burr hole in the angle between the sagittal and lambdoid suture or in front of the coronal suture and lateral to the midline. The extra-length of the intraperitoneal catheter of 30–40 cm allows free motion (the catheter changes its position innumerable times) and compensates for the patient's growth in the first decade

incision and replaced by a thread that is used to pull through the peritoneal catheter. After a burr hole in the parieto-occipital angel or 1 cm in front of the coronal suture and laterally to the midline, the ventricular is introduced with its tip in the frontal horn, the ICP measured, and CSF for culture, protein, and cells collected. Afterward, the ventricular catheter is connected with an intervening Rickham ventriculostomy reservoir and the chosen valve with the peritoneal catheter. After a transverse incision of the fascia of the rectus muscle and longitudinal spreading of its fibers, the peritoneal catheter is introduced in the abdominal cavity for 30–40 cm that allows free motion and sufficient length for the first decade of life. In contrast to sutures to fix the reservoir and the sites of connection safely, the peritoneal catheter is not restraint by sutures. The incisions are carefully closed in two and four layers, respectively.

Shunts are prone to the following **complications**:

1. Lifelong **shunt dependence** in most of the patients; only about 10 % of the patients become shunt-independent with shunts used in former times.
2. **Shunt failure (dysfunction)**. A prognosis for the individual patient is difficult; the history of a straightforward shunt implantation without time delay is one of several prognostically favorable factors. Possible results are as follows: 0.15 shunt revision per patient per year observation time; after 7 and 12 years has 60 and 53 %, respectively, of a shunt population, zero or one shunt revision experienced; and the remainder patients had 2 or more shunt revisions.

The **main causes of shunt dysfunction** are ventricular or central catheter obstruction by debris or in small or slit ventricles and growth of the body length (with final localization of the end of the peritoneal catheter outside the peritoneal cavity) or disconnection of parts of the shunt system. Less frequent causes are abdominal CSF pseudocyst, failure of the valve due to technical properties or unintentional changes of adjustable valve systems by MRI, distal or proximal catheter migration, localized trauma to the shunt, and complications in alternative methods such as in ventriculopleural or gallbladder shunt.

The **abdominal CSF pseudocyst** is mostly caused by shunt infection (occurrence 0.7–4.5 %) and only rarely due to silicone allergy (due to loose, unbounded silicone oil) that leads to adhesions between the intestinal loops by connective tissue and compartmentalization of the drained CSF as a pseudocyst. Clinically,

abdominal pain and distension is combined with signs of shunt dysfunction. The same proceeding is indicated as in shunt infection. After cure, reimplantation of a new ventriculoperitoneal shunt is often possible, or another distal route must be chosen. In case of allergy, systems with extracted silicone must be used.

3. **Shunt infection**. Shunt infection is mostly introduced by surgery with *Staphylococcus epidermidis* as the most frequently observed germ. Less frequently is colonization of shunts by puncture of the reservoir, after ulceration of the overlying skin in very young infants, or during septicemia. It may be combined with shunt dysfunction.

By appropriate surgery, it is possible to keep the infection rate as low as ≤1 % of interventions. Shunt infection is treated at best by removal of the shunt, external ventricular drainage, and systemic and, if needed, by topic antibiotics. Reinsertion of a new shunt after clearance of the CSF infection is possible within 10 days to 2–3 weeks. The results of implantation of shunts impregnated by antibiotics to avoid infection are only partially convincing.

4. **Overdrainage** is one of the main problems in shunt surgery and is caused by siphon effect in upright position.

In **slit ventricle syndrome (SVS)**, overdrainage of the ventricles by the commonly used shunts in the past becomes symptomatic at different times after shunting in infancy. Overdrainage is not only recognizable by an SVS but also primarily by asymptomatic radiological findings such as small or slit ventricles (ventricular volume below the normal value for age and sex or ventricles not or only recognizable as minute structure) and diminished skull growth (low modulus). Clinically, the head circumferences fall gradually below the 50 %.

SVS is characterized by intermittent, more or less dramatic and threatening episodes of severe headache, heliophobia, varying degrees of lethargy, and/or nausea and vomiting in an otherwise healthy child. In a shunt population, up to two thirds have small or slit ventricles on neuroimaging, but only a part of them had an SVS (1–37 %).

The differential diagnosis includes low CSF pressure syndrome combined with a sensitivity to low CSF pressure, intermittent shunt dysfunction, and/or cerebral vasomotor instability similar to migraine. The same disorders occur probably one behind the other or combined in the same patient and episode.

The aim of diagnostic work-up is mainly to exclude complete or partial obstruction of the ventricular catheter by shuntogram (no entry of contrast into the ventricles or only a trace), neuroimaging (enlargement of slit ventricles occurs only delayed if at all), and ICP recording by the Rickham reservoir (no or false-negative recording due to encapsulation of the catheter tip). In addition, careful clinical examination including fundoscopy and optic nerve ultrasound is unreplaceable tools.

Except for complete ventricular catheter obstruction and/or life-threatening increased ICP, delayed surgery should be performed whenever possible with preliminary application of i.v. infusion, steroids, analgetics (or antimigrainous drugs), and Trendelenburg's position. Shunt revision includes replacement of the valve and, if needed, of the ventricular catheter. Prophylaxis by implantation of a new generation of valves at the time of the primary shunt is superior to the former. The new generation of valves (hydrostatic and programmable valves, antisiphon devices, and variable-resistance and so-called flow-regulated valves) overcome or lessen the overdrainage of the former differential pressure valves but are combined with the drawbacks of significant risks of shunt insufficiency.

Epilepsy is observed in up to one fifth of a shunt population. Because it is mostly a sequel of the cause of hydrocephalus and not of its treatment, it is not a typical shunt complication. On the other hand, exacerbation of epilepsy or its deterioration may be a sign of shunt dysfunction.

Neuroendoscopic treatment of hydrocephalus may include aqueductal stenosis and fourth ventricle outlet obstruction, isolated fourth ventricle hydrocephalus, complex compartmentalized hydrocephalus, and hydrocephalus caused in congenital intracranial cysts. It is contraindicated in communicating hydrocephalus. The proof of open subarachnoid spaces may be difficult even by modern neuroimaging (cine flow MRI, if not available, lumbar air encephalography instead of flow studies with isotopes or contrast), for instance, in secondary aqueductal stenosis after hemorrhage, meningitis, long-term shunting, or due to the hydrocephalus itself.

The aim of treatment, the applicable procedures, and the results are different for the quoted pathologies. In **isolated aqueductal stenosis** or fourth **ventricle outlet obstruction**, the endoscopic third ventriculostomy (ETV) creates a communication to the basal subarachnoid spaces and cisterns. The success rate depends on the age and probably on the etiology, for example, worst outcome in patients younger than 3 months and with another than a simple idiopathic aqueductal stenosis, and amounts to ≥70 % with ≥1 year of age. **In distal membraneous aqueductal stenosis # and isolated fourth ventricle hydrocephalus**, aqueductoplasty (or interventriculostomy) with stenting in the latter may be considered which allows an unrestricted flow and equalizes the pressure difference between the ventricles.

For complex compartmentalized hydrocephalus, the option is elimination of multiple shunt systems that is achieved by fenestration between isolated intraventricular compartments and the ventricles. The success rate is 60 % and more with the best results in unilateral (monoventricular) hydrocephalus. **In hydrocephalus caused by congenital intracranial cysts**, their expanding and obstructive effect is eliminated by ventriculocystomy or cystocisternostomy with fair results.

The **drawbacks of neuroendoscopic techniques** are a significant learning curve, inadvertent bleedings, and neurological deficits, for instance, temporary or permanent oculomotor paresis or disconjugated gaze, reclosure of the created communications, for example, with the need of a secondary ETV, and pitfalls due to an insufficient information from the work-ups.

After neuroendoscopic treatment, **long-term follow-ups** are necessary by neuroimaging and clinically because the presence of a functional stoma is not always equal to a significant clinical recovery. On the other hand, the symptoms may improve and do not always completely resolve. After surgery, the ventricular volume falls to a lower value than preoperatively, and stabilization of the volume of the ventricles is achieved within 3–6 months, although it does not return to normal values for age and sex. In case of persistent or recurrent symptomatology and/or persistently increased (as preoperatively) or increasing ventricular volume, reclosure or insufficiency of a functional stoma must be considered. Unfortunately, the long-term effect of moderately enlarged ventricles on the outcome has not yet been studied thoroughly, and exacerbation of hydrocephalus with acute neurological deterioration has been observed after minor head injury in the same way as in compensated hydrocephalus.

Prognosis
It depends on the cause and stage of hydrocephalus as well as on the care and experience of the involved surgeons for the primary surgery and the long-term follow-ups.

In up to two thirds of the patients with isolated hydrocephalus, a normal intelligence (school performance, neuropsychological tests) can be observed with independent lifestyle. Thirty percent of the patients can be educated for practical tools of daily life, and less than 10 % are dependent on somebody else's help (personal hygiene, food intake, locomotion, and body position).

The prognosis is possible at school age in 90 %. Neuropsychological tests are necessary prior to the choice of the career or the job due to a possibly reduced performance in special fields. In **connatal hydrocephalus** (head circumference at term above the normal values), up to 53 % will have no mental deficit # and the remainder different degrees of mental retardation.

2.2   Constitutional Macrocrania (Benign Familial Macrocephaly)

Occurrence, Clinical Significance
Frequent constitutional macrocrania is observed in some sibs and specific regions. It is diagnosed in up to two thirds of children allocated to a tertiary center for work-up of a too large head.

- Severe pathology may be considered due to the large head by parents and general practitioner.
- On the other hand, macrocrania may be observed sometimes in syndromes, hamartomas, encephalopathies, metabolic disorders with brain involvement, and skeletal dysplasias such as achondroplasia.
- Genetic or familial constitutional microcrania exists by analogy with constitutional macrocrania.

In **constitutional microcrania**, the neurocranium is well-proportionate to the face. The head circumference is below or close to the second percentile and below the percentile of the body length, and there is a normal intelligence. Constitutional microcrania is an important differential diagnosis of microencephalia. Occasionally, it is associated with benign external hydrocephalus.

Clinical Presentation
The history yields often members of the same family with large heads. *The large head is adjusted to the face but not necessarily to the body length. The head circumference lies above or close to the 98th percentile and runs parallel with it, although short-term increases above the individual growth curve may be observed for several reasons #. The head circumference of one of the parents is often above the normal values, and photographs of family members may demonstrate macrocrania.*

Differential Diagnosis, Work-Up Examinations
The differential diagnosis may be clinically difficult if the head circumference does not increase harmoniously. In addition to the differentiation from the pathologies quoted in this chapter, the disorders listed under clinical significance must be considered in case of abnormal findings in history, general and neurological examinations, or in neuropsychological tests and their course.

In infants with open fontanel, ultrasound allows to exclude some of the major causes of macrocrania. Later and on follow-up, MRI (or CT) excludes most of the differential diagnoses and reassures parents and other involved people. Nevertheless, clinical follow-up including the course of neuropsychological development is indicated together with the common medical checkups.

Prognosis

The prognosis is excellent. During pregnancy, descendants of members with familial macrocephalia need special consideration of the head size of the unborn patient and if large of their parturition.

2.3 Intraventricular (Periventricular/Intraventricular) Hemorrhage of the Newborn (in Prematurity)

Occurrence

In contrast to the intracranial hemorrhage (IVH) of the newborn at term that occurs less frequently and mostly after birth injury (for instance, after instrumental delivery and less often in platelets and coagulation disorders, its general prevalence is 5–6 per 10,000 live births), the so-called **intraventricular hemorrhage** is observed in the immediate postpartal period in 40 % and more of premature infants (≤35 gestational week and <1,500 g) and in the newborn small for date.

The originally germinal matrix, periventricular hemorrhage can be divided into four grades of which mainly grade III and IV with intraventricular hemorrhage and ventricular dilatation and parenchymatous hemorrhage, respectively, are of clinical significance in the context of macrocephaly #.

Clinical Significance

- Intraventricular hemorrhage may lead to death and to neuropsychological deficits of the surviving patients. In the extremely low-birth-weight infants (<1,000 g), about 35 % will die, and only 5–30 % of the

surviving will have a normal neuropsychological outcome.
- Up to 50 % and more premature newborns with intraventricular hemorrhage may develop ventriculomegaly of different degree; the most severe ventricular dilatations occur significantly in grade III and IV intraventricular hemorrhages.
- Most of the ventriculomegalies are transitory, but their clinical significance is not well-established, and less than 10–15 % (and more in the extremely low-birth-weight infants) with intraventricular hemorrhage develop posthemorrhagic hydrocephalus within the neonatal period or delayed after 1/2–2½ years after temporary stabilization or regression of the initial ventriculomegaly.
- Posthemorrhagic hydrocephalus is mostly communicating. Nevertheless, combined or isolated aqueductal stenosis or closure of the fourth ventricle outlets may be observed as well.

Clinical Presentation

The clinical presentation of the **intraventricular hemorrhage** is unspecific and depends on the magnitude of hemorrhage. *Apathy or stupor, convulsions or tremulousness, in- or decreased muscle tone, apneic spells or need for artificial ventilation, bulging anterior fontanel, paleness and anemia are possible symptoms and signs.*

In **transitory ventriculomegaly**, the observed ventricular dilatation is stable or regressive, and *the increase of head circumference is less than 2 cm per week, and clinical signs are not demonstrable.*

In **progressive hydrocephalus**, the observed ventricular dilatation is increasingly combined *with some of the unspecific signs quoted above or with signs of increased intracranial pressure such as tense and prominent anterior fontanel. The abnormal increase of head circumference (≥ 2 cm or more per week) lags typically behind in relation to the ultrasound findings of the developing posthemorrhagic hydrocephalus in the premature infant.*

These criteria are somewhat arbitrary like a working hypothesis, and the transition from transitory ventriculomegaly to progressive hydrocephalus may occur insidiously and only be confirmed by follow-up.

Work-Ups

To recognize a possible peri- and intraventricular hemorrhage, all neonates at risk (premature and low-birth-weight infants at term) must be followed by ultrasound in regular intervals. In case of a probable posthemorrhagic hydrocephalus, MR or CT is indicated. In case of equivocal clinical and sonographic findings or if the former neuroimaging is not available, a ventricular tap by the anterior fontanel with measurement of the intraventricular pressure (and examinations of the CSF leukocytes and cultures) is a useful adjunct. Amplitude-integrated EEG activity is an example of continuous functional cerebral monitoring (increased discontinuity of background activity and onset of nearly isoelectric pattern) that precedes abnormal sonographic and clinical signs and can be used for the indication of surgical intervention.

Therapy

In the early stage of progressive ventriculomegaly with hematohydrocephalus, an external ventricular drainage (EVD) is indicated to avoid secondary brain damage by the increased intraventricular pressure and to evacuate the hemorrhagic CSF. By proper handling of the EVD and collection of the CSF, there is no time limit #. Less useful alternative methods are subgaleal shunt, serial punctures of a subgaleal reservoir, or lumbar punctures.

The possible negative role of transitory ventriculomegaly for the functional outcome, the development of posthemorrhagic hydrocephalus in intraventricular hemorrhages, and their avoidance by appropriate measures is still a matter of debate. Nevertheless, the normal intraventricular pressure in premature infants is lower than in neonates at term and estimated to be zero cm water or less.

In early hydrocephalus, a ventriculoperitoneal shunt should be performed, whereas in delayed hydrocephalus with proven isolated aqueductal stenosis, an ETV is a reasonable alternative.

Prognosis

The prognosis of intraventricular hemorrhage depends on the stage and the gestational age, and birth weight of the patient. In posthemorrhagic hydrocephalus, the time of continuous normalization of the ICP by different measures and the number of shunt complications are additional prognostic factors. On the other hand, spontaneous arrest of shunted hydrocephalus may occur after several years occasionally.

2.4   Catch-Up Growth of Head Circumference

Occurrence

An abnormal growth of head circumference may be observed in the period of maximum brain growth (first trimenon) after severe illnesses, malnutrition, artificial respiration, and in preterm infants or with low birth weight for date. Sometimes, it may be combined with a prominent and tense anterior fontanel and other signs of increased intracranial pressure typical for this age group.

Clinical Significance

- If the quoted accompanying disorders and/or their treatment are not considered, the abnormal increase of head circumference is interpreted as a presenting symptom of a severe underlying pathology, and work-ups are performed; ultrasound is sufficient under these circumstances.

Prognosis

The abnormal head growth returns to normal values for the individual patient within months provided the development is normal.

2.5 Congenital Intracranial Cysts

Occurrence, Types, Cyst Volumes

Due to prenatal investigations with ultrasound and MRI, an increased number of congenital intracranial cysts are recognized (>1:17,000 fetuses). Significant new informations can be gained by regular pre- and postpartal long-term follow-ups of such patients that differ from those of previous retrospective studies with variable conditions of admission. They concern the occurrence, distribution of types and locations, and natural history of congenital intracranial cysts.

In a cohort of postnatally symptomatic congenital cysts, about 50 % are arachnoid cysts (malformative intracranial cysts), 35 % are Dandy-Walker malformations, and 15 % are porencephalic cysts. In contrast to the former entities of congenital intracranial cysts that have a developmental origin, the latter are mostly prenatally acquired pathologies. The greatest volumes may be encountered in arachnoid cysts (mean volume for the convexity type 100 ml), followed by porencephalic cysts (mean volume 90 ml) and Dandy-Walker cysts (mean volume 50 ml). The remainder cysts reveal a mean volume of < or >20 ml. If measured, there is often a CSF pressure difference between cyst and ventricular system (by a mean value of 60 mm H_2O).

Clinical Significance

- Two thirds of the symptomatic congenital intracranial cysts are diagnosed in the first year of life and 50 % of these in the neonatal period, mostly due to macrocrania or hemimacrocephaly combined with signs of increased ICP.
- Congenital intracranial cyst is a potpourri of different disease entities (namely, the three main groups and additional pathologies) and of different types of the same disease entity. Therefore, their clinical presentation and natural history, treatment, and prognosis may differ considerably.
- An increasing number of intracranial cyst are recognized already in the second half of pregnancy that puts enormous pressure on the obstetrician and the attending pediatrician and/or surgeon (fetal board) from the involved parents.
- On the other hand, the increasing knowledge gained by careful prenatal investigations and postnatal follow-ups or autopsies allows more differentiated recommendations about the unborn patient and for its parents.

Disease Entities

Arachnoid cysts (malformative intracranial cysts): They arise in the second half of pregnancy as a hypoechogenic mass of variable size. The adjacent normal brain and/or ventricles are often shifted or lifted up. Two thirds of the cysts are supratentorial #, and one third are infratentorial including the incisural (dumbbell-shaped) cysts #. The most frequent types are interhemispheric and retrovermian cysts, respectively. Three fourths of the cysts do not increase in size during pregnancy, whereas 20 % increase. Although >10 % are combined with ventriculomegaly, only a small portion develops hydrocephalus during pregnancy.

On the other hand, nearly 30 % of the prenatally recognized arachnoid cysts become symptomatic after birth, among other things due to an increase of the cyst or due to hydrocephalus in early infancy. Hydrocephalus may be due to obstruction (posterior fossa cysts), due to displacement or trapping of parts of the ventricles, and due to additional involvement of the arachnoid space (communicating hydrocephalus).

In symptomatic arachnoid cysts, there is a significant peak in the two first years of life, although they can be observed throughout the whole childhood. They have no or only an insufficient communication with the arachnoid space. In some of the cysts, an intermittent symptomatology is possible due to spontaneous regression and regrowth by cyst rupture or changing communication.

Signs of increased ICP often combined with macrocrania are the leading symptoms in more than 50 % and are recognized mainly in infancy, about 30 % have focal signs corresponding to the cyst, and more than 15 % have seizures. In up to 15 %, arachnoid cysts are discovered by chance by CT for different reasons or in same proportions *after head injury. In the latter group, several previously silent arachnoid cysts, for example, middle cerebral fossa (temporobasal) cysts, become symptomatic due to an impact on or a rupture of the cyst (<10 % of the patients) with intralesional, subarachnoidal, or subdural hematoma or due to simple cyst emptying.*

Some clinical features need special attention: **hemimegalencephaly** (convexity and middle fossa cysts) with temporal bulging and possible exophthalmos in the latter; **large posterior fossa**, gait disturbances, and truncal ataxia (posterior fossa cysts including cysts of the cerebellopontine angle) with eighth (hearing loss, tinnitus, or Meniere's disease), seventh nerve palsy, or hemifacial spasms in the latter. Optic atrophy, visual field defects, and hypopituitarism occur in sellar cysts. In **bobble-head doll syndrome**, there is a rhythmic head bobbing in toddlers during walking that disappears in recumbent position. The causative cystic lesion in the region of the dilated third ventricle is often a suprasellar arachnoid cyst that leads to an intermittent obstruction of the foramina of Monro.

The frequency, pattern of symptoms, and their great variation are explained in part by the preference of Sylvian fissure (middle cerebral fossa) and cerebellomedullary types (posterior or posterolateral cerebellar surface) of arachnoid cysts (35 and 15 %), cerebral convexity #, and sellar cysts (each >10 %). Interhemispheric and quadrigeminal plate cysts are the less frequently observed arachnoid cysts. Asymptomatic arachnoid cysts are encountered in 1 of 1,000 adult autopsies.

Dandy-Walker malformations (Dandy-Walker cyst and variant or complex): This group of, at first glance, similar malformations occurs in 1 of 25,000–35,000 live births. With the advent of new neuroimaging techniques, efforts have been made to define true Dandy-Walker malformation (Dandy-Walker cyst #) with regard to a safer prognostication by the following features: A large median posterior fossa cyst which communicates largely with the fourth ventricle, an upward displaced tentorium, an anterolateral displacement of seemingly normal cerebellar hemispheres, and a vermis which is either rotated,

raised, small, and comes in contact with the tentorium (partial agenesis of the cerebellar vermis), or a malformed and dysplastic vermis.

The latter feature allows differentiation of two prognostic groups. Dandy-Walker complex includes a wide variety of similar malformations that fit not to the described features and have not uniform prognoses.

Hydrocephalus occurs in 70–100 % of the two prognostic groups of true Dandy-Walker malformation. A major challenge of Dandy-Walker malformation combined with hydrocephalus is a possible compartmentalization of the fourth ventricle and its cyst from the supratentorial ventricular system by a primary or secondary aqueductal stenosis or insufficiency with the development of isolated fourth ventricle hydrocephalus. In contrast to the arachnoid cysts, numerous associated central nervous system and systemic malformations (cardiovascular, urogenital, intestinal, facial, and extremities) or genetic disorders are observed in Dandy-Walker malformations. All may have an impact on survival and the necessary treatment options whereas the cerebral anomalies (excluding hydrocephalus) and genetic disorders on the neuropsychological prognostication.

Clinically, most of the true Dandy-Walker malformations are recognized in the neonatal period or in the first year of life due to the bossing of the posterior fossa (if looked for precisely on clinical examination #) and/or macrocrania combined with signs of increased intracranial pressure. Later or with the development of an isolated fourth ventricle hydrocephalus, subtle or distinct (delayed motor development and ataxia), and sometimes life-threatening posterior fossa signs can occur which may simulate a malignant posterior fossa tumor.

In **porencephalic cysts**, a focal deficiency within the cerebral parenchyma is filled with fluid, and most of these congenital cysts communicate with the lateral ventricle. True congenital forms are restricted to one vascular territory (often absence of the middle cerebral artery). In the more frequently, later in pregnancy acquired forms, anoxemia, intracerebral hemorrhage #, and theoretically ventricular puncture, closed head injury, and penetrating wounds of the brain are possible causes. With the advent of ultrasound and MRI applied in pregnancy, their development can be observed prior birth, for instance, after a large intracerebral hemorrhage of the fetus which ends up later with a porencephalic cyst. In general, such intrauterine events need postnatal follow-ups and the symptomatic ones treatment.

Some of them exert a mass effect on follow-up by an enormous increase of their size and/or an insufficient communication with the ventricle with shifting of the midline and compression of the brain and the adjacent ventricles.

Clinically, macrocrania or hemimacrocephaly # combined with signs of increased intracranial pressure (possibly associated with bulging and thinning of the skull overlying the cyst), lateralizing signs corresponding to the involved brain area (hemiparesis or focal seizures which can be lessened or disappear after decompression), and unspecific signs such as apathy, irritability, and failure to thrive can be observed. In addition, often delay of mental and motor development is observed.

By the distribution and the shape of the defect, and by the finding of an avascular area, a differentiation between the two forms of porencephalic cyst is sometimes possible.

Differential Diagnosis, Work-Ups

The differential diagnosis includes other, less frequently symptomatic congenital intracranial cysts such as subcallosal cysts (septum pellucidum cyst, cavum vergae, and cavum velum interpositum cyst), neuroepithelial cysts (colloid cyst of the third ventricle), Rathke's cleft cyst, and acquired cystic lesions such as chronic subdural hematoma and hygroma, leptomeningeal cyst, hydatid cysts, and cystic tumors.

The **septum pellucidum cyst** is mostly communicating with the ventricles. It may be a cause of concern because it is found on neuroimaging in about 80 % of full-term neonates. Because septum pellucidum cyst is found by chance only in 10 % of adults, most of them disappear with time and are asymptomatic. Rarely recurrent headache and vomiting in children can be caused by a not or only insufficiently communicating septum pellucidum cyst that leads to intermittent obstruction of the CSF flow from the lateral ventricles by a ball-valve mechanism with biventricular hydrocephalus. The **cavum vergae cyst** is either a large septum pellucidum cyst with posterior expansion or a solitary cavum of the latter site. **Cavum velum interpositum** is a rostral extension of the quadrigeminal plate cistern and may point to an obstruction of CSF flow at the site of the interpeduncular and chiasmatic cistern.

The work-up examinations include CT and MRI; the former is replaced increasingly by MRI because it allows a more precise delineation and definition of the individual intracranial cyst, for instance, in Dandy-Walker malformation, with sagittal planes and T2-weighted images, and may replace the former dynamic studies of CSF flow with contrast or isotopes in arachnoid cysts by visualization of flow phenomena, for example, in the differentiation of a posterior fossa cyst from a large cisterna magna.

Depending on the type of recognized congenital intracranial cyst, further work-up examinations become necessary to exclude possible CNS or systemic malformations and genetic disorders.

Therapy, Prognosis

Surgery is indicated in symptomatic congenital intracranial cysts in which the symptoms and signs are related to the cyst and can disappear after surgery. Preventive surgery in large or enlarging asymptomatic cysts is a matter of discussion (elimination of expansive and/or obstructive effect with the aim to provide normal development of the involved adjacent brain structures). It should be considered at least in young infants in whom normalization is possible as shown in hemimacrocephaly and local bossing with thinning of the skull and in older children, in whom electrophysiological examinations and psychological testing demonstrate abnormalities.

The available treatment options are shunting (cyst or ventriculoperitoneal shunt, or double shunt), open surgery with microscopic resection of the cyst, fenestration, and establishment of a communication to the ventricles, cisterns, or subarachnoid space, and endoscopic surgery with fenestration to the ventricles and/or cisterns. For the last procedure using stereotactic guidance or a neuronavigation system, success rates up to 70–80 % have been reported that may be possible also in long-term shunting.

Each treatment option has advantages and disadvantages. Shunting is associated with possible revisions, shunt dependency, and the insertion of a cyst tube may be tricky due to the tight cyst membrane. Open surgery may be difficult and combined with major complications, and reclosure of fenestration occurs commonly in childhood.

Probably, each case needs an indication for a specific treatment option, and each of them should be available and, if necessary, be combined in succession until precise indications are available based on large numbers and the principle of evidence-based medicine.

Prognosis depends on the group and type of congenital intracranial cyst. Except for some cases with long-lasting symptomatology, additional congenital anomalies, or acquired perinatal pathology, there is a normal development in arachnoid cysts (90 %). In Dandy-Walker malformations, the more frequently observed group with only partially agenetic vermis has a normal development in a similar percentage as in arachnoid cysts, whereas the group with dysplastic vermis or the variant forms reveals retardation in all or in a changing number, respectively. Almost all patients with porencephalic cyst have some degree of psychomotor retardation.

In a cohort of arachnoid cysts with either shunts (1/3) or open surgery, the symptomatology disappeared or improved, and the cyst was not any more visible or smaller in about three fourth of the cases, and there was a positive trend between reduction of the cyst size and outcome. In a cohort of congenital intracranial cysts with 80 % shunts, a normal psychomotor development and/or normal school placement were achieved in about 60 %, and delayed psychomotor development and/or special school requirement, or marked psychomotor development and/or inability to attend school in about 40 %. Although there was a reduction of the cyst volume in at least two thirds (most strikingly for the convexity

arachnoid cysts and porencephalic cyst by 55 and 41 %, respectively), no uniform pattern of correlation with outcome could be ascertained.

2.6 Subacute and Chronic Subdural Hematoma (Hygroma)

Occurrence, Etiopathogenesis
This type of subdural hematoma # occurs mostly in the first 2 years with a peak incidence between 1 and 6 months of life and preferred in boys because the acute or repeated trauma receives no attention and/or may be accompanied by less dramatic symptoms than in the other age groups. It is less frequent than the former figures of hydrocephalus and spina bifida or as constitutional macrocrania. In the older literature, more than 50 % of the small children with chronic subdural hematoma had no history of birth or another accidental trauma. Neglected or only conservatively treated acute subdural hematoma is an important cause of chronic subdural hematoma according the newer literature.

A population-based study tells that still 53 % of serious or fatal traumatic brain injuries in the first 2 years of life are because of child abuse. Two inflicted brain injuries in 10,000 children ≤2 years of age in North Carolina and 0.13 shaken infants in 1,000 live births in Switzerland with a mortality of 16 % are the available data about head injury in battered child syndrome. These data also permit an estimation of the prevalence of chronic subdural hematoma independent of the possible causes.

Clinical Significance
- The cause of chronic subdural hematoma may be an inflicted traumatic brain injury, especially if a history of a reasonable injury is missing.
- Chronic subdural hematoma may lead to death if it is not recognized or too late and in up to one to two thirds to severe neuropsychological deficits depending on the cause.
- Early diagnosis and treatment of chronic subdural hematoma interrupts additional

spontaneous, inflicted, or accidental hemorrhages and improves therefore the prognosis.

Clinical Presentation

Specific symptoms and signs for chronic subdural hematoma do not exist. *It is rather the history of an infant who is not doing well: anorexia, failure to thrive, intermittent low-grade fever, and resistance to be cuddled in the arms of the attending nurse. Or the combination of the following symptoms and signs that are ambiguous per se and arranged according to their frequency in a large cohort of children: convulsions, fever of different types, vomiting and hyperactive reflexes (≥50 %), restlessness, irritability, or apathy, tense, prominent anterior fontanel, anemia, and large head (about 40–30 %). In at least one fifth of the cases, abnormal fundoscopic findings are observed; the mainly asymmetric retinal hemorrhages are characteristic of subdural hematoma as is the change of the skull shape into a squared or "box-like" form with biparietal bossing #.*

Periods of loss or clouding of consciousness or stupor in the history in up to two thirds of the cases point to an initial or repeated blow(s) to the head. Beyond infancy, signs of increased intracranial pressure become prominent; nevertheless, lateralizing neurological signs are often missing.

Differential Diagnosis

It includes **subdural fluid collections** such as **those due to bacterial meningitis**, and if the findings of neuroimaging are considered as well, **subarachnoid fluid collections of different etiopathogenesis**.

In the former situation, the large fluid collections (>10–15 ml) are yellow, clear or cloudy, bloody or purulent (subdural empyema), follow with time the same pathoanatomical course as in subdural hematoma with membrane formation, and reveal their identity by persistent fever in spite of adequate antibiotic treatment of meningitis, by irritability, and failure to thrive. External drainage or rarely open surgery is necessary to cure large and symptomatic postinfectious subdural fluid collection.

To the latter belong to the **benign extracerebral fluid collections (extraventricular hydrocephalus)** that may be observed in infancy beyond the neonatal period by macrocrania (head circumference >90th percentile with increased growth velocity) and possibly by a squared forehead. In 10–15 % of the cases, there is a motor delay of varying degree. On neuroimaging, enlargement of the anterior subarachnoid soaces that includes the interhemispheric and Sylvian fissures, possibly a mild ventricular dilatation specifically of the frontal horns, and no increased signal intensity on T1-weighted MRI is seen. Rarely, clinical signs of increased ICP (such as tense anterior fontanel, irritability, setting sun phenomenon), acute or subacute abnormal head growth, and arrest of motor development may be observed. Medical treatment (acetazolamide and furosemide) or in case of failure even temporary EVD is indicated in such patients. In general, improvement of motor delay and decreased head growth occur after 1–2 years of age and mild developmental delay in <10 %. Benign external hydrocephalus may be complicated by acute subdural hematoma.

Work-Ups

They include ultrasound, MRI, or CT, and subdural puncture with examination of the subdural fluid.

The latter may be performed for diagnostic and/or therapeutic reasons. Today, it is replaced by MRI and surgery, respectively. If a subdural puncture must be performed, some precautions must be taken: meticulous asepsis, punction lateral to the edge of the anterior fontanel through the coronal suture, and fluid should be allowed to drip from the needle (no use of a syringe).

Ultrasound or more precisely MRI allows to recognize the subdural hematoma, its laterality, and site (in infancy, 80–85 % are bilateral and mostly frontoparietal and interhemispheric), its composition and stage, the width of the subdural space, a possible ventriculomegaly, and some differentiation from other fluid collections. The resolution of the subdural hematoma, the establishment of cerebral atrophy, or progressive communicating hydrocephalus (in about 10 %) can be demonstrated by postoperative radiological follow-up,

Additional examinations include the current status of development, ophthalmological and neurological findings. If a battered child syndrome is suspected, a throughout clinical and radiological search for corresponding findings and confrontation with the caregivers are necessary.

Therapy

Infants with head injury and only small acute subdural hematomas on neuroimaging need clinical and radiological follow-up because it may lead after an early stage of apparent resorption of the hematoma with widening of the subdural space to gross chronic subdural hematoma within 2–4 months.

In the past, treatment was started with repeated daily subdural taps over 2–3 weeks and more up to dryness with reported success in three fourth of the cases with chronic subdural hematoma.

When the subdural fluid gets clear and the protein level is less than 250 mg%, a bi- or unilateral subduroperitoneal shunt with a common distal part, a purpose-designed subdural catheter, and a low pressure valve is performed or alternatively beyond early infancy a subduropleural shunt with or without valve. The whole system should be removed within 6 months because resolution of the hygroma occurs in a few months and the subdural catheter becomes adherent afterward, must be left behind, and may be a source of complications.

Alternatively, burr hole, minicraniotomy, endoscopic washout, or continuous external subdural drainage is proposed. Temporary EVD has been proposed either as intermediate measure until the subdural fluid gets clear or instead of shunting (as definitive treatment in >90 %). Because the time of resolution is variable in chronic subdural hygroma and the risks of infection of the EVD increase with time, a closed system and aseptic handling are necessary.

Today, craniotomy with membrane stripping is less frequently performed because there is questionable evidence that the mechanical constriction leads to brain damage #.

According to the current opinions, prognosis depends more on the cause(s) of the chronic subdural hematoma of infancy than on the treatment with good outcome in two thirds and moderate to severe disability in one third.

2.7   Encephalopathies, Metabolic Disorders with Brain Involvement

Occurrence, Etiopathogenesis

Encephalopathies of different causes such as toxic, metabolic, anoxemic, traumatic, and inflammatory may lead to increased growth of head circumference of minor degree in infants and small children.

Examples of metabolic disorders are the mucopolysaccharidoses, GM2-gangliosidoses, and glutaraciduria type I. Macrocrania develops by two mechanisms: storage of metabolites in brain and skull with increase of volume and/or brain damage with secondary atrophy and dilatation of the subdural space that becomes prone to hematoma and hygroma in minor head injury.

Clinical Significance, Clinical Presentation

- The quoted pathologies with macrocrania are infrequent disorders. Nevertheless, they may have a differential diagnostic and/or prognostic significance in the individual case. The prognostic significance increases if they are combined with hydrocephalus.

In **glutaraciduria type I**, an increasing head size belongs to the first signs of the disorder, the corresponding clinical (microencephalic macrocrania, possible retinal hemorrhages) and CT findings (dilatation of subdural space with hematoma and hygroma) must be differentiated from battered child syndrome, and the chronic subdural hematoma needs possibly surgical treatment. In **Hurler's disease** (as one of the seven types of mucopolysaccharidoses) and **Tay-Sachs' disease** (GM2-gangliosidosis), macrocrania is just one of several other signs, for example, typical features (gargoylism) and hepatomegaly in the former and neurological signs including loss of developmental milestones in the latter. Macrocrania is caused by storage of the corresponding metabolites. In **Hurler's disease**, the thickened leptomeninx and small subarachnoid cysts lead additionally to progressive hydrocephalus that needs shunting.

Red flags that refer to the possibility of such causes of macrocrania are the history of such encephalopathies or familiality of such metabolic disorders, arrest or loss of further neuropsychological development, facial dysmorphia, and other organ involvements.

2.8 Achondroplasia (Chondrodysplasia)

Occurrence

Achondroplasia is the most frequent bone dysplasia, is mostly due to a de novo mutation, and has an autosomal dominant inheritance.

Clinical Significance

- Disproportionate or absolute macrocrania is common.
- Macrocrania may be caused by megalencephaly, excessive growth of the calvaria, and/or hydrocephalus.
- Hydrocephalus is present in up to 50 %. It is mostly a communicating hydrocephalus with stable ventricular size and without clinical signs of increased ICP. It is caused by venous congestion (due to jugular foramen and thoracic inlet obstruction) and/or by obstruction of the basal cisterns and the fourth ventricle outlets (due to distortion of the brain stem).
- The communicating hydrocephalus may get superimposed by an intermittent and/or progressive hydrocephalus due to aqueductal stenosis (following dynamic changes of brain morphology such as tectal beaking) in up to 20 %.
- Up to 75–80 % have or develop chronic pneumopathy for different reasons.
- Up to 50 % have or develop neurological complications, among other things due to compressive cervicomedullary or multisegmented syndrome

(mostly in the third and fourth decade) or cervical myelopathies (mostly in young children).

Clinical Presentation

There is a disproportionate dwarfism combined with rhizomelic, short limbs (mean body length in adulthood 125 cm). The large brachycephalic head displays a narrow cranial base and a sunken root of the nose #. In addition, a small thoracic cavity is combined with a thoracolumbar kyphoscoliosis and with crura vara.

The head circumference lies above or close to the 98th percentile or at a higher percentile than the body length. On follow-up, the head circumference parallels the normal values at a higher level. In case of progressive hydrocephalus of infancy, the slope takes an acute upward turn. In general, all symptoms are progressively worsening with age.

Differential Diagnosis, Work-Ups

The differential diagnosis includes other disorders which lead to macrocrania, particularly in infancy, to dwarfism, and to similar symptoms and signs as in achondroplasia.

Work-ups are necessary in every case right from the start and or if the child becomes symptomatic during the clinical long-term follow-up: cranial CT and MRI including the craniocervical junction, for instance, in case of suspected progressive hydrocephalus or compressive cervicomedullary syndrome. Because the ICP may be increased in moderately dilated ventricles in spite of absence of clinical signs, continuous ICP measurement allows recognition of such cases. Somatosensory evoked responses allow identification of early ongoing compressive syndromes.

Therapy, Prognosis

For the indication of treatment of hydrocephalus, there are two options: either shunting only in case of symptomatic hydrocephalus or by checking for increased ICP. Surgery is indicated in ICP >15 mmHg and/or pressure waves in symptomless cases with moderately increased ventricular size. In craniocervical and other compressive syndromes, decompressive surgery is indicated; it must consider in the former situation the venous congestion in the region of the cranial base.

The prognosis of the individual case depends not only on the time and effectiveness of treatment of hydrocephalus but also on the general intellectual outcome of achondroplasia. Although most of the patients have at worst only a slight delay of psychomotor development and a normal IQ with mild cognitive defects without evidence of progression, up to 10–20 % display a significant delay in psychomotor development and low IQ values. In general, life expectancy is reduced in achondroplasia.

Webcodes

The following webcodes can be used on www.psurg.net for further images and data.

201 Hydrocephalus, macrocrania	213 CT, preterm newborn, grade IV intraventricular hemorrhage (IVM)
202 Hydrocephalus, pathological head circumference	214 External ventricular drainage, IVM
203 Setting sun sign	215 Hemispheric supratentorial arachnoid cyst
204 Valve chamber before	216 Combined supra-/ infratentorial arachnoid cyst
205 And after compression	217 Dandy-Walker cyst
206 Sonography, hydrocephalus	218 Dandy-Walker malformation, occipital bossing
207 MRI, hydrocephalus before	219 Perinatal intracranial hemorrhage
208 And CT after shunt implantation	220 Porencephalic cyst
209 24 h CSF pressure, in arrested hydrocephalus	221 Chron. subdural hematoma
210 And in shunt-dependent hydrocephalus	222 Chron. subdural hematoma, biparietal bossing
211 Kindergarten child, normal development	223 Subdural space, elongated bridging vein
212 Constitutional macrocrania, course of head circumference	224 Macrocrania, achondroplasia

Bibliography

Section 2.1

Garel C, Luton D, Oury J-F, Gressens P (2003) Ventricular dilatations. Childs Nerv Syst 19:517–523

Iskandar BJ, McLaughlin C, Mapstone TB et al (1998) Pitfalls in the diagnosis of ventricular shunt dysfunction: radiology reports and ventricular size. Pediatrics 101:1031–1036

Kraus R, Hanigan WC, Kattah J, Olivero WC (2003) Changes in visual acuity associated with shunt failure. Childs Nerv Syst 19:226–231

Mc Auley D, Paterson A, Sweeney L (2009) Optic nerve sheath ultrasound in the assessment of paediatric hydrocephalus. Childs Nerv Syst 25:87–90

McClinton D, Carraccio C, Englander R (2001) Predictors of ventriculoperitoneal shunt pathology. Pediatr Infect Dis J 20:593–597

Moutard ML, Kieffer V, Feingold J, Kieffer F, Lewin F, Adamsbaum C, Gélot A, Campistol i Plana J, van Bogaert P, André M, Ponsot G (2003) Agenesis of corpus callosum: prenatal diagnosis and prognosis. Childs Nerv Syst 19:471–476

Oi S (2003) Diagnosis, outcome, and management of fetal abnormalities: fetal hydrocephalus. Childs Nerv Syst 19:508–516

Papaiconomou C et al (2004) Reassessment of pathways responsible for cerebrospinal fluid absorption in the neonate. Childs Nerv Syst 20:29–36

Straussberg R, Amir J, Varsano I (1993) Knee-chest position as a sign of increased intracranial pressure in children. J Pediatr 122:99–100

Walker M (2005) Looking at hydrocephalus: where are we now, where are we going? Childs Nerv Syst 21:524–527

Arnold Chiari Malformation

Shane Tubbs R, Jerry Oakes W (2004) Treatment and management of the Chiari II malformation: an evidence-based review of the literature. Childs Nerv Syst 20:375–381

Steinbock P (2004) Clinical features of Chiari I malformation. Childs Nerv Syst 20:329–331

Shunt Surgery

Aschoff A, Benesch C, Kremer P, Fruh K, Hashemi B, Kunza S (1995) How safe are hydrocephalus valves? a critical review on 240 examples tested in vitro. Eur J Pediatr Surg 5(Suppl I):49–50

Hashimoto M, Yokota A, Urasaki E, Tsujigami S, Shimono M (2004) A case of abdominal CSF pseudocyst associated with silicone allergy. Childs Nerv Syst 20:761–764

Jain H, Natarajan K, Sgouros S (2005) Influence of the shunt type in the difference in reduction of volume between the two lateral ventricles in shunted hydrocephalic children. Childs Nerv Syst 21:552–558

Khalil BA, Sarsam Z, Buxton N (2005) External ventricular drains: is there a time limit in children? Childs Nerv Syst 21:355–357

Lüdemann W, Rosahl SK, Kaminsky J, Samii M (2005) Reliability of a new adjustable shunt device without the need for readjustment following 3-Tesla MRI. Childs Nerv Syst 21:227–229

Nadkarni TD, Rekate HL (2005) Treatment of refractory intracranial hypertension in a spina bifida patient by a concurrent ventricular and cisterna magna-to-peritoneal shunt. Childs Nerv Syst 21: 579–582

Pollack IF, Albright AL, Adelson PD (1999) A randomized, controlled study of a programmable shunt valve versus a conventional valve for patients with hydrocephalus: Hakim-Medos Investigator Group. Neurosurgery 45:1399–1408

Spennato P, O'Brien DF, Fraher JP, Mallucci CL (2005) Bilateral abducent and facial nerve palsies following fourth ventricle shunting: two case reports. Childs Nerv Syst 21:309–316

Endoscopic Surgery

Bruwer GE, van der Westhuizen S, Lombard JC, Schoeman JF (2004) Can CT predict the level of CSF block in tuberculous hydrocephalus? Childs Nerv Syst 20:183–187

Figaji AA, Fieggen AG, Peter JC (2005) Air encephalography for hydrocephalus in the era of neuroendoscopy. Childs Nerv Syst 21:559–565

Fritsch MJ, Kienke S, Mehdorn HM (2004) Endoscopic aqueductoplasty: stent or not to stent? Childs Nerv Syst 20:137–142

Koch D, Wagner W (2004) Endoscopic third ventriculostomy in infants of less than 1 year of age: which factors influence the outcome? Childs Nerv Syst 20:405–411

Nowoslawska E et al (2003) Effectiveness of neuroendoscopic procedures in the treatment of complex compartmentalized hydrocephalus. Childs Nerv Syst 19:659–665

St George E, Natarajan K, Sgouros S (2004) Changes in ventricular volume in hydrocephalic children following successful endoscopic third ventriculostomy. Childs Nerv Syst 20:834–838

Section 2.2

Ghods E, Kreissl A, Brandstetter S, Fuiko R, Widhalm K (2011) Head circumference catch-up growth among preterm very low birth weight infants: effect on neurodevelopmental outcome. J Perinat Med 39:579–586

Vargas JE, Allred EN, Leviton A et al (2001) Congenital microcephaly: phenotypic features in a consecutive sample of newborn infants. Pediatrics 139:210–214

Section 2.3

Heep A, Engelskirchen R, Holschneider A, Groneck P (2001) Primary intervention for posthemorrhagic hydrocephalus in very low birthweight infants by ventriculostomy. Childs Nerv Syst 17:47–51

Scavarda D, Bednarek N, Litre F, Koch C, Lena G, Morville P, Rousseau P (2003) Acquired aqueductal stenosis in preterm infants: an indication for neuroendoscopic third ventriculostomy. Childs Nerv Syst 19:756–759

Tsitouras V, Sgouros S (2011) Infantile posthemorrhagic hydrocephalus. Childs Nerv Syst 27:1595–1608

Section 2.4

Williams J, Chir B, Hirsch NJ, Corbet AJS, Rudolph AJ (1977) Postnatal head shrinkage in small infants. Pediatrics 59:619–622

Section 2.5

Ciolkowski MK (2011) Cavum velum interpositum, cavum septum pellucidum and cavum Vergae: a review. Childs Nerv Syst 27:2027–2028; author reply 2029

Godano U, Mascari C, Consales A, Calbucci F (2004) Endoscope-controlled microneurosurgery for the treatment intracranial fluid cysts. Childs Nerv Syst 20:839–841

Klein O, Pierre-Kahn A, Boddaert N, Parisot D, Brunelle F (2003) Dandy-Walker malformation: prenatal diagnosis and prognosis. Childs Nerv Syst 19:484–489

Oberbauer RW, Haase J, Pucher R (1992) Arachnoid cysts in children: a European co-operative study. Childs Nerv Syst 8:281–286

Pierre-Kahn A, Sonigo P (2003) Malformative intracranial cysts: diagnosis and outcome. Childs Nerv Syst 19:477–483

Pirotte B, Morelli D, Alessi G, Lubansu A, Verheulpen D, Fricx C, David P, Brotchi J (2005) Facial nerve palsy in posterior fossa arachnoid cysts: report of two cases. Childs Nerv Syst 21:587–590

Tirakotai W, Schulte DM, Bauer BL, Bertalanffy H, Hellwig D (2004) Neuroendoscopic surgery in intracranial cysts in adults. Childs Nerv Syst 20:842–851

Tsuboi Y, Hamada H, Hayashi N, Kurimoto M, Hirashima Y, Endo S (2005) Huge arachnoid cyst of the posterior fossa: controversial discussion for selection of the surgical approach. Childs Nerv Syst 21:259–261

Zamponi N, Rychlicki F, Triguani R, Polonara G, Ruggiero M, Cesaroni E (2005) Bobble head doll syndrome in a child with third ventricular cyst and hydrocephalus. Childs Nerv Syst 21:350–354

Section 2.6

Aoki N (1990) Chronic subdural hematoma in infancy. Clinical analysis of 30 cases in the CT era. J Neurosurg 73:201–205

Eidlitz-Markus T, Shuper A, Constantini S (2003) Short-term subarachnoid space drainage: a potential treatment for extraventricular hydrocephalus. Childs Nerv Syst 19:367–370

Galaznik JG (2011) A case for in utero etiology of chronic SDH/effusion of infancy. J Perinatol 31:220–222

Hellbusch LC (2007) Benign extracerebral fluid collections in infancy: clinical presentation and long-term follow-up. J Neurosurg 107(2 Suppl):119–125

Hwang SK, Kim SL (2000) Infantile head injury, with special reference to the development of chronic subdural hematoma. Childs Nerv Syst 16:590–594

Kombogiorgas D, Sgouros S (2005) Removal of subdural-peritoneal shunts in infants. Childs Nerv Syst 21:458–460

Lin CL, Hwang SL, Su YF, Tsai LC, Kwan AL, Howng SL, Loh JK (2004) External subdural drainage in the treatment of infantile chronic subdural hematoma. J Trauma 57:104–107

Matson DD (1969) Subdural hematoma. In: Matson DD (ed) Neurosurgery of infancy and childhood, 2nd edn. Charles C Thomas, Springfield

Section 2.7

Staba SL, Escolar ML, Poe M et al (2004) Cord-blood transplants from unrelated donors in patients with Hurler's syndrome. N Engl J Med 350:1960–1969

Strauss KA, Puffenberger EG, Robinson DL, Morton DH (2003) Type I glutaric aciduria, part 1: natural history of 77 patients. Am J Med Genet C Semin Med Genet 121C(1):38–52

Section 2.8

Erdincler P, Dashti R, Kaynar MY, Canbaz B, Ciplak N, Kuday C (1997) Hydrocephalus and chronically increased intracranial pressure in achondroplasia. Childs Nerv Syst 13:345–348

Rollins N, Booth T, Shapiro K (2000) The use of gated cine phase contrast and MR venography in achondroplasia. Childs Nerv Syst 16:569–577

Ruiz-Garcia M et al (1997) Early detection of neurological manifestations of achondroplasia. Childs Nerv Syst 13:208–213

Unconsciousness and Altered States of Consciousness

Unconsciousness and altered states of consciousness are of important clinical significance due to their frequency and many and diverse possible causes. For graduation of altered states of consciousness, the following terms may be used: clouding of consciousness, delirium, stupor, and coma ###. The most important causes of unconsciousness or altered states of consciousness are quoted in Table 3.1, as far as they are important for the pediatric and other surgeons and marked according to their frequency of occurrence.

The Glasgow Coma Scale (GCS) has been developed for patients with head injury with the aim to obtain an objective and reproductive clinical tool for quantification of altered consciousness and determination of the degree of brain injury by its course. It became soon necessary to adapt the GCS for small children and infants (Table 3.2) and to apply it to the other disorders leading to impaired consciousness. In addition, the correct assignment of maximum 15 points may be hindered by additional abnormal findings such as eyelid swelling or paresis and therapeutic measures, for example, intubation and relaxation.

The type of respiration (apnea, irregular and incomplete respiration, intermittent apnea, central hyperventilation, Cheyne-Stokes respiration), skeletal movements (decerebrate or decorticate rigidity #), and ocular or pupillary movements [oculocephalic reflex, doll's head eye phenomenon, and caloric stimulation – direct and consensual pupillary

Table 3.1 Differential diagnosis of unconsciousness and altered states of consciousness

Head injury (central nervous system injury)
- Cerebral concussion
- Syndrome of cerebral concussion in children
- Cerebral contusion
- Epidural hematoma
o Acute subdural and intracerebral hematoma
o **Fat embolism, fat embolism syndrome**
- **Convulsion attacks, epilepsy**
- **Shunt dysfunction, acute exacerbation of native hydrocephalus**
- **Septic disorders and disorders with blood volume deficit**
- Blood volume shock
- Obstructive ileus
- Secondary peritonitis

Spontaneous intracranial hemorrhage
- Vascular malformations
o Cerebrovascular accident
o Cerebral venous thrombosis
o Primary and secondary coagulation disorders

Pediatric disorders
- Metabolic disorders
- Intoxications (alcohol, drugs)
- Cerebral tumors and other intracranial masses and cysts
- Central nervous infections (meningitis, encephalitis, subdural empyema)
- Drowning and near drowning, accidental hypothermia, smoke inhalation
- Hypoxic attacks
- Cardiovascular insufficiency (anoxia)

Table 3.2 Classification of the severity of head injury according to three aspects of behavior (Glasgow Coma Scale) for adults or small children and infants

	Adults	Small children and infants <2 years	Points
Eye opening	Spontaneous	Spontaneous	4
	To call	To sound	3
	To pain	To pain	2
	Absent	Absent	1
Best verbal response	Oriented	Social smile, ocular pursuit and fixation, recognition of family members	5
Nonverbal communication	Disoriented Confused	Above-mentioned reactions inconstant, cries but consolable	4
	Inappropriate coherent	Can be awakened inconstantly, motor irritability, no drinking or eating	3
	Incomprehensible	Cannot be wakened up, motor restlessness	2
	Absent	Absent	1
Best motor response	Obeys commands	Idem	6
	Localizes pain	Idem	5
	Withdraws	Idem	4
	Reflex flexion	Idem	3
	Reflex extension	Idem	2
	Absent	Idem	1
Maximum number of points			15

light reflexes and pupillary width in mm and possible difference – corneal reflex] belong to the qualitative evaluation of the neurological condition (cortical and brain stem function).

At the scene of the accident, respiration, airways, and circulation must be evaluated and maintained together with a preliminary history about possible indications of diabetes, acute inflammatory process, epilepsy, drug intoxication, CSF shunt insufficiency, or head injury.

It is possible to decide together with the neurological and general examination, if the findings of an altered state of consciousness are:

• Caused by a metabolic disorder
• Due to a rapidly progressive mass lesion
• Due to a nonprogressive disorder of impaired consciousness

The necessary drugs must be administered before the transport to the tertiary center.

3.1   Head Injury

Occurrence, Causes, Clinical Significance
At least 1:100 0- to 14-year-old children sustain a significant head injury in developed countries.

The causes depend largely on the age of the child; trauma to the mother before and at birth in newborns; **falling over or from a height**; **motor vehicle accidents** as occupants, pedestrian, cyclist, or driver in older children; and **battered child syndrome** (BC, mostly in small children ≤2 years of age #) in infants and toddlers; and increasingly injuries in leisure activities, sports, and matches in schoolchildren and adolescents.

The clinical significance is as follows:
• The large number of involved youngsters.
• Brain injury strikes an age group of growth, development, and maturation that has a diminished potential of recovery especially in infancy and small children.
• Repeated minor or moderate head injuries in team games receive often little attention, are ignored completely, and may lead to significant permanent deficits if not considered.
• In the single case, severe head injury means an enormous suffer for parents and involved patient and great expenditure on treatment and rehabilitation, and expense of the public or private health-care services.

3.1.1   Cerebral Concussion

Definition, Pathophysiology

Cerebral concussion means a short-term disturbance of cerebral function after head injury that
is often but not always followed by complete
recovery and does not leave any long-term pathoanatomical findings in the brain according to the
current knowledge except for sports concussion
(process of delayed axotomy that may be followed by permanent damage).

Initial unconsciousness of maximum 15 min
that is followed by a period of drowsiness of
maximum 1 h is a diadactic description of cerebral concussion and trial to differentiate it from
cerebral contusion (Fig. 3.1). On the other hand,
the initial unconsciousness has not been observed
or did not occur with the classic clinical presentation and therefore has been recognizable only by
an expert eye.

Cerebral concussion may occur in any of
the causes of head injury and may be combined

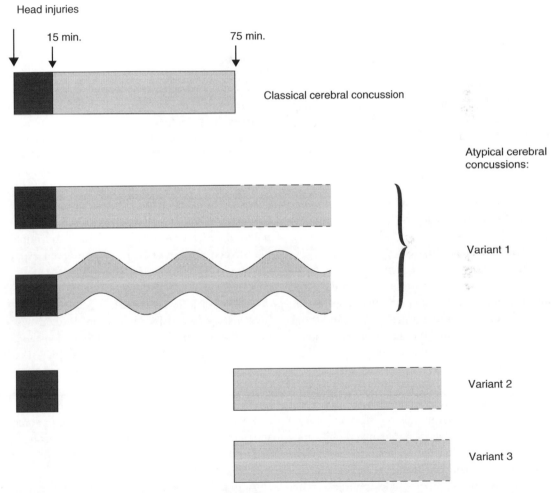

Fig. 3.1 Types of cerebral concussion. The *top row*
shows a possible definition of the most severe form of the
classic cerebral concussion with maximum unconsciousness (*black*) of 15 min that is followed by clouding of consciousness (*gray*) of maximum 1 h. The four *lower rows*
illustrate different forms of atypical cerebral concussion
that are mainly observed in children: Observed (*black*) or
not obvious initial unconsciousness is followed immediately or after a symptom-free interval (*white*) by clouding
of consciousness (*gray*) and/or transient neurological
signs for more than 1 h that disappear after 12–24 h later
without sequels

or not with signs of the associated head contusion such as contusional marks, abrasions, and lacerations of galea and face; it must be taken as starting point that the acute blow combined with braking or acceleration of the head is only of moderated degree and does not occur repeatedly as in severe head injury due to motor vehicle incident. Therefore, a so-called minor head injury (cerebral concussion) is in the fore.

Occurrence

Cerebral concussion belongs together with signs of head contusion to the most common injuries of a large pediatric emergency care department. Every sixth pediatric surgical patient has a head injury.

Clinical Significance

- Cerebral concussion is a very frequent disorder.
- Behind a supposed cerebral concussion, a severe form of head injury may be hidden or may present as syndrome of cerebral concussion in children.
- Repeat head injury in sports may lead to permanent disorder with irreversible damage.

Clinical Presentation

Often a **history** of the sequence of the accident and the posttraumatic course until consultation of the primary care provider or emergency department is possible in minor head injury. In schoolchildren, antero- and retrograde *amnesia* and a period of abnormal behavior permit an estimation of the length and severity of altered consciousness that would be possible otherwise only by an unbroken observation from the beginning of the head injury. Although the information from accompanying people or the involved child may be incomplete, a first estimation of the severity of injury is possible. The length of retro- and to a lesser degree of the anterograde amnesia is more significant than the altered consciousness for prognostication.

Mostly, no altered state of consciousness or only minor grade # is observed at **clinical examination** *(GCS 12–15). Nevertheless, often*

signs indicative of cerebral concussion are present such as contusional marks, abrasions, and lacerations. The neurological and general examination is very important although often normal and may used as starting point for early clinical follow-up and exclusion of associated trauma, for example, blunt abdominal trauma. During examination, neurovegetative signs are often observed such as vomiting, paleness, or starts sweating.

The **observation of minor traumatic brain injuries** (mTBI) **in sports** by side line observation, afterward systemic evaluation, and neuropsychological tests has produced new and substantial informations about minor head injury in adults and teenagers in which velocity and force are transmitted directly or indirectly by the face and neck to the head. The **symptomatology** is observed immediately or delayed in the first few days and disappears mostly within 7–10 days. *It includes confusion, amnesia, and not necessarily unconsciousness, symptoms like headache, dizziness, double vision, or tinnitus, signs like clouded consciousness, disorders of equilibrium, coordination, concentration, or competition and changes of personality such as inadequate emotional reactions, and possibly pathological test results.* In addition to simple mTBI, **complex mTBI** may be observed especially if several injuries have occurred in the past or if the present injury occurs in the recovery period of a former mTBI. It is characterized by a history of possibly longer unconsciousness (>1 min) or cognitive deficits and by persistence after 7–10 days. Mainly in complex mTBI, a so-called second **impact syndrome** may be observed in the period of recovery consisting of brain edema, possible intracranial hematoma, and even death and occurring in <4 %. In some sports (boxing, football), permanent deficits have been observed after repeat mTBI (psychomotor deficits up to dementia).

Accordingly, both types of mTBI are treated differently, stepwise beginning of training after 7–10 days in simple and further work-up with neuropsychological tests and neuroimaging and absence from sports for much longer time in complex mTBI.

3.1.2 Syndrome of Cerebral Concussion in Children (Delayed Encephalopathy)

Occurrence, Causes

A clinical presentation of cerebral concussion that differs from the classic presentation occurs in 9–50 % of small and schoolchildren with minor head injury.

Several terms and attempts at an explanation have been applied to understand the wide variety of clinical presentation of this disorder specific to children. They include terms such as **syndrome of cerebral concussion in children, (post)traumatic stupor, delayed encephalopathy, traumatic twilight state, and amaurosis fugax**.

It is possible that the symptomatology is based on a migraine accompagnée in some of the children triggered by the trauma to the brain and rarely on a state of absence epilepsy or amnestic episode. Delayed encephalopathy cannot be explained in every case with an equivalent of epilepsy if its frequent occurrence is considered.

Clinical Presentation

The large variety of symptoms and signs and their fluctuation and fleeting reminds the observer of a chameleon.

The course of unconsciousness and altered state of consciousness can be divided into three types for didactic reasons: **Type 1**: *Initial unconsciousness is followed by a period of different length with a continuous or fluctuating state of altered consciousness ###*; **Type 2**: *The initial unconsciousness is followed by a symptom-free interval and after it by a period of different length with a continuous or fluctuating state of altered consciousness ####*; **Type 3**: *Initial unconsciousness does not occur or has not been observed. After a symptom-free period of different length, a state of altered consciousness starts for a different length* (Fig. 3.1).

According to our experience, the children can be waked up for a short moment in the periods with altered state of consciousness, but it is possible that waking up is impossible even with painful stimuli for a short time. *The whole disorder is often accompanied by fleeting vegetative and/or neurological symptoms and signs.* The vegetative signs may rarely become life-threatening (e.g., apneic attack), and the neurological signs are many and diverse: neuromuscular system: localized hypertonia, right-left differences of the reflexes, pyramidal signs, pareses #, focal epileptic attacks with possible generalization, disorders of coordination, etc.; eyes: anisocoria, convergence deficit, dilated and nonreacting pupils to light, deviation conjugée, nystagmus asf.; focal symptoms: amaurosis, aphasia, signs of the posterior fossa as tendency to fall. *The described signs, their fluctuation, and fleeting lead to a colorful and dynamic disorder that disappears usually completely within 24 h at latest except for the neurovegetative signs which may last 2–3 days.*

Differential Diagnosis, Work-Ups

If the mechanism of head injury and clinical presentation of cerebral concussion is known, no other disorder must be considered. Differentiation is more difficult, if a history of trauma is not known, the cerebral concussion is combined with early epilepsy, or it manifests as delayed encephalopathy. In such cases, an epidural hematoma or cerebral contusion should not be missed.

The significance of **plain x-ray** in head injury is controversial especially if applied routinely in every patient except he needs immediate CT. Restriction of overuse is possible, if plain x-ray is only performed in the plane of expected fracture and in specific indications such as suspected depressed skull fracture or child abuse, in patients with CSF shunts, or an age of 0.6–2.0 years (because of the increased risk of fracture).

The use of **CT** for all head injuries is also controversial due to radiation and expensive costs if applied in large number of patients. The early CT does not exclude a developing intracranial hematoma and generates a wrong safety. Indications are severe head injury (GCS ≤8), penetrating and open head injury, suspected mass lesion or intracranial hematoma, and other types of head injury. CT can be avoided in a majority of minor head injuries by careful clinical evaluation and continuous follow-up on the emergency department or ICU for 24 h.

EEG changes are observed in about 50 % of the children with minor head injury (slowing EEG activity), and routine EEG is not indicated

Table 3.3 Criteria for supervision of children with cerebral concussion for 24 h as outpatient or for 2–3 days as inpatient

- History of amnesia, observation of unconsciousness, or a severe traumatic impact
- Unconsciousness or clouding of consciousness at initial examination or on follow-up
- Any skull fracture independent of history and state of consciousness
- Syndrome of cerebral concussion in children
- Difficulty of assessment of the circumstances of the head injury and role for the present case, for example, suspected battered child syndrome

except for specific disorders such as status epilepticus.

Treatment, Prognosis
The indication of supervision as outpatient for 24 h in the emergency department or inpatients for 2–3 days is controversial. Criteria for supervision can avoid the pitfalls of rigorous discharge of all children with head injury at home after CT has been performed and classified as normal. A missed epidural hematoma, cerebral contusion, or delayed encephalopathy leaves a great weight of the responsible medical staff and does a great damage to the hospital's reputation. Otherwise the treatment is symptomatic.

The criteria for supervision that are listed in Table 3.3 are recommendations of which the distance of the tertiary center from the patient's home, the availability of a car, the reliability of the parents, and a clear communication are important aspects.

The **outcome** of cerebral concussion is usually favorable. Nevertheless, indications of a posttraumatic syndrome can be observed in 30–50 % of the patients that include mainly neurovegetative, psychoorganic symptoms, and school problems. Even if these deficits are preexisting in some of the patients or are caused by the study design, the primary care provider should consider their possibility after minor head injury.

3.1.3 Skull Fractures

Skull fractures occur in minor and severe traumatic brain injury (TBI).

3.1.3.1 Linear Fractures of the Calvaria

Occurrence
Linear skull fractures and sutural diastases have a peak incidence in small children especially at the ages 0.6–2.0 years with up to 25 % fractures in TBI #.

Clinical Significance
- Linear skull fractures lead to gross subperiosteal hematoma that may be accompanied by anemia and even shock in small children.
- Transverse parietotemporal fractures, fractures extending into the superior sagittal or transverse sinus, or foramen magnum #, and lambdoid sutural diastasis are at risk for venous and arterial extra- or subdural supra- and/or infratentorial hematoma and sinus thrombosis.
- Those extending into the paranasal or mastoid sinuses are at risk for CSF leak and meningitis.
- Broad linear skull fractures in small children may be a sign of growing skull fracture.

Clinical Presentation
In small children, the presenting sign is large subperiosteal hematoma #. It may be the first sign of a minor TBI after a few days if a fall has been overlooked or not attracted the necessary attention. It may be interpreted as depressed skull fracture on palpation because the central liquefaction yields together with a peripheral wall of coagulated blood the impression of a dent.

The majority of skull fractures are identified by routine plain skull x-ray # or CT. Occasionally, a parietal sagittal suture mimics skull fracture #.

Treatment, Prognosis
Linear skull fractures need no further work-up or treatment except for suspected growing or depressed skull fracture and heal within several months. Blood replacement is necessary in fractures with anemia, and those fractures that are at risk for intracranial hematoma must be considered in the guidelines of early follow-up.

3.1.3.2 Depressed Skull Fractures

Pathoanatomy, Causes

Depending on the age-specific elasticity of the skull, special types of depressed skull fractures are observed: ping-pong or celluloid ball fracture in newborns #, greenstick fracture in young children, and typical depressed skull fracture in teenagers with absent, incomplete, or complete break of the skull continuity. Depressed skull fractures occur at birth or thereafter by a circumscribed force or blow (e.g.) or severe TBI.

Clinical Significance

- Depressed skull fracture ≥0.5 cm exerts some pressure on the brain and distorts the esthetical appearance.
- Deeply depressed and comminuted skull fractures are often combined with dural and brain laceration.
- Compound (open) fractures need emergency wound debridement with removal of all foreign bodies including skull pieces and repair of dural and brain laceration, antibiotics, and blood transfusion. Cranioplasty is performed delayed and electively.

Clinical Presentation

Depressed skull fractures are not always recognized by clinical examination # because the visible and palpable dent may be effaced by edema and hematoma soon after the accident and remains so for a few days.

Work-Ups

The majority of depressed skull fractures are recognizable by plain skull x-ray especially in tangential projection #. Deeply depressed, comminuted #, and compound fractures need CT including bone window for delineation of intracranial lesions and extension of depression.

Treatment, Prognosis

Ping-pong and simple depressed skull fractures need elevation that can be performed using a burr hole adjacent to the depression. If the dura has a bluish tinge, it must be opened for exclusion of a subdural hematoma.

If dura laceration is suspected especially in deeply depressed and comminuted fractures, the depressed bone must be removed, and the dura and brain inspected and repaired (the former by sutures or a periosteal or artificial flap). Reimplantation of the removed bone after debridement and creation of small pieces is possible in small and schoolchildren even in larger defects.

The prognosis depends on a possible laceration or contusion of the brain. The outcome is uneventful in simple depressed skull fracture.

3.1.3.3 Basal Skull Fractures

Basal skull fractures can be suspected clinically but need radiological work-up for confirmation, specification, and precise location.

Clinical Significance

- Basal skull fractures may lead to cranial nerve and sensorial deficit (e.g., facial nerve paresis or hearing and smell loss [tearing of olfactory nerves]).
- Possible combination with dural tear causing CSF leak with rhino- or otorrhea that leads possibly to recurrent meningitis if not recognized.
- Parasagittal basal skull fracture may lead to diabetes insipidus

Clinical Presentation

The following signs are indications of basal skull fracture arranged in order of evidence: *Rhinorrhea* (uni- or bilateral dural tear above the cribriform plate, sphenoid ridge, and crista galli or sella turcica) #, *otorrhea* (dural tear above the anterior or less frequently posterior petrous ridge) #, *postauricular* (Battle's sign #), *extraocular muscle sheet #*, or *subconjunctival hematoma* (raccoon sign #), and *uni- or bilateral hematoma of orbit #* (the latter sign also occurs after direct blow to the orbit or injury of frontal skull and galea). The CSF leak is recognizable by direct observation or by collection of a clear fluid on a swab that displays a reddish ring at its periphery if CSF is intermingled with blood.

Work-Ups

They include CT with small slices of the skull base including inner and middle ear, channel of optic nerve, etc., scintiscan for confirmation and location of suspected CSF leak (presence of significant radioactivity on intranasal swabs), possible air on plain skull x-ray (fracture of paranasal and mastoid sinuses), and consultation of ENT and other specialists.

Treatment, Prognosis

It consists of prophylactic antibiotics at least in CSF leak or middle ear involvement. Overt and persistent CSF leak especially rhinorrhea needs uni- or bilateral transethmoidal closure of the dural tear with fascia lata graft(s). Involvement of the middle and inner ear needs ENT assessment and possibly operative treatment.

Recovery does not occur in every cranial nerve and sensorial deficit, whereas spontaneous closure of CSF leaks may be possible.

3.1.3.4 Fractures of the Facial Skeleton

Clinical Significance

- Except for gross involvement of the midfacial soft tissue, nasal deformity and epistaxis, and injuries of lips, gums, and teeth, fractures of the facial skeleton may be overlooked (e.g., minor chin laceration in mandibular fracture ##).
- Fracture of the facial skeleton may lead to deficit of binocular vision and nasal respiration, malocclusion, and masticatory disorder.

Clinical Presentation

Impaired ocular motility or impaired nasal respirations are signs of a fracture of the orbit or the nasal skeleton, respectively, and difficulties to open the mouth of maxilloalveolar or mandibular fracture.

Work-Ups, Treatment, Prognostication

They need assessment by different specialists especially by ENT and plastic and reconstructive surgeons who perform preliminary and permanent measures in relation to the TBI.

3.1.4 Cerebral Contusion

Occurrence, Definition

About 15–20 % of all children with head injury sustain a cerebral contusion of variable grade. The most severe types are mainly recruited from motor vehicle accidents or battered child syndrome. By definition, cerebral contusion is characterized by an irreversible defect of cerebral structures.

Clinical Significance

- Severe cerebral contusion is responsible for the mortality of head injury # and invalidity with prolonged rehabilitation.
- In contrast to the primary insult of the brain caused by the mechanism of the accident, the secondary brain damage by hyp- and anoxemia and hypovolemia can be influenced or prevented by rapid and appropriate resuscitation.

Clinical Presentation

It depends largely on the type of brain damage that has been occurred together with cerebral concussion, namely, single or multiple focal and/ or diffuse brain damage.

A **severe head injury** is defined *by a GCS ≤8 after stabilization of the vital body functions and additionally by the following findings*:
- Neurological findings
- Findings of neuroimaging
- Intracranial pressure and its course
- Coagulation disorders
- The posttraumatic clinical course

In the acute stage, it is often difficult to recognize focal neurological deficits.

The quoted description contrasts with less **severe types of cerebral contusion** in which *the state of altered consciousness is less severe (GCS 9–12) and less focal lesions are recognizable*. In some of such cases, a continuous transition of the clinical presentation may be observed with that of cerebral concussion or delayed encephalopathy.

Differential Diagnosis, Work-Ups

The diagnosis is usually clear except for insolated cases with neither a history nor external signs of trauma to the head or in battered child syndrome.

Early epilepsy can influence the assessment of the severity of head injury in slight and moderate types of cerebral contusion similar to cerebral concussion. The observations of the eyes and specifically of the pupils # are very important, for instance, unilateral mydriasis including consideration of its differential diagnosis.

Treatment, Prognosis

In severe head injury, clinical examination is accompanied by evaluation and resuscitation: It is very important to check immediately airways, respiration including cervical spine, circulation including heart, possible sites of gross hemorrhage, and other life-threatening injuries to avoid a secondary brain damage and because of the frequency of single and multiple associated injuries (severe head injury is accompanied by a multisystemic organ injury in about 50 %). At the site of injury, intubation and ventilation, venous cannulation, and fluid replacement should be performed whenever possible. After stabilization of respiration and circulation or combined with it, extraction of blood samples for standardized examinations, including coagulation studies and blood testing for transfusion, and radiological imaging can be performed: lateral cervical spine, chest, and abdominal plain x-ray including pelvis and CT of the skull, brain, and cervical spine, and depending on suspected chest and abdominal trauma of the trunk. In severe head injury, the basal cisterns and other CSF spaces are obstructed, and intraventricular, subarachnoidal, and multiple small parenchymatous bleedings are present.

In less severe head injury, some of the quoted examinations can be left out depending on the clinical presentation.

Treatment and follow-up on the ICU is necessary in about one third of the cases. It permits **neurointensive care** in GCS ≤ 8 with continuous recording and treatment of increased ICP by different tools. A central venous catheter, an arterial line, and if possible, an intraventricular catheter for ICP measurement and CSF drainage are necessary. CSF drainage, mild hyperventilation (not below PCO_2 <30 mmHg), and boluses of mannitol (serum osmolality ≤ 320 mOsmol) belong to the treatment of increased ICP. If these measures fail, barbiturate coma, profound hypocarbia (PCO_2 <30 mmHg), hypothermia (temperature >30 °C), controlled lumbar subarachnoid drainage, and large decompressive craniectomy are applied. Large decompressive craniectomy is a controversial method and needs a minimal defect of 10-cm diameter, and no real data exist in the literature relating to the efficacy and safety in the other methods. Controlled lumbar subarachnoid drainage needs open basal cisterns.

Clinical Course, Prognosis

During the **acute posttraumatic period** that lasts 10–14 days or more, several specific **complications** may occur especially in severe head injury: diffuse or localized brain edema, intracranial bleedings, convulsive attacks, syndrome of inappropriate ADH secretion (SIAD), diabetes insipidus, coagulation disorders, and complications of cranial fractures.

In the severe head injury, the possible complications are only partly recognizable by the clinical course because the state of the patient is considerably altered by the measures of the neurointensive care. Therefore, radiological imaging and laboratory tests play together with attention and expertise of the medical staff a greater role.

The **intermediate and late posttraumatic period** in the rehabilitation department permits a retrospective grading of the severity of head injury by the posttraumatic course. According to Lange-Cosack, six grades of severity of the head injury can be differentiated of which unconsciousness of 1–24 h means grade IV, of 24 h to 7 days grade V, and of >7 days grade VI. The last two groups have been considered as severe head injury. Although the treatment of secondary brain damage has significantly improved since 30–40 years ago, the mortality of severe head injury is still 20–30 %. The newer Glasgow outcome scale has five grades of which grades 1 and 2 correspond to permanent vegetative state (coma vigile #) and grade 5 complete recovery. Two thirds of the patients belong after neurointensive care to the group 4 or 5. Nevertheless, the individual grade of invalidity is larger, if the initial age and different special fields are considered. The same applies to moderate and slight types of cerebral contusion.

In <10 % of all children with cerebral contusion, a late epilepsy develops mainly in the first 1–2 years after trauma and in <3 % a posthemorrhagic hydrocephalus (usually in the first 2–3 weeks or weeks to months after the accident).

3.1.5   Epidural Hematoma

Occurrence, Pathoanatomy

Epidural hematoma occurs in 1–3 % of children with head injury and less frequently in infancy.

In contrast to adult patients, the sources of hemorrhage are in children (especially in small children) not only the meningeal arteries or one of their branches but also veins or bone marrow of the skull, and signs of impaction may occur late in spite of large hematomas with anemia because the open sutures and subcutaneous propagation of the hematoma permit initial compensation.

Occasionally, epidural hematomas come to the clinical attention after 24 h (subacute) or within the first week after trauma (chronic epidural hematoma). About 90 % of all epidural hematomas concern the supra- and 10 % the infratentorial compartment.

Clinical Significance

- Already slight injuries may lead to epidural hematoma by an appropriate local impact.
- Isolated epidural hematoma has a good prognosis, if the hematoma is evacuated immediately, and not significant contra- or ipsilateral focal cerebral contusion has occurred.

Clinical Presentation

Relatively slight injury may lead to epidural hematoma, for example, a blow from a puck in ice hockey or a fall on the edge of a piece of furniture. The accompanying cerebral concussion or only focal cerebral contusion explains why >80 % of the children have a GCS of >8 (this does not apply to uncal herniation).

Of the classic triad:

- *Lucid interval*
- *Mydriasis*
- *Hemiparesis*

The lucid interval has minor significance in children. A lucid interval after an initial unconsciousness occurs only in one third, and the signs of impaction (decrease of level of consciousness – contralateral or less frequently ipsilateral spastic hemiparesis – paresis of abducens and oculomotor nerves – respiratory and cardiac arrest) manifest less clearly and in an irregular order.

In addition to a contusional mark of the skull corresponding to the site of impact, headache, vomitus, papillary asymmetry, paleness, and bradycardia, the course of the level of consciousness has a major significance.

Schematically, the following courses of altered consciousness are possible (Fig. 3.2): *Without initial unconsciousness, a gradual decrease of consciousness develops after minutes to hours up to coma (1); the patient is unconscious from the beginning and remains so (2); after initial clouded consciousness, the patients wakes gradually up and remains awake the whole time (3); the patient remains awake the whole time (4); and the patient displays a disorder of consciousness consisting of three parts: initial unconsciousness, intermediate part of a lucid interval, and progressive clouding of consciousness.*

Insidious types of epidural hematoma are infratentorial epidural hematoma with possible rapid deterioration, epidural hematoma of the infant with anemia, possible shock, and gross external hematoma as possible clinical presentation, frontal epidural hematoma in the older child with obstinate headache that has never been experienced by the patient before.

Differential Diagnosis, Work-Ups

Cerebral concussion, cerebral contusion, and delayed encephalopathy depending on the clinical presentation of these disorders.

CT should be performed in the faintest suspicion, for example, considerable occipital fracture. Epidural hematoma can be missed by CT in its early stage. In selected infants (young patients

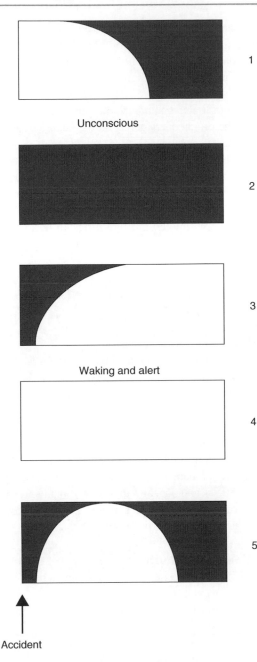

Fig. 3.2 Five different courses of the state of consciousness are observed in the child with epidural hematoma: *1* the child is initially awake, but after that, there is more and more clouding of consciousness; *2* following head injury, the child retains clouding of consciousness or unconsciousness; *3* the child has initially clouding of consciousness and wakes up after that; *4* the child remains always awake; *5* after initial short unconsciousness, the patient exhibits a symptom-free interval that is followed by secondary progressive deterioration

with thin skull bones), the diagnosis of epidural hematoma is possible by ultrasound #.

Hb and blood tests for transfusion are necessary, especially in infants.

Treatment, Prognosis

Craniotomy is usually indicated and consists of raising a skin and bone flap over the site of the hematoma that is based in the temporal region #. The coagulated hematoma is evacuated by smooth lavage, and the disrupted meningeal artery or their branch is clipped. The bone and skin flap are closed with absorbable single sutures.

The outcome is good except for delayed recognition and surgery, or contrecoup cerebral contusion with possible neurological deficit and posttraumatic epilepsy. In delayed cases, death or cerebral damage due to impaction is possible.

3.1.6 Subdural and Intracerebral Hematoma

Occurrence

Although acute subdural or intracerebral hematoma # occurs already prenatally and in young children in the context of head injury (birth injury, accidental or inflicted trauma) and with a clinical presentation similar to those of older children because of the acute mass lesion, some subdural hematomas remain undetected in their acute state and manifest in their subacute (3 days to 3 weeks) or chronic state (>3 weeks). In toddlers and schoolchildren, subdural or intracerebral hematoma is usually a part of a severe head injury.

Clinical Significance

- The acute subdural or intracerebral hematoma occurs usually in the context of a significant head injury and is a sign of severe head injury.
- In battered child syndrome of young children, the acute stage of subdural hematoma may escape its recognition for several reasons.
- In newborns with difficult labor, an acute subdural or intracerebral hematoma must be considered, if sudden or gradual deterioration is observed immediately after birth.

Clinical Presentation

Acute subdural or intracranial hematoma *manifests by a persistently altered or deteriorating state of consciousness*, by *new localizing signs and symptoms of herniation, deterioration of the biological and laboratory data*, or *abnormal findings of subsequently or regularly performed radiological imaging*.

In the daily praxis, isolated acute subdural hematoma manifests hardly without any signs of moderate to severe cerebral contusion in contrast to the epidural hematoma.

Acute subdural hematoma of the neonate or infant that is often caused by shaking leads to seizures, clouded consciousness, retinal hemorrhage, and a GCS on admission that corresponds either to a moderate (9–12) or a severe (≤8) and rarely to a mild head injury (13–15). More than one third need craniotomy for evacuation of blood clot. More than 80 % of those with nonoperative treatment develop within 4 weeks (15–80 days) a chronic subdural hematoma.

Exception of the quoted clinical presentation with possible moderate or mild presentations are **isolated intracerebral hemorrhages** that occur in the depth of brain due shearing forces at any age and **newborns with birth injury** that leads to tearing of the tentorium, sutural dehiscence, and hemorrhage from the deep and superficial veins and sinuses. *After a period of no or minimal symptoms of hours to 3 days, respiratory distress symptom, convulsions, a tense fontanel, opisthotonus, shock, and anemia develop*. CT displays **uni- or bilateral subdural hematoma over the hemispheres, in the posterior interhemispheric cleft or infratentorially**.

Differential Diagnosis, Work-Ups

It includes spontaneous intracranial hemorrhage in which no injury has occurred and the symptom and signs develop rapidly.

CT shows a subdural or intracerebral hematoma, its size, extension, and a possible space-occupying effect.

Treatment, Prognosis

In case of significant mass lesion, **urgent craniotomy**, evacuation of the hematoma, and blood stanching are indicated. Especially in newborns and infants, an underlying coagulation disorder must be recognized and treated before surgery. Evacuation of acute subdural hematoma by burr hole(s) and lavage may be possible in specific cases of the neonatal period or infancy.

The prognosis depends on the degree of associated brain damage and correlates with the initial GCS. In the quoted acute subdural hematoma of the young child, about two thirds have a good outcome, one third display moderate or severe disability, and at least 5 % die in the acute stage, and in the quoted birth injuries, prognosis is worse.

3.1.7 Child Abuse, Battered Child Syndrome (BC)

Definitions, Occurrence

Child abuse encompasses physical maltreatment (battered child syndrome), emotional or sexual abuse, and the most common neglect.

The stated figures of maltreated children are lower than in reality because of underreporting. Two to three percent of children <18 years of age experience in the United States some form of abuse. The majority of them are younger than 4–5 years of age (75–80 %), and one third to 40 % are infants. A parent, related caretakers, or someone known is mostly the abuser, but foster parents are also at risk.

Clinical Significance

- Child abuse and specific BC occur in every socioeconomic class.
- BC must be considered in the differential diagnosis of every injury, especially in infants and toddlers with unusual skin lesions, fractures, and/or severe head injuries. More than 50 % of subdural hematomas in children ≤2 years are due to a shaken infant syndrome.
- At least 10 % of involved children sustain severe or life-threatening injuries and 1‰ dies.
- Recurrence rate is high, and BC becomes even worse if maltreatment is not recognized early.
- Surviving children may suffer from mental and physical handicaps or maltreat their own children later.

Clinical Presentation

The **history** must consider possible risk factors leading to child abuse, the circumstances of consultation, and stated explanations of the presented injuries: Parenteral and child-related risk factors are among other things: (1) unemployment, disturbed partnership, overwork, toxicomania, or psychosis of the caretaker; (2) retardation, feeding difficulties (poor appetite, difficulties in sucking and swallowing), unwanted pregnancy, or prematurity of the involved child; (3) consultation occurs often delayed, at unusual times, and many medical professionals are contacted instead of the family doctor; (4) the informations about the cause of the injuries are vague, do not correspond to severity of the findings, and change in time and content if asked for at different times.

The evaluation of the **clinical findings** *must consider the whole body, and neglected appearance or malnutrition may be observed. They concern the* **skin** *including the body apertures and external genitals, bones of the whole skeleton, chest and abdomen, and central nervous system.*

Although a single lesion may be present, often multiple lesions of different ages are present. No dermatosis causes such a polymorphous appearance like former battering. Ecchymoses, contusional marks, hematomas, excoriations, and lacerations occur at sites that are not accessible to the small child, display shapes which are not caused by common age-related injuries, and are often in a neglected condition. Face, buttock, and external genitals, belly, feet, and hands may be scalded, or the skin is burned, for example, marks of cigarette.

In contrast to the less frequent **blunt abdominal trauma** with possible contusional marks after use of violence, brain injuries and **fractures of the skeleton** are not necessarily recognizable by local findings. Fractures may be suspected because of refusal to walk but the whole spectrum of multiple fractures of different ages of healing and of specific types and locations become only visible by a skeletal surview.

Clouded consciousness up to coma, convulsions, apneic attacks, and retinal hemorrhages are indications of the mostly **severe head injuries**.

Differential Diagnosis, Work-Ups

It encompasses traumatic and nontraumatic disorders of the skin (e.g., scalds or coagulation disorders, hematological or solid tumors), skeletal system (e.g., osteogenesis imperfecta), brain (e.g., primary intracranial hemorrhage), sequel of cardiorespiratory resuscitation, or blunt abdominal trauma (e.g., due to motor vehicle accident).

If battered child syndrome is suspected due to specific data of the history or clinical findings at clinical examination, the following work-ups should be performed:

- Written documentation of history and clinical findings supplemented by photographs.
- Skeletal surview including extremities, skull, spine, and trunk.
- Precise neurological, ophthalmological, and if needed other specific examination that includes fundoscopy with photographic documentation.
- Hematological work-up including coagulation studies.
- Depending on the clinical findings and those of the quoted work-ups, CT in acute and MRI in chronic condition of the brain, ultrasound and CT of the abdomen, etc., should be performed.

Simultaneously, repeated and specific inquiries are necessary of parents and possibly involved people by members of the BC team.

Diagnostic is either characteristic and specific findings, or confession of the abuser, or both.

The **skeletal surview** shows multiple fractures in different stages of healing, fractures of unusual location (multiple dorsal rib fractures), or specific fractures such as subperiosteal hematoma recognizable by a faint calcification 2 weeks after the injury, dislocation of a small piece of the metaphysis of long bones, and damage of the epiphyseal line.

CT and MRI display usually signs of **severe head injuries** such as cerebral contusion, subarachnoid hemorrhage, and the most common subacute and chronic subdural hematoma that is caused by violent shaking (shaken infant syndrome) or most likely by a mechanism in which the trunk is held and the back of the head is struck against a surface.

Impact and/or sudden acceleration and/or deceleration lead to rotational forces. They cause global shearing injuries that are responsible for brain atrophy like the visible chronic subdural hematoma. Hemorrhages may lead to posttraumatic hydrocephalus. Fundoscopy displays retinal hemorrhages in 47–100 % that are often asymmetric; their distribution correlates with the patterns of acute and evolving regional cerebral parenchymal injury patterns.

Ultrasound and CT of the abdomen demonstrate in order of decreasing frequency hemoperitoneum, hematoma of the duodenal or intestinal wall, intestinal perforation, and contusion of pancreas (with posttraumatic pancreatitis and pancreatic pseudocyst). Traumatic rupture of kidney, spleen, or liver occurs less frequently.

Treatment, Prognosis
It consists (1) of coordination and performance of treatment of the injuries by the responsible pediatrician or pediatric surgeon and (2) of evaluation of history, clinical findings, work-up examinations, and inquiries by the BC team with regard to child abuse, confrontation with the parents and initiation of psychological advice, report to civil authorities, and possibly support in implementation of measure of the civil authorities such as temporary or permanent removal of the child from its home.

The responsible physician should not be a member of the BC team. However, complete and reciprocal exchange of informations is essential. Health professionals must report suspicion of child abuse or neglect to civil authorities in the United States and Canada, whereas this is only inevitable in severe, life-threatening cases or permanent, severe handicap, repeated battering, and if the parents have a psychiatric disorder or toxicomania in other countries, for example, Switzerland. It is important to know that the majority of involved parents are not criminals but people who need our help to overcome their risk factors and to avoid further battering.

Prognosis depends on the severity and duration of battering and the type of injury.

Severe brain injury is the most common cause of death (>15 up to >25 %) followed by delayed diagnosis of blunt abdominal injury. The damage to the brain is also responsible for the neurological disability and posttraumatic epilepsy; only one third has a good outcome and two thirds have a moderate to severe disability in school age, part of physical disability may be due to cortical visual loss, detachment of the retina, hemianopia, or damage to the epiphyseal line of long bones.

3.2   Convulsive Attacks and Epilepsy

Occurrence, Clinical Significance
Convulsive attacks and epilepsy may be an important cause of unconsciousness or altered consciousness. The reader is referred to the neuropediatric literature.

In relation to head injury, convulsive attacks or epilepsy have the following clinical significance:
- **Early epilepsy** occurs in head injury frequently, concerns the first 7 days after trauma, and is observed in cerebral concussion, depressed skull fracture with or without recognizable cerebral concussion, or moderate or severe cerebral contusion.

  Because of the symptomatology of early epilepsy, minor head injury may be assessed as more severe, especially if early epilepsy occurs shortly after the injury and due to the postictal sleep.
- Convulsive attacks occur also after the interval of 7 days or posttraumatic epilepsy sets up (especially after open or penetrating head injury, depressed skull fracture with dural laceration, fractures of the skull base, intracranial hematomas, and grade V or VI [Lange-Cosack] cerebral contusion)
- Convulsive attacks in severe head injury may turn into an epileptic state that impairs the level of consciousness. If the epilepsy is not recognized, the cerebral contusion is misinterpreted as deteriorating (e.g., absence epilepsy).
- Head injury may be caused by a convulsive attack. It must be considered especially if other people have not observed the patient.

Treatment

Early epilepsy is usually treated for 1 week with anticonvulsants. Prophylactic treatment of children at risk is not meaningful because development of posttraumatic epilepsy cannot be prevented by it. Especially in the second to fourth situation quoted above, a neuropediatrician must be consulted for work-up and treatment.

3.3   Fat Embolism Syndrome, Fat Embolism

Occurrence, Clinical Significance

Although fat embolism syndrome has not gained much attention in the pediatric age group, it occurs in children as well. The fat embolism syndrome is observed in motor vehicle accidents with fractures of the long bones, extended soft tissue injury including contusion or burns, and without an overt trauma, for example, in necrotizing pancreatitis.

It must be differentiated from **fat embolism** that is caused by microembolism of bone marrow components during orthopedic surgery (e.g., intramedullary nailing) and leads to cardiovascular complications up to cardiac arrest during surgery.

- Fat embolism syndrome involves also the brain. It leads to secondary altered states of consciousness.
- Specific measures can prevent a fatal outcome with possible death.

Clinical Presentation

In addition to the less common peracute fat embolism, fat embolism syndrome occurs mostly between 36 and 72 h after the injury and as pulmonic or systemic clinical presentation.

Tachy- and dyspnea, cyanosis, tachycardia, and fever (>39 °C) are signs of the pulmonic form. If the child is already ventilated, deterioration of the ventilatory parameters, hypoxia of the blood gas analyses, and diffuse opacity of the chest x-ray are the manifestations of the disorder (adult respiratory distress syndrome).

In systemic forms, qualitative and quantitative impairment of consciousness are in the fore (delirium or progressive clouding of consciousness). About one third have inguinal and shoulder girdle petechial bleedings. Fundoscopy, urinalysis (albumin- and hematuria, fat droplets), decrease of Hb and thrombocytes may be useful tools.

Differential Diagnosis

In case of a corresponding history and respiratory signs (e.g., cyanosis, hypoxia), fat embolism syndrome must be considered in the differential diagnosis. Lung contusion leads immediately to restriction of lung function and shock lung after the time of onset of fat embolism syndrome. In secondary deterioration of consciousness, an intracranial hematoma must be considered.

Treatment

It considers the complex pathophysiology in which embolism of fat droplets is only a partial aspect:

- Prevention and treatment of shock.
- Supervision of respiration and their laboratory parameters combined with optimal oxygenation and, if needed, with artificial ventilation.
- Early osteosynthesis of instable fractures and prevention of a permanent immobilization in the supine position by measures of physiotherapy.
- In intraoperative fat embolism, 100 % oxygenation, positive inotropic medication, and cautious fluid replacement are indicated.
- If these therapeutic principles are applied early, fatal outcome can be prevented with good recovery.

3.4   Shunt Dysfunction, Decompensation of Native Hydrocephalus

Occurrence, Clinical Significance

Today, progressive hydrocephalus gets either shunted or treated by endoscopy (e.g., third ventriculostomy). Obstruction of the shunt or ventriculostomy leads to signs of shunt insufficiency or increased ICP depending on the completeness and the time in which complete obstruction is achieved. Altered state of consciousness may also occur in compensated hydrocephalus without or with a shunt that does not function any more. The clinical significance is as follows:

- Altered level of consciousness means a life-threatening condition in a patient with CSF shunt or compensated hydrocephalus.

Clinical Presentation

Alteration of consciousness is initially not in the foreground of shunt insufficiency or decompensation of the hydrocephalus. The main symptomatology includes headache, vomitus (in the morning and recurrent), paleness, and bradycardia. In young infants, irritability and tense fontanel in a quiet and upright held child are more frequent.

Fluctuations of the altered consciousness and increasing, permanent clouding of consciousness are the signs of imminent cerebral herniation.

Signs of shunt insufficiency are numerous, variable, and extend from hardly recognizable signs to a peracute life-threatening presentation. The sunset phenomenon occurs also in shunted hydrocephalus of any age (Parinaud syndrome # as life-threatening sign). The causes of the variation of clinical presentation are the speed, site, and completeness of obstruction (quick vs. slow, central vs. peripheral, and incomplete vs. complete obstruction), and the degree of shunt dependency. Slit ventricle syndrome has a high shunt dependency.

Deep unconsciousness #, opisthotonus, bradycardia, oculomotor, and pupillary paresis (uncal herniation) are signs of extreme mortal danger #.

Differential Diagnosis, Work-Ups

Depending on the history, other possible causes of altered level of consciousness, headache, or vomiting are imaginable. In shunt patients, the possibility of shunt dysfunction must always be considered until the proof of the contrary. Signs of a symptomatic Dandy-Walker cyst, Arnold-Chiari II anomaly, or another cause of a space-occupying disorder without or with associated shunt dysfunction may be misleading.

Fundoscopy (papilledema, retinal hemorrhages, increase of caliber, and pulsations of the retinal vein) and palpatory check of the valve chamber (the chamber is or remains flat after compression ##) are useful clinical skills.

Additional examinations are best performed in a tertiary center and include CT, ICP determination in the supratentorial compartment (**no** lumbar puncture), shuntogram with fluoroscopy, and plain x-rays of skull including neck, thorax, or abdomen.

Treatment, Prognosis

If necessary, relief of the increased ICP is possible by direct punction of the shunt reservoir or along the central catheter of the ventricle. Permanent cure is only possible by shunt revision with replacement of the obstructed part and the valve by a programmable system.

If the diagnosis is not delayed and surgery is performed immediately, the outcome is good. Otherwise, the patient may die or survive with deficits, for example, diminished visual field and acuity.

In slight and chronic form of shunt insufficiency, revision can be performed electively the next day.

3.5   Disorders with Septicemia or Blood Volume Deficit

Shock due to blood volume deficit, advanced obstructive ileus, secondary peritonitis, and other disorders associated with septicemia or blood volume deficit belong to this group.

Clinical Significance

- Shock due to traumatic blood volume deficit, obstructive ileus, and secondary peritonitis in intestinal perforation with shock due to septicemia and blood volume deficit may lead in advanced stages to apathy, confusion, and clouded consciousness.

  It is important that the underlying cause is recognized in such situations without delay in spite of altered consciousness.

3.6 Spontaneous Intracranial Hemorrhage

Definitions, Occurrence, Causes

Spontaneous (primary or nontraumatic) intracerebral hemorrhage is observed more frequently than pure spontaneous subarachnoid hemorrhage. Subarachnoid hemorrhage in aneurysm is associated with frontobasal or bleeding in the region of the lateral fissure only in about 10 %. Arteriovenous malformations, cavernous malformations, venous angiomas, and aneurisms belong to the most common causes of primary intracerebral and/or subarachnoid hemorrhage in children. Coagulopathies, primary and metastatic brain tumors including leukemias, arterial hypertension, or vasculitis also belong to the possible causes. Finally, cocaine (smoking of "crack" cocaine) and amphetamine must be considered as cause in adolescents being on drugs.

Clinical Significance

- It is very important to consider this differential diagnosis, mainly if no injury has occurred and the altered consciousness and/or focal neurological deficit starts immediately and is associated with or without sudden onset headache.
- Intracerebral hemorrhage due to arteriovenous malformation is four times more frequently than subarachnoid bleeding due to aneurysm.

Clinical Presentation

Severity and presentation depend on the location and magnitude of intracerebral hemorrhage. *Chronic headache, seizures, or progressive dementia and focal neurological signs are possible unspecific presentations. Sudden onset of severe headache and vomiting are followed by rapidly progressive neurological deficits and/or clouding of consciousness up to coma are the most life-threatening and common specific presentations. Congestive heart failure and a cranial bruit are possible presentation in newborns.* The clinical presentation of aneurysms may be less dramatic with *headache, meningism, photophobia, and focal neurological signs, but clouding or loss of consciousness may also occur. They may bleed after a minor head injury.*

Differential Diagnosis, Work-Ups

It includes other causes of the quoted clinical presentation. In spontaneous intracerebral hemorrhage, the history yields no significant trauma but possible indications of the mentioned causes. The clinical presentation of aneurysm may be mixed up with meningitis. Isolated headache reminds of migraine.

CT is used as screening tool and later angio MRI or angiography for recognition of the cause and precise site of hemorrhage. Spinal tap for confirmation of subarachnoid hemorrhage may be useful in less dramatic aneurysm. The arteriovenous malformations display a tangle of dilated vessels with one or more arterial feeders and one or more veins with outflow to the superficial or deep venous system or to the dural sinuses. The mass lies in the brain parenchyma, is wedge-shaped, and points toward the ventricle.

Aneurysms occur on peripheral distal artery branches, are frequently large, and tend to arise without a true neck from a parenteral vessel. Cavernous angiomas are progressive, bluish, and lobulated masses filled with blood, and venous angiomas are dilated medullary veins with radial arrangement around a central vein.

Treatment, Prognosis

The children need neurointensive care to stabilize the metabolism, to treat the cause (such as coagulation disorders or arterial hypertension), to prevent the secondary brain edema and increased intracranial hypertension (tentorial herniation or CSF obstruction by displacement of brain parenchyma), and to perform angio MRI or angiography.

Superficial expanding hematoma needs evacuation, whereas deep hematomas (brain stem, thalamus, and basal ganglia) are not amenable to surgery.

Children with severe symptomatology need complete resection of the arteriovenous malformation as soon as possible without or with preoperative endovascular embolization of the feeding arteries in large AVM, or radiosurgical obliteration in small and deep forms (the procedure is effective only within 1–2 years with risk of rebleeding and local edema). Surgery should also be considered in children with minor symptoms and signs because the risk of major bleeding is about 4 % and the mortality rate about 1 % per year without treatment. The vein of Galen malformations and fistulas are difficult to manage although urgent treatment becomes necessary in newborns or infants (due to congestive heart failure or progressive neurological deficit). Endovascular procedures are superior without or with ligation of the feeding vessels to surgery.

Aneurysm needs surgical clipping with special consideration of the peculiarities of childhood aneurysm. Cavernous angiomas need resection in symptomatic cases (seizures, recurrent focal hemorrhages), whereas venous angiomas need removal of rare hematomas but not of the venous channels due to the risk of venous infarctions.

Posthemorrhage or death is possible. The sequels depend on the location and size of the hemorrhage and secondary brain damage. The hemorrhage leaves a cavity and scar as possible cause of epilepsy.

3.7   Pediatric Disorders

Metabolic disorders, hypoxic attacks, CNS infections, brain tumors, intoxications, cardiovascular insufficiency belong to this group.

Clinical Significance
- These disorders and spontaneous intracranial hemorrhage belong to the responsibility of pediatricians, neuropediatricians, and intensive care physicians.

It is important for the pediatric surgeon to consider such disorders in the differential diagnosis of unconsciousness and altered consciousness and specifically intoxications with **drugs or alcohol in teenagers**. The latter disorders are increasingly associated with trauma (e.g., motor vehicle accident as drivers) and sole disorder (e.g., clouded consciousness or psychotic state in intoxication with Cannabis sativa).

3.8   Conversion Disorders

The trial to cope with acute head injury may lead to conversion disorders. It concerns the acute minor head injury and subacute period after severe trauma to the brain. The clinical presentation and duration of such conversion disorders are different in the two conditions, depend on the individual patient, and are characteristic for children.

In **severe head injury**, the awakening child responds to an unbearable situation by a *pseudo-permanent vegetative state that is characterized by apathy, akinesia, and mutism, and lasts for several days, weeks, or even longer*. This presentation has a differential diagnostic, diagnostic, and therapeutic significance: It may be mixed up with coma vigile and lead to an incorrect prognostication. Its recognition and treatment needs specific experience and skills.

Minor head injury may lead in toddlers and preschool children to a similar reaction as quoted for severe head injury and in teenagers to disorders with variable neurological and sensorial deficit or with excitation. *Examples are paresis of the extremities or hearing loss that is not in accordance with the common pattern observed in head injury and yields no organic cause on work-up examination.* The deficits last hours to few days and disappear spontaneously and completely and sometimes by gradual amelioration. Such conversion disorders have mainly a differential diagnostic significance because the head injury may be assessed as more severe or the excited teenager is judged to be on drugs.

Webcodes

The following webcodes can be used on www. psurg.net for further images and data.

301 Clouded consciousness, GCS 13	320 Plain skull x-ray, comminuted depressed-skull fracture
302 Stupor, GCS 10	321 Unilateral rhinorrhea
303 Coma, GCS 5	322 Otorrhea, swab with CSF/blood
304 Decorticate rigidity	323 Battle sign
305 Battered child syndrome, head injury	324 Muscle sheet hematoma orbit
306 Cerebral concussion, GCS <15	325 Raccoon sign
307 Delayed encephalopathy,	326 Unilateral hematoma orbit
308 Fluctuating state of altered	327 Laceration chin with
309 Consciousness	328 Underlying mandibular fracture, left collum
310 Delayed encephalopathy, after 24 h	329 Uncal herniation, cerebral contusion
311 Temporary ankle paresis	330 Pre-existing anisocoria
312 Types of calvarial fractures, infancy	331 Permanent vegetative state
313 CT, linear fracture, extending into foramen magnum	332 Ultrasound, epidural hematoma
314 Large subperiosteal hematoma in	333 Intraop. finding, epidural hematoma
315 Parieto-occipital skull fracture	334 Parieto-occipital intracerebral hematoma
316 Parietal sagittal suture	335 Parinaud syndrome, shunt dysfunction
317 Celluloid ball fracture, neonate	336 Coma, shunt dysfunction
318 Depressed skull fracture, small child	337 Uncal herniation, shunt dysfunction
319 CT, celluloid ball fracture	338 Valve chamber before
	339 And after compression, shunt dysfunction

Bibliography

Sections 3.1.1–3.1.2

Amar AP, Aryan HE, Meltzer HS, Levy ML (2003) Neonatal subgaleal hematoma causing brain compression: report of two cases and review of the literature. Neurosurgery 52:1470–1474; discussion 1474

Chadwick DL, Bertocci G, Castillo E, Frasier L, Guenther E, Hansen K, Herman B, Krous HF (2008) Annual risk of death resulting from short falls among young children: less than 1 in 1 million. Pediatrics 121:1213–1224

Kaiser G (1978) Die acute posttraumatische Phase bei leichteren Formen von Schädel-Hirn-Verletzungen (The acute posttraumatic phase in milder forms of craniocerebral lesions in the child). Z Kinderchir 24:303–312

Luerssen TG (1998) Central nervous system injuries. In: O'Neill JA Jr et al (eds) Pediatric surgery, vol I, 5th edn. Mosby, St Louis

Vu TT, Guerrera MF, Hamburger EK (2004) Subgaleal hematoma from hair braiding: case report and literature review. Pediatr Emerg Care 20:821–823

Section 3.1.3

Becker DB, Cheverud JM, Govier DP, Kane AA (2005) Os parietale divisum. Clin Anat 18:452–456

Kos M, Luczak K, Godzinski J, Rapala M, Klempous J (2002) Midfacial fractures in children. Eur J Pediatr Surg 12:218–225

Section 3.1.4

Rekate HL (2001) Head injuries: management of primary injuries and prevention of secondary damage. Childs Nerv Syst 17:632–634

Sections 3.1.5–3.1.6

Gupta SN, Kechli AM, Kanamalla US (2009) Intracranial hemorrhage in term newborns: management and outcomes. Pediatr Neurol 40:1–12

Loh JK, Lin CL, Kwan AL, Howng SL (2002) Acute subdural hematoma in infancy. Surg Neurol 58:218–224

Section 3.1.7

Bariciak ED, Plint AC, Gaboury I et al (2003) Dating of bruises in children: an assessment of physicians accuracy. Pediatrics 112:804–807

Dube SR, Anda RF, Felitti VJ et al (2001) Childhood abuse, household dysfunction, and the risk of attempted suicide throughout life span: findings from the adverse childhood experiences study. JAMA 286:3089–3096

Duhaime AC, Gennarelli TA, Sutton LM, Schut L (1988) The "shaken baby syndrome": a misnomer? J Pediatr Neurosci 4:77–86

Duhaime AC, Christian C, Moss E, Seidl T (1996) Long-term outcome in infants with shaking-impact syndrome. Pediatr Neurosurg 24:292–298

Gilbert R, Widom CS, Browne K, Fergusson D, Webb E, Janson S (2009) Burden and consequences of child maltreatment in high-income countries. Lancet 373:68–81

Gilles EE, Mc Gregor ML, Levy-Clarke G (2003) Retinal hemorrhage asymmetry in inflicted head injury: a clue to pathogenesis? J Pediatr 143:494–499

Harris BH, Stylianos S (1998) Special considerations in trauma: child abuse and birth injuries. In: O'Neill JA Jr et al (eds) Pediatric surgery, vol I, 5th edn. Mosby, St Louis

Keenan HT, Runyan DK, Mashall SW et al (2003) A population-based study of inflicted traumatic brain injury in young children. JAMA 290:621–626

Kemp AM, Dunstan F, Harrison S, Morris S, Mann M, Rolfe K, Datta S, Thomas DP, Sibert JR, Maguire S (2008) Patterns of skeletal fractures in child abuse: systematic review. BMJ 337:a1518. doi:10.1136/bmj.a1518, Comment in: BMJ (2008); 337:a1398, a2279

Labbé J, Caouette G (2001) Recent skin injuries in normal children. Pediatrics 108:271–276

Miller R, Miller M (2010) Overrepresentation of males in traumatic brain injury of infancy and in infants with macrocephaly: further evidence that questions the existence of shaken baby syndrome. Am J Forensic Med Pathol 31:165–173

Reijneveld SA, van der Wal MF, Brugman E et al (2004) Infant crying and abuse. Lancet 364:1340–1342

Section 3.3

Aebli N, Rocco P, Krebs J (2005) Fettembolie – eine potentiell tödliche Komplikation während orthopädischen Eingriffen (Fat embolism – a potentially fatal complication during orthopaedic surgery). Schweiz Med Forum 5:512–518

Forster C, Jöhr M, Gebbers J-O (2002) Fettembolie und Fettembolie-Syndrom. Schweiz Med Forum 2:673–678

Hulman G (2000) The pathogenesis of fat embolism. J Pathol 176:3–9

Levy D (1990) The fat embolism syndrome. A review. Clin Orthop 261:281–286

Section 3.4

Dickerman RD, McConathy WJ, Lustrin E, Schneider SJ (2003) Rapid neurological deterioration associated with minor head injury in chronic hydrocephalus. Childs Nerv Syst 19:249–251

Section 3.6

Del Zoppo GJ, Mori E (1992) Hematological causes of intracerebral hemorrhage and their treatment. Neurosurg Clin N Am 3:637–658

Greene RM, Kelly KM, Gabrielsen T, Levine SR, Vanderzant C (1990) Multiple intracerebral hemorrhages after smoking 'crack' cocaine. Stroke 21:957–962

Kazui S, Naritomi H, Yamamoto H, Sawada T, Yamaguchi T (1996) Enlargement of spontaneous intracerebral hemorrhage: incidence and time course. Stroke 27:1783–1787

Sutton LN (1998) Central nervous system tumors and vascular malformations. In: O'Neill JA Jr et al (eds) Pediatric surgery, vol I, 5th edn. Mosby, St Louis

Conspicuous and/or Abnormal Head Shape

Abnormal head shape attracts attention of parents and physicians mainly in neonates and infants because the hair does not cover the deformity as later in life. On the other hand, the family becomes used to the abnormal head shape with time.

After discussion of the head that is too large in chapter "macrocrania," remain the causes of deviation from the normal shape of the neurocranium such as abnormal proportions or right-left asymmetry without or with involvement of the facial skeleton.

Because **craniosynostoses** (premature closure of one or more sutures) are in the fore of interest due to the possibility of surgical correction, the other causes of conspicuous or abnormal head shape are explained in the differential diagnosis of the single craniosynostoses and listed in Table 4.1.

It is worth asking for known familial skull deformities and for perinatal disorders in the **history.** On **clinical examination,** the head of the patient should be inspected from front, behind, both sides, and the top, and measured: head circumference, skull index, and interpupillary (interorbital) and intercanthal distances (if hyper-, hypotelorism, or telecanthus is suspected). In every case, general, neurological, and developmental examination should be performed as well as body measurements.

The skull index is determined as follows: maximum temporoparietal width divided by maximum fronto-occipital length $\times$ 100. Normal values for the horizontal skull plane are 70–80 (or 76–81 %) and <70 (<76 %) means dolichocephaly and >80

Table 4.1 Differential diagnosis of conspicuous and/or abnormal head shape

Dolichocephaly
- Sagittal synostosis
- Dolichocephaly (normal variation of skull shape)
- Dolichocephaly of prematurity
o Sagittal synostosis in hypophosphatemic rickets
o Birth molding[a]
o Multiple-suture synostosis[a]
o Craniofacial dysostosis (syndromic craniosynostosis)[a]
- Macrocrania
o Bathrocephaly
o Posterior fossa cyst

Anterior brachycephaly and plagiocephaly
- Bicoronal synostosis
- Unicoronal synostosis
- Brachycephaly (normal variation of skull shape)
o Postural anterior brachy- and plagiocephaly
- Positional anterior brachy- and plagiocephaly
- Other forms of deformational anterior brachy- and plagiocephaly

Trigonocephaly
- Metopic synostosis
o Syndromic metopic synostosis
o Treacher Collins syndrome

Posterior brachycephaly and plagiocephaly
- Bilambdoid synostosis
- Unilambdoid synostosis
- Brachycephaly (normal variation of skull shape)
- Deformational posterior brachycephaly and plagiocephaly
o Contralateral posterior fossa cyst

Oxycephaly, any ab- or normal head shape, cloverleaf skull deformity
- Multiple-suture a synostosis
- Syndromic a synostosis

G.L. Kaiser, *Symptoms and Signs in Pediatric Surgery,*
DOI 10.1007/978-3-642-31161-1_4, © Springer-Verlag Berlin Heidelberg 2012

Table 4.1 (continued)

o Familial microcephaly

o Microencephaly

o Disorders of Chap. 1

[a]Multiple-suture synostosis, syndromic craniosynostosis, and birth molding may be a differential diagnosis of every conspicuous and/or abnormal head shape

(or >81 %) brachycephaly (flat front or back head), plagiocephaly means skewness of the head or oblique head for which oblique cranial length ratio ≥106 % is a measure.

Values above correspond to a brachycephalic and values below to a dolichocephalic head shape.

In contrast to earlier times, the appearance of the children brings increased attention to the parents and neighbors. Therefore, only scientifically sound informations by the primary care provider or a tertiary center may reassure the parents in contrast to some information in the Internet crammed full with information and without the possibility of counter questions.

Occurrence

Premature closure of a single or of multiple suture(s) without or with involvement of the splanchnocranium (craniofacial dysostoses) occurs approximately in 1 per 2,500 births.

Clinical Significance

• Different functional impairments may be observed in some craniosynostoses and aesthetic impairment with possible psychosocial consequences in almost all.

• Surgical correction is possible in many with less expenditure and better results if performed in infancy.

Pathophysiology Pathogenesis

The current opinion on this matter makes it easier to understand the clinical presentation and the concepts of treatment. In contrast to the epiphyseal growth plates, the sutures are not primary sites of calvarial growth. Growth rather takes place by a continuous remodeling process with breakdown and rebuilding of the single calvarial bone. The suture passes normally through different stages from loose to tight fibrous tissue with

functional closure in the second decade and osseous closure in adulthood. In craniosynostosis, closure of the sutures occurs too early (prematurely) and is combined with structural alterations that are seen by the naked eye and histologically dependent on the suture localization.

The growth of the neurocranium and its directions depends on the brain growth and its velocity that is larger prenatally and in the first half of infancy than in the second half and later. In contrast, the growth in craniosynostosis is inhibited in the direction perpendicularly to the closed suture and increased as compensatory mechanism in the not involved sutures. In all craniosynostoses, the cranial base, the midface, and the mandible are primarily and/or secondarily involved, too.

Clinical Presentation

Depending on the involved suture(s), different abnormal skull shapes result. In spite of similar common features of the patients with the same type of craniosynostosis, no case is equal to the other due to the variability of time and completeness of closure of the involved suture(s).

The order of fusion of the single sutures and its completeness is important for the final skull shape if multiple sutures are closed. The skull shape may change after birth if closure has not been already finished at all involved suture sites and if only one suture is considered by surgery.

The main types of craniosynostosis are depicted in Figs. 4.1, 4.2, and 4.3.

4.1 Single Suture Synostosis

4.1.1 Sagittal Synostosis

Occurrence

Sagittal synostosis is the most frequently encountered single suture synostosis in all operative populations. It occurs in 0.2–1.0 % of newborn infants. Most cases of sagittal synostosis are recognizable at birth.

Clinical Presentation

The narrow dolichocephalic skull disfigures the appearance of the patient mainly by its

Fig. 4.1 Drawings of the main types of premature closure of the cranial sutures. The *black line* corresponds to one or several closed suture(s). *1*: lateral view and view from the *top* of the skull in synostosis of the sagittal suture

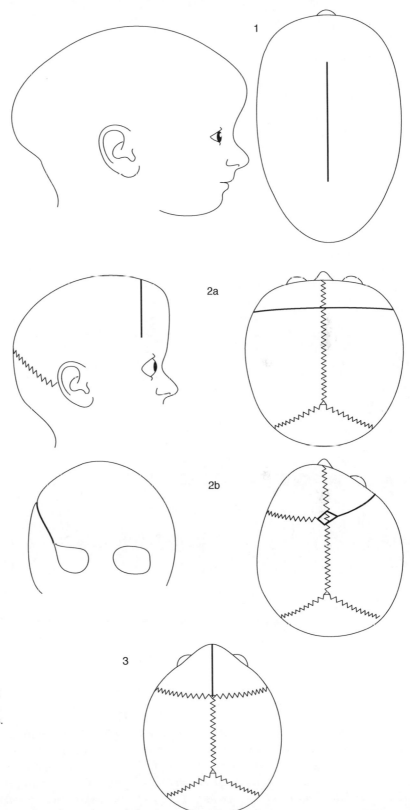

Fig. 4.2 Drawings of the main types of premature closure of the cranial sutures. The *black line* corresponds to one or several closed suture(s). *2a*: lateral view and view from the *top* of the skull in bilateral coronal synostosis. *2b*: view from the *front* and the *top* of the skull in unilateral (*right*) coronal synostosis. *3*: view from the *top* of the skull (bird's eye view) in frontal (metopic) synostosis

Fig. 4.3 Drawings of the main types of premature closure of the cranial sutures. The *black line* corresponds to one or several closed suture(s). *4a*: lateral view and view from the *top* of the skull in bilateral lambdoid suture synostosis. *4b*: view from the *top* in unilateral (*right*) lambdoid suture synostosis. *5*: lateral view of the skull in closure of multiple sutures (oxycephaly as one variety of closure of multiple sutures). *6*: view of the skull from the *top* in an example of a complex abnormality of the skull without closure of a suture

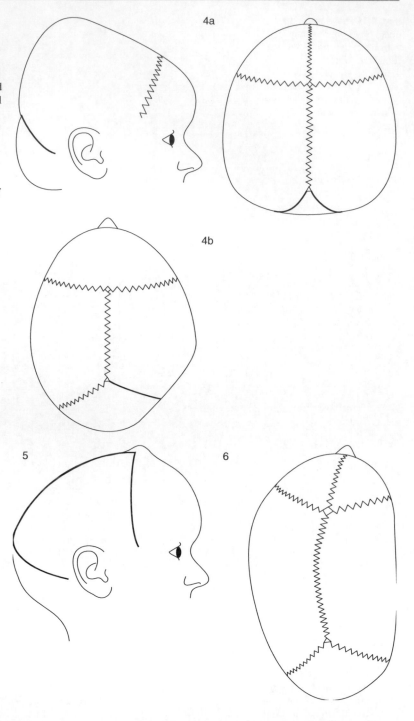

combination with a distinctly prominent fore- and back head # and a small and high brow in relation to the normally wide face (Fig. 4.1 number 1). The latter finding leads sometimes to a pear-like contour of the face #.

The fused suture is visible and palpable as osseous ridge #. The anterior fontanel is often closed. Rarely, a wormian bone can occupy the anterior fontanel giving the appearance of a closed fontanel. *In early stages, it is impossible to move the adjacent parietal bones against each other.*

The head circumference is often in the upper percentiles and the skull index below the normal value of 70–80. The extracranial venous system is prominent, especially on crying. Occasionally, parasutural craniotabes is (are) palpable in younger and small osseous defects in older infants #.

Because a wide spectrum of minor anomalies may be observed in one fourth and major malformations in the same range as in the general population, careful general examination is necessary in sagittal synostosis as well as in all single and multiple craniosynostoses. The distribution of body length shows a shift toward short infants in comparison with the normal distribution, and a thrombocytosis ($>500 \times 10EE9/L$) is seen preoperatively in about one third.

The following functional impairments may be observed:

- Complicated birth is observed in about one third due to impairment of head molding of the sagittal suture. Sagittal (and metopic) synostosis is (are) more likely to develop in twins compared with singletons.
- Minimal signs of increased intracranial pressure (irritability with frequent crying, vomiting without recognizable cause, and sleep disorders, which disappear after surgery, and occasionally papilledema), early signs of possible cerebral palsy, and rarely of psychomotor retardation may be observed altogether in up to one third of the patients.
- Increased ICP (>15 mmHg prior or at surgery) occurs in more than 10–25 %.
- Increased postoperative risk for headache (>10 %).
- Increased risk of learning disorders regardless of surgical status.
- Trend toward myopia due to the elongated ocular bulb.
- Trend toward malocclusion.

Whereas the former impairments are mainly observed in infancy prior surgery, cephalgia, learning disorders, myopia, and malocclusion become more significant in school age and adolescence, respectively.

Children with sagittal synostosis differ not in global or specific indicators of cognitive and psychomotor development from demographically matched comparison infants in the first year of life and after surgery, in the second year of life. On the other hand, schoolchildren operated on in infancy for scaphocephaly have no marked problems of cognition and behavior except for verbal conceptual thinking and reasoning and auditory short-term memory in which they score less than a control group. Schoolchildren after linear "strip" craniectomy with minimal bone removal and resembling somehow to untreated scaphocephaly display in 50 % a reading and/or spelling learning disability and the mean verbal IQ that is significantly higher than the mean performance IQ (the full-scale IQ fell in the normal range of the general population). In contrast to sagittal synostosis of infancy, delay in mental development and learning disorders occur with increasing frequency in sagittal synostosis with diagnosis beyond infancy (1 % with <90 Brunet-Lézine development quotient in infants vs. 10 % in older children), other single-suture synostoses especially in bilateral coronal and metopic synostosis, multiple-suture synostosis, and craniofacial dysostoses. This applies also for patients with increased ICP in general, and the longer craniosynostosis has been left untreated. It has been shown that children of small sample size with nonsyndromic unicoronal synostosis, metopic, and sagittal synostosis with early or late surgery (75 %) or no surgery (25 %) obtain developmental quotients within the normal range in infancy. But the rates of retardation may increase relative to normative expectations as children mature and a high rate of learning disorders can be identified. The above quoted normal developmental data for sagittal synostosis and those for different single sutures in the sentence above in infancy have been recently questioned. In a fairly large cohort of infants with all types of untreated single synostosis, the overall scores were significantly lower than normative data in mental and psychomotor developmental indices and in the receptive and expressive language scales. The developmental risk is therefore greater than previously thought.

The **long-term developmental correlates and outcomes in single-suture synostosis** are still a matter of discussion. They are mentioned here because recent research refers admittedly not exclusively to sagittal synostosis because cases of trigonocephaly, uni- and bicoronal, and lambdoid synostosis are often quoted together. For infants with a single-suture synostosis, there may be a greater developmental risk than previously believed (expressed especially by the psychomotor and less by the mental developmental index, and by receptive and expressive language scales) and independent of maternal IQ and socioeconomic status. One year after surgery, improvement of the psychomotor but not of the mental developmental indices may be observed in some. At the beginning of school age, cognitive, speech, and/or behavioral abnormalities can be found in about half of the children with operated nonsyndromic craniosynostoses (with the lowest rate in sagittal and highest rate in bicoronal types). During school age, the global intelligence is normal in almost all of the nonsyndromic craniosynostoses with former surgery. But different learning disorders may be found in one third up to 50 % of the patients regardless of surgical status. On the other hand, it is unknown if these problems are minimized by early surgery and if the quoted patients with surgery had an adequate procedure for decompression of a possibly increased ICP.

Work-Ups, Differential Diagnosis

The clinical diagnosis is confirmed by plain AP and lateral skull x-ray and/or finally by CT. In addition to the so-called sutural signs (effacement or disappearance of the suture #, parasutural sclerosis), the characteristic abnormal head shape and, in some patients, signs of increased ICP (increased convolutional markings ["silver beaten" skull] and diastasis of the still open sutures) are depicted.

The x-rays are used for differential diagnosis and as starting point for prospective follow-ups with precise evaluation of remodeling of the skull after surgery.

The differential diagnosis includes **normal variations** of the skull shape (dolichocephalic individuals) and **dolichocephaly of prematurity**

in which the skulls are often elongated and small with indices below 70 #. Whereas the former do not have all the specific morphological characteristics of sagittal synostosis and remain so, the latter's skull changes into a normal shape within 3–4 months if development is normal. In both diagnoses, both parietal calvaria are movable against each other at any time in early infancy. A special issue is **sagittal synostosis in hypophosphatemic rickets**. It occurs in up to 50 % of x-linked hypophosphatemic rickets and related diseases. The shape of the skull may be somewhat less typical, and scaphocephaly may be absent in some. In addition, the disease may have negative influence on postoperative reossification. In the neonatal period, **skull deformation by birth molding** must be considered in the differential diagnosis as in each type of craniosynostosis. Overlapping of the calvarial bones and spontaneous resolution of the deformity within the neonatal period are the typical signs of birth molding.

If the single features of sagittal synostosis are considered, several differential diagnoses arise: **macrocrania** in head circumference with values in the upper limit of normality, **posterior fossa cyst** # (Dandy-Walker malformations, arachnoid cyst) or **bathrocephaly** in prominent back head, and some types of **craniofacial dysostosis** or **multiple-suture synostosis** with priority of the sagittal synostosis followed by prominent fore- and/or back head. In bathrocephaly, buckling of midline calvaria concerns either the back head # or the posterior vertex.

4.1.2 Coronal Synostoses (Bi- and Unilateral)

Occurrence

Bicoronal synostosis is observed as non- or as syndromic brachycephaly. The former is observed in about 15 % with a subgroup of FGFR P250R mutation. Unicoronal synostosis occurs in about 25 % of the operated cases.

Clinical Presentation

In **bilateral coronal synostosis**, *the brachycephalic skull shows an upright ascending front* *with hardly recognizable vault # (Fig. 4.2 number 2a) and insufficiently covered bulbi that leads to proptosis or exophthalmos # of different degree. An osseous rim of the coronal suture is less often observed than in sagittal synostosis, and dimension of involvement of the peripheral part of the suture and of the adjacent basal sutures differs from case to case.* HC is often in the lower percentiles and skull index higher than 80.

In **unilateral coronal suture**, *facial asymmetry is obvious, and the deformity is the most grotesque type of anterior plagiocephaly. The contour of the involved orbit is displaced to the lateral side and backward #; the view from the top (bird's eye view) exhibits an effacement of the ipsilateral brow in contrast to the prominent brow of the contralateral side, and the roof of the ipsilateral orbit is underdeveloped on the lateral side with partially visible orbital bulb #. Often, there is a scoliotic curvature of the vertical midline axis of the face with concavity to the involved side. The ipsilateral eye fissure is wider, and the horizontal axis of the eye corners deviates from the horizontal axis of the mouth angles on the involved side. Occasionally, an ocular torticollis is encountered on the side of the coronal suture.* Secondary disorders of growth include the contralateral face and cranial base as well (Fig. 4.2 number 2b).

Functional Impairments
- In bilateral coronal synostosis, signs of increased ICP, early signs of possible cerebral palsy, and of delay of psychomotor development occur more frequently than in sagittal synostosis, especially in craniofacial dysostoses that are often combined with insidiously and gradually developing hydrocephalus and possibly with mental retardation.
- Exophthalmos with possible keratitis due to insufficient lid closure, possible loss of visual acuity and visual field defect due to increased ICP, or stenosis of the optic nerve channel.
- The above-mentioned impairments are less frequently observed except for exophthalmos and possible keratitis in unilateral coronal synostosis.
- But, beyond the age of 6 months, strabismus with or without amblyopia and absent binocular vision, astigmatism of one or both eye(s), and

hypermetropia are frequent findings (strabismus in one third and astigmatism in 40 %) and relate with the unilateral maldevelopment of the orbit. Half of the patients with strabismus develop ocular torticollis.
- Malocclusion is another impairment due to the oblique chewing plane in unicoronal synostosis in non- or too late operated cases that is true as well in bicoronal synostosis for other reasons.

Work-Ups, Differential Diagnosis
Plain AP and lateral skull x-rays show some characteristics of bi- and unilateral coronal synostosis which are not present in other forms of brachycephaly or unilateral plagiocephaly and allow the differential diagnosis.

In **bicoronal synostosis**, the abnormal shape of the brachycephalic skull with upright and high front, shallow orbits, and short anterior cranial fossa correspond to the clinical presentation. In addition, the steepness of the anterior fossa is recognizable by the pathognomonic obliquity of the orbits in the anteroposterior and by the elevation of the sphenoid wings in the lateral projection.

In **unicoronal synostosis**, the abnormal shape of the corresponding anterior cranial segment is less well depicted, but absence of the sphenoid wing in projection of the middle of the orbital contours and its elevation with formation of the so-called harlequin eye sign in the AP # and the elevation of the corresponding sphenoid wing # in the lateral projection are pathognomonic.

CT with 3D reconstruction considers individual variations and specific questions such as diameter of optic channel or middle and inner ear anatomy in craniofacial dysostoses, and permits preoperative planning and objective comparison with the postoperative results. In unicoronal synostosis, there is a deviation of the midline anterior fossa angle from the 0° to 180° midsagittal line of more than 5–10°.

The differential diagnosis includes **normal brachycephalic variation of skull shape, multiple-suture synostosis**, and **craniofacial dysostoses** in bicoronal, and **postural #, positional #, other forms of anterior plagiocephaly** and **complex deformities of the skull without**

synostosis (Fig. 4.3 number 6) in unicoronal synostosis.

Familiality and absent clinical and radiologic characteristics of bilateral coronal synostosis are indications of a **normal variation of skull shape**. In **multiple-suture synostosis**, additional characteristics of the skull concerning shape and suture signs allow differentiation clinically, on plain x-ray and CT. **Craniofacial dysostoses** may be characterized by data of the history (familiality), of the clinical examination (typical features and combination with characteristic associated malformations), and of different work-ups.

The "back to sleep" campaign to prevent sudden infant death in the early 1990s of American Academy of Pediatrics led to an increase of babies with nonsutural posterior plagiocephaly and brachycephaly which is mostly an asymmetrical brachycephaly. After this time, the following percentages of the natural history of posterior plagio- and brachycephaly have been obtained by longitudinal observation of a normal population at 6 weeks, 4, 8, 12, and 24 months of life: 16, 19.7, 6.8, and 3.3 % infants with nonsutural deformity for which supine position was the most important risk factor. That the supine sleep position tends to mold the skull into a more brachycephaly and the prone sleep position into a dolichocephalic form mainly in the first 3 months of life has been demonstrated as well. The nonsutural deformity can be corrected by putting early the infants in a prone position or to either side when they are awake. In the second trimester, an orthotic helmet is more effective. It diminishes the cephalic indices >81 by a mean of 2 % and those >90 by a mean of 4 % during treatment from the age 5–9 months. For severe cases with cephalic indices >90 before and after 6 months of age, craniectomy of the lambdoid sutures combined transposition osteotomy of the back can be offered which yields even better results. The percentages of 6.8 and 3.3 % tell that the deformity does not disappear spontaneously beyond infancy in all.

Mainly data of the history (causes and evolution of plagiocephaly), absent clinical and radiological characteristics of unicoronal synostosis, specific signs of nonsutural anterior plagiocephaly, and the possibility of resolution by medical treatment permit differentiation in **postural or positional anterior plagiocephaly**.

4.1.3   Metopic Synostosis (Trigonocephaly, Frontal Synostosis)

Occurrence, Pathology

Trigonocephaly is observed in less than 15 % of operated craniosynostoses; if mild forms are included, the percentage is somewhat higher. In contrast to the other sutures, normal osseous closure occurs earlier at the age of 2–3 years. The intracranial volumes may be smaller than average for age-correlated normal values and in up to one fifth, synostosis of other sutures is present.

Clinical Presentation

Independent of severity of premature fusion of the frontal suture, the common feature is a more or less visible and palpable osseous ridge in the midline of the forehead # (Fig. 4.2 number 3).

In moderate and severe forms, *a keel-like deformity (trigonocephaly) of the brow, a deficient lateral supraorbital rim combined with temporal narrowing, and medialized orbits (hypotelorism with diminished intraocular distance) are visible* #; the former signs are best seen from a bird's eye view and the latter from the front. The typical appearance of the face results from elevation of the lateral canthi.

In mild forms, a heel-shaped forehead, depressed temples, and slight hypotelorism are observed, but most parents bother about the somewhat prominent osseous midline ridge. The recognition of mild forms may be difficult if the parents are not concerned on it, and yet important because some of them may become symptomatic beyond infancy (with language and motor delay, and behavioral abnormalities), exhibit distinctly elevated ICP values, and show some amelioration after decompressive cranioplasty.

Functional Impairment

- Psychomotor and mental retardation may occur in less than 20 % up to one third depending on the references and is observed in nonoperated and operated patients as well. Distinctly increased ICP and papilledema are observed occasionally.
- The role of hypotelorism for the development of the visual system is not yet sufficiently

evaluated in trigonocephaly. Analogously with unilateral coronal synostosis, occurrence of strabismus and astigmatism with possible influence on (binocular) vision must be considered.

- In preschool and school age, nonsyndromic trigonocephaly is associated with a high frequency of developmental, educational, and behavioral problems (more than 30 %) regardless of surgical status and severity of the trigonocephaly, and more than 10 % have a distinct mental delay.

Work-Ups, Differential Diagnosis

Plain AP and lateral skull x-rays show closure of the metopic suture, some hypotelorism, and ovoid orbits with parallel medial borders and inverse longitudinal axis. CT with 3D reconstruction permits a precise grading of severity of trigonocephaly and preoperative planning.

Further work-ups are necessary to exclude syndromic forms such as Opitz C syndrome and others, inherited forms, or forms with spontaneous mutation.

Syndromic metopic synostosis and **Treacher Collins syndrome** are the main differential diagnoses of nonsyndromic metopic synostosis. **In Treacher Collins syndrome (mandibulofacial dysostosis or Franceschetti syndrome)**, the narrow and slender forehead reminds of trigonocephaly although craniosynostosis does not belong to this syndrome. The midface hypoplasia is combined with mandibular hypoplasia and leads frequently together with other possible anomalies to airway obstruction that needs often early intervention. Antimongoloid slanting palpebral fissures, lower eyelid coloboma, and malformations of the auricles are the typical facial features.

4.1.4 Lambdoid Synostosis (Bi- and Unilateral)

Occurrence Lambdoid synostosis is the less frequent craniosynostosis in most series (<5 %) if only the cases are considered who have complete ossification of the lambdoid sutures.

In addition, circumstantial evidence exists of the occurrence of so-called **uni- or bilateral functional synostosis** # of the lambdoid suture.

(1) In ±5 % of infants with presumably positional posterior deformities, there is no improvement of the mostly severe unilateral or bilateral flattening in spite of expectant and nonoperative treatment. (2) In such cases, the following findings are recognizable: a dent at the site of the closed posterior fontanel where the back head does never rest in supine position, often bilateral flattening of the back head with one side more involved than the other (even in cases with seemingly unilateral flattening), craniotabes of the adjacent parietal and occipital bones like in rickets with corresponding thinning and holes on plain x-rays and CT #, osseous ridge of the inner table over the lambdoid sutures at surgery # with various stages of premature ossification of the sutures on histological examination, frequent combination with mild to moderate asymmetric prominent ears. (3) The increased levels of TGF-β 2 and 3 at the sutural sites may be an indicator of advanced sutural closure on a genetic basis and/or due to prolonged external pressure against the sutures leading to functional synostosis of the lambdoid suture.

Clinical Presentation

The brachycephalic skull of **bilateral lambdoid synostosis** has *a flat (like cutoff) and often asymmetric back head. The site of greatest flattening does not correspond to the usual resting site. In addition, there is a compensatory widening of the posterior parietal regions and a tower-shaped disfigurement of the back head* # (Fig. 4.3) *number 4a.*

In contrast to the mostly closed and retracted posterior fontanel, the anterior fontanel is open and often too wide for the age. The calvarial bones adjacent to the lambdoid sutures are not movable against each other, and the suture itself is prominent. HC is often in the lower percentiles and skull index distinctly above 80.

In **unilateral lambdoid synostosis**, the already described disfigurement is unilateral, but compensatory growth involves the contralateral side like in unilateral coronal synostosis. In addition to the view from both sides, the view from the vertex and from behind is particularly important: *In contrast to the view from the ipsilateral side with occipital flattening, the contralateral* *side is prominent and round viewed from the contralateral side. The vertical view shows ipsilateral occipital flattening and occipitomastoid bossing and contralateral parietal bossing. In relation to the contralateral ear, the ipsilateral ear is displaced posteriorly. The contours of the head display a trapezium-shaped skull. Seen from behind, the contours of the head display a contralateral parietal and an occipitomastoid bossing laterally, an ipsilateral interior tilt of skull base, and displacement of the ear* (Fig. 4.3 number 4b).

Work-Ups, Differential Diagnosis
They include plain x-rays in lateral and Town projection, and CT with 3D reconstruction with the important axial plane of the skull base. In addition to the suture signs such a total or partial loss, osseous bridging, and parasutural sclerosis and roundish osseous defects, the axial CT slices allow differentiation from posterior deformational brachycephaly and plagiocephaly by the arrangement of the basal skull structures and in the latter by a deviation angle of the posterior fossa midline from the 0–180° midsagittal line by more than 5–10°.

The differential diagnosis includes deformational posterior brachycephaly and plagiocephaly, multiple-suture synostosis, and craniofacial dysostosis with involvement of the lambdoid suture. In case of trapezoid head shape on bird's eye view, unicoronal craniosynostosis combined with either an ipsilateral deformational posterior plagiocephaly or a unilambdoid synostosis or anterior and ipsilateral posterior deformational plagiocephaly must be considered in the differential diagnosis.

Deformational brachy- and plagiocephaly (brachy- and plagiocephaly without synostosis) #: It is observed frequently (>3.3:1,000 live births and up to two thirds of admitted infants with plagiocephaly) and is possibly due to intrauterine constraint (postural brachy- and plagiocephaly), due to postnatal positioning (positional brachy- and plagiocephaly) such as supine position (to prevent sudden infant death), due to any ordered position, for example, after shunting of neonates to prevent pressure sore of the scar, due

to purposeful head binding, due to congenital muscular torticollis, Klippel-Feil syndrome, or due to an ocular disorder torticollis.

Deformational brachy- and plagiocephaly is mostly an occipital flattening. The posterior brachycephaly is often asymmetric with one side more involved than the other. In deformational posterior plagiocephaly, the ipsilateral ear is advanced, and the ipsilateral frontal region is prominent leading to the impression of a seemingly contralateral anterior plagiocephaly. The bird's eye view yields a parallelogram shape of the axial head contour. The growth of face and cranial base, the cognitive and psychomotor development, and the eyes may be involved as well, the latter by astigmatism.

Treatment is medical, either by passive and active corrective positioning or by an orthotic helmet with resolution of the deformity as long as the increase of HC is in the steep part of growth curve corresponding to the brain growth in infancy. Improvement of the deformities occurs to a much lesser degree beyond 6 months of age. Some deformities are still present in adulthood.

Bi- and unilateral lambdoid synostoses may be a part of **multiple-suture synostosis** or **craniofacial dysostosis**; in the latter disorder, deformational brachy- or plagiocephaly must be considered also as additional cause due to psychomotor retardation with prolonged supine position.

4.2   Multiple-Suture Synostosis (Pansynostosis)

Occurrence, Pathology
Multiple-suture synostosis in which at least two different sutures are closed is an infrequent type of craniosynostosis and amounts to less than 5 % of nonsyndromic synostoses.

Cranial sutures may prematurely close in various combinations more or less at the same time or in different order of time that applies particularly to syndromic multiple-suture synostoses. The term "oxycephaly" refers to a pointed appearing vertex corresponding to the site of the anterior fontanel where compensatory calvarial growth has been possible last and is used differently in the literature.

Clinical Significance
- Multiple-suture synostosis is often combined with symptomatic increased intracranial pressure and, if not treated, followed by neuropsychological deficits.
- In syndromic multiple-suture synostoses, progressive hydrocephalus is often an additional pathology.
- Discovery of multiple-suture synostosis may be delayed by months to years in patients with harmonious closure of multiple sutures leading to normal skull shape, in syndromic multiple-suture synostoses with long intervals between closure of the single sutures, or in cases presenting initially as nonsyndromic single-suture synostosis.

Clinical Presentation
In contrast to single-suture craniosynostoses, different abnormal head shapes or even a normal head shape is possible depending on the primarily involved suture(s).

In **oxycephaly**, *the head is either abnormal high (turricephalic) and conical with a pointed vertex at the side of the closed anterior fontanel or any abnormal head shape is combined with a pointed bony deformity at the same site #* (Fig. 4.3 number 5).

In **nonsyndromic multiple-suture synostosis following repair of a single suture,** the initial head shape depends on the involved suture and may be altered on follow-up. This disease entity is observed in at least 1 % of operated nonsyndromic craniosynostoses and may occur in nonoperated cases as well. The clinical manifestation occurs 1 to several years after the initial operation either by overt signs of increased ICP or in seemingly asymptomatic patient with papilledema that emphasizes the need for long-term follow-ups.

In **harmonious multiple-suture synostosis**, *the head has a normal shape*, and the diminished skull growth is *possibly demonstrated by abnormally low percentiles of head circumference values in relation to the initial values or to the body length.*

In **cloverleaf skull** (triphyllocephaly, kleeblattschädel deformity) # with preferred premature closure of the sagittal and lambdoid suture, *the disproportionate, vertical, and anterior bulging of the parasagittal and frontal region, and the lateral bulging of the temporal region lead to a trilobular appearance of the skull if viewed from the front and the top.*

Cloverleaf skull occurs either as isolated malformation or associated with craniofacial dysostoses (Crouzon, Apert, Pfeiffer, Carpenter syndrome), with parietal sagittal synostosis, or thanatophoric dwarfism. The severe forms of cloverleaf skull are often a sign of syndromic craniosynostosis and combined with a grotesque constriction ring of the lambdoid-squamosal or of another zone. The clinical presentation of each patient is unique. Very frequent signs are beaked nose, low-set ears, high forehead, short midface and depressed premaxillary region, and proptosis or exophthalmos. In addition, stillbirth or neonatal death, moderate to severe mental retardation, syndactyly of the fingers and toes, dysostosis multiplex, restricted joint motility, and abnormal vertebral size and shape may be present.

Differential Diagnosis, Work-Ups
It includes mainly the differentiation between **nonsyndromic** and **syndromic forms of multiple-suture synostosis**, their specification, and the precise determination of the involved sutures. In harmonious multiple-suture synostosis, **constitutional microcrania** or **microencephaly** # must be considered; in the latter case, a disproportion between normal splanchno- and low neurocranium is observed, and the head circumference has been too small already at birth. In case of signs of increased ICP, accompanying **progressive hydrocephalus** and postoperative **reclosure of the fused sutures** are possible differential diagnoses.

Plain anteroposterior and lateral skull x-rays result in preliminary informations, but only CT with 3D reconstruction demonstrates the precise diagnosis and the closed sutures including the recognition of possible intracranial and other malformations.

4.3   Syndromic Craniosynostosis (Craniofacial Dysostosis)

Occurrence, Causes

In syndromic craniosynostosis, single- or multiple-suture synostosis is associated with craniofacial syndromes. The different types occur in about 1:100,000 live births or even more rarely. They account for roughly one third of all operated craniosynostoses. Most of them have an autosomal dominant or recessive inheritance or occur due to spontaneous mutations. Crouzon, Apert, and Pfeiffer syndrome and the rare Muenke, Jackson-Weiss, and Beare-Stevenson syndrome belong to the FGFR gene family (mutations of the fibroblast-growth factor-receptor genes 1, 2, and/or 3). Other craniosynostoses with known genes concern the Boston-type craniosynostosis, bicoronal synostosis with FGFR3 P250R mutation, and the Saethre-Chotzen syndrome. In addition, craniosynostosis occurs in more than 150 syndromes as occasional malformation.

Clinical Significance

- Early recognition of craniofacial dysostoses and precise classification are indispensable for prognostication, therapeutic planning, and family consultation.
- Prevention of secondary damage by early nonsurgical and/or surgical intervention against the numerous possible functional disorders such as airway obstruction and sensorial and mental deficit is necessary.
- Strengthening of acceptance of such children by the parents and of the self-esteem of both by continuous and close care, appropriate nonsurgical measures, and reconstructive surgery up to adulthood by a craniofacial team and an experienced representative are very important.

Clinical Presentation

The different craniofacial dysostoses have mostly common features such as maxillary hypoplasia, ocular hypertelorism and proptosis, extracranial anomalies, and several functional disorders such as airway obstruction and feeding difficulties, deficits of the sensory organs, delays of motor and mental development, malocclusion, and aesthetic impairment. In addition, at least 40 % of children with Crouzon, Pfeiffer, and Apert syndrome have hydrocephalus that is progressive mainly in the former two. The recognition of hydrocephalus in these syndromes may be difficult because classic signs may be absent and progressive ventricular dilatation becomes mostly evident after decompressive surgery. Clinically, the syndromes differ from each other by a combination of characteristic craniofacial findings and/or the occurrence of specific extracranial anomalies. Most have been described by the authors who were leaving their marks on these syndromes.

Differential Diagnosis, Work-Ups

In addition to the already quoted craniofacial dysostoses, the following disorders must be considered either due to possible craniosynostosis (Antley-Bixler and Baller-Gerold syndrome) or due to craniofacial abnormalities (Greig cephalopolysyndactyly, Treacher Collins, Strickler, Shprintzen, and fetal alcohol syndrome).

The work-up includes throughout clinical examination, plain x-rays, cephalometry with multivariant analysis, CT with 3D reconstruction, evaluation of specific organs, for example, middle and inner ear, and genetic investigations (interpretation of pedigrees, molecular diagnosis). Variability of expression, broad overlap of symptoms, and occasional absence of signs that are considered as obligatory for a specific syndrome may render the diagnosis difficult but not impossible if additional examinations are applied.

In **Crouzon syndrome**, there are typically no extracranial malformations. Five percent of all craniosynostoses recognized at birth belong to Crouzon syndrome.

Ocular proptosis and hypertelorism, variable degrees of *hypoplasia of the maxilla, curved parrot-like nose and inverted V (ogival) shape of the palate, mouth breeding due to upper airway obstruction* (in one third, e.g., by nasomaxillary retrusion leading to rhinopharyngeal "atresia" with possible sleep apnea)*, otological malformations, and hearing loss, class III malocclusion, fusion of cervical vertebrae C2/C3, and fusion of cranial and facial sutures* belong to the main features.

Three fourth of the cases are inherited, the remainder spontaneous mutations. *Shallow orbits and proptosis* # are the most constant features of Crouzon syndrome that has an autosomal dominant inheritance with variable expression, although clinically normal appearing patients occur. A rare type of Crouzon syndrome is combined with acanthosis nigricans.

The degree and age of onset of **craniosynostosis** is variable from single- to multiple-suture synostosis with bicoronal synostosis the most frequently observed type. The same is true for hydrocephalus that occurs more frequently than in Apert syndrome.

In **Apert syndrome** (acrocephalosyndactyly), shallowness of the orbits is less striking in spite of the same main cranial findings as in Crouzon syndrome. Characteristic features of the face # are *flatness, supraorbital horizontal groove, small nose, asymmetric upper eyelid ptosis, downslanting of the palpebral fissure, and narrow palate with median groove and possible clefting* (30 %). Otological structural anomalies and hearing loss (30 %) are frequent findings similar to Crouzon syndrome. Characteristically, *a thick gingiva, teeth disorders, and teeth development delay belong to the Apert syndrome; the latter finding corresponds to general growth that shows a trend of increasing delay with increased age.*

The extracranial anomalies include mainly cutaneous and/or osseous syndactyly of the fingers and toes (second, third, and fourth) with partial or total fusion #, and broad distal phalanges of the thumbs and great toes with valgus position. Except for very rare cases, *osseous syndactyly of the distal phalanges of the hands is an obligate universal feature of Apert syndrome.* There is an increased risk of additional nonskeletal malformations and *severe acne at puberty.* Most of the cases are fresh mutations with a recurrence risk of 50 % in the offspring.

In **craniosynostosis**, the coronal suture is mostly involved that leads together with a roundish brain to a short anteroposterior diameter of the skull with a high flat fore- and back head. Frequent mental retardation of Apert syndrome must be considered in prognostication.

In **Saethre-Chotzen syndrome**, *brachycephaly* with high forehead due to a very frequent **bicoronal synostosis** is a typical sign. Characteristic features of the face are *a low-set frontal hairline, asymmetry with deviation of the nasal septum, ptosis of the eyelids, and downslanting palpebral fissure, prominent ear crus extending from the helical root across the concha, and large and late closing fontanels.*

The observed syndactyly is usually partial and concerns the second and third fingers and the third and fourth toes. Typical are *brachydactyly, with small distal phalanges and broad thumbs, and great toes.* Short clavicles with distal hypoplasia and *developing fusions of the vertebral bodies and their posterior element C2–C3 beyond the age of 2 years* on x-ray are frequent findings of the syndrome. The latter possibility calls for preoperative radiological evaluation of the cervical spine.

Saethre-Chotzen syndrome is an autosomal dominant inherited disorder with a wide variance of expression. Therefore, variable features may be observed in the same family.

In **Pfeiffer syndrome**, Cohen type 1, the classic Pfeiffer syndrome must be differentiated from Cohen types 2 and 3. The former consists of **single-suture synostosis** (mostly bicoronal synostosis with minor turricephaly), *mild degree of midfacial hypoplasia with relative prognathism, exorbitism, and hypertelorism, broad thumbs and great toes with radial or medial deviation, and partial soft tissue syndactyly of the hands and feet.* The *nose is small with a low bridge, and the palpebral fissures display antimongoloid upslanting.* Hearing loss and otological structural anomalies are very frequent findings.

In contrast to type 1 with autosomal dominant inheritance and good long-term prognosis, types 2 and 3 are fresh mutations, have grotesque deformations, and have untreated a poor prognosis with possible death in infancy.

Except for head shape and different degree of hydrocephalus – *type 2 with* **cloverleaf skull** *and severe hydrocephalus and type 3 with* **turricephaly or another head shape** due to multiple-suture synostosis and *variable degree of hydrocephalus – both types show severe* *maxillary hypoplasia with orbitostenosis and exorbitism, intracranial anomalies, upper airway obstruction, limb and vertebral anomalies (without consistent pattern, e.g., Arnold-Chiari malformation), with possible blindness, hearing loss, and chronic hypoxemia.* In addition, choanal atresia and laryngotracheal anomalies are quoted in type 2 and elbow ankylosis (radiohumeral synostosis) in type 3.

In **Carpenter syndrome**, brachycephaly or another conspicuous head shape due to variable coronal, sagittal, and lambdoid **synostosis,** *shallow supraorbital ridges and lateral displacement of the inner canthi*, and different skeletal anomalies are observed; the latter include mainly *brachydactyly of the hands with clinodactyly, partial syndactyly, and camptodactyly. Hypogenitalism and obesity* are other features of the Carpenter syndrome with autosomal recessive inheritance.

4.4   Treatment

4.4.1   Indication

It is important to know that no spontaneous correction of the deformity occurs in the natural history of any craniosynostosis #.

In **single-suture synostosis** (sagittal, unicoronal, frontal, and lambdoid synostosis), the main indication is aesthetic although increasing data on possible functional impairment arise. In all types, cases with increased ICP do occur (17 % with distinctly and 38 % with borderline increased ICP [>15 and 10–15 mmHg]) #. Some of the patients have minimal sign of increased ICP that disappear after surgery, and many exhibit localized radiological signs of increased ICP. On long-term follow-up, learning disorders are observed in sagittal and mental deficiencies in frontal and lambdoid synostoses, and serious ocular symptoms in unicoronal synostoses. Therefore, the indication may be preventive or curative in some of the cases.

In **multiple-suture synostosis** (bicoronal synostosis is assigned to this group for practical purposes), the indication is functional due to the

frequent occurrence of increased ICP and other functional disorders, and often aesthetic.

In **syndromic craniosynostosis**, the indication is always aesthetic due to the mostly grotesque deformation and equally functional due to the frequency of increased ICP and the numerous possible and sometimes life-threatening disorders.

4.4.2   Risks

The main anesthesiological and surgical risks are in all three groups hemorrhage, specific major and moderate to minor intraoperative complications, bradycardia in case of orbital manipulations, need for postoperative pulmonary ventilation, infections, CSF leaks, insufficient reossification with permanent skull defects, problems associated with biomaterials, and insufficient correction or recurrence of the deformity.

More than 90 % of the patients require, independent on the length of surgery, a perioperative **blood transfusion**, more than 50 % need 50–100 %, and up to 20 % more than 100 % of the estimated blood volume. The use of a cell saver may be useful in this respect. To the **major complications** (in up to 3 %) belong sudden massive hemorrhage, air embolism, and failing vagolysis in oculocardiac reflex, and to the **moderate to minor complications** airway problems (difficult intubation, dislocation or obstruction of the tracheal tube) and circulatory problems (under- and overtransfusion, secondary coagulation disorders). The needs for **postoperative pulmonary ventilation** (in <10 %) are very young age, major intraoperative complications, long-lasting surgery, and upper airway obstruction (mostly in craniofacial dysostoses).

For several reasons, universally obligatory figures of the risks are not available (differently mixed patient cohorts, recent improvements, not published data). Whereas residual skull defects and problems associated with biomaterials are increasingly solvable, **insufficient corrections and recurrences** are still a matter of concern. In single-suture synostosis, reoperation is necessary in less than 10 % and in multiple-suture synostosis or craniofacial dysostosis in about one fourth

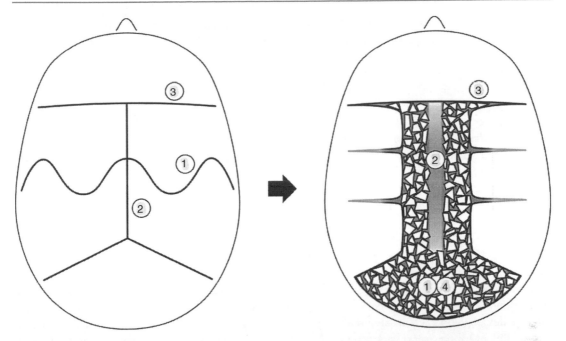

Fig. 4.4 Surgery in sagittal synostosis. The drawing on the left side displays: *1*: the wavy coronal skin incision to avoid that the somewhat hairless scar lies not in a line over the vertex; *2*: the site of the closed sagittal suture; and *3*: the site of the open coronal suture. The drawing on the *right side* shows the different steps of craniectomy: After removal of a 6-cm wide strip from the vertex including the fused sagittal suture, a triangle of bone behind the coronal sutures *3*: and the bone of the occipital region are removed from the site of major occipital bossing including the former posterior fontanel and lambdoid sutures *1*. In addition, the parietal bones are incised in a vertical direction. The large bone defect is closed with small pieces of the removed bone like a mosaic *4*: except for a 0.5–1-cm midline zone at the site of the former fused sagittal suture. *2*: this method is performed in infancy; it allows continuous remodeling of the skull shape in a period of largest growth and leaves no skull defects behind

(e.g., missing effacement of the dead space due to slow brain expansion and growth as in Apert syndrome).

4.4.3   Surgery

In all **single-suture synostoses**, linear craniectomy is mostly insufficient for normalization of head shape and prevention or relief of functional disorders. Out of the numerous procedures quoted in the literature including the endoscopic craniectomy and cranial vault distraction, vertex craniectomy including occipital bossing and vertical incisions of the remaining calvaria is sufficient for cranial vault reconstruction if performed in the first half of infancy in case of **sagittal synostosis**. The large skull defects are covered with small pieces like a mosaic (Fig. 4.4). In older children

(>1 year), major calvarial reconstruction may become necessary for relief of a possible increased ICP and correction of abnormal head shape. In uni- or bilateral **lambdoid synostosis**, the back head is reconstructed after large resection of the involved sutures by large flaps taken from the posterior parietalia which are rotated and reinserted according to their most prominent bulge and by small pieces of bone. In **frontal and uni- or bilateral coronal synostosis**, a frontoorbital advancement must be performed (in unicoronal synostosis sometimes unilaterally) with reconstruction of the adjacent frontal and temporoparietal region by removed bone pieces which are repositioned and fixed with resorbable miniplates and osteosutures.

In **multiple-suture craniosynostosis**, the procedure depends on the age of the patient and the shape of the head. The optimal procedure should include removal of all involved sutures and sufficient decompression of the brain, prevention of reclosure of the sutures during the period of maximum brain growth, persistent skull defects, and guarantee a normal head shape. In neonates and young infants, brain decompression and safety has priority over aesthetic reconstruction. Therefore, surgery in two stages may become necessary.

In **syndromic craniosynostosis**, often advancement procedure is necessary, and the possibility of multiple-suture synostosis must be considered in operative planning as well as the reduced growth potential of the midface, and the multiple possible functional disorders (e.g., tracheostomy in obstruction of the upper airways). Therefore, staged procedures are necessary depending on the age and the actually necessary steps (e.g., correction of malocclusion at puberty after eruption of permanent teeth by midface osteotomies), and distraction osteotomy may be a useful adjunct for the splanchnocranium.

4.5   Prognosis

The assumption that early correction of **single-suture craniosynostosis** has a positive effect on global developmental functioning has not been supported by the recent clinical research. However, there is a two to three times increased risk for single-suture synostosis of retardation later in life and of a variety of learning disorders regardless of surgical status. On the other hand, it is unknown if these problems are minimized by early surgery and if the quoted patients with surgery had an adequate procedure for decompression of a possibly increased ICP. Difficulties arise to apply the data of these studies about learning disorders for the clinician because their occurrence varies between one third and half of such patients, they have not a constant pattern of learning disorder, and they refer to a relatively small number of patients and mostly to sagittal synostosis.

Intermediate and long-term results of all fields of the single-suture synostoses are not yet available in a substantial number of publications and/or patients.

In *sagittal synostosis and similarly in osseous and functional lambdoid synostosis*, **the aspect of head shape** is completely (in 81.5–91 %) or nearly completely (in the remainder percentage) normalized; the distribution of head circumferences and skull indices, and the radiological findings become normal and remain so in the long term ##. Correction of the shape takes place by a lessened growth velocity in length (sagittal synostosis) and breadth (lambdoid synostosis) in the early months after surgery. In addition, the facial aspect changes distinctly ## as well as the skull base (significant correction of the increased orbital angle in both types of synostosis toward normalization). A substantial proportion of sagittal and lambdoid synostosis profits from surgery **functionally**: more than two thirds of the neurological abnormalities (mostly signs of increased ICP or early signs of CP, present in one third before surgery for sagittal synostosis) and more than half of the neurological abnormalities disappear (mostly developmental delay and signs of increased ICP, present in 50 % before surgery for lambdoid synostosis).

In *frontal and unicoronal synostosis*, the **early and intermediate results** are mostly quoted as good to excellent on qualitative evaluation. But quantitative evaluation shows that complete normalization is not achieved at 1 year postoperatively (for instance, in ipsilateral dysmorphology of unicoronal synostosis). The percentage of needed reoperations (<10 %) may be taken as an indication for the quality of the reconstructed **head shape**. In contrast to unicoronal synostosis which presents the least complications concerning mental development and increased ICP, in frontal synostosis, **mental retardation** may be observed in up to one third and mild neurological abnormalities in up to 50 % on follow-up. On the other hand, **ocular problems** such as strabism and astigmatism can be reduced by a factor 3 or 2, respectively, by early surgery of unicoronal synostosis in the first half of infancy.

In **multiple-suture synostosis**, the developmental and **intellectual outcome** is good if decompressive surgery has been performed early in infancy. The aesthetic outcome is less favorable if the reoperation quote is considered which is similar to that of syndromic craniosynostosis.

The prognosis in **syndromic craniosynostosis** concerning **mental performance** depends on the specific syndrome and its expression, on possible associated functional disorders and their timely and appropriate treatment, on possible associated multiple-suture synostosis, hydrocephalus, and CNS malformations, and on still unknown factors. Up to three fourths may be of normal global intelligence although intellectual function is significantly lower in syndromic than in nonsyndromic craniosynostoses. For prognosis of the final **skull shape**, the specific syndrome and its expression, the possible multiple-suture synostosis and/or hydrocephalus, and on a large scale, the corrective growth potential of the skeleton especially of the splanchnocranium are very important # #. The reoperation quote for insufficient results is up to 25 %.

Webcodes

The following webcodes can be used on www. psurg.net for further images and data.

401 Dolichocephaly	420 Bone holes
402 Narrow forehead	421 Inner osseous ridges
403 Osseous ridge	422 Posterior turricephaly
404 Parasutural defects	423 Plagiocephaly
405 Disappearance of suture	424 Oxycephaly
406 Prematurity	425 Cloverleaf skull
407 Posterior fossa cyst	426 Microencephaly
408 Bathrocephaly	427 Shallow orbits, Crouzon
409 Brachycephaly	428 Face features, Apert
410 Exophthalmos	429 Apert hands
411 Facial asymmetry	430 Natural history
412 Bird's eye view	431 Pre-/postoperative ICP
413 "Harlequin eye" sign	432 Preoperative x-ray
414 Sphenoid wing elevation	433 Postoperative x-ray
415 Plagiocephaly	434 Preoperative face
416 Plagiocephaly	435 Postoperative face
417 Frontal ridge	436 Preoperative x-ray
418 Trigonocephaly	437 Postoperative x-ray
419 Flat back head	

Bibliography

General: Genetics, Functional Loss, Hydrocephalus, Radiological Imaging

Baranello G, Vasco G, Ricci D, Mercuri E (2007) Visual function in nonsyndromic craniosynostosis: past, present, and future. Childs Nerv Syst 23: 1461–1465

Collmann H, Sörensen N, Krauss J (2005) Hydrocephalus in craniosynostosis: a review. Childs Nerv Syst 21: 902–912

Lehman S (2006) Strabismus in craniosynostosis. Curr Opin Ophthalmol 17:432–434

Passos-Bueno MR, Serti Eacute AE, Jehee FS, Fanganiello R, Yeh E (2008) Genetics of craniosynostosis: genes, syndromes, mutations and genotype-phenotype correlations. Front Oral Biol 12:107–143

van der Meulen J, van der Vlugt J, Okkerse J, Hofman B (2008) Early beaten-copper pattern: its long-term effect on intelligence quotients in 95 children with craniosynostosis. J Neurosurg Pediatr 1:25–30

Weber J, Collmann H, Czarnetzki A, Spring A, Pusch CM (2008) Morphometric analysis of untreated adults skulls in syndromic and nonsyndromic craniosynostosis. Neurosurg Rev 31:179–188

Section 4.1 Single-Suture Synostosis, Functional Evaluation, Intracranial Pressure

Becker DB, Petersen JD, Kane AA, Cradock MM, Pilgram TK, Marsh JL (2005) Speech, cognitive, and behavioral outcomes in nonsyndromic craniosynostosis. Plast Reconstr Surg 116:400–407

Cohen SR, Persing JA (1998) Intracranial pressure in single-suture craniosynostosis. Cleft Palate Craniofac J 35:194–196

Cohen SR, Cho DC, Nichols SL, Simms C, Cross KP, Burstein FD (2004) American Society of Maxillofacial Surgeons Outcome Study: preoperative and postoperative neurodevelopmental findings in single-suture craniosynostosis. Plast Reconstr Surg 114:841–847; discussion 848–849

Hukki J, Saarinen P, Kangasniemi M (2008) Single suture craniosynostosis: diagnosis and imaging. Front Oral Biol 12:79–90

Kapp-Simon KA (1998) Mental development and learning disorders in children with single-suture craniosynostosis. Cleft Palate Craniofac J 35:197–203

Kapp-Simon KA, Leroux B, Cunningham M, Speltz ML (2005) Multisite study of infants with single-suture craniosynostosis; preliminary report of presurgical development. Cleft Palate Craniofac Surg J 42:377–384

Mouradian WE (1998) Controversies in the diagnosis of craniosynostosis: a panel discussion. Cleft Palate Craniofac J 35:190–193

Panchal J, Amirsheybani H, Gurwitch R, Cook V, Francel P, Neas B, Levine N (2001) Neurodevelopment in children with single-suture craniosynostosis and plagiocephaly without synostosis. Plast Reconstr Surg 108:1492–1498; discussion 1499

Section 4.1.1 Sagittal Synostosis

Agrawal D, Steinbok P, Cochrane DD (2006) Pseudoclosure of anterior fontanelle by wormian bone in isolated sagittal synostosis. Pediatr Neurosurg 42: 135–137

Albright AL, Towbin RB, Shultz BL (1996) Long-term outcome after sagittal synostosis operations. Pediatr Neurosurg 25:78–82

Arnaud E, Renier D, Marchac D (1995) Prognosis for mental function in scaphocephaly. J Neurosurg 83: 476–479

Currarino G (2007) Sagittal synostosis in X-linked hypophosphatemic rickets and related diseases. Pediatr Radiol 37:805–812

Deleon VB, Richtsmeier JT (2009) Fluctuating asymmetry and developmental instability in sagittal craniosynostosis. Cleft Palate Craniofac J 46:187–196

Gewalli F, da Silva Guimaraes-Ferreira JP, Sahlin P, Emanuelsson I, Horneman G, Stephensen H, Lauritzen CGK (2001) Mental development after modified π procedure: dynamic cranioplasty for sagittal synostosis. Ann Plast Surg 46:415–420

Kaiser G (1988) Sagittal synostosis – its clinical significance and the results of three different methods of craniectomy. Childs Nerv Syst 4:223–230

Kaufman BA, Muszynski CA, Matthews A, Etter N (2004) The circle of sagittal synostosis surgery. Semin Pediatr Neurol 11:243–248

Magge SN, Westerveld M, Pruzinsky T, Persing JA (2002) Long-term neuropsychological effects of sagittal craniosynostosis on child development. J Craniofac Surg 13:49–104

Schmelzer RE, Perlyn CA, Kane AA, Pilgram TK, Govier D, Marsh JL (2007) Identifying reproducible patterns of calvarial dysmorphology in nonsyndromic sagittal craniosynostosis may affect operative intervention and outcome assessment. Plast Reconstr Surg 119:1546–1552, Comment in: Plast Reconstr Surg (2008) 121:335–336

Speltz ML, Endriga MC, Mouradian WE (1997) Presurgical and postsurgical mental and psychomotor development of infants with sagittal synostosis. Cleft Palate Craniofac J 34:374–379

Virtanen R, Korhonen T, Fagerholm J, Viljanto J (1999) Neurocognitive sequelae of scaphocephaly. Pediatrics 103:791–795

Section 4.1.2 Coronal Synostosis

Arnaud E, Meneses P, Lajeunie E, Thorne JA, Marchac D, Renier D (2002) Postoperative mental and morphological outcome for nonsyndromic brachycephaly. Plast Reconstr Surg 110:6–12; discussion 13

Denis D, Genitori L, Bolufer A, Lena G, Saracco J-B, Choux M (1994) Refractive error and ocular motility in plagiocephaly. Childs Nerv Syst 10:210–216

Ehret FW, Whelan MF, Ellenbogen RG, Cunningham ML, Gruss JS (2004) Differential diagnosis of trapezoid-shaped head. Childs Nerv Syst 41:13–19

Gupta PC, Foster J, Crowe S, Papay FA, Luciano M, Traboulsi EI (2003) Ophthalmological findings in patients with nonsyndromic plagiocephaly. J Craniofac Surg 14:529–532

Keller MK, Hermann MV, Darvann TA, Larsen P, Hove HD, Christensen L, Schwartz M, Marsh JL, Kreiborg S (2007) Craniofacial morphology in Muenke syndrome. J Craniofac Surg 18:374–386

Lo LJ, Marsh JL, Pilgram TK, Vannier MW (1996a) Plagiocephaly: differential diagnosis based on endocranial morphology. Plast Reconstr Surg 97:282–291

Lo LJ, Marsh JL, Kane AA, Vannier MW (1996b) Orbital dysmorphology in unilateral coronal synostosis. Cleft Palate Craniofac J 33:190–197

Selber JC, Brooks C, Kurichi JE, Temmen T, Sonnad SS, Whitaker LA (2008) Long-term results following fronto-orbital reconstruction in nonsyndromic unicoronal synostosis. Plast Reconstr Surg 121: 251e–260e

Tomlinson JK, Breidahl AF (2007) Anterior fontanelle morphology in unilateral coronal synostosis: a clear clinical (nonradiographic) sign for the diagnosis of frontal plagiocephaly. Plast Reconstr Surg 119: 1882–1888

Section 4.1.3 Metopic Synostosis

Anderson PJ, Netherway DJ, Abbott A, David DJ (2004) Intracranial volume measurement of metopic craniosynostosis. J Craniofac Surg 15:1014–1016; discussion 1017–1018

Aryan HE, Jandial R, Ozgur BM, Hughes SA, Meltzer HS, Park MS, Levy ML (2005) Surgical correction of metopic synostosis. Childs Nerv Syst 21:392–398

Greenberg BM, Schneider SJ (2006) Trigonocephaly: surgical considerations and long term evaluation. J Craniofac Surg 17:528–535

Kelleher MO, Murray DJ, Mc Gillivary A, Kamel MH, Alleutt D, Earley MJ (2006) Behavioral, developmental, and educational problems in children with nonsyndromic trigonocephaly. J Neurosurg 105(5 Suppl): 382–384

Mendonca DA, White N, West F, Dover S, Solanki G, Nishikawa H (2009) Is there a relationship between the severity of metopic synostosis and speech and language impairments? J Craniofac Surg 20:85–88; discussion 89

Shimoji T, Tomiyama N (2004) Mild trigonocephaly and intracranial pressure: report of 56 patients. Childs Nerv Syst 20:749–756

Section 4.1.4 Lambdoid Synostosis

Graham JM Jr, Kreutzman J, Earl D et al (2005a) Deformational brachycephaly in supine-sleeping infants. J Pediatr 146:253–257

Graham JM, Gomes M, Halberg A et al (2005b) Management of deformational plagiocephaly: repositioning versus orthotic therapy. J Pediatr 146:258–262

Huang CS, Cheng HC, Lin WY, Liou JW, Chen YR (1995) Skull morphology affected by different sleep positions in infancy. Cleft Palate Craniofac J 32:413–419

Huang MHS, Mouradian WE, Cohen SR, Gruss JS (1998) The differential diagnosis of abnormal head shapes: separating craniosynostosis from positional deformities and normal variants. Cleft Palat Craniofac J 35:204–211

Hutchison BL, Hutchison LAD, Thompson JMD et al (2004) Plagiocephaly and brachycephaly in the first two years of life: a prospective cohort study. Pediatrics 114:970–980

Kadlub N, Persing JA, da Silva Freitas R, Shin JH (2008) Familial lambdoid craniosynostosis between father and son. J Craniofac Surg 19:850–854

Kane AA, Lo LJ, Vannier MW, Marsh JL (1996) Discrete, measurable, etiology-specific mandibular dysmorphology in unicoronal synostosis and plagiocephaly without synostosis. Cleft Palate Craniofac J 33:418–423

Kelly KM, Littlefield TR, Pomatto JK, Ripley CE, Beals SP, Joganic EF (1999) Importance of early recognition and treatment of deformational plagiocephaly with orthotic cranioplasty. Cleft Palate Craniofac J 36:127–138

Lin KY, Nolen AA, Gamprer TJ, Jane JA, Opperman LA, Ogle RC (1997) Elevated levels of transforming growth factors beta 2 and beta 3 in lambdoid sutures from children with persistent plagiocephaly. Cleft Palate Craniofac J 34:331–337

McComb JG (1991) Treatment of functional lambdoid synostosis. Neurosurg Clin N Am 2:665–672

Section 4.2 Pansynostosis

Blount JP, Louis RG Jr, Tubbs RS, Grant JH (2007) Pansynostosis: a review. Childs Nerv Syst 23:1103–1109

Hudgins RJ, Cohen SR, Burstein FD, Boydston WR (1998) Multiple suture synostosis and increased intracranial pressure following repair of a single

suture, nonsyndromal craniosynostosis. Cleft Palat Craniofac J 35:167–172

Scott JR, Isom CN, Gruss JS, Salemy S, Ellenbogen RG, Avellino A, Birgfeld C, Hopper RA (2009) Symptom outcomes following cranial vault expansion for craniosynostosis in children older than 2 years. Plast Reconstr Surg 123:289–297; discussion 298–299

Section 4.3 Syndromic Synostosis

Anderson PJ, Hall CM, Evans RD, Hayward RD, Harkness WJ, Jones BM (1997) The cervical spine in Saethre-Chotzen syndrome. Cleft Palate Craniofac J 34:79–82

Cantrell SB, Moore MH, Trott JA, Morris RJ, David DJ (1994) Phenotypic variation in acrocephalosyndactyly syndromes: unusual findings in patient with features of Apert and Saethre-Chotzen syndromes. Cleft Palate Craniofac J 31:487–493

Carinci F, Avantaggiato A, Curioni C (1994) Crouzon syndrome: cephalometric analysis and evaluation of pathogenesis. Cleft Palate Craniofac J 31:201–209

Kaloust S, Ishii K, Vagervik K (1997) Dental development in Apert syndrome. Cleft Palate Craniofac J 34:117–121

Manjila S, Chim H, Eisele S, Chowdhry SA, Gosain AK, Cohen AR (2010) History of the Kleeblattschädel deformity: origin of concepts and evolution of management in the past 50 years. Neurosurg Focus 29(6):E7

Moore MH, Abbott AH (1996) Extradural deadspace after infant fronto-orbital advancement in Apert syndrome. Cleft Palate Craniofac J 33:202–205

Moore MH, Cantrell SB, Trott JA, David DJ (1995) Pfeiffer syndrome: a clinical review. Cleft Palate Craniofac J 32:62–70

Witt PD, Hardesty RA, Zuppan C, Rouse G, Hasso AN, Boyne P (1992) Fetal kleeblattschädel cranium: morphologic, radiographic, and histologic analysis. Cleft Palate Craniofac Surg J 29:363–368

Sections 4.4–4.5

Clayman MA, Murad GJ, Steele MH, Seagle MB, Pincus DW (2007) History of craniosynostosis surgery and the evolution of minimally invasive endoscopic techniques: the University of Florida experience. Ann Plast Surg 58:285–287

Cohen SR, Pryor L, Mittermiller PA, Meltzer HS, Levy MI, Broder KW, Ozgur BM (2008) Nonsyndromic craniosynostosis: current treatment options. Plast Surg Nurs 28:79–91

Da Costa AC, Walters I, Savarirayan R, Anderson VA, Wrennall JA, Meara JG (2006) Intellectual outcomes in children and adolescents with syndromic and nonsyndromic craniosynostosis. Plast Reconstr Surg 118:175–181; discussion 182–183

Jarrahy R, Kawamoto HK, Keagle J, Dickinson BP, Katchikian HV, Bradley JP (2009) Three tenets for staged correction of Kleeblattschädel or cloverleaf skull deformity. Plast Reconstr Surg 123:210–318

Moylan S, Collee G, Mackersie A, Bingham R (1993) Anaesthetic management in paediatric craniofacial surgery: a review of 126 cases. Paediatr Anaesth 3:275–281

Okkerse JM, Beemer FA, de Jong TH, Mellenbergh GJ, Vaandrager JM, Vermeij-Keers C, Heineman-de Boer JA (2004) Condition variables in children with craniofacial anomalies: a descriptive study. J Craniofac Surg 15:151–156; discussion 157

Perkins JA, Sie KCY, Milczuk H, Richardson MA (1997) Airway management in children with craniofacial anomalies. Cleft Palate Craniofac J 34:135–140

Persing JA (2008) MOC-PS(SM) CME article: management considerations in the treatment of craniosynostosis. Plast Reconstr Surg 121(4 Suppl):1–11

Salyer KE (2000) Distraction osteogenesis vs. craniofacial osteotomy. J Craniomaxillofac Surg 28(Suppl 1):62

Williams JK, Ellenbogen RG, Gruss JS (1999) State of the art in craniofacial surgery: nonsyndromic craniosynostosis. Cleft Palate Craniofac J 36:471–485

Malformations of the Face Visible from the Outside

5.1 Orofacial Clefts

Occurrence

Cleft lip (alveolus) palate is the most common malformation of the face (80 %), whereas facial clefts or lip fistulas are encountered less frequently.

The prevalence of all orofacial clefts is 1.7:1,000 live births of which at least two thirds are isolated malformations and the remainder belong to chromosomal aberrations or syndromes. All orofacial clefts come to two thirds of the major congenital craniofacial defects.

Clinical Significance

- At least 1:1,000 live births has one of the different forms of cleft lip (alveolus) palate.
- Ethnic susceptibility is different (1:400–500 in Asians, 1:750–900 in Caucasian, and 1:1,500–2,000 in Africans).
- Esthetical appearance and several functions such as sucking or chewing, speech, and hearing may be involved.
- Many need long-term follow-up and treatment until the end of growth.
- Last two topics including vision concern also facial clefts and to a lesser degree lip fistulas.

5.1.1 Cleft Lip (Alveolus) Palate

Occurrence, Forms, Pathoanatomy, Causes

The following forms are observed in order of frequency:

1. Unilateral and bilateral, partial and complete cleft lip (alveolus) = UCL/BCL
2. Combinations of the two forms = UCLP/BCLP
3. Partial and complete cleft palate (Fig. 5.1) = CP

   Syndromic types of cleft lip (alveolus) palate occur in up to 15 % #. Among other things, >19 syndromes exist with frequent (>50 %) and >171 syndromes with occasional association with clefts. Clefts may also be associated with major or minor anomalies.

Only a part of the visible anomaly consists of tissue defect and hypoplasia. The remaining findings are secondary sequels, for example, asymmetrical muscular activity or disproportionate growth of the involved osseous structures of the face and jaw #.

The causes are multifactorial and include genes and environment, although transmission of clefts occurs rarely in a simple Mendelian fashion. To the environmental factor belong cigarette smoke, folic acid deficiency, anticonvulsants, alcohol, and other drugs that have prophylactic implications. In all clefts, a wide variability of expression is observed.

Clinical Presentation

*In **unilateral partial or total cleft lip** (alveolus) ##, the cupid's bow is absent on the ipsilateral side. In total forms, the philtrum of the ipsilateral half of the upper lip and the anterior floor and aperture of the nose are partially absent and displaced to the ipsilateral side by the miming muscles which are recognizable as a bulge of the*

Fig. 5.1 Drawing of the main types of cleft lip palate. *Black* = tissue adjacent to the cleft(s). *Left picture* at the *top*: bilateral partial cleft lip with involvement of the alveolus (marked with a notch). The significance of minor involvement of the alveolus is that anomalies of the milk and permanent teeth may be observed. *Right picture* at the *top*: subtotal cleft palate with view to the roof of the oral cavity = palate. The cleft lies in the midline, concerns the total soft palate, and most of the hard palate with the edges of the vomer in direction of the nasal cavity. Picture at the *bottom*: right total cleft lip (alveolus) palate, for example, a combination of a cleft of the lip, alveolus, and palate; notice the position and diastasis of the right alveolus and the missing floor of the right nose. In addition, a minor form of a cleft lip alveolus with preserved floor of the left nose is present on the left side of the patient

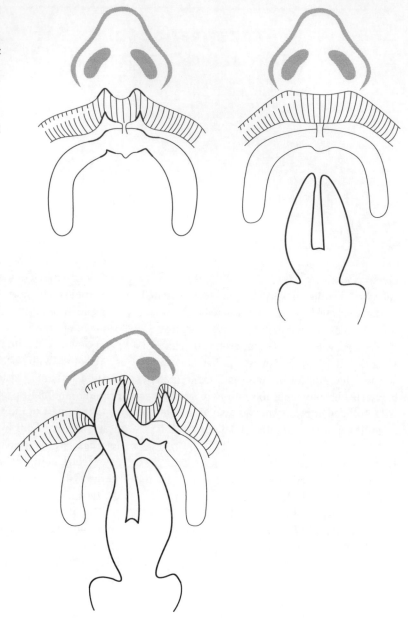

nasolabial muscles because they do not insert in the midline structures. The ipsilateral wing of the nose is deformed and screwed up as well in partial cleft lip; in total forms, the nasal bridge is in addition inclined to the contralateral side.

A **cleft of the alveolus** # is not obligatory. It occurs as a small, hardly visible notch or as large cleft of the alveolar process and arch which is lateralized also on the ipsilateral side and permits a view in the nasal cavity.

Bilateral partial or total cleft lip (alveolus) ## is either symmetrical or asymmetrical. A midline and hypoplastic remnant of the upper lip and the premaxilla with its alveolar process remain; the nasal bridge is short, and in case of a bilateral cleft alveolus, the premaxilla may grow *grotesquely to the front. Therefore, the alveolar arch is interrupted and not harmonious.*

The **partial or total cleft palate** *## lies always in the midline and extends to the premaxillary behind the alveolar arch. In total cleft palate, the examiner of the oral cavity recognizes two nasal cavities divided by the nasal septum. Isolated cleft of the uvula may be a sign of submucous cleft palate #; a whitish or bluish midline strip of the velum, a palpable notch of the posterior limit of the osseous palate, and disproportionate movements of the velum on pronunciation confirm the diagnosis.*

In case of **uni- or bilateral cleft lip (alveolus) palate** *##, a combination of the described findings is found; nevertheless, right-left asymmetry of the degree of clefting and oblique position of the septum may lead to confusing findings; because the cleft palate runs after a midline course on both sides along the premaxilla to a paramedian position of the cleft alveolus and lip, the impression of a bilateral cleft palate arises on inspection of the oral cavity.* In total uni- and bilateral cleft lip palate, there is a displacement of the maxillary segments: The greater segment is often rotated outward, sometimes the lesser segment is rotated toward the midline and behind the greater segment with normal position, and only rarely both segments are in a normal position in unilateral forms; on the other hand, the two buccal segments are nearly always rotated toward the midline leaving insufficient place for the premaxilla. *Unrestricted growth of the premaxilla leads to a symmetrical or asymmetrical kinked position in front of the buccal segments.*

Functional disorders associated with cleft lip (alveolus) palate: The initial disturbance of **food intake** (sucking and swallowing), **respiration**, and **failure to thrive** is caused by a deficient ability to suck and produce a vacuum and depends on the severity of the individual cleft. If they occur for a prolonged time, Pierre-Robin sequence # or syndromic cleft must be considered.

Mainly in the presence of a cleft palate, **acquisition of speech** may be delayed and abnormal; in addition to a diminished and pathological function of the structures that are important for speech, for example, velopharyngeal competence, impaired ventilation of the middle ear with subsequent chronic-recurrent **otitis** adds to the difficulties of speech acquisition by the **hearing deficit**.

Number, position, and structures of the **teeth adjacent to the cleft** may deviate from normality in milk and permanent teeth. Because of that and of an abnormal growth of the maxillary segments in relation to each other and to the mandible, occlusion is often abnormal; **malocclusion** impairs not only the ability to bite and chew and puts the maxillary joint under strain, but it impairs also the esthetical appearance of the face. Deviation of the nasal septum may restrict **respiration through the nose**.

Differential Diagnosis Work-Ups

It includes the facial clefts, especially the vertical and oblique forms, and syndromic clefts.

Work-ups are initially not necessary because the diagnosis cleft lip (alveolus) palate is a clinical diagnosis. Exceptions are syndromic types and single severe associated malformations. Usually genetic consultation is performed for parents and the patient with possible molecular genetic exams depending on the formulation of a question.

Treatment, Prognosis

A multidisciplinary approach by a cleft lip palate team is necessary. Follow-ups and treatment should be conducted by different specialists from birth until adolescence who play a different role depending on the age and the current problems of the patient (oral, plastic, and maxillofacial surgery, otorhinolaryngology, orthodontics, prosthodontics, and pediatric dentistry, speech/language evaluation and treatment, nursing, genetics, social work, and psychology).

Before and immediately after birth, **information of the parents** by a medical person who represents the cleft palate team is indispensable as well as **nursing advice** for handling of the newborn (e.g., for breast feeding # or use of a presurgical appliance for feeding in complete cleft lip palate).

Cleft lip and palate repair are the first surgical interventions and may be combined with ear microscopy, paracentesis, and tube drainage of the middle ear.

Cleft lip closure is best performed at the age of 3 months (there is no evidence for a repair performed at an earlier time). Triangular flap technique (Tennison), rotation-advancement flap technique (Millard), functional cheilorhinoplasty (Delaire) ######, and their modifications display similar results in expert hands. Surgery should include restoration of the perinasal and perioral muscular anatomy and some type of primary nasal reconstruction. Presurgical orthopedics in general and nasoalveolar molding specifically is controversial except in wide cleft lip and palate in which surgical closure is facilitated.

Cleft palate closure is best performed between 7 and 15 months to achieve an appropriate balance between possible maxillary growth restriction and optimal speech development. Whereas one-stage repair is performed mostly in North America, some centers in Europe prefer two-stage repair closure with delayed closure of the hard palate to avoid any maxillary growth restriction.

The commonly used two methods are the two-flap palatoplasty (von Langenbeck) and the double-opposing Z-plasty (Furlow). In both methods, some push-back of the velopharyngeal muscles is integrated, in the former, by combination with the intravelar veloplasty (Kriens) or as Veau-Wardill-Kilner technique.

The two main methods differ somewhat with more hypernasality (without) and maxillary growth restriction (with push-back) in the former and more fistulas in the latter depending on the individual communications. The minimal rate of fistulas is for both techniques ≥3 %.

Speech therapy starts at the age of 3 years. Depending on the results of continuous evaluation and of the result of nasopharyngeal endoscopy, some type of **velopharyngoplasty** is performed around 7 years of age and/or **repair of palatal fistula** (preschool age) if so localized and large enough to interfere with language development and cause significant oronasal regurgitation. In the past, velopharyngoplasty became necessary in

greater than one third of cleft lip palate patients with <10 % recurrences.

At the same time, eruption of the permanent incisors is observed that need **orthodontic treatment** until correction for their displacement. It is followed by supervision until most of the upper permanent teeth have erupted. Children with complete cleft lip palate and cleft lip alveolus may need secondary **bone grafting** (not primary to avoid damage to the canine tooth) that is performed >11 years of age with aim to stabilize the maxillary arch (prevention of transverse collapse) and for covering of the roots of the teeth adjacent to the alveolar cleft. Further ortho- and prosthodontic treatment is performed from 11 to 17 years with retention until 19 years.

After puberty with the end of nasal growth, **secondary (septo)rhino- and cheiloplasties** are performed and, if needed, **maxillary advancement surgery** for correction of residual malocclusion and abnormal profile. Overall maxillary advancement surgery has decreased to 1 % (in the past ≥20 % in the whole population and ≤50 % in cleft lip palate patients).

The aim of cleft lip palate treatment is normalized aesthetic appearance including profile of the face and mimic expression at conversational distance, an intact primary and secondary palate, a normalized speech, language, and hearing, patency of nasal airway, class I occlusion with normal masticatory function, normal dental and periodontal findings, and normal psychosocial development.

Although randomized prospective controlled trials with comparative data (multicenter studies, normal individuals) are lacking to a great extent, the experience of many centers shows that these aims are increasingly achieved for the most part although no single cleft is equal to the other.

5.1.2   Other Orofacial Clefts

Forms

Oro- and craniofacial clefts are divided into specific forms, each of which has a number according to Tessier's anatomical classification

Fig. 5.2 Drawing of the observed orofacial clefts according to the anatomical classification of Tessier for facial, craniofacial, and laterofacial clefts. The distribution of the clefts with an odd number on the left side and those with an even number on the right side of the presented child allows a clear survey. Orofacial clefts can be observed as incomplete or complete, unilateral or bilateral clefts and clefts in combination with cleft lip palate or other orofacial clefts

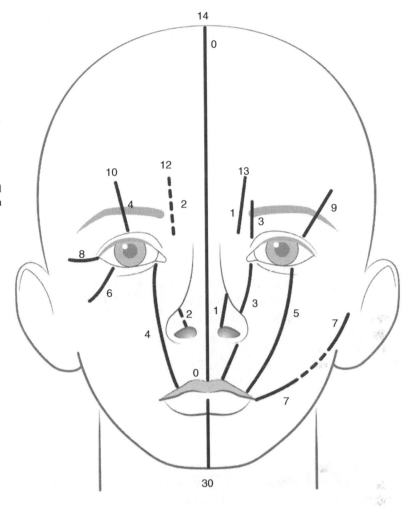

(numbers 0–30). The cleft numbers 30 and 0–7 are orofacial clefts (Fig. 5.2), although some of them may extend above the palpebral fissure, and the remainder numbers are craniofacial cleft above the palpebral fissure. A simpler classification differentiates three groups depending on the facial axis of the cleft into transverse (the clefts start at the angle of the mouth and extend in direction of the tragus), oblique (the clefts extend and diverge from the nasal aperture in direction of the forehead or temple), or vertical clefts (the clefts extend and diverge from the lateral third of the upper lip in direction of the lower eyelid and orbit).

Important is a possible involvement of the facial soft tissues and osseous structures that concerns: nose, etc. ; neurocranium and CNS, and may lead in all to anatomic deficiencies and functional disturbancies.

The slightest form of a transverse facial cleft is unilateral macrostomy in which the angle of the mouth is widened. Partial forms of vertical clefts with an intact nasal wing and of oblique forms with a cleft of the nasal wing may be mixed up with a common cleft lip palate. In general, the risk of involvement of other siblings by this or the clefts quoted below is only 3–5 %.

5.1.2.1   Lateral Facial Cleft (Commissural Cleft)
Occurrence Pathoanatomy

The lateral facial cleft (number 7) is the second most common orofacial cleft (>1:5,000 live births). It may be a part of hemifacial microsomia or Goldenhar syndrome. The facial cleft is rarely inherited and occurs in 10 % bilateral.

The observed anomalies of hemifacial microsomia syndrome # arise from the first and second branchial arches, the intervening first pharyngeal pouch and branchial cleft, and temporal bone forerunners, and are usually incomplete in number and degree of expression with *macrostomia* as slightest expression of number 7 cleft observed in the majority of patients.

Clinical Significance
- In case of a lateral facial cleft, it must be looked for signs of hemifacial microsomia.
- Lateral facial cleft and hemifacial microsomia syndrome are relatively frequent anomalies and may lead to functional deficits in esthetical appearance and hearing.

Clinical Presentation
The lateral facial cleft extends from the commissure to the tragus. *The lateral facial cleft presents mostly as macrostomia or as a cleft of up to 3 cm length # (with interruption of orbicularis and buccinator muscle), occasionally as skin depression along the cleft line, and rarely as complete cleft.*

In **hemifacial microsomia**, auricular anomalies (from a small auricle to residual skin tags), absent external auditory canal, and middle ear anomalies (with possible hearing loss), ipsilateral underdevelopment of maxilla, zygoma, temple, and mandible (mainly condylar region), ipsilateral underdevelopment of facial, masticatory, palatal, and tongue muscles, and first branchial cleft sinus tract (starting from the external auditory canal and ending below the body of the mandible). The syndrome may be associated with vertebral/rib anomalies, eye/eyelid, and CLP in ≤10 %.

Differential Diagnosis Work-Ups
It includes other disorders that include some features of the hemifacial microsomia syndrome. Evaluation by CT (bones), MRI (soft tissues), and ENT examination is the main work-ups.

Treatment, Prognosis
It includes plastic surgery for macrostomia (Z-plasties combined with tissue excision and prevention of obliteration of the mouth angle), onlay grafts for underdeveloped bone especially mandible (split-rib grafts) and soft tissues (esthetical correction of cheek deficit), and otological surgery for auricular and hearing deficit. The inner ear is usually not involved, and velopharyngeal deficit must not be expected.

The prognosis depends on the severity of lateral facial cleft and macrostomia syndrome and the possibilities of reconstructive surgery.

5.1.2.2 Oblique Facial Clefts
The nasoocular cleft, the medial and lateral oroocular cleft, and mixed forms belong to the oblique facial clefts.

The **nasoocular form** #### starts *from the lip (if the maxilla is involved from a gap between median and lateral incisor) and extends lateral to the nose to the lower eyelid or includes the nasal wing with clefting or hypoplasia and dislocation in a superior direction and involvement of the lacrimal duct.* The **oroocular form** ##### starts *from the lip* (lateral to the peak of cupid's bow, if the maxilla is involved from a gap between cuspid and first molar tooth) *and extends along the nasolabial fold to the inner canthus or lower eyelid, or from the mouth angle to the orbit* (lateral canthus or lower eyelid).

Depending on the severity of these clefts, only the skin is partially involved or the underlying soft tissues and bones including the eyelid. Incomplete closure of the eyelids due to the lower eyelid defect must be considered in these cases with risk of keratitis.

Treatment consists of sparse skin and tissue excision and multiple Z-plasties including reconstruction of the lower eyelid.

5.1.2.3 Median Cleft Lip (Number 0)
Median cleft lip is a rare, sporadic disorder and is observed in <1:100 live births with cleft lip palate. *If incomplete, it occurs as isolated type or as part of an orofacial-digital syndrome, and if*

complete, as two different syndromes and isolated disorder. It presents with a spectrum of severity from a vermilion notch and double frenulum to a complete median upper lip cleft.

The complete forms occur with hypotelorism, hypertelorism, or a normal interpupillary distance. The former two belong to specific entities:

If the median cleft lip is combined with hypotelorism, usually cerebral anomalies (cerebrum without hemispheres and with a monoventricle) and deficit of the median soft tissue and osseous structures (absence of columella # and prolabium, of crista galli, ethmoid, nasal, and premaxillary bones, and nasal septum) are present. The median cleft lip with hypotelorism is also called (alobar or lobar) **holoprosencephaly** or **arhinencephaly** #. Severe forms of this syndrome do not survive beyond infancy. Major surgery should not be performed except for surviving individuals with less severe types. Binderoid complete cleft lip/palate has a similar appearance (with hypotelorism) but no holoprosencephaly, an intact ethmoid, crista galli, and nasal bone. The same applies to formes with different degrees of hypoplasia of vomer, septum, lips, and normal interpupillary distance.

In median cleft lip combined with hypertelorism, the syndrome is associated in its most severe variety with telecanthus, bifid nose (that consists of diastatic parts and a wide bridge of the nose), cleft palate, inferiorly displaced V-shaped hairline, and defects of the frontal bone (cranium bifidum occultum). In **medial cleft face syndrome or frontonasal dysplasia**, hypertelorism may be only sign at the other end of the spectrum of severity. It has a good survival and mental development #, although the esthetical appearance may be alarming at the first glance. The differential diagnosis of less severe forms of frontonasal dysplasia includes **median cleft lip and bifid nose** in which the anomalies are restricted to the midface. The median cleft lip (the cleft is widest at the vermilion margin of the upper lip) is combined with a bifid nose (the "cleft" extends to columella and nasal tip with a widening of these structures or to the nasal bridge and root with corresponding widening [the nasal bones are cleft]), a cleft of the premaxilla (duplication of frenulum, wide gap between medial incisors), and possible hypertelorism (combined with gross extension of bifid nose).

Treatment of frontonasal dysplasia and median cleft lip and bifid nose needs a team approach and includes early closure of lip and palate and reconstruction of the nose followed by direct approach of hypertelorism in the former and lip and possibly premaxilla and nose reconstruction by approximation of the nasal skeleton and skin resection and correction of hypertelorism depending on its degree and type.

Prognosis depends on the severity of the syndrome and the reconstructive possibilities.

5.1.2.4 Median Cleft of the Lower Lip (Mandibular Cleft)

A median cleft of the lower lip is an extremely rare anomaly. *A cord of connective tissue leads from the cleft through the mandible to the jugulum, and the tip of the tongue is adherent to the cleft lip.*

Treatment consists of a triangular excision of the cleft including the connection to the tongue and closure of lip and tongue. In early surgery, the two parts of the mandible are adapted in the midline by sutures after scarification of their cleft surfaces or by bridges of an osseous graft.

5.2 Nasal Clefts

5.2.1 Median and Lateral Nasal Clefts

Median nasal clefts are characterized by a *shallow groove of the nasal tip or nasal bridge and root depending on the extension of the cleft.* The midline nasal skeleton is diastatic, and the septum may be divided. Associated hypertelorism is possible. *The esthetical appearance corresponds to a broad and clumsy nose.*

In the **lateral nasal cleft**, a *triangular tissue defect of the nasal wing is visible with possible extension of a shallow furrow to the inner canthus* and associated meningocele at the root of the nose.

Treatment of median nasal cleft needs mobilization of the medial parts of the cartilage of the nasal wing and possibly of the nasal bone, approximation of them, and closure of the partially resected skin with/without a bone graft for the nasal bridge.

Surgery of lateral clefts needs sparse triangular excision of the skin adjacent to the defect and closure without or with a composite craft from the auricle depending on its size. Watertight closure of the meningocele is performed at the same time.

5.3 Congenital Fistulas of the Face

5.3.1 Congenital Lip Fistulas

Occurrence

Congenital lip fistulas are observed more frequently combined with common cleft lip palate than as isolated disorder (Van der Woude Syndrome).

Clinical Presentation

The funnel-shaped pits occur *in pairs on either side of paramedian lower lip at the dividing line between the vermilion and inner side of the lip #*.

Impairment consists of continuous secretion and unattractive appearance of the associated bulges at the site of the fistulas and their openings. The differential diagnosis must consider congenital fistulas of the upper lip between vermilion and nose #.

Treatment

Excision must consider the bulges, sinus tract, and the glands within the inner side of the lower lip that must be excised completely.

5.3.2 Congenital Fistulas of the Nose and Auricle

Congenital fistulas of the nose and auricle are dealed with in Chaps. 1 and 7.

Webcodes

The following webcodes can be used on www.psurg.net for further images and data.

501 Syndromic cleft lip (trisomy 13)	516 Before skin closure (lip closure)
502 Unrestricted growth in BCL (premaxilla)	517 Position of the alveolar segments before
503 Partial unilateral cleft lip (UCL)	518 And after surgery of BCLP
504 Total UCL	519 UCL before
505 Unilateral total cleft lip alveolus	520 And after surgery
506 Partial bilateral cleft lip (BCL)	521 Rudimentary signs of hemifacial microsomia
507 Total BCL	522 Commissural cleft
508 Partial cleft palate (CP)	523 Oblique nasoocular cleft (number 3)
509 Total CP	524 Oblique oroocular cleft (number 5)
510 Submucous cleft palate	525 Absence of columella
511 UCLP (unilateral cleft lip palate)	526 Median CL with hypotelorism
512 BCLP (bilateral cleft lip palate)	527 Median CL with hypertelorism, slight form
513 Pierre Robin sequence	528 Congenital lower lip fistulas
514 Preoperative feeding plate	529 Congenital lip fistulas upper lip
515 Muscle sutures (lip closure)	

Bibliography

General: Radiological Imaging, Fetal Surgery

Robson CD, Barnewolt CE (2004) MR imaging of fetal head and neck anomalies. Neuroimaging Clin N Am 14:273–291

Wagner W, Harrison MR (2002) Fetal operations in the head and neck area: current state. Head Neck 24:482–490

Section 5.1.1

Armour A, Fischbach S, Klaiman P, Fisher DM (2005) Does velopharyngeal closure pattern affect the success of pharyngeal flap pharyngoplasty? Plast Reconstr Surg 115:45–52; discussion 53

Campbell A, Costello BJ, Ruiz RL (2010) Cleft lip and palate surgery: an update of clinical outcomes for primary repair. Oral Maxillofac Surg Clin North Am 22:43–58

Coleman JR Jr, Sykes JM (2001) The embryology, classification, epidemiology, and genetics of facial clefting. Facial Plast Surg Clin North Am 9:1–13

Exalto N, Cohen-Overbeek TE, van Adrichem LN, Oudesluijs GG, Hoogeboom AJ, Wildschut HI (2009) Prenatally detected orofacial cleft. Ned Tijdschr Geneeskd 153:B316

Farmand M (2002) Lip repair techniques and their influence on the nose. Facial Plast Surg 18:155–164

Friede H (2007) Maxillary growth controversies after two-stage palatal repair with delayed hard palate closure in unilateral cleft lip and palate patients: perspectives from literature and personal experience. Cleft Palate Craniofac J 44:129–136

Kim SK, Cha BH, Lee KC, Park JM (2004) Primary correction of unilateral cleft lip nasal deformity in Asian patients: anthropometric evaluation. Plast Reconstr Surg 114:1373–1381

Marcusson A (2001) Adult patients with treated complete cleft lip and palate. Methodological and clinical studies. Swed Dent J Suppl 145:1–57

Marsh JL (2004) The evaluation and management of velopharyngeal dysfunction. Clin Plast Surg 31: 261–269

Molsted K (1999) Treatment outcome in cleft lip and palate: issues and perspectives. Crit Rev Oral Biol Med 10:225–239

Mulliken JB (2000) Repair of bilateral complete cleft lip and nasal deformity—state of the art. Cleft Palate Craniofac J 37:342–347

Piffko J, Meyer U, Joos U (2002) Possibilities and limitations in evaluating treatment concepts in lip-jaw-palate clefts. Mund Kiefer Gesichtschir 6:49–52

Posnick JC, Ricalde P (2004) Cleft-orthognathic surgery. Clin Plast Surg 31:315–330

Pryor LS, Lehman J, Parker MG, Schmidt A, Foy L, Murthy AS (2006) Outcomes in pharyngoplasty: a 10-year experience. Cleft Palate Craniofac J 43: 222–225

Salyer KE, Genecov ER, Genecov DG (2004) Unilateral cleft lip-nose repair—long-term outcome. Clin Plast Surg 31:191–208

Section 5.1.2

Allam KA, Wan DC, Kawamoto HK, Bradley JP, Sedano HO, Saied S (2011) The spectrum of median craniofacial dysplasia. Plast Reconstr Surg 127:812–821

Benhammou A, Jazouli N, Kzadri M, Benhammou M (2006) Median cleft of the tongue, the lower lip and the mandible. Rev Stomatol Chir Maxillofac 107:41–43

Eppley BL, van Aalst JA, Robey A, Havlik RJ, Sadove AM (2004) The spectrum of orofacial clefting. Plast Reconstr Surg 115:101e–114e

Hunt JA, Hobar PC (2003) Common craniofacial anomalies: facial clefts and encephaloceles. Plast Reconstr Surg 112:606–615; quiz 616, 722

Section 5.2

Shewmake KB, Kawamoto HK Jr (1992) Congenital clefts of the nose: principles of surgical management. Cleft Palate Craniofac J 29:531–539

Section 5.3

Schinzel A, Kläusler M (1986) The Van der Woude syndrome (dominantly inherited lip pits and clefts). J Med Genet 23:291–294

Part II
Neck

Torticollis

The term "torticollis" may be defined narrowly or widely: In a narrower sense, it means **congenital muscular torticollis**; in this case, the sternomastoid muscle is involved and leads to a tilt of the head to the affected, a torsion to the contralateral side, and a chin elevation (Fig. 6.1).

In wider sense, torticollis includes all abnormal postures of the head: head tilt, face turn, and chin elevation or depression as single or combined features. This general term is important for a comprehensive differential diagnosis of congenital muscular torticollis because it is an abnormal head posture which attracts attention at the first glance in clinical practice.

A careful history and clinical examination including specific clinical skills are crucial for a preliminary differential diagnosis. Depending on the results, additional examinations must be performed. But the former serve not only for the differential diagnosis but also for follow-up and checking of the applied therapeutic measures if they are combined with standardized and reproducible methods of clinical examination and with corresponding quantitative results.

The leading symptom "torticollis" is often not very prominent or even absent in the newborn with the so-called congenital muscular torticollis. Instead, a **tumor of the sternomastoid muscle** # is visible. Accordingly, additional presenting symptoms may be present in torticollis seemingly or really as follows; in some of these, connections exist with specific disorders:

- Stiffness of the neck
- Sternomastoid tumor

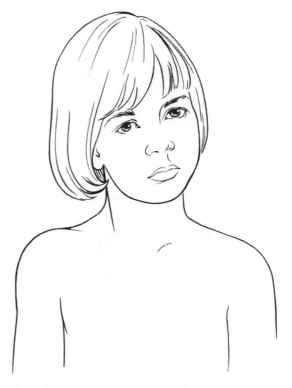

Fig. 6.1 The drawing of this schoolgirl illustrates the three primary characteristics of congenital muscular torticollis. (1) Inclination of the head to the involved right side. (2) Rotation of the head to the left not involved side. (3) Protrusion of the fibrotic and shortened right sternomastoid muscle like a string. These characteristics are not always clearly recognizable

- Plagiocephaly and/or facial hemihypoplasia (asymmetry)
- Shoulder elevation and/or scoliosis of the cervical spine

G.L. Kaiser, *Symptoms and Signs in Pediatric Surgery*,
DOI 10.1007/978-3-642-31161-1_6, © Springer-Verlag Berlin Heidelberg 2012

Table 6.1 Differential diagnosis of torticollis

Congenital torticollis

- Congenital muscular torticollis[a] and sternomastoid tumor
- Postural torticollis
- Klippel-Feil syndrome
- o Other congenital malformations of the cervical spine (hypermotility, instability),[a] basilary invagination, atlantoaxial, and atlantooccipital instability

Acquired torticollis

- Acute torticollis (wryneck)
- Traumatic torticollis:
  Subluxations, luxations, ligamentous ruptures, fractures of atlas, dens, and lower cervical spine
- o Grisel syndrome
- Atlantoaxial rotatory subluxation (fixation)
- o Sandifer syndrome[b]
- Ocular torticollis[b]:
  Congenital paralytic squint or nystagmus, after craniofacial injury, or in craniosynostosis
- o Torticollis in pneumomediastinum, ventriculoperitoneal shunt, etc.
- Neurogenic torticollis[b]:
  Posterior fossa, cervical cord, or spine mass, Chiari malformations, syrinx, etc.
- o Medicamentous torticollis[b]
- o Psychogenic torticollis[b]

For the differential diagnosis of sternomastoid tumor, see Tumors and Tumor-like Masses and Fistulas of the Neck
[a]Congenital torticollis is mostly chronic or may develop sometimes after birth slowly or acutely
[b]In acquired types of torticollis, often an acute onset is observed because it is initially not always paid attention to or it seems chronic or chronic recurrent in some of the causes

- Tumors and tumor-like masses of the neck (e.g., lymphangioma)
- Vomiting (e.g., gastroesophageal reflux)

A continuous transition can be observed between acute malposition of the head and torticollis existing for a long time. Nevertheless, the differentiation between acute onset of torticollis and chronic forms of torticollis permits a limitation of the differential diagnoses to a few disorders; the same is true, if the age of the patient is also considered. In Table 6.1, differentiation between congenital and acquired forms of torticollis is used as additional aid. The congenital torticollis is often chronic or develops slowly or peracutely sometime after birth. In acquired torticollis, often an acute

onset is observed. But torticollis seems in some of the causes as chronic or chronic recurrent because it is not paid attention to at the beginning.

6.1 Congenital Forms of Torticollis

6.1.1 Congenital Muscular Torticollis

Cause

The cause and pathogenesis of congenital muscular torticollis remains vague although complicated births occur more frequently than in the average newborn. Though, congenital muscular torticollis must be present already before birth and the hypothesis of intrauterine compartment of one or less frequently both (<10 %) sternomastoid muscles are an attractive explication.

Clinical Significance

- Congenital muscular torticollis is often combined with difficult birth such as assisted breech birth, instrumental deliveries, and cesarean section (≥50 %); early gross motor delay (<1/3 in which absent prone position seems to play a major role); and developmental hip dysplasia (>10 % that needs treatment). Mainly, the latter two disorders must be considered on follow-ups.
- It leads to positional plagiocephaly, facial hemihypoplasia by growth inhibition (both in infancy), shoulder elevation, and cervical scoliosis to maintain the eyes in a horizontal plane.
- If not treated early in infancy, therapy becomes more difficult with less favorable results.

Clinical Presentation

The clinical presentation is either a sternomastoid tumor (<2/3) or a muscular torticollis (>1/3) when seen at less than 1 year of age (#).

In **sternomastoid tumor** *that becomes visible and/or palpable in the neonatal period, there is a painless and hard mass with a diameter of 1–3 cm and gradual continuation in both directions of the muscle. It occurs not only in the distal part of the muscle but also in the middle or proximal third or may be less prominent and involve the whole muscle.*

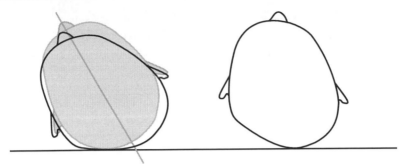

Fig. 6.2 Drawing of the contours of the head from the top during torsion to the left (*left figure*) and in straight position (*right figure*). As a secondary sequel of congenital muscular torticollis with preferred torsion of the head to the left in right-sided congenital muscular torticollis (predominant torsion by the normal contralateral left-sided sternomastoid muscle), there is a parieto-occipital flattening on the left side. This positional plagiocephaly displays a partially baldhead with diminished growth of hair at the side of flattening and may be combined with a contralateral frontal plagiocephaly

It shows initially no or less distinct feature of a muscular torticollis, and only head turn and not head tilting may be visible. Mandibular hypoplasia of the same side may be an early sign in the neonate. The sternomastoid tumor disappears in round 50 % within a few months and mostly by 1 year.

Due to its frequency (0.4–1.3 % of all newborns), sternomastoid tumor is the most frequently observed mass in the neonatal period and may be mixed up with a neoplastic mass because it may initially increase in size.

In **congenital muscular torticollis**, *the sternomastoid muscle is short, tight, and prominent like a string or cord (#). On palpation, there is either a localized or long-distance fibrosis. Rotation is restricted on the involved side as well as tilting to the contralateral side, and the chin is somewhat depressed (cock-robin posture (#)).*

Secondary changes may follow both clinical presentations: **Plagiocephaly** that is best seen by a view from above develops on the occiput of the contralateral side. It may also occur on the forehead of the involved side (Fig. 6.2). In **hemihypoplasia** of the face, the axes of the eyes and of the mouth converge on the involved side with a shorter midface (#). Compensatory shoulder elevation (#) and **cervical scoliosis** enable horizontal eye movements and balancing (#).

Reasons for referral are not only a mass of the neck or head tilt but also quite frequently a plagiocephaly or facial asymmetry and other secondary changes.

Clinical Skills, Work-Ups

After evaluation of the spontaneous head position, the child is examined in supine position (Fig. 6.3): Head and neck are held freely by the hand of the examiner, and both sternomastoid muscles are palpated simultaneously and compared with each other. The determination of restriction of rotation

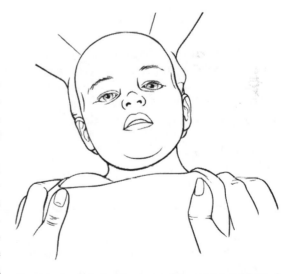

Fig. 6.3 Instead of testing a possibly restricted sideward inclination for quantifying the restriction of motion, determination of the possible rotation of the involved side in comparison to the normal side is a better tool. The normal rotation of the head amounts for both sides to 80–90° down to the surface of the bed. The achieved value is a good measure for the severity of torticollis and is reproducible. Therefore, the natural history and a possible benefit of therapy can be quantitatively tested

on the involved side is a more reliable and precise method of examination than the evaluation of the restriction of head tilt. The normal range of rotation to one side is 90°, and the larger the restriction, the more there is muscular involvement (#). Photographic documentation of the spontaneous head position enables also a precise evaluation of facial hemihypoplasia by measurement of the vertical distance between the horizontal intercanthal line and the mouth angle line on both sides or by measurement of the angle between the two lines #. In addition, plagiocephaly may be outlined on photographs taken from above and documented for follow-up #.

In the last years, ultrasound of the sternomastoid muscle and comparison with the contralateral normal muscle has been introduced. It includes echogenicity, texture, transverse and longitudinal extension of involvement, measurement of transverse diameters, and grouping according to the severity of findings. A significant correlation exists between clinical and sonographic findings. In contrast to the severe findings (type III and IV) without any change of the types, the findings in types I and II are dynamic with the possibility of deterioration or normalization.

Other additional examinations are only necessary if the clinical diagnosis is uncertain or another cause is suspected. Rarely, congenital muscular torticollis may be combined with torticollis of another origin, for example, with Klippel-Feil disease or ocular torticollis.

Natural History

Sternomastoid tumor and muscular torticollis in infancy may disappear without functional or aesthetic sequels in some patients. On the other hand, muscular torticollis that resolves after one of the two types of clinical presentation may recur without any chance of spontaneous healing after infancy. Precise figures are not available about the natural history because of the lack of prospective, randomized studies.

Differential Diagnosis

The frequency of the numerous possible differential diagnoses (Table 6.1) depends on the age (newborns and infants vs. toddlers and schoolchildren). Although the clinical presentation may be similar

to the torticollis of congenital muscular torticollis, onset and appearance of the abnormal head position is often determined by its cause.

Treatment, Prognosis

Because it is impossible to preclude spontaneous resolution in the individual case and early treatment is indispensable for good results, every patient should be treated.

Physiotherapy with active or passive stretching exercises is the **medical treatment** of choice in children less than 1 year of age. The results of other methods such as plaster or cap brace treatment and botulinum toxin injection and methods of alternative medicine are less evident and may be used as additional measures. Physiotherapy may be applied for maximum 6 months as follows:

- In slight forms of congenital torticollis (restriction of rotation <15°): active exercises (positioning and stimulation) in a way that the infant corrects the restriction of movements by himself.
- In moderate or severe forms (restriction of rotation 15–30° and >30°, respectively): passive exercises (manual stretching) by experienced physiotherapists. Others recommend exclusively manual stretching performed by cooperative and instructed parents what is sensible in countries with restricted resources and large catchment areas but holds the risk of muscle lesions by too forceful movements.

The **indications of surgery** are as follows:

- Infants with moderate or severe congenital muscular torticollis who do not respond to medical therapy within 6 months (persistent restriction of movement and/or absent resolution or development of plagiocephaly and facial hypoplasia)
- Patients with clear congenital muscular torticollis beyond the age of 1.0–1.6 years and with an equivocal diagnosis of congenital muscular torticollis after exclusion of another cause
- Patients with torticollis of another cause combined with congenital muscular torticollis after treatment of the former

Standard surgery consists of transverse incision of the skin, division of both heads of the sternomastoid muscle and of the corresponding anterior and posterior fascia with continuation in the fascia of the posterior neck triangle (#), or alternatively of middle-third transection of the sternomastoid muscle.

Modifications belong either to the group of less or minimally invasive surgery such as subcutaneous tenotomy or transaxillary subcutaneous endoscopic release or to the group of extended surgery in schoolchildren such as biterminal (bipolar) tenotomy without or with subperiosteal lengthening at its mastoid insertion or total resection procedure. Bipolar myotomy may be considered in advanced cases of schoolchildren.

On the other hand, acceptable results may be obtained with the standard technique combined with postoperative plaster treatment and physiotherapy.

Prognosis depends largely on the age at beginning of treatment, on the initial clinical group, and on the initial rotational deficit. With presentation and start of physiotherapy in early infancy, less than 10 % need surgery on follow-up. Beyond the age of 1.0–1.6 years, the majority of children need surgery for optimal cure.

6.1.2 Postural Torticollis

Cause
In postural torticollis, familiality and abnormal intrauterine position of the fetus may be observed. The term "transient cerebromotorial syndrome" tries to explain its spontaneous recovery in infancy.

Clinical Significance
- Postural torticollis is the most frequent differential diagnosis of congenital muscular torticollis in infancy (15–25 % in a population of less than 1 year of age referred for torticollis).
- It does not need such intensive physiotherapy or even surgery as in moderate and severe types of congenital muscular torticollis and always subsides during infancy.

Clinical Presentation
In postural torticollis, *neither a sternomastoid tumor nor a localized tightness is encountered although head tilt and torsion may be observed early after birth and similar to congenital muscu-*

lar torticollis with measurable restriction of rotation. Because hypertonia of the sternomastoid muscle may be palpable and/or plagiocephaly and facial hypoplasia can be observed, the initial differentiation from a congenital muscular torticollis may be difficult #.

Differential Diagnosis
A positive history, the observation of right-left asymmetric posture and movement patterns, rotational restriction in the lower range, and normal findings of ultrasound permit a preliminary diagnosis that is confirmed by uneventful resolution of final assessment scoring.

Treatment
Medical treatment with corrective *positioning* and stimulation of the involved muscles is often sufficient. But follow-up till complete resolution is necessary.

6.1.3 Klippel-Feil Syndrome

Pathology
It consists of congenital, mainly cervical fusions of the vertebrae and numerous, possible spinal and extraspinal anomalies.

Clinical Significance
- The recognition of Klippel-Feil syndrome and its differentiation from other forms of torticollis is very important due to the inherent, mainly neurological complications that may occur spontaneously, after minor or major injury or therapeutic manipulations such as intubation.
- The possibility of associated malformations in Klippel-Feil syndrome as quoted below and the occurrence of Klippel-Feil syndrome not recognized hitherto in such anomalies must be considered.

Clinical Presentation
A triad of short neck, low posterior hairline, and abnormal head posture combined with restricted head movement points to Klippel-Feil syndrome.

But only the restricted motility is observed in more than 50 % of the patients.

Torticollis is present since birth and does not progress in otherwise asymptomatic children. The cervicovertebral anomalies may be suspected on careful inspection and palpation of the neck.

Chronic neck or back pain and neurological symptoms may develop on follow-up or are recognized at first presentation.

Klippel-Feil syndrome may be associated with genitourinary (<2/3, e.g., unilateral renal agenesis), otorhinolaryngological (30 %, e.g., deafness), cardiovascular (>10 %), ocular, facial (e.g., cleft palate), and skeletal anomalies. The latter include abnormalities of the skull including the facial and basal skeleton, the spine (e.g., congenital or compensatory scoliosis in >2/3), and Sprengel's deformity (30 %, #).

Differential Diagnosis, Work-Ups
Mainly, the differential diagnoses of restricted neck movement and of vertebral anomalies must be considered.

Work-ups are decisive in the diagnosis of Klippel-Feil syndrome. The x-ray of the cervical spine in two projections should include the craniocervical junction and whole cervical spine. C2–C3, C5–C6, and atlantooccipital fusions are mostly seen. Cinematical studies confirm possible instabilities above the fused segments. MRI and CT demonstrate more precisely the pathoanatomical structures of the spine including those of the cervicomedullary junctions and of the cervical spinal cord (syrinx, diastematomyelia, tethered cord, and secondary lesions such as compression, vascular disruption or dissection, canal stenosis, disc prolapse, and other degenerations). They are particularly useful for delineation of the clinical types and risk groups, on follow-up (progressive deformities), and in acutely or chronically symptomatic cases for the explication of the symptoms and for the most appropriate treatment.

The most frequently observed clinical type II exhibits one or two fused segments that are unstable further up and often combined with hemivertebrae, and/or atlantooccipital fusion. Type I consists of extended cervical and upper thoracic and type III of cervical, lower thoracic, and

lumbar fusions. The three main risk groups are patients with instable fusion pattern, with craniocervical anomalies, and with (cervical) canal stenosis.

Work-up examinations should also exclude some of the possible major or important associated anomalies at first presentation and on follow-up such as cardiovascular and urogenital anomalies by ultrasound and deafness or scoliosis by corresponding examinations in the so-called asymptomatic cases (except for restriction of neck movement).

Treatment, Prognosis
Physiotherapy, advice of parents and patient including written handout for medical staff and sport officials, and regular clinical follow-ups are necessary and, if needed, posterior cervical fusion, anterior or posterior decompression (including internal stabilization if necessary), and/or decompressive laminectomy becomes mandatory in children with progressive deformities and/or symptoms.

The prognosis depends on the age and the cause of presentation, on the risk group and clinical type, and the presence and type of associated malformations as well as on the quality of follow-up and treatment options.

6.1.4   Other Malformations of the Cervical Spine

Pathology, Causes
Hypermotility, instability, and subsequent subluxations concern either isolated or combined the craniocervical junction, the connection between atlas and axis, C2 and C3, or C3 and C4.

These movement disorders are due to osseous defects, dysplasias, or diseases and/or due to a primary or secondary laxity of the ligaments and/or properties of the young child. Subsequent subluxations occur spontaneously, after injuries, or following inflammations.

Clinical Significance
• The possibility of hypermotility and instability of the cervical spine must be considered mainly in **Down syndrome**, in **disproportionate dwarfism**, and **rheumatic diseases**;

- In newborns or older children with symptoms of brainstem or upper cervical spinal cord and nerves, it must be looked for such malformations of the cervical spine.

Clinical Presentation

Acute or repeated painful and fixed abnormal head positions in patient with the quoted malformations or diseases

Possible types of pathologies are **basilary invagination** in which the odontoid peg enters the foramen magnum (tip of the dens ≥4–5 mm above the auxiliary McGregor line), the **atlantoaxial** (atlantoaxial distance >4 mm), and the **atlantooccipital instability**.

Differential Diagnosis, Work-Ups

It includes acute nontraumatic torticollis (wryneck), Grisel syndrome, and atlantoaxial rotatory subluxation.

Therapy, Prognosis

Patients with known hypermotility and instability as quoted above need avoidance of contact sport and protection against common neck injuries including while doing sports and on therapeutic manipulations such as intubation and positioning for surgery.

In case of acute or repeated subluxation, subtle closed reduction and operative stabilization must be performed. It must be combined with decompressive surgery in case of space-occupying effect on the underlying nervous structures.

In hypermobility of C2–C3 or C3–C4 (dislocation >4 mm in the lateral projection) are those disorders of clinical significance with painful limitation of motion and spasticity of the neck muscles.

6.2   Acquired Forms of Torticollis

6.2.1   Acute Nontraumatic Torticollis (Wryneck)

Occurrence, Cause

Wryneck is a frequent disorder that occurs mostly together with an inflammatory process in the head and/or neck region. Occasionally, a minor neck trauma is mentioned to explain the complaints or no cause is recognizable. The inflammatory process leads to irritation of the sternomastoid muscle, other muscles, or structures what causes in turn an abnormal position to lessen the pain.

Clinical Significance

- Acute nontraumatic torticollis is a common disorder.
- The underlying pathology may be more important than the wryneck and should be recognized and treated.
- In acute torticollis, the initial clinical presentation may be similar to a severe neck injury, Grisel syndrome, an atlantoaxial rotatory subluxation, or another cause of a torticollis, and these most important differential diagnoses should be considered always.

Clinical Presentation

The acute nontraumatic torticollis starts abruptly and disappears or lessens within 1–2 days. Movement from the abnormal head position is typically painful. The head is turned with the occiput to the affected side by the spastic sternomastoid muscle and the chin to the contralateral side.

In case of prolongation or recurrence, either the actual cause of torticollis is not recognized or the underlying inflammation of wryneck is not recognized and treated.

Work-Ups, Differential Diagnosis

Plain x-rays of the cervical spine are confusing in wryneck due to the abnormal head position and may lead to misinterpretation (e.g., calcification of the intervertebral discs is either insignificant or due to a former inflammatory disease) and only necessary if a significant and relevant trauma or another cause is suspected according to the history and the clinical findings or if the clinical presentation remains unchanged for 1 week or longer. In the typical wryneck, atlantoaxial rotatory subluxation is not usually present, and it is not necessary to obtain dynamic CT.

Otherwise, the search for an underlying inflammatory process such adenotonsillitis, otitis, sinusitis, respiratory tract infection, lymphadenitis of the neck, or retropharyngeal abscess must be looked for that may be overt or occult.

Therapy, Prognosis

Treatment of wryneck consists of a soft collar, analgetics, and medical treatment of the underlying cause. But follow-up is mandatory within 1 week by the family doctor and further work-up in case of persistence of clinical presentation.

6.2.2 Traumatic Torticollis (Cervical Spine Injuries)

Occurrence, Causes

In children with injuries of the spine, the cervical spinal column is a preferred site and here the region of the atlantoaxial articulation, and combinations with preexisting anomalies of the spine may occur (see Sects. 6.1.3 and 6.1.4).

Birth injuries (those of head and neck occur in 9.5 per 1000 live-births, 16.5 % include the neck of whom one third concerns the brachial plexus), battered child syndrome, falls (among other things by diving in shallow waters), road accidents with multisystemic organ injury, and transmission of the force from the head to the cervical spine are possible causes.

Clinical Significance

- Injury to the spinal cord and nerves is possible in each case of cervical spine injury.
- Missed cervical spine injuries.

Clinical Presentation

In each child with acute torticollis, neck pain, and/or restricted head movement, a significant and relevant trauma must be excluded at first by history and clinical examination. Occipital headache, neck stiffness, and resistance against extension of the neck may be additional signs. The child holds anxiously the head with the hands.

In chronic torticollis, obstinate neck pain, and restricted neck movements with a fixed head position, a former cervical injury as possible cause must be considered and excluded as well.

The causes of atlantoaxial instability after trauma may be atlantoaxial rotatory subluxation, ligamentous rupture, or atlantoaxial fracture with or without dislocation.

Pathoanatomical Types

Subluxations and luxations concern mainly the atlantoaxial joint, the atlantooccipital junction, and in combination with fractures the remainder cervical spinal column. The spinal cord is put more at risk by **rupture of the transverse ligament** (on lateral x-ray of the cervical spine distance between atlas and dens >5 mm or direct visualization by MRI) than by fracture of the dens. In severe injuries, **the transition C2–C3** is a preferred site; **the ligamentous ruptures are here combined with osseous detachments** of the anterior lower edge of the vertebral body and of the secondary ossification centers.

Fractures of the atlas are a typical example of indirect force to the cervical spine by a blow on the head. The fracture runs through the lateral mass, the posterior arch (or the synchondrosis), or concern as ringlike fracture both parts of the atlas (for diagnosis, CT is needed). In younger children, **dens fractures** are observed at the site of the not yet ossified synchondrosis below the upper articulating facets (the lateral x-ray of the spine demonstrates inclination of the dens and the anteroposterior open mouth radiography the fracture; unfortunately, hyperplastic dens or odontoid ossicle may lead to misinterpretation). In the less frequent **fractures of the lower cervical spine**, there is a rupture of the posterior ligaments combined with detachment of osseous parts of the articulations (on lateral x-ray of the spine increased distance between the spinous process) and depression of the anterior upper edges of the vertebral bodies. The fractures of the secondary ossification centers at the lower edge of the vertebral body that are easy to recognize in teenagers (type III with detachment of the most anterior part and type I with continuous division) may occur in the first decade as well; due to the still absent ossification, the same fracture can only be suspected in the lateral projection by dislocation of the adjacent vertebral bodies or due to a prevertebral soft tissue swelling in less severe cases and much later by an abnormal position of the secondary ossification centers.

Work-Ups

They include anteroposterior and lateral x-ray of the cervical spine in neutral position and depending on history, clinical, and radiological findings of the former plain x-rays (#), CT and/or MRI with specific techniques. An anteroposterior open mouth radiography and cineradiography in lateral projection are additional options.

In plain x-ray of the spine, misinterpretation may occur in case of flattened contours of the vertebrae in their anterior upper part, due to an absent lordosis, by a prevertebral soft tissue swelling, and especially in the so-called **pseudoluxation of C2–C3**. The latter radiological finding is a normal variation in childhood and occurs in up to 20 % of the patients. In addition, modifications of ossification or sequels of former injury or disease must be considered.

Therapy, Prognosis

Although not all children with traumatic torticollis need surgery, evaluation and treatment should be performed in a tertiary care center in every case of (suspected) severe injury of the spine with and without spinal cord involvement, and the hard collar should not be removed before the type of injury is recognized, and the danger of secondary neurological complication is excluded.

The treatment includes immobilization and surgical procedures such as decompression, reduction, fixation, fusion, and/or arthrodesis.

Prognosis concerning long-term recovery or neurological and functional deficits, and pain depends on the specific type of cervical spine injury and spinal cord involvement.

6.2.3   Grisel Syndrome

Pathology, Causes

Grisel syndrome is a rotatory subluxation of the atlantoaxial joint due to an acquired ligamentous laxity. It is unrelated to trauma and occurs after infectious or inflammatory processes. One of the lateral joints of the atlas shifts forward and downward on the body of the axis.

Specifically, it is observed in upper respiratory tract infection, cervical adenopathies, pharyngitis, adenotonsillitis, tonsillar or retropharyngeal abscess, otitis, parotitis, or after head and neck surgery such as adenotonsillectomy, velopharyngoplasty, mastoidectomy, excision of neck tumors, or choanal atresia repair.

Clinical Significance

• If Grisel syndrome is recognized early and treated appropriately, the prognosis is usually excellent. Otherwise, permanent deformity and neurological deficit may occur, and surgery becomes necessary instead of medical treatment.

Clinical Presentation

In the course of infections of the head and/or neck region that may seem insignificant, is even not noticed, or several days after surgery in the same region, *the child develops* in addition to possible symptoms of the primary cause *neck pain, neck stiffness, torticollis in cock-robin position, and reduced and painful neck mobility. Or similar symptoms are present postoperatively from the beginning and persist more than 3–4 days. On palpation, the spinous process of the axis deviates in the same direction of rotation, the ipsilateral sternomastoid muscle is spastic, and the head cannot be turned beyond the midline in the contralateral direction of the involved muscle. In case of chronification, permanent neck deformity and pain are present.*

Differential Diagnosis, Work-Ups

The differential diagnosis includes a not recognized or not reported neck trauma including a possible traumatic subluxation by surgery or positioning (the latter must be considered in Grisel symptomatology from the first day after surgery), a wryneck, and atlantoaxial rotatory subluxation of other etiology.

In the lateral x-ray of the cervical spine, the distance between the odontoid process and the anterior part of the atlas is >4–5 mm (in general, interpretation of the plain x-rays may be difficult due to the abnormal head position). Static CT with 3D reconstruction demonstrates a more precise pathoanatomical relation between the involved parts of the atlantoaxial joint for instance rotatory abnormalities and the degree of subluxation (Fielding classification) but may fail in differentiating normal rotation from atlantoaxial rotatory subluxation, what is overcome by a somewhat troublesome dynamic CT for children.

Therapy, Prognosis

It includes appropriate antibiotics in case of an infectious disease, analgetics, and muscle relaxants; Holter; or skeletal traction for several days (in prompt diagnosis, a short trial of neck immobilization may be sufficient, because spontaneous reduction is possible), thereafter physiotherapy and immobilization for several weeks (e.g., soft collar).

In chronic Grisel syndrome, surgical reduction and cervical fusion may be necessary.

Nevertheless, long-term traction may be successful in some children.

Down syndrome or the application of monopolar electrocautery must be considered as risk factors for the development of Grisel syndrome.

6.2.4 Atlantoaxial Rotatory Subluxation or Fixation

Pathology, Causes

In atlantoaxial rotatory subluxation, there is a unilateral malrotation of the atlas compared with the axis without or with anterior or posterior displacement of the atlas. If it is irreducible, the term fixation instead of subluxation is used.

According to Fielding and Hawkins, the disorder can be classified into four types of different severity: In type I, there is a rotatory fixation without displacement; in types II and III, the rotatory subluxation is combined with anterior displacement of the atlas by 3–5 and >5 mm, respectively; and in type IV, with posterior displacement. Except for children and/or congenital or acquired laxity of the ligaments, rupture of the ligaments is needed for types II–IV.

Possible causes are minor or major injuries of the cervical spine, the same causes as in Grisel syndrome (about one third of all patients), congenital abnormalities and anatomical variants, or combinations of such causes. It occurs mainly in toddlers up to teenage and may be observed spontaneously as well.

Clinical Significance

- Delay of recognition of atlantoaxial rotatory subluxation leads to chronic intractable pain and neither spontaneously nor by conservative treatment to a reducible rotational tilt of the head.
- Damage to the cervical spinal cord and the spinal nerves is possible in severe types of atlantoaxial rotatory subluxation.

Clinical Presentation

Acutely occurring and visible, abnormal head position which may present as typical "cock-robin" posture as in congenital muscular torticollis. In contrast to the latter, the sternomastoid muscle is neither shortened nor tight but may become hypertonic on the contralateral side. Efforts to correct manually the abnormal head position are painful.

In subacute and chronic (>3 months after the onset) forms, the neck pain becomes intractable and the abnormal head position fixed.

Differential Diagnosis, Work-Ups

The atlantoaxial rotational subluxation may initially be interpreted as an acute nontraumatic torticollis (wryneck). Connections or combinations exist with other injuries of the cervical spine, congenital types of torticollis, and Grisel syndrome.

Plain ap and lateral x-ray of the cervical spine and dynamic CT or 3D CT are considered as sufficient for the diagnosis and grading by some (shift of the odontoid peg to one side and lateral mass of the atlas appearing wider and close to the midline, or increased atlantoodontoid distance, anterolisthesis of the atlas, and malrotation of the atlas relative to the axis in the former, and the sign of articulating facet displacement of lateral atlantoaxial joint in neutral position or rotational fixation or asymmetry in rotary position in the latter examination).

On the other hand, the following work-ups may be used as alternative methods depending on the available resources and the expected lesions: an open mouth radiography with eccentric position of the odontoid peg, cineradiography in lateral position (during attempted neck rotation movement of the posterior aches of atlas and of the axis as unit and not independently), static CT (recognition of types II–IV, of additional fractures, or of atlantooccipital subluxation, but no differentiation between type I, wryneck, and normal children with head held in rotation), and MRI for soft tissue differentiation, for example, transverse ligament rupture or spinal cord damage.

Therapy, Prognosis
It includes closed reduction by skeletal traction, retention by a hard collar, and physiotherapy. In immediate diagnosis, minimally 24 h of traction may be sufficient or even several days of hard collar with spontaneous reduction. In case of recurrence after conservative treatment or of irreducibility, atlantoaxial C1–C2 fusion is indicated which is necessary in about 30 %.

Whereas closed reduction is possible in up to 90 % within several days independent of duration of subluxation, retention is possible afterward only in up to 60 % that is true mainly for chronic and/or type III subluxation. In dynamic CT, there is a correlation between grouping of severity and length and intensity of treatment. In the chronic group, facet joint deformity and >20° lateral inclination of the atlas in 3D CT are signs of recurrence.

6.2.5 Sandifer Syndrome

Pathology, Occurrence
Sandifer syndrome is a combination of torticollis with gastroesophageal reflux and dystonic body movements. It is an infrequent disorder but occurs in up to 5 % of children with torticollis. The etiopathogenesis is still unclear, and the observed gastroesophageal reflux may be different from the common reflux disease in some of the patients.

Clinical Significance
- Sandifer syndrome is often misinterpreted as neuropsychiatric disorders such as epilepsy, evaluated by several specialists with needless investigations and suffering, and often diagnosed and treated with delay.
- The early recognition of Sandifer syndrome leads to a prompt relief of the symptomatology by medical or surgical treatment.

Clinical Presentation
The Sandifer syndrome is observed at any age between infancy and adolescence and rarely even in adulthood. The older patients have often a history of complaints since many years.

In contrast to reflux, torticollis may develop only with time. Instead of shortness and tightness, spasticity of the sternomastoid muscle is present.

The abdominal symptoms are those of gastroesophageal reflux. Esophagitis is encountered in up to two thirds and according to the case reports, often of severe degree and combined with anemia (#). Thoracic hernia is observed more frequently than in common reflux.

The dystonic body movements belong to the paroxysmal nonepileptic events with a proportion of 15 %. The EEG is normal except for patients with a probably independent seizure disorder. The dystonic body movements are described in the literature as atypical seizures or abnormal body movements and take place in the paroxysmal form as attacks with irritability, head and eye version, extensor spasm, rectus abdominis contraction, and dystonic posture.

Work-Ups, Differential Diagnosis
They include in order of most probable abnormal findings esophagogastrography (#), esophagogastroscopy with biopsy (#), and 24-h pH-metry with up to two thirds in the former two and of one third in the latter examination(s). Due to the observed dysmotility of the esophagus, manometry is a useful adjunct if available. In addition, neurological consultation is necessary to exclude a seizure disorder.

The differential diagnoses are the same as in the common gastroesophageal reflux, chronic torticollis, and paroxysmal nonepileptic events, for example, conversion disorders that are observed in schoolchildren and teenagers.

Treatment
Because of the often long-standing and severe type of gastroesophageal reflux, surgery is the preferred method.

6.2.6   Ocular Torticollis

Causes
Different ophthalmological disorders may lead to abnormal head posture: paralytic or restrictive pathologies of ocular movement, visual field defects, and nystagmus. Maintenance of binocular vision and avoidance of diplopia is just one of the possible pathophysiological mechanisms leading to an abnormal head position.

In infancy, congenital paralytic squint and nystagmus (which have a vestibular origin) are common causes of ocular torticollis, and independent on age, reduced function of the superior oblique muscle occurs most frequently. Ocular torticollis after head injury and birth trauma or combined with unilateral coronal synostosis (#) are possible disorders which lie within the scope of this book.

Clinical Significance
- Ocular torticollis should be excluded in every torticollis without a clear cause because it can be diagnosed precisely only by sophisticated ophthalmological examination and the abnormal head posture can only be resolved or improved by an appropriate treatment (e.g., extraocular muscle surgery).

Clinical Presentation, Work-Ups
Except for a positive family history (e.g., congenital nystagmus) or *a conspicuous history of the patient* (e.g., former head injury with cranial nerve deficit or frontoorbital deformity), *the clinical features may not differ grossly from those of a common congenital muscular torticollis or a postural torticollis*. Each of the three components including chin elevation or depression or in combination may occur. *Although the range of neck movement is usually normal in ocular torticollis*, the age of clinical presentation may differ from that of congenital muscular torticollis, and a tight sternomastoid muscle may be found occasionally as well.

Ocular torticollis is diagnosed by 3-step testing. As screening, the monocular occlusion test and later the sit-up test with resolution of the torticollis in supine position have been recommended; unfortunately, their value is restricted because they do not work in long-standing ocular

torticollis and if the pathophysiological mechanism is not a prevention of diplopia.

Therapy
Early referral to an experienced ophthalmologist is necessary for evaluation and treatment of specific ocular disorders. Improvement or resolution of torticollis is possible by extraocular muscle surgery in some.

6.2.7   Torticollis in Pneumomediastinum and Other Disorders

Pathology, Causes
Acute torticollis in pneumomediastinum and acute or chronic torticollis in patients with ventriculoperitoneal shunt are examples of relatively rare and often not considered causes of acquired abnormal head position. The pneumothorax may be caused by an injury to the trachea or by airway leaks in asthma, attacks of coughing, vomiting, and hyperventilation, for example, during sporting activities, and by snorting crack cocaine.

Clinical Significance
- Acute torticollis may be a red flag pointing to an underlying important cause which is not recognized at first if not looked for disorders like pneumomediastinum.
- Chronic torticollis may be resolved by treatment of the underlying cause if recognized immediately as in patients with long-term ventriculoperitoneal shunt.

Clinical Presentation
In pneumomediastinum, *swelling of the neck with effacement of the contours may be visible. Palpation and auscultation of the pathognomonic crunching sound in the soft tissue of neck and chest lead to the often unexpected diagnosis of pneumomediastinum* if there are no obvious complaints such as neck pain or dyspnea and the specific history does not consider possible neck injury, attacks of coughing, retching, vomiting, or hyperventilation during sport, or other disorders (asthma, cocaine abuse).

In shunt patients, the pain caused by the implantation of the peritoneal catheter leads to *inclination of the head to the involved side for several days to lessen the pain.* In long-term patients, the peritoneal catheter is enclosed by a so-called pseudo-epithelium with calcification at its internal side, loses its sliding property, and gets too short in relation to the growth of body length. *It becomes visible and palpable as a prominent and hard string bending the neck to the involved side.* Acute and chronic torticollis may occur in similar conditions of neck surgery.

Work-Ups, Differential Diagnosis
Chest x-ray including the neck confirms the air in the neck and chest wall soft tissue and mediastinum. Tracheobronchoscopy may demonstrate the site of air leak; it is mostly unnecessary, because the leaks heal spontaneously. More important is the evaluation of the underlying cause.

The differential diagnoses are those of acute (or chronic) acquired torticollis.

Therapy, Prognosis
Treatment of torticollis is expectative and corresponds to treatment of the underlying cause. In chronic torticollis of the patient with ventriculoperitoneal shunt, evaluation of its function is necessary followed by exchange or removal of the peritoneal catheter depending on the results. In both disorders, treatment is followed by resolution of torticollis.

6.2.8   Neurogenic Torticollis

Pathology, Causes
In neurogenic torticollis, the stiff neck and head tilt is a possible sign of a neurological disorder such as a mass of the posterior fossa, the cervical cord, or spine with or without epidural extension (e.g., posterior fossa tumor, arachnoid cyst, tuberculoma, cysticercosis, eosinophilic granuloma), an abnormality (e.g., Chiari malformations, syringomyelia, isolated fourth ventricle hydrocephalus), or another pathoanatomical entity. One possible mechanism of neck stiffness and

torticollis in posterior fossa mass is irritation and stretching of the dura.

Clinical Significance
- Torticollis may be the only presenting symptom in neurogenic torticollis initially.
- If this type of torticollis is not recognized as neurogenic, inappropriate treatment is performed and a mostly life-threatening disease is recognized delayed with possible deterioration of its prognosis.

Clinical Presentation
In contrast to congenital muscular torticollis, *the abnormal head position occurs acutely* and is not always prominent. *For relief of his pain, the child maintains a fixed and usually rigid position with head tilt and rotation. Flexion of the spine leads to severe pain, and the patient resists actively to any movements.*

In a large cohort of posterior masses consisting mostly of astrocytoma, medulloblastoma (#), and ependymoma, neck stiffness and torticollis is observed in about 10 % as initial and only presenting symptom. This percentage is somewhat higher in a large group of supra- and infratentorial brain tumors at the time of diagnosis (14 % in all and 20 % in the subgroup with <2 years of age). But nearly 90 % of all have two or more symptoms and signs at the moment of final diagnosis.

Work-Ups, Differential Diagnosis
Neurogenic torticollis must be considered in every child with acquired torticollis, especially in case of the described clinical presentation and if additional neurological symptoms are present. Therefore, a precise history and clinical and neurological examination is absolutely necessary, and CT and/or MRI is the next step.

The differential diagnoses are mainly those of acquired torticollis.

Treatment and Prognosis
Both topics including the indications depend on the specific neurological disorder. In case of posterior fossa tumor, age, site, and type of neoplasm are important factors of prognosis that may be

improved by a prompt diagnosis with further reduction of the mean prediagnostic symptomatic interval of about 2 months in brain tumors of children in Central Europe.

6.2.9 Medicamentous Torticollis

Acute or chronic torticollis may be observed in neuroleptic-induced dystonia as one of the several simultaneously or consecutively occurring symptoms and signs. In addition to neuroleptics, fentanyl (morphine-like analgetic), isoniazid (tuberculostatic), and other drugs may lead to torticollis. A history of treatment with neuroleptics, strong analgetics, or tuberculostatics and the presentation of distinct extrapyramidal symptoms in case of neuroleptics and fentanyl explain possible torticollis. Stopping of responsible drugs and anticholinergics alleviates torticollis.

6.2.10 Psychogenic Torticollis

Diagnosis
Diagnosis is possible on condition that the following points are met:
1. The torticollis occurs in specific situations with normal head position in the meantime, and the child has a psychopathology or a psychiatric disorder of which shyness is the most probable.
2. The clinical examination of the neck is normal.
3. Other causes of torticollis are excluded.

Webcodes

The following webcodes can be used on www.psurg.net for further images and data.

601 Tumor sternomastoid muscle	610 Outline of plagiocephaly
602 Infant with muscular torticollis	611 Division of sternomastoid muscle
603 Stringlike prominence sternomastoid muscle	612 Postural torticollis
604 Cock-robin posture	613 Right-sided Sprengel's deformity
605 Left-sided hemihypoplasia	614 Lateral x-ray cervical spine
606 Right-sided shoulder elevation	615 Contrast swallow, thoracic hernia
607 Cervical spine scoliosis	616 Esophagoscopy, esophagitis
608 Restriction of rotation	617 Ocular torticollis, left coronal synostosis
609 Measurement in hemihypoplasia of the face	618 MRI medulloblastoma

Bibliography

Sections 6.1.1–6.1.2

Arslan H, Gündüz S, Subasi M, Kesemenli C, Necmioglu S (2002) Frontal cephalometric analysis in the evaluation of facial asymmetry in torticollis, and outcomes of bipolar release in patients over 6 years of age. Arch Orthop Trauma Surg 122:489–493

Ballock RT, Song KM (1996) The prevalence of nonmuscular causes of torticollis in children. J Pediatr Orthop 16:500–504

Beasley SW (1998) Torticollis. In: O'Neill JA et al (eds) Pediatric surgery, vol 1, 5th edn. Mosby, St. Louis

Cheng JC, Tang SP (1999) Outcome of surgical treatment of congenital muscular torticollis. Clin Orthop Relat Res 362:190–200

Cheng JCY et al (2000a) The clinical presentation and outcome of treatment of congenital muscular torticollis in infants – a study of 1086 cases. J Pediatr Surg 35:1091–1096

Cheng JC, Metreweli C, Chen TM, Tang S (2000b) Correlation of ultrasonographic imaging of congenital muscular torticollis with clinical assessment in infants. Ultrasound Med Biol 26:1237–1241

Cheng JC, Wong MW, Tang SP, Chen TM, Shum SL, Wong EM (2001) Clinical determinations of the outcome of manual stretching in the treatment of congenital muscular torticollis in infants: a prospective study of eight hundred twenty-one cases. J Bone Joint Surg Am 83-A:679–687

Shim JS, Noh KC, Park SJ (2004) Treatment of congenital muscular torticollis in patients older than 8 years. J Pediatr Orthop 24:683–688

Stassen LF, Kerawal CJ (2000) New surgical technique for correction of congenital muscular torticollis (wry neck). Br J Oral Maxillofac Surg 38:142–147

Sudre-Levillain I, Nicollas R, Roman S, Aladio P, Moukheiber A, Triglia JM (2000) Sternocleidomastoid inflammatory pseudotumors of muscle in children. Arch Pediatr 7:1180–1184

Tien YC, Su JY, Lin GT, Lin SY (2001) Ultrasonographic study of coexistence of muscular torticollis and dysplasia of the hip. J Pediatr Orthop 21:343–347

Wei JL, Schwartz KM, Weaver AL, Orvidas LJ (2001) Pseudotumor of infancy and congenital muscular torticollis: 170 cases. Laryngoscope 111:688–695

Yu CC, Wong FH, Lo LJ, Chen YR (2004) Craniofacial deformity in patients with uncorrected congenital muscular torticollis: an assessment from three-dimensional computed tomography imaging. Plast Reconstr Surg 113:23–33

Section 6.1.3

Nabib MG et al (1985) Klippel-feil syndrome in children: clinical features and management. Childs Nerv Syst 1:255–263

Section 6.1.4

Sharma A, Gaikwad SB, Deol PS, Mishra NK, Kale SS (2000) Partial aplasia of the posterior arch of the atlas with an isolated posterior arch remnant: findings in three cases. AJNR Am J Neuroradiol 21:1167–1171

Sections 6.2.1–6.2.2

Ballock RT, Song KM (1996) The prevalence of nonmuscular causes of torticollis in children. J Pediatr Orthop 16:500–514

Fielding WJ, Hensinger RN (1984) Fractures of the spine. In: Rockwood CA et al (eds) Fractures in children, 3rd edn. Lippincott, Philadelphia

Merian M, Jeannneret B (2005) Der Schiefhals des Kindes, eine Bagatelle? (Torticollis, a simple disease?). Schweiz Med Forum 5:472–474

Ogden JA (1990) Spine. In: Ogden JA (ed) Skeletal injury in the child, 2nd edn. Saunders, Philadelphia

Rang M (1983) Spine and spinal cord. In: Rang M (ed) Children's fractures, 2nd edn. Lippincott, Philadelphia

Staheli LP (1992) Spine. In: Staheli LT (ed) Fundamentals of pediatric orthopedics. Raven, New York

Swischuk LE (1977) Anterior displacement of C2 in children: physiologic or pathologic? Radiology 122:759–763

Section 6.2.3

Fernandez Cornejo VJ, Martinez-Lage JF, Piqueras C, Gelabert A, Poza M (2003) Inflammatory atlanto-axial subluxation (Grisel's syndrome) in children: clinical diagnosis and management. Childs Nerv Syst 19:342–347

Meek MF, Hermens RAEC, Robinson PH (2001) La maladie de grisel: spontaneous atlantoaxial subluxation. Cleft Palate J 38:268–270

Ortega-Evangelio G, Alcon JJ, Alvarez-Pitti J, Sebastia V, Juncos M, Lurbe E (2011) Eponym: Grisel syndrome. Eur J Pediatr 170:965–968

Yu KK, White DR, Weissler MC, Pillsbury HC (2003) Nontraumatic atlantoaxial subluxation (Grisel syndrome): a rare complication of otolaryngological procedures. Laryngoscope 113:1047–1049

Section 6.2.4

Fielding WJ, Hawkins RN (1977) Atlanto-axial rotatory fixation. J Bone Joint Surg Am 59-A:37–44

Martinez-Lage JF, Martinez Perez M, Fernandez Cornejo V, Poza M (2001) Atlanto-axial rotatory subluxation in children: early management. Acta Neurochir (Wien) 143:1223–1228

Merian M, Jeanneret B (2005) Der Schiefhals des Kindes, eine Bagatelle? (Torticollis, a simple disease?). Schweiz Med Forum 5:472–474

Pang D (2010) Atlantoaxial rotatory fixation. Neurosurgery 66(3 Suppl):161–183

Park SW, Cho KH, Shin YS, Kim SH, Ahn YH, Cho KG, Huh JS, Yoon SH (2005) Successful reduction for paediatric chronic atlantoaxial rotatory fixation (Grisel syndrome) with long-term halter traction: case report. Spine (Phila Pa 1976) 30:E444–E449

Subach BR, McLaughlin MR, Albright AL, Pollack IF (1998) Current management of pediatric atlanto-axial rotatory subluxation. Spine (Phila Pa 1976) 23:2174–2179

Tschopp K (2002) Monopolar electrocautery in adenoidectomy as a possible risk factor for Grisel's syndrome. Laryngoscope 112:1445–1449

Tsirikos AI, Chang W, Shah SA et al (2003) Acquired atlantoaxial instability in children with spastic cerebral palsy. J Pediatr Orthop 23:335–341

Weisskopf M, Naeve D, Ruf M, Harms J, Jeszenszky D (2005) Therapeutic options and results following fixed atlantoaxial rotatory dislocation. Eur Spine J 14:61–68

Section 6.2.5

Ramenofsky ML (1986) Gastroesophageal reflux: clinical manifestations and diagnosis. In: Ashcraft KW, Holder TM (eds) Pediatric esophageal surgery. Grune and Stratton, Orlando

Section 6.2.6

Caputo AR, Mickey KJ, Guo S, Wagner RS, Reynolds K, DeRespinis PA, Deluca JA (1992) The sit-up-test: an alternate clinical test for evaluating pediatric torticollis. Pediatrics 90:612–615

Velez FG, Clark RA, Demer JL (2000) Facial asymmetry in superior oblique muscle palsy and pulley heterotopy. J AAPOS 4:233–239

In: Amador LV (ed) Brain tumors in the young. Charles C Thomas, Springfield
Turgut M et al (1995) Acquired torticollis as the only presenting symptom in children with posterior fossa tumors. Childs Nerv Syst 11:86–88

Section 6.2.7

Deckel B et al (1996) Torticollis: an unusual presentation of spontaneous pneumomediastinum. Pediatr Emerg Care 12:352–353
Singh G, Kaif M, Ojha BK, Chandra A, Cronk K, Nakaji P (2011) Torticollis as a late complication of ventriculoperitoneal shunt surgery. J Clin Neurosci 18:865–866

Section 6.2.9

Dehring DJ, Gupta B, Peruzzi WT (1991) Postoperative opisthotonus and torticollis after fentanyl, enflurane, and nitrous oxide. Can J Anaesth 38:919–925
Inada T, Yagi G (1996) Current topics in neuroleptic-induced extrapyramidal symptoms in Japan. Keio J Med 45:95–99
Vinkers DJ, Schols D, van Harten PN (2010) Long-term use of cocaine and late-onset torticollis. Prog Neuropsychopharmacol Biol Psychiatry 34:425–426
Yamada S, Suzuki T, Oe K, Serada K (2010) Case of acute dystonia during epidural droperidol infusion to prevent postoperative nausea and vomiting. Masui 59:238–241

Section 6.2.8

Tomita T (1983) Statistical analysis of symptoms and signs in cerebellar astrocytoma and medulloblastoma.

Tumors and Tumor-Like Masses and Fistulas of the Neck

The symptoms and signs that lead to medical consultation or further work-up examinations after careful clinical examination (often performed for other reasons) are a visible and/or palpable **mass** and/or **fistula of the neck**.

The history and precise clinical examination have a high significance for the differential diagnosis of these two leading signs. The **midline** or **lateral location**, the properties, and the history of the lesion (**congenital** or **acquired**) make it possible to assign them to a preliminary differential diagnosis as listed in Table 7.1 and to confirm it by additional examinations such as ultrasound, MRI/CT, fine needle aspiration, or fistulography.

Nevertheless, congenital pathologies may manifest themselves later during childhood or even in adulthood, and some acquired lesions have preferred ages of manifestation. In this chapter, some typical pathologies that concern the face and mouth region are mentioned here for the sake of simplicity. Mediastinal masses may continue to the neck and be considered by mistake as primary neck tumors (e.g., congenital neurogenic tumors of the posterior mediastinum).

On the other hand, neck processes may extend as far as the mediastinum (e.g., retrosternal goiter).

7.1 Congenital Midline Pathologies (Fig. 7.1)

7.1.1 Thyroglossal Duct Cyst

Occurrence, Pathology

Together with the second branchial anomalies, the thyroglossal duct cyst is the most frequent congenital malformation of the neck in which surgery is indicated. It is mostly observed in the first two decades of life # and becomes visible for the first time in infancy. Nevertheless, one third is not recognized until adulthood.

The thyroglossal duct cyst originates from the former thyroglossal duct which starts at the site of the latter foramen cecum and is a precursor of the thyroid gland. The cyst may develop somewhere between the tongue and the jugulum, and the whole way in front of it; remnants of thyroglossal duct may be encountered, especially at the level of the hyoid bone and in front or at the back of it.

Table 7.1 Differential diagnosis of tumors and tumor-like masses and fistulas of the neck

Midline pathologies	Lateral pathologies
Congenital malformations	
• Thyroglossal duct cyst	• Second branchial anomalies
o Dermoid and epidermoid cyst	o First branchial cleft anomalies
o Congenital midline cervical cleft	o Piriform sinus fistulas
o Ectopic thyroid or thymic tissue	• Cystic lymphangioma
• Congenital goiter and teratoma	• Salivary glands pathologies
o Plunging ranula	(Hemangioma or lymphangioma, ranula)
	• Sternomastoid tumor
	• Neck and preauricular tags
	• Preauricular fistula
	o Tumors of the mouth
	o Phlebectasia of the jugular vein
Acquired lesions	
o Lymph node disorders	•Lymph node disorders
• Thyroid pathologies	
o Primary hyperparathyroidism	o Salivary glands pathologies
• Mediastinal masses	• Mediastinal masses

Clinical Significance

- The growing cyst impairs the child's appearance.
- Recurrent infections of the cyst are possible with subsequent fistulization and frequent recurrences after surgery.
- Carcinoma may develop in the cyst already in childhood (<1 %, mainly medullary carcinoma).

Clinical Presentation

The thyroglossal duct cyst becomes visible as a *painless, more or less midline swelling mostly at the level of the hyoid bone* (of the remainder cysts, one fourth is located above and less below) #. Intralingual localization occurs in <10 %, and cysts adjacent to or within the thyroid gland are even more infrequent and are one of the differential diagnoses of an unilocular cyst or a cold lesion of the thyroid gland.

Clinical Skills

Examination is performed at best with a roll under the neck and reclination of the head. On palpation, *the overlying skin is movable, the mass is cystic or less often tender, and has the size of a hazelnut up to of the size of a plum*. On swallowing a glass of water or sticking out the tongue, *the mass is moving with the hyoid bone*.

In case of cyst infection, the described local findings are blurred and overlapped by inflammatory signs #. The frequency of an associated sinus tract depends on the prevalence of infection what again depends on the catchment area and the medical attention.

Work-Ups, Differential Diagnosis

Because the clinical diagnosis of thyroglossal duct cyst is possible by an experienced surgeon in only about two thirds of children, additional examinations are necessary especially if history and/or clinical findings are not typical. Ultarsound yields additional confirmation of the clinical diagnosis. Scintiscan is only mandatory in suspected hypothyroidism, absent thyroid tissue in the normal location, and of exceptional or uncertain clinical or sonographic findings.

The differential diagnosis includes some of the midline pathologies quoted in Table 7.1. Dermoid or epidermoid cysts and enlarged lymph nodes are the most frequent differential diagnoses, whereas median ectopic thyroid tissue is extremely rare (<1 %).

Therapy, Prognosis

If a thyroglossal duct cyst is diagnosed, it should be operated electively by an experienced surgeon. The Sistrunk procedure includes extirpation of the cyst without rupture combined with excision of the midline structures from the cyst to the foramen cecum including the middle portion of the hyoid and the tissue in front and behind of it # #.

Appropriate i.v. antibiotics are necessary in case of infected cyst including needle aspiration if needed. Incision should be avoided whenever possible.

Permanent cure is achieved in nearly 100 % if not one or several of the following risk factors are

Fig. 7.1 The schematic drawing shows the congenital malformations and masses that have to be considered in the differential diagnosis of congenital medial and lateral disorders. *1–4* = Medial disorders. *1*: Thyroglossal duct cyst. *2*: Epidermoid and dermoid cysts. *3*: Congenital cervical midline cleft. *4*: Ectopic thyroid gland. *a–f* = Lateral disorders. *a*: Second branchial anomalies. *b*: Preauricular and neck tags. *c*: Cystic lymphangioma. *d*: Congenital pathologies of the salivary glands. *e*: Ranula and stenosis of caruncula sublingualis. *f*: Ectopic Thymus. *g*: Preauricular fistulas

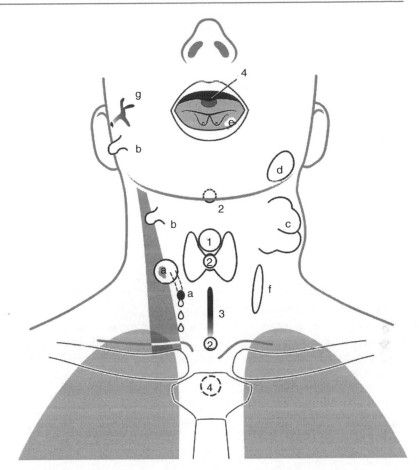

present: former surgery and/or infection(s) without or with abscess incision, cyst lobulation or rupture, and if the Sistrunk principles of surgery have been disregarded.

7.1.2   Dermoid and Epidermoid Cyst

Pathology
Similar to the thyroglossal duct cyst and in contrast to the nearly ubiquitous location of dermoid tumors of the head, dermoid and epidermoid cysts of the neck occur exclusively in the midline.

Clinical Significance
- Dermoid cysts may visibly increase in size.
- They may become infected.
- Dermoid cysts occur relatively frequently and are an important differential diagnosis of

thyroglossal duct cyst (one in five thyroglossal duct cysts).

Clinical Presentation
Differentiation from thyroglossal duct cyst is possible by their *possible submental or jugular location* and to a lesser degree by their *solid to cystic consistency* on palpation independent of its site #. *The skin is usually nonirritant and movable except for a tiny adhesion with the underlying spherical mass* without or with a sinus tract. Except for localizations close to the hyoid bone, additional examinations are not necessary, and the clinical diagnosis is sufficient for the indication of excision.

Therapy, Prognosis
With a transverse incision and complete resection including a small spindle of covering skin without spillage of cyst content, permanent cure can

be expected. Sistrunk procedure is recommended in locations close to the hyoid and histological work-up in every case.

7.1.3 Congenital Midline Cervical Cleft

Pathology

The midline cervical cleft is a remnant of the former superficial connection between the heart buckle and the branchial arches in the early developmental period. Possible associated defects are median cleft of the lower lip and mandible with tongue adhesion, thyroglossal duct or bronchogenic cyst, chest wall defects, and congenital heart disease.

Clinical Presentation

The anomaly consists of *a ventral midline defect of the skin with a cranial skin tag, atrophic mucosal surface like a healing scar, and caudal superficial sinus #. It may be associated with a subcutaneous fibrous cord* and extends from the region of the hyoid bone to the jugulum.

Except for a careful general examination and a photograph, other additional examinations are not necessary.

Therapy

Excision of the rare pathology is indicated for cosmetic, functional, and nursing reasons and should include all abnormal layers of the median cleft neck. Z-plasty techniques should be used to interrupt the longitudinal skin defect after resection and to avoid a scar and contraction along the neck.

7.1.4 Ectopic Thyroid or Thymic Tissue

Pathology

In contrast to the ectopic thyroid tissue that occurs exclusively in the midline or close to it and along the former route of descent, solid or cystic thymic tissue may be encountered nearly everywhere in the neck. Because the preferred sites of thymic tissue are the base of the tongue and the thyroid or its adjacent zone and less often along its route of descent, ectopic thymic tissue is quoted under the congenital midline pathologies.

Three general possibilities of descent exist for thyroid and thymic tissue:

- The thyroid gland or thymus remain exclusively at the site of their origin or somewhere on the route of descent (what is true for 70 % of lingual thyroid tissue and for at least 40 % of ectopic thymus).
- In addition to a normal organ at its normal site, ectopic parts occur somewhere on the route of descent (e.g., in one third of thyroglossal duct cysts or thymic tissue in the neck).
- Far away from their normal site, thyroid or thymic tissue is encountered (thyroid gland in the anterosuperior or thymus in the posterior mediastinum).

Therefore, these pathologies must be included in the differential diagnoses of any neck mass or mediastinal tumor. Because of the occurrence of ectopic thymus, the diagnosis "thymus aplasia" should be used with caution. In case of a clinically suspected lingual thyroid gland, a clinically and sonographically solid mass within or close to a thyroglossal duct cyst, or a mass of the anterior mediastinum, the suspected diagnosis of ectopic thyroid tissue should be confirmed by a positive scintiscan that makes biopsy unnecessary.

Clinical Significance

- Exclusive ectopic thyroid tissue is usually combined with hypothyroidism.
- Hidden ectopic thymic tissue may exclude the possibility of thymus aplasia.
- Ectopic thyroid and to a lesser degree ectopic thymic tissue may be an unusual site of a malignancy.

Clinical Presentation

A *visible and palpable lingual mass, especially at the root of the tongue #;* (a) *solid midline nodule(s) of the neck;* and a *jugular mass with continuation into the mediastinum* are possible clinical manifestations of ectopic thyroid or in the two former sites of ectopic thymus tissue. *Upper airway obstruction, dysphagia, hypersalivation, and oral hemorrhage* are possible additional signs of ectopic lingual tissue, whereas jugular location may lead to an *upper venous inlet obstruction* and intrathoracic sites to an *anterior or posterior mediastinal tumor on chest x-ray.*

In *any solid or cystic mass of the neck #*, ectopic thymus tissue must be considered (it occurs more frequently unilateral and single than bilateral and multiple, its size is more frequently ≤2.5 cm than more, it is located more frequently close to the thyroid gland than above or below it, and pain and compression of the adjacent organs is rarely observed).

Differential Diagnosis, Work-Ups

It includes in case of midline location thyroglossal duct cyst, enlarged lymph nodes, and dermoid cyst and in a lateral location, second branchial anomaly, enlarged lymph nodes, cystic lymphangioma, sternomastoid tumor, and semimalignant or malignant tumor (neurogenic or salivary gland tumor).

Depending on history and clinical findings, ultrasound, MRI, or CT, scintiscan, blood examinations, fine needle aspiration, or diagnostic excision are necessary.

Therapy, Prognosis

In ectopic thyroid tissue, for example, in lingual thyroid, excision (or I^{123} ablation) is only necessary in case of complications as mentioned before or of malignancy, whereas in thymic ectopic tissue of the neck, surgery is usually performed for diagnostic reasons. This is not necessary in case of ectopic thymus tissue in the posterior mediastinum except for suspected malignancy or in some cases of myasthenia gravis.

The prognosis concerning thyroid or thymus function of ectopic tissue is determined by the presence or absence of a normal thyroid gland or thymus at the normal site in the former and to a lesser degree in the latter.

7.1.5 Cervical Teratoma

Pathology

Teratomas are observed in <10 % on the neck and are mostly benign in the neonate.

Clinical Significance

- The cervical teratomas are often large and may hinder normal birth and lead immediately after birth to an RDS or later rapidly to a life-threatening dyspnea,

- Potential lethal outcome prior, during, and after surgery must be considered.

Clinical Presentation

The *often large midline swelling lies superficially close to the thyroid gland, spreads more to one side than the other, has often a nodular appearance, and feels solid and cystic on palpation.* Rarely, only a small mass is present that may be overlooked.

Differential Diagnosis, Work-Ups

Mainly, an obstructive goiter must be considered in the neonate and later an acquired lesion of the thyroid gland.

Ultrasound and CT or MRI are useful to confirm the diagnosis, to define the extension of the mass, and to differentiate it from the other structures of the neck as preoperative measure. In addition, pre- and postoperative determinations of α-fetoprotein, T3, T4, and TSH are recommended.

Therapy, Prognosis

In case of prenatal ultrasound diagnosis, planning of birth and the immediate postnatal period is possible. C-section or intubation after presentation of the head has been proposed by some.

Excision is indicated as soon as possible due to the already present or inherent danger of airway obstruction and the possible malignant degeneration. Whereas the connection to the thyroid gland is usually only superficial, huge long-standing masses may lead to pressure atrophy of the normal structures such as the hypopharynx and larynx and to a difficult resection.

The prognosis is mostly good with permanent cure except for possible cases with severe RDS and difficult intubation or with a huge mass and pressure atrophy.

7.1.6 Congenital Obstructive Goiter

Pathology

Congenital nonobstructive and obstructive goiters are observed in endemic areas. They are caused either by iodide deficit or excess of iodide intake of the mother.

Clinical Significance
- Congenital goiter is combined with hypothyroidism.
- Congenital goiter leads in its obstructive type to a RDS.

Clinical Presentation
In obstructive goiter, *a huge collar-like mass that involves the upper part of the neck # leads to a hyperextended head, stridor, and dyspnea*. In the nonobstructive type, the thyroid gland is larger than usually in the newborn.

Differential Diagnosis, Work-Ups
It includes mainly cervical teratoma. Screening test and TSH are initially necessary. In obstructive goiter, ultrasound may be useful.

Therapy, Prognosis
In case of obstructive goiter, in addition to the application of L-thyroxine, resection of the isthmus and tracheotomy may become necessary.

7.2   Acquired Midline Pathologies
(Fig. 7.2)

7.2.1   Thyroid Pathologies

Clinical Significance
- In general, thyroid pathologies of children have a different clinical significance than of adults because they occur less frequently and have different age prevalences dependent on the different pathologies.

Clinical Presentation
From a surgical point of view, the following findings are in the foreground of clinical presentation:
(a) *A diffuse swelling of the thyroid gland that is present already at birth or more frequently and that develops as a slowly progressive goiter mainly at puberty.*
(b) *A diffuse swelling of the thyroid gland combined with nodes from the beginning or with nodes developing later.*
(c) *Formation of a solitary or multiple firm node(s) within or close to the normal thyroid or within or close to the goiter.*
(d) *No recognizable local findings are present in the thyroid region.*

Differential Diagnosis
In general, the history including the age of clinical manifestation and the local and general findings are important tools in the differential diagnosis.

Variation (a) is characteristic of goiter due to either iodine deficit or iodine excess such as caused by endemic iodine deficit without supplementation, enzymic defect, or pre- or postnatal drugs.

Congenital (obstructive) goiter (an increase in size over the usual slight enlargement of the newborn) and goiter at puberty belong to this group as well as **sporadic goiter**. In addition, **Graves' disease** beyond the age of 3 years #, **chronic lymphocytic thyroiditis** (Hashimoto's disease) beyond 6 years, and the rare **subacute thyroiditis (DeQuervain)** must be considered.

Variation (b): A recognizable **multinodular goiter** is developing primarily or secondarily for the same pathologies as in variation (a) and also may be combined with thyroid dysfunction (more frequently with hypothyroidism).

Variation (c): In case of a clinically suspected **solitary thyroid nodule** or of two or more nodules, a relatively frequent thyroid malignancy must be considered as first problem. Although solitary thyroid nodules are observed mainly in adults, a **thyroid carcinoma** is present in one fourth to half of such cases in the second half of the second decade. The second problem related to a solitary thyroid nodule concerns thyroid function. In this respect, hyperthyroidism such as in toxic nodule is observed in children infrequently.

The differential diagnosis of a seemingly solitary nodule includes:
- Thyroid carcinoma including Hürthle cell lesion
- Multinodular goiter
- Colloid cyst
- Follicular adenoma

Fig. 7.2 The schematic drawing shows the acquired disorders that have to be considered in the differential diagnosis of acquired medial and lateral disorders. *1–3* = Medial disorders. *1* Submental, parathyroid, and supraclavicular (not quoted in the drawing) lymphomas. *2*: Goiter, multinodular goiter, and thyroid neoplasms. *3*: Mediastinal tumor with extension in the neck. *a–b* = Lateral disorders. *a*: Submandibular, deep-cranial cervical, and other lateral (not quoted in the drawing) lymphomas. *b*: Acquired disorders of the salivary glands

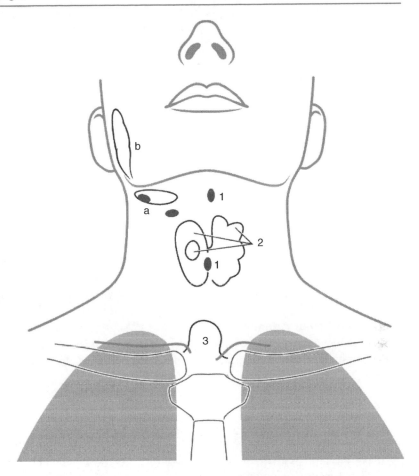

- Hashimoto's disease (chronic lymphocytic thyroiditis) with prominent lobulation
- Subacute thyroiditis (DeQuervain) with wandering inflammatory nodules
- Unilaterally enlarged thyroid lobe
- Enlarged lymph nodes other than in thyroid carcinoma
- Dermoid cyst, thyroglossal duct cyst, ectopic thymic tissue, and third or fourth branchial abnormalities

7.2.1.1 Thyroid Carcinoma

Pathology

In about 80 % of the children, papillary carcinoma is observed. Follicular, anaplastic, and medullary carcinoma or lymphoma occurs much less frequently. Medullary carcinoma accounts for less than 10 % of thyroid malignancies of which one fourth is inherited.

Clinical Significance

- Every solitary or multiple nodular mass of the thyroid especially in a female teenager should be considered as a thyroid malignancy until the proof of the contrary.
- In case of hereditary thyroid medullary carcinoma, children not yet manifesting cancer can be cured permanently by prophylactic thyroidectomy.

Clinical Presentation

The history may result in a former radiation of the neck or the head or kindreds with familial thyroid carcinoma or **syndrome of multiple endocrine neoplasms**. Rarely, such a history is gathered in a patient without any overt signs of thyroid cancer.

The most frequent complaint is *a before not existing mass in the neck which corresponds on closer examination to (a) solitary or multiple thyroid nodule(s). The mass may be firm or hard and irregular on palpation* # and corresponds clinically to involved central lymph nodes and/or to the thyroid cancer. In advanced cases, hoarseness of the voice and difficulties with swallowing are reported. In such cases, pulmonary metastasis may be detected by chest x-ray.

7.2.1.2 Goiter and Multinodular Variation

Although sporadic and endemic goiter appears as **multinodular variation** # in only in 5–10 %, the actual figure is much higher if nodules below the minimally palpable size of 1.0–1.5 cm are considered and ultrasound is performed #. Therefore, one of the most common causes in seemingly solitary thyroid nodule is colloid cyst as part of a multinodular goiter.

7.2.1.3 Follicular Adenoma

Follicular adenoma as cause of a solitary thyroid node is often a benign disorder #, although follicular carcinoma may occur rarely in children.

7.2.1.4 Thyroiditis

In **Hashimoto's disease** which is one of the most common causes of acquired hypothyroidism beyond the age of 6 years, *the initially slowly growing and asymmetric goiter develops later into different possible manifestations such as a hypothyroid goiter*. In the rarely seen **DeQuervain's subacute thyroiditis,** *the thyroid becomes asymmetric and tender, and swallowing may be painful.*

In case of acute suppurative thyroiditis, third or fourth branchial anomaly must be considered as underlying cause.

Variation (d): This possibility includes children not yet involved in manifest thyroid cancer but in familial thyroid medullary carcinoma or in **syndrome of multiple endocrine neoplasms** (MEN IIA or IIB) by autosomal dominant inheritance. All of these patients will develop thyroid medullary carcinoma sooner or later in childhood (or adulthood) in 100 %. This type of medullary carcinoma is often multifocal, bilateral, more aggressive, and amounts to one fourth of all medullary carcinomas.

In MEN IIA, the obligatory thyroid medullary carcinoma is combined with pheochromocytoma

in 50 % and with hyperparathyroidism in 15–30 % of the patients that appear in adolescence or later. In MEN IIB, thyroid medullary carcinoma occurs already early in infancy and hyperparathyroidism is unusual; other possible features include ganglioneuroma throughout the gastrointestinal tract, marfanoid habitus, and delayed puberty. The characteristic mucosal ganglioneuroma of the lips and tongue are occasionally red flags of an underlying MEN IIB syndrome.

General Clinical Skills

While the examiner is sitting behind the movable and hyperextended head, the region of the thyroid and the whole neck is inspected and palpated with the fingers of both hands comparing each side with the other. The borders, consistency, motility, and tenderness of the thyroid are assessed, as well as the presence of possible solitary or multiple node(s) in and beside it and eventually reevaluated by repeated small swallows of fluid.

General Differential Diagnosis, Work-Ups

All thyroid and midline pathologies of the neck belong to the differential diagnosis of a specific thyroid disorder and rarely, to a third or fourth branchial anomaly, specifically in **acute suppurative thyroiditis** on the left side.

The **work-ups** include thyroid tests (T4, T3, TG, TSH, thyroid antibodies), ultrasound, scintiscan # (Tc99m, I^{123}), and fine needle aspiration and biopsy (FNA). TSH (thyroid-stimulating hormone), T4 (thyroxine), and T3 (triiodothyronine) levels are of specific interest in hyper- (e.g., toxic nodule or Graves' disease) and in hypothyroidism (e.g., in Hashimoto's disease). TG (thyroglobulin) is used in follow-up of thyroid cancer. Scintiscan is used in suspected hyperthyroidism (some of the goiters, Graves' disease, and toxic nodule #) and on follow-up after treatment of thyroid cancer.

In case of suspected thyroid cancer and/or solitary thyroid nodule, the work-up is started with **TSH and ultrasound**: The former excludes hyperthyroidism. Admittedly, the latter is not useful for differentiation between malignant tumor and benign lesion, but it defines the origin of a neck mass, its relation to the thyroid, and its size. In case of normal or increased TSH and/or suspected malignancy, **fine needle aspiration with cytology** is performed (it should be performed under sedation or in general anesthesia and under sonographic guidance by a experienced examiner and pathologist). Four possibilities are encountered: identification of a macrofollicular or microfollicular lesion, of a carcinoma, or of elements without follicular tissue. In case of microfollicular lesion or carcinoma, surgery is performed (in case of microfollicular lesion, the prevalence of carcinoma is 5–10 %, primary lobectomy is performed with continuation to a total thyroidectomy in case of recognizable or histologically proven cancer by frozen sections). In the remainder situations, reevaluation is necessary in children, although the demonstration of a macrofollicular lesion as equivalent of a benign lesion has a specificity (erroneously <5 % positive) and sensitivity (erroneously <5 % negative results) of more than 95 %.

In case of suspected familial thyroid medullary carcinoma or MEN IIA or IIB or for the examination of members of such families, polymerase chain reaction gene amplification should be performed for identification of pathological mutations in the RET oncogene in chromosome 10 and 11. The same applies to sporadic cases with thyroid medullary carcinoma due to possible fresh mutations. Pentagastrin-stimulated calcitonin determinations are used for follow-up of such patients.

Therapy, Prognosis
Possible indications of thyroid surgery include neonatal obstructive goiter, multinodular and diffuse goiter, Graves' disease, solitary thyroid nodule, thyroid carcinoma, and non-thyroid pathologies within or close to the thyroid. In these cases, not only indications of adulthood, for example, goiters with airway obstruction, dysphagia, hyperthyroidism, or substernal extension or with possibly neoplastic lesion should be considered but also specific needs of childhood such as long life expectancy or treatment options not suitable for this age group.

In **thyroid papillary carcinoma**, treatment includes total thyroidectomy and excision of the lymph nodes of the central compartment (VI,

delphic lymph nodes) and thyroid hormone replacement.

Lymphadenectomy of other compartments is only performed in expected spread. Adjuvant I^{123} ablation is indicated in patients with high risks dependent on age, type of carcinoma, and TNM stage, for example, increased T3 and T4 levels, and TN1M1. On the other hand, residual tumor and recurrences should be resected in childhood if they are palpable or surgically accessible.

Depending on the risk level (that is determined by the type of RET germline mutations), **hereditary thyroid medullary carcinoma** is treated within the first 6 months, up to the fifth year of life, up to the tenth year of life, or at the time of first elevated pentagastrin-stimulated calcitonin level by total thyroidectomy and central lymph node dissection.

The prognosis of papillary carcinoma is quoted as excellent in childhood except for children below 10 years of age with extension to the larynx and trachea and metastatic disease (the overall 10-year survival in adults with metastatic disease is 40 %).

The same is true for inherited thyroid medullary carcinoma with prophylactic thyroidectomy, whereas the prognosis is poor in children with overt thyroid medullary carcinoma.

Long-term follow-up includes clinical examination, ultrasound, serum thyroglobulin, I^{123} scintiscan, and other examinations according to the possible courses of the disease and to the different consensus algorithms.

7.2.2 Primary Hyperparathyroidism

Occurrence, Pathoanatomy
In contrast to the more common secondary hyperparathyroidism, primary hyperthyroidism is unusual in children and includes the more frequent solitary adenoma (up to two thirds of the cases) and the less common hyperplasia mainly in MEN 1 syndrome.

Clinical Significance
- Diagnosis of primary hyperparathyroidism is often delayed due to the unspecific symptomatology and because it is not considered or

occurs at genetic work-up in familial disorders or endocrine syndromes (MEN 1 and MEN 2A).

- Significant morbidity is usually present at clinical diagnosis.
- Malignancies, renal failure, immobilization, vitamin D intoxication, milk alkali syndrome, and hyperthyroidism are more frequent causes of encountered hypercalcemia.

Clinical Presentation
Primary hyperparathyroidism with different main pathoanatomical findings is observed in order of increasing frequency in the following age groups: neonatal period and early infancy, throughout childhood, and adolescence and early adulthood (median age 16.8 years).

The **neonatal manifestation** occurs mostly within the context of a familial inherited disorder and is characterized by *lethargy, irritability, hypotonicity, failure to thrive, and possible polyuria or respiratory distress syndrome*. Chief cell hyperplasia is encountered in all glands.

Manifestation **during the whole childhood** belongs either to familial primary hyperparathyroidism or to a MEN 1 or MEN 2A syndrome and consists of *similar signs as primary hyperthyroidism of adolescence* and/or *possible peptic ulcer syndrome or diarrhea* (Zollinger-Ellison syndrome). One or two parathyroid glands are enlarged in MEN 1, and all display hyperplasia on histological examination, whereas MEN A2 reveals possibly asymmetric cell hyperplasia, and hypercalcemia is present initially only in one fifth.

Fatigue, exhaustion, weakness, anorexia, irritability, polymyopathy, neuropsychiatric symptoms, and signs of end-organ damage (acute pancreatitis, nephrocalcinosis or nephrolithiasis, and hypertension or bone involvement) in ≥40 % belong to the possible symptomatology of **adolescents and young adults**.

Work-Ups, Differential Diagnosis
They encompass serum calcium (hypercalcemia in >90 %), parathyroid hormone (increase in ≥85 %), and radiological imaging with ultrasound and 99 m Tc-tetrofosmin or sestamibi scintiscan for recognition and location of an adenoma.

Additional examinations are calcium-creatinine clearance ratio and urinary calcium reabsorption for differential diagnosis of familial hypocalciuric hypercalcemia (reabsorbption >99 %) and alkaline phosphatase and specific skeletal x-ray in suspected bone involvement.

The differential diagnosis includes (1) disorders with a similar symptomatology and/or hypercalcemia; (2) in addition to the already quoted causes of hypercalcemia, familial hypocalciuric hypercalcemia, idiopathic hypercalcemia of childhood, and hypercalcemia associated with hyperalimentation.

Treatment, Prognosis
Treatment consists of (1) exploration of all glands with biopsy of adenoma and a normal-appearing gland and resection of the adenoma gland after confirmation of hyperplasia and normal tissue, respectively, in the two frozen sections in adolescents with adenoma; (2) total parathyroidectomy and parathyroid autotransplantation in newborns with primary hyperparathyroidism; (3) subtotal parathyroidectomy (3½ glands) or total parathyroidectomy and autotransplantation (forearm, 40–50 mg) in MEN 1 and resection of 1 or 2 enlarged glands in MEN 2A initially; and 4) subtotal parathyroidectomy with preservation of one normal gland and ectomy of thymus and ectopic thymus in grossly symptomatic secondary hyperparathyroidism.

Short-term complications in these types of parathyroid surgery are transient hypocalcemia (>50 %) and transient vocal cord paralysis (<5 %). Long-term results include resolution of hypercalcemia in 94 % and permanent hypocalcemia in <5 %.

7.3   Congenital Lateral Pathologies (Fig. 7.1)

7.3.1   Second Branchial Anomalies

Occurrence, Pathology
Second branchial anomalies are the most frequent variety of abnormal remnants of the branchial

clefts and pouches and occur in >90 %, whereas first branchial anomalies are encountered less frequently (<10 %) and third and fourth branchial malformations are extremely rare. Due to their location away from the midline, they are also called congenital lateral sinuses and cysts. The former account for one fourth and the latter for three fourths if the cases recognized beyond childhood are included. The sinus tract leads to a blind end, continues in an intervening cyst with or without continuation to the tonsillary fossa.

Clinical Significance

- Sinuses may lead to bothering, repeated secretions. Cysts may lead to disfigurement of the neck or to carcinophobia.
- Sinuses and cysts are prone to repeated suppurative infections.
- Sinuses and cysts may be the origin of carcinoma later in life.

Clinical Presentation

In children, a sinus attracts more frequently attention to the parents or the practitioner than a mass. Therefore, some slowly enlarging cysts may be recognized for the first time only in the second decade or even in adulthood. A history of preceding infections of the lateral neck with antibiotic and/or surgical treatment may be traced in both clinical presentations. On the other hand, ongoing infection may efface the typical local findings.

The opening of the sinus tract lies at the anterior border of the sternomastoid muscle in its inferior third #. Sometimes, secretion of an often clear and viscous fluid is observed or may be provoked by gentle expression along the supposed sinus tract #. Occasionally, it can be felt as a solid cord running in a cranial direction from the opening. Sometimes cannulation is possible with a fine probe. The location of the orifice does not permit a differentiation between second and third or fourth branchial anomalies.

In case of a cyst, *a cystic or solid mass is visible indirectly by lifting up the muscle or partially visible at its border or palpable below the upper third of the sternomastoid muscle #.*

Differential Diagnosis, Work-Ups

The main differential diagnoses of a **sinus** are first, third, and fourth branchial anomalies whereas in **cysts,** lymphadenopathy, cystic lymphangioma, sternomastoid tumor #, and relatively rare masses such as cystic ectopic thymus of the lateral neck must be considered.

In the former situation, further work-ups are only necessary in case of deviation of history and local findings such as infections in the region of the mandibular angle or the ear or previous suppurative thyroiditis. Demonstration of the sinus tract by application of contrast is not necessary and may be harmful.

In the latter situation, ultrasound and sometimes MRI is useful to exclude some of the differential diagnoses such as cystic lymphangioma.

Therapy, Prognosis

In second branchial anomalies, surgery is recommended in the second trimenon of infancy or then shortly after recognition of the malformation. Excision is performed by a transverse incision over the cyst. In case of sinus tract with intervening cyst with continuation of the sinus tract to the palatine tonsil, two or more incisions may be necessary including the site of the sinus opening to gain a better overview and to avoid strong traction on the sinus tract #. Dissection should remain close to the wall of the cyst and/or sinus, and incision of the sinus tract should be avoided and advanced in case of cranial continuation up to the tonsillary fossa. In addition, injury to the glossopharyngeal or hypoglossal nerve and to the external or internal carotid artery should be prevented.

In second branchial anomalies, the intervening cyst and sinus tract crosses the arterial bifurcation, the internal carotid, and the adjacent nerves laterally and in front of them, whereas a third branchial anomaly follows a course laterally and behind the internal carotid artery and between the two nerves, what permits a differentiation between the two entities.

A permanent cure is achieved if the anomaly is completely removed and no spillage has occurred.

7.3.2   First, Third, and Fourth Branchial Anomalies

Occurrence, Pathology

First branchial anomalies are observed in less than 10 % of all branchial pathologies; piriform sinus fistulas (third and fourth branchial anomalies) are isolated cases.

First branchial anomalies are remnants of a duplicated external ear channel. They can be described either by two main groups depending on location and relation to the regular external canal, facial nerve, parotis, and other structures or by pathoanatomical characterization of the individual cysts, sinuses, and fistulas.

Third and fourth branchial anomalies have a common localization of the sinus orifice in the piriform sinus. From there, the third branchial anomaly continues as sinus tract to the vicinity of the corresponding thyroid lobe, forms a cyst or ends, or opens in the region of the lateral neck similar to second branchial anomalies. Isolated cyst close to one thyroid lobe is also observed. The sinus tract of the so-called fourth branchial anomaly follows along the trachea up to the aortic arch on the left and up to the brachiocephalic artery on the right side. A supposed continuation to the outside has not been observed so far.

Clinical Significance

- Recognition and treatment of first branchial anomalies may be difficult, especially if they are not considered in the differential diagnosis, and a precise work-up has not been performed.
- Recognition and treatment of the piriform sinus fistulas is even more difficult, and in spite of repeated clinical manifestation, the anomalies are often not recognized until adulthood.

Clinical Presentation

First branchial anomalies must be considered in the following clinical situation, if they are not detected by chance in asymptomatic cases due to specific findings such as *cystic mass or tiny sinus openings*:

- *A history of repeated infections or of previous nonpurulent fluid discharges in the area described below.*
- *Any cutaneous defect including sinus opening, cystic or solid mass, or inflammatory lesion in the neck above the hyoid (e.g., mandibular angle), region of the parotis, periauricular zone #, auricular meatus, external canal, and middle ear including tympanic membrane*

In third and fourth branchial anomalies, a history of repeated upper respiratory tract infections, hoarseness and sore throat, or pain and tenderness in the thyroid region and *findings of acute suppurative thyroiditis or of a cystic mass in this region* are red flags pointing to these anomalies. According to the case reports, the left side is almost always involved.

Differential Diagnosis, Work-Ups

The differential diagnosis depends largely on the location of the encountered infectious complications, mass, or fistula: **Mastoiditis** or infected **preauricular fistula** in post- or preauricular localization, **acute otitis media or externa** in purulent discharge from the ear, **lymphadenitis, or infection of the submandibular gland** in angular location must be considered.

The work-up examinations include for first branchial anomalies precise otological examination and instead of fistulography MRI for delineation of the whole anomaly and the adjacent structures which must be considered during surgery. In piriform sinus fistulas, direct endoscopy of the piriform sinus performed after treatment of infection demonstrates often the corresponding orifice and enables direct visualization of the corresponding sinus tract by contrast, whereas contrast swallow shows less often such a fistula; simultaneous cannulation of the sinus tract by a fine catheter may be useful if surgery is performed immediately after it.

Therapy, Prognosis

In first branchial anomalies, four premises for successful surgery are necessary: precise pathoanatomical knowledge by preoperative work-up; use of magnification, identification, and preservation of the facial nerve; and complete removal of all parts (including parts or all of the parotis if necessary).

In third and fourth branchial anomaly, complete resection can be performed (at least in the former) by different approaches from the neck with the risk of injury to the external branch of the superior laryngeal nerve and recurrent laryngeal nerve; removal of adjacent scar and thyroid tissue is necessary. As alternative method, endoscopic chemical or electrical cautery of the internal openings is recommended. A cyst must be removed from the neck and combined with cauterization of a possible internal opening. A fourth piriform sinus tract should be followed as far as possible, at least to the level of upper thoracic aperture.

Permanent cure is possible if the anomaly is completely removed.

7.3.3 Congenital Preauricular and Neck Tags

Occurrence
Preauricular tags and pits are observed in 5–10 per 1,000 newborns and neck tags less frequently.

Clinical Significance
- Tags bother cosmesis and occur occasionally with severe malformations such as transverse facial cleft.
- Preauricular tags and pits are not combined with an increased risk for urinary tract anomalies but with an increased risk of hearing disorders.

Clinical Findings
In front of the tragus or in the posterior triangle of the neck #, *a uni- or bilateral skin tumor is visible of the size of an orange pip. Occasionally, it has a stalk, or hard pieces are palpable subcutaneously* corresponding to residual cartilage and other dermal abnormalities.

Therapy
For cosmesis, excision of the skin tumor including the island of cartilage is recommended. The principles of plastic surgery should be applied.

7.3.4 Cystic Lymphangioma

Occurrence, Pathology
The numerous and different developmental defects of the lymphatic pathways have one common feature, namely, obstructed or inadequate efferent and dilated proximal afferent channels. Of the main pathoanatomical groups "lymphangioma simplex, cavernous lymphangioma, and cystic lymphangioma," the latter has a specific clinical significance in the head and neck region where the majority with up 75 % of this entity is located. In Africa, cystic cervicofacial lymphangioma is a particular aspect of surgical pathology in children.

Clinical Significance
- Recognition of increased nuchal translucency (so-called cystic lymphangioma) in the first and second or at the beginning of the third trimester by ultrasound is a marker of possible aneuploidy and other malformations.
- Cystic lymphangioma leads mostly to more or less severe disfigurement.
- Depending on its size and involvement of the deep structures such as oral cavity, pharyngeal and/or laryngeal compartments, and mediastinum, cystic lymphangioma may lead to an obstacle to normal delivery, to a life-threatening RDS, or less dramatic obstruction of the upper airways and dysphagia, and a space-occupying mass of the mediastinum.
- Recurrent enlargements of the cystic lymphoma due to spontaneous bleeding, infection, or without such events increase the disfigurement and preexisting symptoms or lead to the first manifestation of cystic lymphoma or to septicemia.
- Severe forms of cystic lymphangioma are often combined with prolonged treatment, permanent complications, and incomplete cure.

Clinical Presentation
The majority of cases are recognizable already in the first 2 years. Preferred sites are the posterior triangle of the neck #, the submandibular region, and the axilla although midline localization may be observed occasionally.

Except for disfigurement, two thirds are otherwise asymptomatic. Symptoms such as *pain or discomfort* arise by sudden enlargement of the cystic mass, either due to spontaneous intralesional hemorrhage or infection or due to expansion by spontaneous accumulation of lymph fluid or provoked by an upper respiratory tract infection.

The enlargement of the mass may return to its original size; *this variability of size is a characteristic feature of the natural history of cystic lymphangioma.*

Large lesions with involvement of the deep structures of the neck may lead to RDS of the newborn or to a less dramatic obstruction of the upper airways and to feeding difficulties in infancy.

The probability of airway compromise or dysphagia can be predicted either by the location above or below the hyoid or by a classification dependent on the volume of the cystic lymphangioma. In contrast to suprahyoidal cystic lymphangiomas with 40 % and more of such cases, dysphagia or airway compromise is unusual in infrahyoidal location. Up to two thirds of type IV cystic lymphangiomas may need tracheostomy and gastrostomy initially and for several months, whereas this is usually not necessary in type I and II cystic lymphangiomas in whom the mass does cross neither the line drawn at the lateral border of the head nor a line through the midline of the body.

The uni- or multilobular mass is cystic and compressible on palpation, and the overlying skin is nonirritant and movable except for infected or neglected cases. In the latter situation, inflammatory signs and tenderness or ulceration effaces the characteristic findings of cystic lymphangioma. *Cystic lymphangioma with a mediastinal part can be suspected in low midline or axillary forms and if they increase with coughing or straining.*

Differential Diagnosis, Work-Ups

Ultrasound has a high diagnostic accuracy in the differential diagnosis of benign cystic lesions of the neck and recognition of cystic lymphangioma and may be used together with intraoperative findings and histology to determine the type of lymphangioma. MRI is indicated in large cystic lymphangiomas and if involvement of deep structures is suspected for determination of the extent and relation to the other structures of the neck and for definition of the type.

The main differential diagnosis is teratoma of the neck and rarely **cystic choriostoma** (=mass with a normal histology at an abnormal location). In infected cystic hygroma, any of the cystic and solid masses of the neck must be considered.

Therapy, Prognosis

Increased **nuchal translucency** observed in 0.7 % of first and second trimester screening is an important marker of possible aneuploidy and other malformations. It is presumably caused by nuchal edema and combined with lymphatic abnormalities in the neck and unfortunately called cystic hygroma in case of massive edema; other terms are septated and nonseptated cyst hygroma. Chromosomal aberrations may be encountered in 40–50 % of fetuses with trisomy 21 and Turner's syndrome, the most common. In spite of the quoted high risk for adverse outcome, it is useful to carry out extensive work-up examinations because normal outcome is possible in at least 50 % of chromosomally normal pregnancies.

The indications for treatment are more or less life-threatening symptoms and signs, complications, disfigurement, and occasionally differential diagnostic considerations.

Surgery should include whenever possible complete resection and avoidance of any damage to vital structures such as the cervical branch of the facial nerve; the accessory, phrenic, recurrent laryngeal, and vagus nerves; and the sympathetic chain. **Primary resection** is indicated in **cervico-mediastinal cystic lymphangioma** without involvement of the deep neck structures #, especially in types I–III cystic lymphangioma of the neck, in cystic lymphangioma below the hyoid, or in cystic lymphangioma with continuation to the mediastinum.

In cervicofacial cystic lymphangioma # especially in cystic lymphangioma above the hypoid or in type IV cystic lymphangioma with involvement of the oral cavity, pharyngeal, and laryngeal structures, the requirement of a tracheostomy and gastrostomy should be evaluated at the beginning and if necessary, be performed. Whereas some of the oral, pharyngeal, and laryngeal parts may be treated by laser, the bulk of the cystic lymphangioma is first treated either by repeated intralesional OK-432 (monoclonal antibody produced by streptococcus pyogenes) sclerotherapy or by percutaneous embolization of Ethibloc (containing a biodegradable protein). In general, OK-432 has no response in 20 % and recurrence occur in 10 % of the cases, and specifically, it is effective in single and macrocystic types and less in microcystic or cavernous types of lymphangioma. **Secondary resection** is only preformed if the cystic lymphangioma remains unchanged, in case of a significant residual mass, or for a specific part of the cystic lymphangioma. In the former situation, several steps of resection restricted to one compartment should be performed.

The prognosis concerning recurrences, cure without permanent sequels, and therapeutic expenditures depends on the size, extension, and composition of the cystic lymphangioma as well as on the time of diagnosis of the cystic lymphangioma, the chosen therapeutic strategy, and the applied methods.

After surgery, recurrences occur mostly at the earliest in the first few months and at the latest within 4 years after surgery. Extension between and around vital structure make it difficult to remove the cystic lymphangioma completely. Whereas only one fourth of the cervicomediastinal cystic lymphangioma needs repeated surgery, the rate of recurrences is much higher in incomplete resection and specifically in cervicofacial cystic lymphangiomas. The complications include mainly seromas or hematomas and less frequently damage to important nerves.

The prognosis known so far depends largely on the reported and therefore available results in addition to the above-mentioned factors: Overall good response in 80 % independent of location has been quoted and response to treatment in only one third of the mixed types of cystic lymphangioma.

7.3.5   Preauricular Fistulas

Occurrence, Surgical Pathology
Uni- and bilateral preauricular fistulas have been observed in 2.6 % of a large number of Japanese schoolchildren. They lie mostly on the anterior part of the external ear and here on the anterior margin of the ascending limb of the helix. But, they occur in about 10 % as well as postauricular fistulas which lie posterior to an imaginary line that connects the tragus with the posterior margin of the ascending limb of the helix (posterior to external auditory canal). Besides simple pits with one simple blindly ending sinus and corresponding gland, complicated fistulas occur with branching sinuses and corresponding glands like a set of antlers.

Clinical Significance
- The majority of preauricular fistulas remains asymptomatic, but some have bothering chronic secretion and repeated inflammations with possible abscess.
- Fistulas may be combined with other malformations of the head in 50 % and with anomalies of the neck in 10 %.

Clinical Findings
A uni- or bilateral (in at least 12–15 %), tiny opening is visible at the already quoted sites. Cannulation is often possible with a fine probe like a hair; it demonstrates the course of the sinus tract.

Work-Ups, Differential Diagnosis
Specific work-up examinations are not necessary if the possible ramification, course, and extension up to the cartilage of the auricle are known. Depending on the history and local findings, a first branchial anomaly must be considered.

Therapy, Prognosis
In symptomatic preauricular fistulas, elective surgery is indicated after antibiotic treatment (abscess incision should be avoided whenever possible). Due to the increased recurrence rate after infection(s) in comparison to native cases, some recommend prophylactic resection.

The classic preauricular fistulectomy should be performed with magnification, including exposure to the entire system of sinus tract and corresponding glands, and resection including a piece of adherent cartilage. It leads in the majority of cases to permanent cure. Recommended modifications include a dual, pre- and retroauricular incision in postauricular fistulas, and a supra-auricular approach instead of standard technique in common preauricular fistulas.

Although much higher recurrence rates are quoted by some, less than 10 % or even less than 5 % relapses can be achieved. Former infection, incomplete resection, and infiltration by local anesthesia are the main causes for recurrences.

7.3.6 Congenital Disorders of the Salivary Glands

Occurrence

Congenital disorders of the salivary gland are relatively rare. With age, there is a continuous transition of such disorders to acquired pathologies.

Clinical Significance

- Pathologies of the sublingual salivary gland may lead to feeding difficulties and less often to upper airway obstruction.
- The parotis and the adjacent region is a preferred site of hemangioma or lymphangioma and less frequently of vascular malformations. All lead to significant disfigurement.
- Carcinophobia of the parents is a matter of fact in both locations.

Clinical Presentation

In case of a so-called **ranula** that corresponds to a developmental retention cyst of the sublingual gland, *a submucous mass of the size of a hazelnut up to the size of a hen's egg is visible on the mouth floor. The cystic and bluishly translucent tumor extends depending on its size lateral to the lingual frenulum or asymmetrically on both sides and may continue below the floor of the mouth and become visible as a more or less midline mass of the neck (plunging ranula). Rarely,* plunging ranula is observed also as neck mass without a visible intraoral part.

In contrast to the **uni- or bilateral stenosis or atresia of the orifice of the sublingual gland** with manifestation in the newborn period or infancy, ranula gets recognizable although not exclusively beyond infancy and preferred in girls. Stenosis (es) of the caruncula sublingualis has (have) a characteristic appearance with *uni- or bilateral cystic dilatation of the Wharton's duct and the adjacent sublingual gland like a bullhorn.*

Differential Diagnosis

It includes mucocele, dermoid or epidermoid cyst, cystic lymphangioma, hemangioma, and vascular malformations. **Mucocele** is a retention cyst of a minor salivary gland with spontaneous or development after an injury, for example, after a bite. It may occur anywhere on the mucosal surface of the mouth and has the shape and the size of a pea.

Unlike the cystic mucocele, the **dermoid cyst** occurs mostly in the midline, displays a yellowish translucence, and is soft and pasty on palpation. **(Cystic) lymphangiomas and hemangiomas** have an asymmetric distribution and characteristic properties of surface and color #.

Clinical Presentation

In case of a congenital swelling of the region of the parotis or submental salivary gland or of a rapid growing mass in the first weeks after birth, the following disorders must be considered:

- Intracapsular parotis hemangioma or less frequently the counterpart in the submental salivary gland
- (Cystic) lymphangioma of the face, parotis, or submental salivary gland
- Sialoblastoma of the parotis, submental salivary gland, sublingual salivary gland, or ectopic salivary gland tissue in the neck

In intracapsular **parotis hemangioma**, *there is often an enormous unilateral swelling of the parotis and involvement of the adjacent regions (bilateral parotis hemangioma occurs in 10–25 %)* #. Because the parotis hemangioma is relatively poor in larger vessels and premonitory cutaneous lesion is present at birth in only half of the cases, the clinical differentiation from cystic or diffuse lymphangioma may be impossible. The hemangioma concerns mostly the superficial parotis lobe and extends in the mimic muscles in front of it. The mass has a spongy consistence on palpation.

*In cystic or diffuse **lymphangioma**, the limits of the mass are less distinct, and it may be a continuous transition in the midfacial region with possible eversion and swelling of the lower lip and downward shift of the corresponding mouth corner. The dynamics of changing volume of the mass, specifically in case of cystic lymphangioma, may be useful to differentiate it from hemangioma.*

*The **sialoblastoma** presents as a congenital nodular or multinodular swelling of the parotis or the submandibular salivary gland (submandibular swelling contiguously to the gland) or develops shortly or within few months after birth with insidious onset and rapid growth.* The biological behavior is variable with the possibility of local recurrences and metastases; it depends partially on the histological pattern of this epithelial tumor. Occasionally, sialoblastoma occurs in ectopic salivary gland tissue somewhere in the cervicofacial region and may be diagnosed in toddlers. Depending on the local findings, conservative surgery with tumor-free margins may be possible although sometimes complete resection of the gland and the corresponding lymph nodes is necessary.

Differential Diagnosis, Work-Ups
A precise history may help to extrapolate the specific course of the different disorders including vascular malformation. But, a differential diagnosis based on the local findings may be difficult or even impossible.

A correct diagnosis is possible with ultrasound including Doppler-flow studies. MRI shows the extension of the mass and enables typifying of a cystic lymphangioma. Surgical biopsy is only indicated in possibly malignant tumor.

Therapy, Prognosis
Ranula is best treated by transoral excision of the ipsilateral sublingual gland with ranula evacuation (in about 10 % complications such as tongue hypesthesia, hematoma, infection,

Wharton's duct injury, or recurrences are observed), whereas **stenosis of the caruncula sublingualis** needs incision including the distal Wharton's duct. In case of **mucocele and dermoid cyst**, complete extirpation is indicated including a spindle of mucous membrane over the cyst.

Treatment options of **parotis hemangioma** include **observation** (with the expectation of natural involution); **medication** of steroids and interferon α-2a or 2b, or **intralesional** steroid **injections**; and early resection or reconstructive surgery in the involutional phase or thereafter. Problems of exclusive pharmacological therapy in the growth phase are numerous although a response rate is reported in up to 90 %. They include treatment over several months with possible side reactions: possible ulceration, hemorrhage, involvement of nearby structures, and congestive heart failure; resistance to medical treatment; unpredictable involution time with attendant psychological sequels to child and parents (complete involution takes several months to years [0.9–10 with a mean of 5.4 years] after reaching the maximal size within the first 6–10 months of life); and the need of reconstructive surgery in about two thirds.

Therefore, **parotidectomy** may be indicated early in case of rapid tumor growth, hemorrhage, ulceration, disfigurement, in resistance to medical treatment, and in the subtype of hemangioma with unusually prolonged growth phase (this **subtype of hemangioma** consists of segmental morphological characteristics and a deep component, that cintinues to grow after 9 months to a mean age of 17 months). The complications of parotidectomy are temporary or permanent facial nerve weakness or paralysis, hematoma, and/or the need of transfusion. Although facial nerve paralysis is quoted in about 10 %, surgery is possible without such sequels except for rare cases of malignancies if the facial nerve and its branches are prepared before excision. To avoid irregularities of the facial contours, musculoaponeurotic fold flaps and allograft dermal matrix for the parotid bed are used by some together with parotidectomy.

Treatment of the less frequent vascular malformations is surgical with possible reconstruction, in case of high-flow types (arteriovenous malformations), combined with embolization. For lymphangioma, see cystic lymphangioma.

7.4 Acquired Lateral Pathologies (Fig. 7.2)

7.4.1 Lymphadenopathies

Clinical Significance

- Visible and/or palpable lymph nodes belong to the most frequent tumor-like masses of the neck.
- Enlarged lymph nodes may point to a pathological process in their drainage area, develop an independent disorder, or are a part of a disease with general lymph node involvement

and early recognized due to the exposed location on the neck.

Pathoanatomy

Lymph nodes occur either close to the midline (e.g., submental, thyroidal, or supraclavicular lymph nodes) or laterally to the midline. Concerning frequency, the latter lymph nodes are clinically more significant.

Although most of the lymphadenopathies are inflammatory disorders, malignant tumors do occur occasionally. In the clinical practice however, the following questions are relevant:

- Are diagnostic measures and/or surgical interventions required?
- Is differential diagnostic evaluation of other pathologies required?

In Fig. 7.3, the different groups of regional lymph nodes are depicted that drain the different

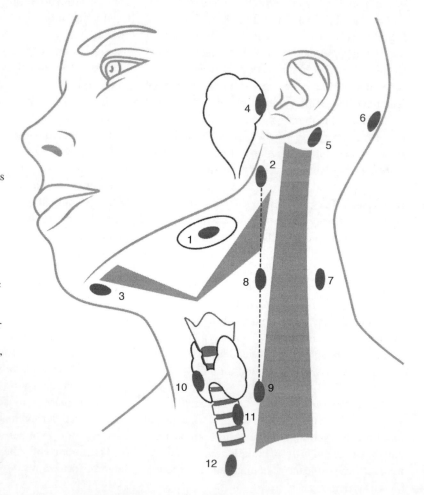

Fig. 7.3 Lymph node groups of the neck. *1* and *3*: Submandibular and submental lymph nodes (I). *4*, *5*, and *6*: Preauricular, retroauricular, and nuchal lymph nodes. *2* (II), *8* (III), and *9* (III): Deep-cervical lymph nodes (jugulodigastric lymph nodes and along the internal jugular vein). *7*: Lymph nodes of the posterior triangle of the neck (accessory lymph node chain, V). *10*, *11*, and *12*: Thyroid, paratracheal (VI), and supraclavicular (VII) lymph nodes. The groups of lymph nodes I–VII correspond to a classification of lymph node metastases of primary head and neck malignancies of adulthood

areas. Most frequently, the submental and profound cervical (jugulodigastric) lymph nodes are involved in children.

Clinical Presentation

The local findings depend on the presence of acute, subacute, or chronic lymphadenitis; of a primarily malignant or metastatic tumor; and on the stage of the disease for which the practitioner is consulted. A history of possible complaints, of general symptoms, and of onset and course of the local findings is useful information for the interpretation of the encountered local findings.

7.4.2 Acute Lymphadenitis

Surgical Pathology

The acute purulent lymphadenitis is limited to one side and a regional group of lymph nodes in contrast to lymphadenites caused by viruses with bilateral involvement of multiple lymph nodes and self-limiting disease. It is caused by penicillin-resistant staphylococci, streptococci A, and other bacteria. The lymphadenitis proceeds to a phlegmonous stage or possibly to abscess, becomes an independent disease process, and the site of portal entry is not recognizable anymore.

Clinical Findings

Often, acute purulent lymphadenitis of the neck is first recognized in the stage of phlegmonous inflammation: *The involved region, for example, the angle of the mandible is diffusely swollen, tender, warmed up, and hard, and differentiation of single lymph nodes is impossible #. Localized redness and fluctuation are signs of abscess in superficial lymph nodes #, whereas persistence of local inflammatory signs and fever in spite of appropriate antibiotic treatment is an indication of an abscess of the deep lymph nodes.*

Differential Diagnosis

In case of unusual presentation or location such as previous or current nonpurulent or relatively nonpurulent discharge or sites like the periauricular, submental, hyoidal, and thyroidal area or along the sternomastoid muscle, first, second,

or third/fourth branchial anomalies; infected dermoid; or thyroglossal duct cyst must be considered. Some of the subacute or chronic lymphadenites closely resemble the clinical findings of acute phlegmonous lymphadenitis with abscess.

7.4.3 Subacute and Chronic Lymphadenitis

Causes

In developed countries, cat scratch disease, atypical mycobacterial lymphadenitis, mononucleosis, toxoplasmosis, tularemia, and less frequently lymphadenitis after BCG vaccination and tuberculous lymphadenitis belong to the subacute and chronic lymphadenitis. Tuberculous lymphadenitis is a frequent disorder in developing countries with endemic tuberculosis.

Clinical Findings

In spite of the typically prolonged duration of the local findings, the single masses may be recognizable as lymph nodes #. They are large, hard, and adherent; the overlying skin may be reddened in spite of absent fever with possible fistulization. Dependent on the site of portal entry or on a possible strewing, the other lymph nodes of the neck may be involved as well.

The **cat scratch disease** is related to contact with a cat. In one fourth of the cases, the scratch or bite concerns the head or neck. In addition to the *initial skin lesion with papules, the corresponding regional lymph node(s) develop(s) within 1–2 weeks an inflammatory mass with possible fistulization and suppuration and are combined with generalized symptoms such a fever and myalgia.*

Spontaneous recovery occurs within 6–8 weeks if no superinfection has been transmitted by the bite. The clinical diagnosis is possible if a typical history is available combined with corresponding local findings. Otherwise, specific staining for the gram-negative Bartonella henselae of punctate or discharge or PCR (=polymerase chain reaction) for DNA analysis are possible diagnostic tools. Excisional biopsy is only necessary in case of chronic draining sinus or ambiguous diagnosis.

In **atypical or nontuberculous mycobacterial lymphadenitis**, mostly small children are involved without signs of systemic illness. *The inflammatory enlargement concerns the submandibular or submental lymph nodes of one side; they are nontender, feel like rubber on palpation, and may develop a draining sinus on follow-up.* Examinations from fine needle aspiration or sinus discharge demonstrate acid-fast bacteria, and culture shows one of the subtypes of atypical mycobacteria. Preferred treatment is excision of the lymph nodes with a spindle of overlying skin and subcutaneous tissue without dissection of the single nods and primary wound closure.

Tularemia occurs in the whole Nordic hemisphere with some endemic regions (e.g., Norway) or epidemic outbursts. Infection with Francisella tularensis (of which biotype A is more virulent than biotype B) comes from rodents and is transmitted by the contact with the skin or a mucous membrane or bites of blood-sucking parasites. Initially, general symptoms such as fever and neck and rheumatic pains are observed followed by local findings depending on the site of portal entry. The oropharyngeal form leads to ulcers in the oral cavity and inflammatory enlargement of the draining lymph nodes in the neck. Within a few days, the adjacent soft tissue becomes grossly swollen, and possibly abscess develops with a clinical presentation similar to acute purulent lymphadenitis. Diagnosis is possible by increased antibodies in the serum and by culture of punctate or discharge. Treatment of choice is Ciprofloxacin and abscess needs incision and drainage.

Tuberculous lymphadenitis is observed mainly in older children. It is a local manifestation of a systemic disease (except for neck location after ingestion of contaminated milk by Mycobacterium bovis. The latter occurs in underdeveloped countries and may lead to tuberculous infection and disease as well). *The enlarged lymph node(s) of the neck may also occur in the posterior triangle or bilaterally. They may be covered by a thin skin with creases and/or develop a draining sinus #.* The clinical diagnosis is based on the history of a previous exposure to a known carrier of tuberculosis (mostly due to Mycobacterium tuberculosis), on possible general symptoms and signs, and on the local findings. The confirmation of the suspected diagnosis by appropriate tests is difficult in children as well as differentiation from atypical mycobacterial lymphadenitis, and chest x-ray demonstrates often no evidence of active disease except for signs of former infection. Diagnostic work-up includes tuberculin PPD skin test, interferon gamma release assays, and examination of nodal tissue by stain and culture for acid-fast bacteria. In tuberculin skin test, a palpable induration of ≥ 5 mm is positive in children (sensitivity and specificity restricted in immunodeficiency or active tuberculosis and after BCG vaccination or infection with atypical mycobacteria). Interferon gamma release assays are not yet sufficiently evaluated in children with extrapulmonary tuberculosis. Treatment is multiagent chemotherapy (initially with three and later with two tuberculostatic drugs over several months). Excision of lymph node(s) is indicated for diagnostic purposes, in case of chronic fistulization, or resistant mycobacteria.

Additional chronic lymphadenites are caused by toxoplasmosis, infectious mononucleosis, HIV, Kawasaki disease, and mucocutaneous lymph node syndrome.

Differential Diagnosis

Depending on the clinical presentation, it includes all the quoted and additional rare subacute and chronic lymphadenites. Infection by **actinomyces** in the head and neck region leads to visible extensive indurations of the soft tissue with multiple fistulization and may be occasionally mixed up with chronic lymphadenitis.

7.4.4 Primary Neoplastic Tumors and Metastases

Pathology

In **primary neoplastic tumors**, in which involvement of the lymph nodes is a part of a systemic disease, neurofibromatosis, Langerhans' cell histiocytoses (lymph node involvement is possible in all three disorders), non-Hodgkin's and Hodgkin's lymphomas and leukemias must be considered. In **metastatic tumors**, neuroblastoma (primary neuroblastoma occurs in the paraspinal region with possible extension to the supraclavicular zone and Horner's syndrome and rarely in the thyroid region in newborns), thyroid carcinoma, and rhabdomyosarcoma with orbital, parameningeal, or superficial sites belong to more common malignancies.

Clinical Presentation

Each of these malignancies may have specific characteristics of the local findings and occurs together with recognizable findings of other organs. *In general, malignant tumors grow rapidly, the involved region is indurated, and the mass attached to skin and adjacent tissues.*

Neurofibromas feel as tubular and rootlike masses under the skin. In **non-Hodgkin's lymphoma**, indolent or dolent and firm lymphadenopathies occur mostly unilaterally in the neck including the supraclavicular region. Nontender and moderately enlarged lymph node(s) is (are) in 90 % the first manifestation of **Hodgkin's disease** and occurs in three fourths in the neck region; the patients are older than 5 years with a peak in adolescence. The primary lymph node metastases of the **thyroid carcinoma** concern the Delphic group and may be the only visible or palpable mass. **Rhabdomyosarcoma** occurs more frequently in the oral cavity than superficially on the neck; therefore, lymph node metastasis may be the first recognized part.

Work-Ups

They depend largely on the history, the local findings, and the suspected cause. In addition to the inflammatory parameters and specific blood and tissue examinations, ultrasound should be performed and, if necessary, MRI or CT and excisional biopsy.

Suspected abscess in acute purulent lymphadenitis is confirmed by sonography that displays signs of lymphadenitis associated with fluid. Inflammatory blood signs, specific tests, stain, and cultures of node tissue are in the foreground in subacute and chronic lymphadenitis. In case of primary or metastatic tumors, work-ups of suspected systemic disease or primary tumor are necessary. Excisional biopsy is often superior to fine needle aspiration especially in young children and if biological work-up is needed.

Therapy, Prognosis

In acute purulent lymphadenitis, incision and drainage is indicated combined with appropriate antibiotics. Incision should avoid damage to the lower branches of the facial nerve, open all abscess cavities, and be performed below the lower jaw. Prolonged antibiotic treatment may be necessary in cases without abscess. In subacute and chronic lymphadenitis, medical treatment is usually indicated. The choice between abscess incision and excisional biopsy must be carefully chosen depending on the specific pathology and purpose.

In suspected malignancy, excisional biopsy of lymph nodes is indicated, if additional examinations do not permit a reliable diagnosis, if excisional biopsy is the minimally possible expenditure for preservation of tissue for biological type sizing, and if a suspicious lymph node persists for several weeks and/or exceeds the size of 3–3.5 cm in diameter. If the excised node is not tumor-free, sticks firmly to the surrounding tissue, and has a size of ≥ 3 cm, the mass is in three fourths combined with extracapsular expansion of the tumor.

Prognosis for permanent and sequel-free outcome is good for acute purulent and most chronic lymphadenites, although in the latter and in some acute phlegmonous types, the course may be protracted with possible scars and contour irregularities left behind. Prognosis in malignancies depends on the individual tumor, its stage, and biological characteristics.

7.4.5 Acquired Pathologies of the Salivary Glands

Occurrence

In relation to acute sialadenitis and to adulthood, chronic inflammatory pathologies and neoplastic tumors of the salivary glands occur in children much less frequently. At least for these disorders, the parotis is with 60 % more frequently involved than the submandibular and sublingual salivary gland. If only a mass of the parotis is considered as leading sign, about one third are infectious or inflammatory lesions, 50 % are benign, and ≥15 % malignant disorders.

Clinical Significance

* Due to the frequently occurring nonsurgical disorders, the risk exists that the rare pathologies are not considered in the differential diagnosis although they need appropriate treatment without delay.

Clinical Presentation

The local sign is **swelling of the involved salivary gland including the perisalivary gland region**. Due to the close vicinity of other structures, it may be difficult to distinguish the salivary gland from structures of extrasalivary origin. In addition, *bilaterality or involvement of two or all salivary glands, pain, abnormal discharge by the corresponding duct, enlargement by mastication and food intake, tenderness, induration or fluctuation on palpation, and abnormalities of the overlying skin are possible. The clinical examination includes inspection of the overlying skin or mucous membrane and duct orifices, bimanual palpation, and provocation of abnormal discharge.*

Specific Disorders

The **acute epidemic parotitis** presents as *painful swelling* and is in more than 50 % bilateral (timely postponed until hours to several days) and may involve the other salivary glands and/or organs. The possibility of an **associated orchitis** and epididymitis (occurring mostly in adolescence) or **pancreatitis** has a differential diagnostic significance, especially, if the per se generalized viral infection presents as monosymptomatic disorder. Therefore, mumps orchitis or pancreatitis must be included in the differential diagnosis of scrotal and testicular swelling or surgical abdomen.

Acute suppurative parotitis is usually *unilateral and is accompanied by pain, swelling, tenderness, possible fluctuation, and inflammatory*

signs of the overlying skin and surrounding tissue. If the submandibular gland is involved, it is an important differential diagnosis of the more frequent acute suppurative submandibular lymphadenitis.

Chronic sialadenites are mainly observed as a part of a systemic disease and, for example, lead to alterations of the glandular structure. In contrast to the commonly observed nonobstructive forms with dilated ducts, salivation is grossly hindered in the less frequent chronic obstructive sialadenites with congenital or acquired stenosis, for example, due to stones or injuries such as bites.

Benign and Malignant Tumors: *The main sign is a slowly or rapidly growing mass and not pain #.* The perisalivary gland region plays not only in the major salivary glands an important role in the clinical presentation but also far away from the original salivary gland # (palate, cheek and tongue, lip and gums, etc.). Of all noninflammatory masses, up to 85 % are hemangiomas or lymphangiomas, and only ≥10 % are solid salivary or perisalivary tumors with a wide variety of histopathological diagnoses and biological behavior. Three fourth are benign and one fourth malignant disorders with a mean age of presentation at 7 years (age range >1–17 years). In the former group, **pilomatrixoma** as perisalivary tumor and **benign mixed or pleomorphic adenoma** belong to the most commonly observed disorders. Adenoma occurs between 5 and 15 years and is solid and firm on palpation. To the latter group belong mucoepidermoid carcinomas and rhabdomyosarcomas as the most frequent types.

Differential Diagnosis, Work-Ups

The differential diagnosis is especially important in tumors and chronic sialadenites. **Traumatic contusions of the facial soft tissue**, especially muscle hematomas, are often mixed up with neoplastic tumors because they resolve only slowly after several weeks and are hard on palpation without distinct margins. A history of significant trauma to the face and short-term clinical and radiological examinations by ultrasound prevent the patient from open biopsy. In general, the differential diagnosis is restricted to the perisalivary and salivary disorders.

In the first step, inflammatory disorders are differentiated from noninflammatory disorders, and the former treated by antibiotics. The second step distinguishes between cystic or solid lesions by clinical examination, sonography, and possibly fine needle aspiration (=FNA). The third step includes MRI, and possibly CT, and FNA that permits differentiation from perisalivary or salivary pathology and is followed in salivary pathology by open biopsy or frozen section during elective surgery. In obstructive sialadenitis, sialendoscopy is superior to sialography or sialo MRI.

Treatment, Prognosis

In chronic sialadenitis, medical treatment and interventional sialendoscopy (sialolithiasis in major glands) or sialectomy must be considered; transoral excision is possible as well if the submandibular gland is involved. The surgical procedures of the neoplasms vary from simple # or wide excision of the mass, superficial or total excision of the salivary gland without/with neck dissection, and surgical biopsy followed by oncological treatment. The prognosis of tumors is excellent except for single malignancies with overall 5- and 10-year survival rates of more than 90 %.

Webcodes

The following webcodes can be used on www.psurg.net for further images and data.

701 Thyroglossal duct cyst	718 Second branchial sinus tract, secretion
702 Thyroglossal duct cyst	719 Second branchial cyst
703 Infected thyroglossal duct cyst	720 Second branchial cyst at surgery
704 Resection of middle hyoid bone	721 First branchial anomaly
705 Thyroglossal duct cyst with continuation to foramen cecum	722 Neck tag
706 Jugular dermoid cyst	723 Cystic lymphangioma, posterior neck
707 Congenital midline cervical cleft	724 Cervicomediastinal cystic lymphangioma

708 Teratoma tongue vs. ectopic thyroid gland	725 Cervicofacial cystic lymphangioma
709 Ectopic thymus of the neck	726 Cystic lymphangioma neck
710 Congenital obstructive goiter	727 Parotid hemangioma
711 Ultrasonography, Graves' disease	728 Phlegmonous lymphadenitis neck
712 Thyroid carcinoma	729 Lymphadenitis with abscess neck
713 Multinodular goiter	730 Chronic lymphadenitis neck
714 Ultrasonography, nodular goiter, and cyst	731 Draining sinus, BCG lymphadenitis
715 Follicular adenoma	732 Mixed pleomorphic adenoma submandibulargland
716 Scintiscan, inactive node left thyroid gland	733 Perisalivary mixed pleomorphic adenoma
717 Second branchial sinus tract, opening	734 Mixed pleomorphic adenoma, simpleexcision

Bibliography

General: Textbooks, Differential Diagnosis

Nicollas R, Guelfucci B, Roman S, Triglia JM (2000) Congenital cysts and fistulas of the neck. Int J Pediatr Otorhinolaryngol 55:117–124

Smith CD (1998) Cysts and sinuses of the neck. In: O'Neill JA Jr et al (eds) Pediatric surgery, vol I, 5th edn. Mosby, St Louis

Section 7.1.1

Horisawa M et al (1991) Anatomical reconstruction of the thyroglossal duct. J Pediatr Surg 26:766–769

Perez-Martinez A, Bento-Bravo L, Martinez-Bermejo MA, Conde-Cortes J, de Miguel-Medina C (2005) An intra-thyroid thyroglossal duct cyst. Eur J Pediatr Surg 15:428–430

Section 7.1.3

Cochran CS, DeFatta RJ, Brenski AC (2006) Congenital midline cervical cleft: a practical approach to Z-plasty closure. Int J Pediatr Otorhinolaryngol 70:553–559

Mendis D, Moss AL (2007) Case series: variations in the embryology of congenital midline cervical clefts. Acta Chir Plast 49:71–74

Section 7.1.4

Bale PM, Sotelo-Avila C (1993) Maldescent of the thymus: 34 necropsy and 10 surgical cases, including 7 thymuses medial to the mandible. Pediatr Pathol 13:181–190

Büyükyavuzi OS, Karnaki I, Akcören Z, Senocak ME (2002) Ectopic thymic tissue as a rare and confusing entity. Eur J Pediatr Surg 12:327–329

Cigliano B, Baltogiannis N, De Marco M, Faviou E, Antoniou D, De Luca U, Soutis M, Settimi A (2007) Cervical thymic cysts. Pediatr Surg Int 23:1219–1225

Statham MM, Mehta D, Wilging JP (2008) Cervical thymic remnants in children. Int J Pediatr Otorhinolaryngol 72:1807–1813

Section 7.1.5

Elmasalme F, Giacomastonio M, Clarke KD, Othman L, Matbouli S (2000) Congenital cervical teratoma in neonates. Case report and review. Eur J Pediatr Surg 10:252–257

Section 7.2.1

Almeida MQ, Stratakis CA (2010) Solid tumors associated with multiple endocrine neoplasias. Cancer Genet Cytogenet 203:30–36

Ardito G, Pintus C, Revelli L, Grottesi A, Modugno C, Vincenzoni C, Fadda G, Perrelli L (2001) Thyroid tumors in children and adolescents: preoperative study. Eur J Pediatr Surg 11:154–157

Bingöl-Kologlu M, Tanyel FC, Senocak ME, Büyükpamukcu N, Hicsönmez A (2000) Surgical treatment of differentiated thyroid carcinoma in children. Eur J Pediatr Surg 10:347–352

Fitze G (2004) Management of patients with hereditary medullary thyroid carcinoma. Eur J Pediatr Surg 14:375–383

Monte O, Calliari LE, Kochi C, Scalisse NM, Marone M, Longui CA (2007) Thyroid carcinoma in children and adolescents. Arq Bras Endocrinol Metabol 51:763–768

Thompson NW, Geiger JD (1998) Thyroid/parathyroid. In: O'Neill JA Jr (ed) Pediatric surgery, vol I, 5th edn. Mosby, St Louis

Section 7.2.2

Biertho LD, Kim C, Wu HS, Unger P, Inabnet WB (2004) Relationship between sestamibi uptake, parathyroid

hormone assay; and nuclear morphology in primary hyperparathyroidism. J Am Coll Surg 199:229–233

Bilezikian JP, Brandi ML, Rubin M, Silverberg SJ (2005) Primary hyperparathyroidism: new concepts in clinical, densitometric and biochemical features. J Intern Med 257:6–17

Kollars J, Zarroung AE, van Heerden J et al (2005) Primary hyperparathyroidism in pediatric patients. Pediatrics 115:974–980

Kurmann A, Schmassmann A, Wildisen A (2006) Pesistierender primärer hyperparathyroidismus und rezidivierende pankreatitis nach der resection eines parathyroi-dea-adenomas (persistent primary hyperparathyroidism and recurrent pancreatitis after resection of a parathyroid adenoma). Schweiz Med Forum 6:1134–1136

Peacock M, Bilezikian JP, Preston S, Klassen PS, Matthew DG, Turner SA et al (2005) Cinacalcet hydrochloride maintains long-term normocalcemia in patients with primary hyperparathyroidism. J Clin Endocrinol Metab 90:135–141

Schweizer I, Meili A, Gemsenjäger E (2005) Kropfknoten mit Polyarthralgie und Myalgie (thyroid node accompanied by polyarthralgia and myalgia). Schweiz Med Forum 5:882–884

Section 7.3.1–7.3.2

Chen Z, Wang Z, Dai C (2010) An effective surgical technique for excision of first branchial cleft fistulas: make-inside-exposed method by tract incision. Eur Arch Otorhinolaryngol 267:267–271

Mantle BA, Otteson TD, Chi DH (2008) Fourth branchial cleft sinus: relationship to superior and recurrent laryngeal nerves. Am J Otolaryngol 29:198–200

Martinez DelPero M, Majumdar S, Bateman N, Bull PD (2007) Presentation of first branchial cleft anomalies: the Sheffield experience. J Laryngol Otol 121:455–459

Neff L, Kirse D, Pranikoff T (2009) An unusual presentation of a fourth pharyngeal arch (branchial cleft) sinus. J Pediatr Surg 44:626–629

Schroeder JW Jr, Mohyuddin N, Maddalozzo J (2007) Branchial anomalies in the pediatric population. Otolaryngol Head Neck Surg 137:289–295

Shrime M, Kacker A, Bent J, Ward RF (2003) Fourth branchial complex anomalies: a case series. Int J Pediatr Otorhinolaryngol 67:1227–1233

Smith SL, Pereira KD (2008) Suppurative thyroiditis in children: a management algorithm. Pediatr Emerg Care 24:764–767

Stenquist M, Juhlin C, Aström G, Friberg U (2003) Fourth branchial pouch sinus with recurrent deep cervical abscesses successfully treated with trichloroacetic acid cauterization. Acta Otolaryngol 123:879–882

Tham YS, Low WK (2005) First branchial cleft anomalies have relevance in otology and more. Ann Acad Med Singapore 34:335–338

Section 7.3.4

Banieghbal B, Davies MRQ (2003) Guidelines for the successful treatment of lymphangioma with OK-432. Eur J Pediatr Surg 13:103–107

Bekker MN, van den Akker NM, de Mooij YM, Bartelings MM, van Vugt JM, Gitten berger-de Groot AC (2008) Jugular lymphatic maldevelopment in turner syndrome and trisomy 21: different anomalies leading to nuchal edema. Reprod Sci 15:295–304

DiLorenzo M, Yazbeck S (1998) Lymphangiomas. In: Stringer MD et al (eds) Pediatric surgery and urology: long term outcomes. Saunders, London

Gedikbasi A, Gul A, Sargin A, Ceylan Y (2007) Cystic hygroma and lymphangioma: associated findings, perinatal outcome and prognostic factors in live-born infants. Arch Gynecol Obstet 276:491–498

Graesslin O, Derniaux E, Alanio E, Gaillard D, Vitry F, Quéreux C, Ducarme G (2007) Characteristics and outcome of fetal hygroma diagnosed in the first trimester. Acta Obstet Gynecol Scand 86:1442–1446

Mulliken JB, Glowacki J (1982) Hemangiomas and vascular malformations in infants and children. A classification based on endothelial characteristics. Plast Reconstr Surg 69:412–420

Okazaki T, Iwatani S, Yanai T, Kobayashi H, Kato Y, Marusasa T, Lane GJ, Yamataka A (2007) Treatment of lymphangioma in children: our experience of 128 cases. J Pediatr Surg 42:386–389

Schuster T, Grantzow R, Nicolai T (2003) Lymphangioma colli – a new classification contributing to prognosis. Eur J Pediatr Surg 13:97–102

Section 7.3.5

Chavez Delgado ME, Castro Castaneda S, Ramirez Jaime GC, de la Rosa AC, Real Choi SJ, Choung YH, Park K, Bae J, Park HY (2007) The variant type of preauricular sinus: postauricular sinus. Laryngoscope 117:1798–1802

Gohary A, Rangecroft L, Cook RC (1983) Congenital auricular and preauricular sinuses in childhood. Z Kinderchir 38:81–82

Kugelman A, Tubi A, Bader D et al (2002) Pre-auricular tags and pits in the newborn: the role of renal ultrasonography. J Pediatr 141:388–391

Marquez E, Gonzalez Fuentes VM (2008) Surgical management and recurrence of congenital preauricular fistula. Cir Pediatr 21:73–78

Yeo SW, Jun BC, Park SN, Lee JH, Song CE, Chang KH, Lee DH (2006) The preauricular sinus: factors contributing to recurrence after surgery. Am J Otolaryngol 27:396–400

Section 7.3.6

Cardin P, Orbach D (2010) Sialoblastoma of salivary glands in children: chemotherapy should be discussed as an alternative to mutilating surgery. Int J Pediatr Otorhinolaryngol 74:942–945

Marucci DD, Lawson K, Harper J, Sebire NJ, Dunaway DJ (2009) Sialoblastoma arising in ectopic salivary gland tissues. J Plast Reconstr Aesthet Surg 62:e241–e246

Mortellaro C, Dall'Oca S, Lucchina AG, Castiglia A, Farronato G, Fenini E, Marenzi G, Trosino O, Cafiero C, Sammartino G (2008) Sublingual ranula: a closer look to its surgical management. J Craniofac Surg 19:286–290

Patel MR, Deal AM, Shockley WW (2009) Oval and plunging ranulas: what is the most effective treatment. Laryngoscope 119:1501–1509

Scott JX, Krishnan S, Bourne AJ, Williams MP, Agzarian M, Revesz T (2008) Treatment of metastatic sialoblastoma with chemotherapy and surgery. Pediatr Blood Cancer 50:134–137

Williams SB, Ellis GL, Warnock GR (2006) Sialoblastoma: a clinicopathologic and immunohistochemical study of 7 cases. Ann Diagn Pathol 10:320–326

Differential Diagnosis Congenital Neck Tumors

Challapalli A, Howell L, Farrier M, Kelsey A, Birch J, Eden T (2007) Cervical paraganglioma – a case report and review of all cases reported to the Manchester Children's tumour registry 1954-2004. Pediatr Blood Cancer 48:112–116

Manolidis S, Higuera S, Boyd V, Hollier LH (2006) Single-stage total and near-total resection of massive pediatric head and neck neurofibromas. J Craniofac Surg 17:506–510

Ustundag E, Iseri M, Keskin G, Yayla B, Muezzinoglu B (2005) Cervical bronchogenic cysts in the head and neck region. J Laryngol Otol 119:419–423

Section 7.4.1–7.4.3

Ellis J, Oyston PC, Green M, Titball RW (2002) Tularemia. Clin Microbiol Rev 15:631–646

Leventhal BG, Donaldson SS (1993) Hodgkin's disease. In: Pizzo PA, Poplack DC (eds) Principles and practice of pediatric oncology. Lippincott, Philadelphia

Margrath IT (1993) Malignant non-Hodgkin's lymphoma in children. In: Pizzo PA, Poplack DC (eds) Principles and practice of pediatric oncology. Lippincott, Philadelphia

Newman KD, Sato TT (1998) Lymph node disorders. In: O'Neill JA et al (eds) Pediatric surgery, vol I, 5th edn. Mosby, St Louis

Piedimonte G, Wolford ET, Fordham LA et al (1997) Mediastinal lymphadenopathy caused by mycobacterium avium-intracellulare complex in a child with normal immunity: successful treatment anti-mycobacterial drugs and laser bronchoscopy. Pediatr Pulmonol 24:287–291

Pranghofer S, Rossi M, Uebelhart T (2004) Tularämie bei Lymphknotenschwellung – Differentialdiagnose der Vergangengenheit? Schweiz Med Forum 4:567–569

Shah JP et al (1993) Cervical lymph node metastasis. Curr Probl Surg 30:273–335

Section 7.4.4–7.4.5

Bentz BG, Hughes CA, Lüdemann JP, Maddalozzo J (2000) Masses of the salivary gland region in children. Arch Otolaryngol Head Neck Surg 126:1435–1439

Fraser GC (1998) Salivary glands. In: O'Neill JA Jr et al (eds) Pediatric surgery, vol I, 5th edn. Mosby, St Louis

Greene AK, Rogers GF, Mulliken JB (2004) Management of parotid hemangioma in 100 children. Plast Reconstr Surg 113:53–60

Marchal F, Dulguerov P (2003) Sialolithiasis management: the state of the art. Arch Otolaryngol Head Neck Surg 129:951–956

Orvidas LJ, Kasperbauer JL, Lewis JE, Olsen KD, Lesnick TB (2000) Pediatric parotid masses. Arch Otolaryngol Head Neck Surg 126:177–184

Prigent M, Teissier N, Peuchmaur M, El-Maleh-Berges M, Philippe-Chomette P, Wolfensberger M (2003) ORL, Hals- und Gesichtschirurgie: Das Endoskop erobert die Speicheldrüse. Schweiz Med Forum 51(52):1269–1272

Part III

Chest

Mediastinal Tumors

8

Mediastinal tumor is a collective term which includes a large number of developmental, inflammatory, and neoplastic masses.

In contrast to the leading symptoms and signs of most other chapters, only a part of the mediastinal tumors manifest themselves clinically, and up to 50 % of the cases are detected by chance on prenatal ultrasound or more frequently on chest x-rays performed for other reasons ##.

In addition, the possible symptoms and signs are many and diverse and are caused by compression (e.g., bronchi or trachea), involvement, or infiltration of the chest wall, the organs of the thoracic cavity, or spinal canal; that means that the precise location of the different disorders is important to a considerable degree for the symptomatology.

Three aspects of mediastinal tumors are important to the clinician:

- Mediastinal tumor is a classic and relatively frequent leading clinical and/or radiological sign in childhood.
- In case of symptoms and signs as listed diagrammatically in Table 8.1, a mediastinal tumor must be always considered as their possible cause.
- Because particular pathologies occur in the majority in a certain compartment of the mediastinum, it is possible to assign findings of ap and lateral chest x-rays or CT slices to a specific diagnosis of the encountered mediastinal tumor. The traditional compartment model depicted in Fig. 8.1 enables the physician to classify mediastinal tumors as disorders of

Table 8.1 Possible symptoms and signs in mediastinal tumors

- Cough, stridor (expiratory and/or inspiratory noisy breathing), cyanosis, orthopnea, tachypnea, and dyspnea with increased expiratory and/or inspiratory time. Respiratory distress syndrome
- Superior vena cava syndrome (=cyanosis of head and neck, neck vein distension, syncope, and cardiovascular collapse). Collateral venous bypass circulation
- Chest, spine, shoulder, and arm pain
- Dysphagia
- Neurological signs: Horner's syndrome #, hoarseness, pareses (diaphragm, paraparesis)
- Circumscribed chest wall deformity (prominence)

the anterior, middle, posterior, and superior mediastinum.

The velocity of onset and the type of symptoms and signs depend largely on the location of the mediastinal tumor, the age of the child, and the velocity of growth. The possible clinical presentation extends from peracute onset of life-threatening RDS and/or cardiovascular collapse to insidious development of pathognomonic signs.

In Table 8.2, the prevalence and location of the relatively frequent and characteristic mediastinal tumors of childhood are quoted, and Table 8.3 yields an overview of all differential diagnoses of childhood mediastinal tumor depending on the mediastinal compartments.

In addition to chest x-rays and CT with contrast, ultrasound, MRI #, bronchoscopy with biopsy and punction, esophagoscopy, and esophagography with fluoroscopy in different directions, echocardiography, scintiscan #, and increasingly thoracoscopy

G.L. Kaiser, *Symptoms and Signs in Pediatric Surgery*,
DOI 10.1007/978-3-642-31161-1_8, © Springer-Verlag Berlin Heidelberg 2012

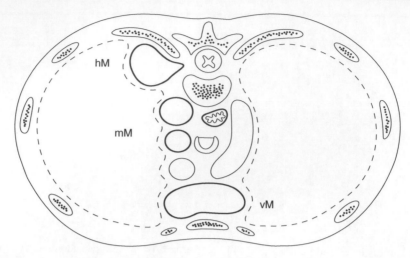

Fig. 8.1 Schematic cross-section for a topographic subdivision of the mediastinum which can be used for classification and radiological differential diagnosis of mediastinal tumors. Most symptoms and signs of mediastinal tumors are unspecific and may be attributed to multiple pathologies. In case of a radiologically visible mediastinal tumor, the site of the mass in the anterior, middle, or posterior mediastinum allows a restriction of the possible tumors and few have to be considered. In the anterior mediastinum (*vM*), there are mainly teratoma, dermoid cyst, and thymic pathologies. Inflammatory and neoplastic lymphadenopathies, bronchogenic cyst, and cystic lymphangioma occur mainly in the middle mediastinum (*mM*). Neurogenic tumors and enteric duplication cysts are mainly encountered in the posterior mediastinum (*hM*)

Table 8.2 Prevalence and location of the relatively frequent mediastinal tumors

• Lymphomas (malignant, inflammatory):	>40 %	Middle/anterior mediastinum
• Neurogenic tumors:	1/3	Posterior mediastinum
• Germ cell tumors (dermoid cyst, teratoma):	7 %	Anterior mediastinum
• Mesenchymal tumors (cystic lymphangioma):	7 %	Anterior/middle mediastinum
• Bronchogenic, enterogenic cysts:	7 %	Middle/posterior mediastinum
• Thymus lesions:	>3 %	Anterior mediastinum

Table 8.3   Differential diagnosis of mediastinal tumors

Anterior and superior mediastinum

• Malignant lymphomas

o Cystic lymphangioma

• Dermoid cyst, teratoma

o Thymic lesions: hyperplasia, neoplastic tumors

o Ectopic thyroid

Middle mediastinum

• Malignant and inflammatory lymphoma

• Bronchogenic cyst

• Pericardial cyst (pericardial effusion and tumor, cardiac tumor)

Posterior mediastinum

• Neurogenic tumors: neuroblastoma, ganglioneuroma, ganglioneuroblastoma, neurinoma, neurofibroma

• Enterogenic cyst

o Neurenteric cyst (combined or isolated)

o Ectopic thymus

are available as diagnostic tools depending on the clinical presentation and suspected diagnosis.

The additional examinations cannot and should not enable a precise diagnosis at all costs; the knowledge of the exact location of the lesion and of its relation to the other organs is just as important as the latter because the optimal interventional access arises from it. In general, the whenever possible elective thoracotomy or thoracoscopy has the aim to achieve confirmation of the suspected diagnosis by histology or resection of the lesion if indicated, to avoid inherent complications of the lesion, and to perform the intervention under optimal conditions.

8.1   Anterior and Superior Mediastinum

Occurrence

The anterior and superior mediastinum is the most frequent location of mediastinal tumors. Only half of them are benign, and they are encountered in the following order of frequency:

- Malignant lymphomas
- Mesenchymal tumors
- Germ cell tumors
- Thymus disorders

Clinical Significance

- The mediastinum is either involved in advanced stages of malignant lymphoma or is the primary site in stage IIIB of non-Hodgkin's or I of Hodgkin's lymphoma. Malignant lymphomas may lead to peracute or even life-threatening clinical presentation in both conditions.
- Cystic lymphangioma as example of mesenchymal tumor may extend to the axilla or the neck and vice versa. Acute clinical manifestation occurs in case of rapid increase of its size due to hemorrhage or lymph accumulation.
- Germ cell tumors have a large variety of histological and biological types. The malignant forms that are located in the mediastinum or the neck have a lower probability of event-free survival than gonadal, retroperitoneal, or sacrococcygeal germ cell tumors.

    Teratomas are prone to complications such as infection or break into pleura, bronchial system, or pericardium.
- The thymus is often large and has a differential diagnostic significance due to the diversity of its shape leading to a variable radiological opacity of the mediastinum mainly in newborns and young infants.

    Reactive or rebound thymus hyperplasia is also a matter of concern after intensive chemotherapy for lymphoma.
- Ectopic thyroid may occur in the superior and ectopic thymus in the posterior mediastinum including the rare occurrence of corresponding pathologies at the same sites.

8.1.1   Malignant Lymphomas

Occurrence, Pathology

The incidence of non-Hodgkin's lymphoma (NHL) and Hodgkin's disease (HD) corresponds to 10–12 new patients a year per one million children under the age of 16 years of whom 60 % have NHL and 40 % HD. About 85 % of mediastinal malignancies in children are malignant lymphomas.

NHL is mostly a diffuse, fast growing tumor of the lymphatic tissue (generalized disease) at the moment of its clinical diagnosis. The three histopathological types "undifferentiated (or small, noncleaved cell) lymphoma, lymphoblastic lymphoma, and the large cell lymphoma" are observed in 40–50 %, 30–40 %, and 15 %, respectively, with different histopathological and pathoanatomical subtypes. The African Burkitt's tumor belongs to the small, noncleaved cell lymphoma and is endemic in equatorial Africa and New Guinea. For clinical purposes, stages I–IV are used for the two most common types (e.g., Murphy's or National Cancer Institute staging system) and for chemotherapeutical stratification and immunological typization.

Hodgkin's disease begins usually in a single lymph node region or a single extra-lymphatic organ or site (stage I) and spreads from one lymph node region to the other. Out of the four histopathological types, the nodular sclerosis type is the most common in children. The Ann Arbor staging system serves for clinical purposes, includes four stages, and uses the involvement of disease on one or both sides of the diaphragm as stages III and IV.

Clinical Presentation

The **NHL** is mainly observed before puberty and in early adolescence. In the lymphoblastic type, the predominant clinical presentation is an anterior mediastinal and/or intrathoracic tumor (in 50–70 %) combined with cervical, supraclavicular, or axillary lymphadenopathy in up to 80 %. The same location is also observed in the other types of NHL albeit in a much smaller percentage. The patient complains of *chest pain, dyspnea, or dysphagia.* They may develop pleural effusions and life-threatening tracheal or bronchial narrowing (with *stridor, cough, dyspnea, and orthopnea*) and/or superior vena cava syndrome (with *cyanosis, swelling, and fullness of the veins of arms, neck, and head*) within days to weeks.

The undifferentiated type of NHL leads in more than 90 % to abdominal tumor or surgical abdomen as leading signs except for the African Burkitt's lymphoma in which diffuse swelling of the jaw is in the foreground in more than 50 %.

Hodgkin's disease is observed beyond the age of 5 years with a peak in adolescence. The leading sign is mostly *a neck mass corresponding to (an) enlarged, painless regional cervical lymph node(s) with a nonirritable overlying skin and persisting over weeks, months, to years*. Primary involvement of axillary or inguinal lymph nodes occurs only rarely. At the moment of clinical diagnosis, more than 50 % to two thirds have an *anterior mediastinal mass or hilar lymphadenopathy #*, and one third general symptoms such as weight loss, fever, and night sweats (in staging, A means without and B with general symptoms).

Differential Diagnosis, Work-Ups
A malignancy must be considered if the mediastinal tumor is very large, leads to pleural effusion, and airway or cardiovascular compromise is imminent. Sarcomas; malignant germ cell or thymus tumor; metastatic tumors, for example, neuroblastoma; and inflammatory processes must be considered particularly.

Work-ups start with a careful clinical examination of all visible and/or palpable lymph node regions and sites of lymphatic tissue, followed by complete blood count including platelets and full coagulation screen, serum liver function tests, electrolytes, BUN, creatinine, and possible markers for prognostication such as LDH.

For diagnosis and biological characterization of the tumor, sufficient tissue must be available which should be gathered with minimal trauma to the child and tissue: lymph node biopsy in **Hodgkin's disease** and bone marrow aspiration and biopsy, thoracocentesis or abdominal paracentesis, lumbar puncture, or peripheral lymph node biopsy in **NHL**. Only exceptionally, tissue biopsy is necessary by anterior mediastinotomy (Chamberlain procedure) or minimal laparotomy; alternatively, tissue biopsy by thoracoscopic or laparoscopic techniques is performed if available.

The imaging techniques are used for diagnostic and mainly for staging purposes and include chest pa/lateral x-rays, thoracic and abdominal CT with i.v. (and peroral) contrast (quantification of tumor size in mediastinal tumor may be used for prognostication), and scintiscan and MRI, echocardiogram, and PET for specific questions. Laparotomy in Hodgkin's disease has lost its significance for staging and splenectomy.

Therapy, Prognosis
The treatment of **NHL** is multiagent chemotherapy according to histopathology-specific protocols. Surgery is restricted to peripheral lymph node biopsies or minimal invasive procedures for lymph node or tissue biopsies, vascular access for rehydration or dialysis, and ureteral stenting by cystoscopy in tumor lysis syndrome. In addition, surgery is indicated in case of abdominal complications and in abdominal NHL with predominant intestinal involvement that is strictly localized.

The treatment of **Hodgkin's disease** is radiation for stage I and IIA in older children and chemotherapy or a combination with radiation for the remaining patients and for all with stage IIB and higher stages. Surgery is indicated for peripheral lymph node biopsy, rarely for staging laparotomy (if radiation is considered as single therapy), and thoracotomy or thoracoscopy in case of residual mediastinal mass after combined therapy in HD or rebound thymic hyperplasia after chemotherapy in HD and NHL.

Long-term and event-free survival is >80 % in most histological subtypes of childhood NHL (5-year EFS 85 % with less favorable results in mediastinal B-cell and in anaplastic lymphomas. Long-term and event-free survival is >90 % of childhood Hodgkin disease (5-year survival 96 %, 5 % with no remission or relapse after initial response and less favorable results for stage IV and mediastinal disease.

8.1.2   Mesenchymal Tumors

Occurrence, Pathology
Mesenchymal tumors are the second most frequent disorder of the anterior mediastinum and

include a wide variety of pathologies as listed below in order of their frequency:

- Lymphangioma (cystic lymphangioma, lymphangioma simplex, mixed lymphangiohemangioma)
- Lipoma (lipoma, lipoblastoma, liposarcoma)
- Rhabdomyosarcoma
- Hemangioma, vascular malformations
- Fibroma, fibrosarcoma

Clinical Significance

- In the differential diagnosis of a mass of the anterior mediastinum, a large diversity of possible mesenchymal disorders must be considered.

Clinical Presentation

In general, symptoms and signs of an anterior mediastinal mass can be observed if the quoted disorders attain a particular size or grow rapidly as in malignant neoplasms or cystic lymphangioma.

The cystic lymphangioma # *becomes symptomatic if there is a sudden increase due to spontaneous hemorrhage or lymph accumulation or if an extension into the neck or axilla is or becomes visible*. Extension to the cervicothoracic epidural space by the intervertebral foramina has also been described with formation of epidural hematoma. This rare example emphasizes the possible expansion of cystic lymphangioma between all intra- and extrathoracic structures with a large variety of possible clinical signs and surgical implications. Excision may be followed by chylothorax.

Lipomatous tumors are the second most common disorders of mesenchymal tumors and include lipoma, lipoblastoma, and liposarcoma. Lipomas are encountered mostly beyond infancy and lipoblastoma up to 5 years. The latter entity is composed of whitish appearing, immature fat what grows rapidly either localized or diffusely and may recur after possibly incomplete resection. Liposarcoma is a specific type of soft tissue sarcoma with possible recurrences and metastases that needs complete resection and chemotherapy.

Rhabdomyosarcoma occurs not only in the anterior mediastinum but also in the chest wall and or in the paraspinal region with possible extension to the spinal canal.

Differential Diagnosis, Work-Ups

It includes the other pathologies of the anterior and middle mediastinum, but those of the adjacent chest wall must be considered as well. On work-up, MRI with i.v. contrast application adds significant information about the characteristics and extension of the quoted disorders.

Therapy, Prognosis

The role of surgery and the other therapeutic modalities depends on the specific disorder. In general, complete resection must be achieved if feasible. Except for rhabdomyosarcoma, soft tissue sarcomas, and some (cystic) lymphangiomas, permanent cure is possible.

8.1.3   Germ Cell Tumors (Dermoid Cyst, Teratoma, and Other Germ Cell Tumors)

Occurrence, Pathology

Germ cell tumors belong similar to the mesenchymal tumors to the second most common tumors of the anterior mediastinum, and the mediastinum is the second most frequent site of extragonadal germ cell tumors. Germ cell tumors are derived from fetal germ cells. They are a heterogeneous group of tumors and contain (1) germinoma that has a similar histology to dysgerminoma in the ovary and to seminoma in the testis; (2) dermoid cyst, teratoma, and embryonic carcinoma; (3) yolk sac tumor (entodermal sinus tumor) and choriocarcinoma; and (4) mixed germ cell tumors that contain multiple histological types. The proportion of the different types depends on the involved organ or site. Five to ten percent of the germ cell tumors occur in the mediastinum or neck. The majority of them are either dermoid cysts (with two) or teratoma (with three germ layers) in up to 80 %. One fourth of teratoma is immature. The remainder germ cell tumors belong to the four groups mentioned above.

Clinical Significance

- Dermoid cysts and teratomas are sometimes in spite of their remarkable size relatively symptomless and may occasionally lead to severe and life-threatening complications.

• On the other hand, malignant types of germ cell tumors are severely symptomatic and have the worst prognosis in comparison to the other extragonadal and gonadal germ cell tumors.

Clinical Presentation
Some of the benign dermoid cysts and teratomas may be detected by fetal ultrasound or shortly after birth due to *an RDS and/or an asymmetric prominence of the chest wall ##*. Although recognition of dermoid cysts and teratomas is reported in all ages, the mean age of diagnosis in the third trimenon of infancy means that *most of them are symptomatic* for a longer time and contrasts with the malignant types of germ cell tumors which lead *rapidly to dyspnea, wheezing, cough, chest pain, fever, anorexia, and weight loss*.

Due to alpha-fetoprotein and beta-human chorionic gonadotropin secretion, *signs of precocious puberty* may be observed in benign and malignant germ cell tumors. The association between **Klinefelter's syndrome** and germ cell tumor leads in 20–25 % of it to seeming precocious puberty masking the diagnosis of Klinefelter's syndrome.

Occasionally, germ cell tumors lead to severe complications such as infection and/or perforation into the pleural cavity, bronchial tree, or pericardium with presenting signs of *purulent pleuropneumonia, hemoptysis, or heart failure*.

Differential Diagnosis, Work-Ups
The differential diagnosis includes all possible pathologies of the mediastinum, especially of the anterior and middle mediastinum. In every case of **pleural empyema** or **purulent pleuropneumonia**, a mediastinal tumor must be considered as underlying cause.

Chest x-ray in two planes, CT with i.v. contrast, and determination of infectious and biological markers (AFP, β-HCG, LDH, and PALP [placental alkaline phosphatase]) belong to the obligatory work-up examinations, whereas bone scan, MRI, cardioechogram, PET/CT, and karyotyping (in suspected Klinefelter's syndrome) are used if needed. The chest x-rays demonstrate a roundish

opacity of the anterior mediastinum with asymmetrical expansion to one hemithorax. If coarse-grained, central or peripheral calcifications, or primitive teeth are visible in the mass #, the diagnosis of dermoid cyst or teratoma is confirmed.

Therapy
Complete excision is indicated in all benign germ cell tumors either by sternotomy ##, thoracotomy, or thoracoscopy. In malignant germ cell tumors, meticulous staging (e.g., of the regional lymph nodes) and complete resection is indicated in low stages followed by platinum-based and possibly multiagent chemotherapy, and tumor biopsy in high stages followed by chemotherapy and second look resection of residual tumor (that may contain mature teratoma tissue) after completion of chemotherapy. Throughout histological examination is necessary in every case, especially in teratoma # and mixed germ cell tumors as well as long-term follow-ups by clinical and radiological examination and determination of biological markers.

Prognosis
In general, prognosis in germ cell tumors depend on the age (first vs. second decade), the site (gonadal and extragonadal vs. mediastinal), the histological type(s) (e.g., dermoid cyst vs. mixed germ cell type), and the stage (stages I–IV for extragonadal germ cell tumors, stages I and II vs. III and IV).

The overall survival of extracranial germ cell tumors is 91 % and the event-free survival 88 % at 10 years. In the mediastinum, the prognosis for benign germ cell tumors is excellent. The 3-year survival rate is 100 % for stages I and II and only somewhat more than 60 % for stage IV and relapses of malignant germ cell tumors.

8.1.4 Thymic Pathologies

Occurrence
The incidence of thymic pathologies depends on the reported figures of individual institutions or on their sum, on whether only neoplastic tumors are included or thymic hyperplasia as well, and if

all pediatric tumors of the mediastinum are considered or only those of the anterior mediastinum, for example, thymic pathologies account for 2–3 % of all mediastinal tumors or 4–15 % of all tumors of the anterior mediastinum are thymic neoplasms. If all cases of neonatal thymic hyperplasia and rebound thymus hyperplasia are included (of which the majority is only considered in the differential diagnosis of mediastinal tumors and thereafter discarded from surgery), the real prevalence of thymic pathologies is much higher.

Clinical Significance
- Thymus hyperplasia of the newborn and young infant has a differential diagnostic significance.
- The same is true for older children with the less frequent reactive (or rebound) thymic hyperplasia after chemotherapy of malignant lymphoma.
- Thymic cyst may present as symptomatic space-occupying lesion or as sign of a possible malignancy.
- Although infrequent, most thymic epithelial neoplasms are malignant and have a bad prognosis.

Clinical Presentation
Thymus hyperplasia is a frequent radiological finding on chest x-ray performed in neonates and young infants for respiratory tract symptoms. Although often large, *thymic hyperplasia is never a cause of symptoms and signs*. Because only part of the thymus is depicted by pa and lateral chest x-rays and its shape is very variable, differential diagnostic delineation from other mediastinal masses and organs may be difficult but not impossible if CT with i.v. contrast is performed or steroids are applied as in older days.

Thymic hyperplasia becomes significant in the differential diagnosis if it persists # beyond the age of 2 years, if it reappears after spontaneous resolution, and if it manifests as nodular form.

Rebound thymic hyperplasia is observed 2–12 months after completion of chemotherapy in malignant lymphomas or during maintenance chemotherapy. The thymus regrows to a mean diameter of 4 cm. PET/CT allows differentiation from a still active malignancy.

Thymic cysts are either congenital or acquired. The former are residuals of a thymopharyngeal duct and the latter a sequel of an inflammatory process or a combination with a malignant tumor (thymoepithelial tumors, Hodgkin's disease, germ cell tumor).

At least 50 % of them are recognized as incidental finding by chest x-rays performed for other reasons. The remainder may lead to signs of an anterior mediastinal mass due to its size or a rapid increase of its volume.

The differential diagnosis includes after radiological imaging dermoid cyst, cystic lymphangioma, mesothelial, and hydatid cyst. If chest x-rays and contrast CT have been performed, additional examination by transthoracic ultrasound is useful because rarely atypical CT findings may mimic a solid tumor. The typical CT findings of a thymic cyst are a homogeneous mass with low density with a capsule and a connection with a residual thymus. The presence of a uni- or a multilocal cyst with possible septa does not allow differentiation between congenital or acquired cyst. On the other hand, an inhomogeneous mass is observed in thymic cyst combined with a malignancy.

The **thymic epithelial tumors** include in order of their frequency thymoma, thymic carcinoma, or thymic carcinoid. **Thymoma** # consists of epitheloid cell and lymphocytes. The dignity of the thymoma is mainly defined by its clinical behavior (stages II: infiltration of the capsule and fat, III: infiltration or metastases of the adjacent organs, and IV: remote metastases). The epithelial **thymic carcinoma** is characterized by cytological anaplasia and as thymic epithelial-like carcinoma associated with **Epstein-Barr virus**. HIV infection in children predisposes to thymic epithelial tumors.

Occasionally, thymoma is recognized in an early stage: Nodular thymic hyperplasia, thymic cyst, or rarely thymoma is encountered if surgery is performed due to a persistent thymic hyperplasia or for other reasons. Mostly, the thymic epithelial tumors are encountered due to a large mass of the anterior mediastinum leading to rapidly progressive orthopnea and dyspnea and signs of superior vena cava syndrome in teenagers.

Differential Diagnosis, Work-Ups
Differentiation of the different thymic pathologies from each other may be difficult if the single pathologies or variants are combined.

Work-ups are the same as in germ cell tumors concerning imaging. MRI allows a better description of thymic parenchyma than CT, and transthoracic ultrasound may be useful in suspected cystic lesions.

Therapy, Prognosis
In case of **malignancy,** complete thymectomy is indicated by sternotomy, anterolateral thoracotomy, or thoracoscopy (combined with chemotherapy and/or possibly radiation if needed), whereas in **benign pathologies** such as nodular hyperplasia, benign thymic cyst, and thymolipoma, partial resection should be considered. In **thymic hyperplasia**, the indication of surgery may arise in the nodular type, in persistency beyond 2 years of age, in resistance to steroids, or reappearance of thymic hyperplasia after spontaneous involution.

Thymectomy may be useful in children with **myasthenia gravis**. The autoimmune disease leads to intermittent failure of postsynaptic neuromuscular transmission with fluctuant weakness of cranial and skeletal muscles. One fourth of all cases belong to the juvenile form. The treatment is medical with the anticholinesterase blocker pyridostigmine, and total thymectomy may be indicated beyond 5 years of age in case of generalization or progression (with increasing drug requirements). Postoperatively, possible respiratory insufficiency must be considered (ventilatory support, plasmapheresis). With thymectomy, the chance of remission is several times increased. Prognosis depends on the length of the disease and the histological findings. In adults, only 10–15 % has a normal thymus and the remainder mostly follicular thymus hyperplasia or thymoma in 10–20 %.

Malignant thymic pathologies have a bad prognosis because they are recognized often in an advanced stage.

8.2　Middle Mediastinum

The middle mediastinum is the least often involved part in mediastinal tumors. The following disorders are encountered arranged in order of their occurrence:

- Inflammatory and neoplastic adenopathy
- Bronchogenic cyst
- Pericardial cyst (pericardial effusion, pericardial or cardial tumor)

8.2.1　Inflammatory and Neoplastic Adenopathy

Readers are referred to Chapters 7.4.1–7.4.3 and Chapter 8.1.1.

8.2.2　Bronchogenic Cyst

Occurrence, Pathology
Bronchogenic cysts are remnants of bronchial tree tissue developing from the ventral foregut and amounts together with the less frequent enterogenic cysts (visceral duplications) to less than 10 % of all mediastinal tumors. They are encountered along the whole tracheobronchial tree in the mediastinum, perihilar, intrapulmonic, and paraesophageal location and rarely in other sites (neck, head, back, and infradiaphragmatic). Bronchogenic cysts may rarely communicate primarily with the bronchial tree or somewhat more frequently secondarily due to perforation.

Clinical Significance
- Bronchogenic cysts are prone to several complications such as more or less rapid increase in size, infection, hemorrhage, and/or perforation into the tracheobronchial tree or mediastinum with sudden death, respiratory distress syndrome, hemoptysis, and less dramatic thoracic symptoms such as thoracic pain. Malignant degeneration has also been described.
- Bronchogenic cyst belongs to the possible differential diagnosis of masses of the middle

and posterior mediastinum and of disorders of the respiratory tract or lung.

Clinical Presentation
Bronchogenic cyst may be suspected by prenatal ultrasound.

It depends on the *age* of the child and *site* of the bronchogenic cyst: In infants and young children, symptoms and signs of different degrees of airway obstruction are observed, whereas bronchogenic cysts of the older child manifest with pneumonia or less overt thoracic signs if they become symptomatic at all.

In central bronchial cyst (=mediastinal with tracheal and preferentially left main stem bronchial involvement), *recurrent cough, wheezing, and fever up to respiratory distress syndrome are recorded with generalized or unilateral expiratory and inspiratory stridor on clinical examination.* In peripheral bronchogenic cysts (=perihilar and intrapulmonic site of bronchi), *only half of the children become symptomatic with signs of recurrent bronchitis or pneumonia, and segmental or lobar dullness to percussion and absent breathing sounds.*

In general, *the recurrent character of the thoracic signs* should draw attention to a possible bronchogenic cyst. Probably less than half of the bronchogenic cysts are either detected incidentally by chest x-ray # or not at all during childhood and adulthood.

Work-Ups, Differential Diagnosis
Bronchogenic cysts are often suspected in plain chest x-ray, and the diagnosis is confirmed by CT. Differential diagnosis includes disorders that lead to stenosis of the tracheobronchial system (tracheobronchial stenosis) or to localized pneumonia or emphysema (foreign body, bronchus adenoma).

Treatment, Prognosis
Open or thoracoscopic enucleation of central bronchial cysts is indicated if the diagnosis is confirmed by CT even if they are not symptomatic because of the inherent possible complications #. The peripheral form is difficult to recognize, the pleura must be incised, and the cyst must be prepared without any damage to the adjacent bronchus. Permanent cure is the role if the cyst is completely resected.

8.2.3   Pericardial Cyst

Occurrence, Pathology
Pericardial cysts are observed in less than 1 % of mediastinal tumors. They are benign mesothelial cysts originating from the pericardium and lie in or adjacent to the pericardium on the right side of the heart or in the cardiophrenic sulcus.

Clinical Significance
• Most of the pericardial cysts have only a differential diagnostic significance.

Clinical Presentation
Some of the cysts are detected by prenatal ultrasound in the second half of pregnancy and may disappear spontaneously till birth. The majority of pericardial cysts are detected incidentally by chest x-ray and further work-up.

Differential Diagnosis, Work-Ups
It includes all mediastinal cysts in case of prenatal recognition by ultrasound. Postnatally, echocardiogram and CT confirm a pericardial cyst that has been suspected on chest x-ray including its location. Occasionally, a cystic lymphangioma or a **pericardial effusion** may be mixed up with a pericardial cyst. The latter may be a sign of an **intrapericardial or cardial tumor** such as cystic lymphangioma, hemangioma, rhabdomyoma, or teratoma.

Therapy
Resection or unroofing of the pericardial cyst is performed by anterolateral thoracotomy or thoracoscopy if necessary (large or symptomatic pericardial cyst or equivocal finding).

8.3   Posterior Mediastinum

The posterior mediastinum is the second most frequently involved part of the mediastinum. The following pathologies are encountered in order of frequency:
• Neurogenic tumors: neuroblastoma, ganglioneuroma, and ganglioneuroblastoma Schwannoma and neurofibroma

- Enteric and neurenteric cysts
- Miscellaneous disorders: mesenchymal and other tumors, infectious, granulomatous pathologies, parasitoses, and other congenital malformations.

Depending on the precise location of the disorder, dignity, and natural course, many masses may only become symptomatic if they reach a large size because a large space is available in the posterior mediastinum without embarrassment of vital structures.

8.3.1 Neuroblastoma

Occurrence, Pathology

Each year, 7–8 new cases are detected in one million children under the age of 16 years or 1 child out of 8,000–10,000 children suffer from neuroblastoma. More than 20 % of the neuroblastomas concern the mediastinum either as primary tumor in its posterior compartment # or as secondary tumor from another site by metastatic lymph nodes in the middle mediastinum.

Clinical Significance

- The mediastinum is after the retroperitoneum, the second most frequent site of neuroblastoma with 20 %, and neuroblastoma is altogether the most frequent neurogenic tumor of the mediastinum.
- In contrast to other masses of the posterior mediastinum, for example, ganglioneuroma, neuroblastoma is recognized earlier due to its rapid and infiltrating growth, general signs, and possible effects of catecholamines and other by-products.

Clinical Signs

The general signs and those resulting from by-products include *weight loss and failure to thrive, fever and paleness (anemia), refusal to walk (skeletal pain) and spontaneous hemorrhages (increased bleeding diathesis), and flushing, sweating, or intractable diarrhea.*

More specific signs are *dysphagia, thoracic and respiratory signs, neurological signs such as ipsilateral Horner's syndrome and iris heterochromia* (involvement of upper mediastinum, neck, or both compartments), *paraparesis* (involvement of thoracic spinal canal), *dancing eye syndrome*, and palpable *neck mass* (extension to the neck).

Differential Diagnosis, Work-Ups

It must consider all masses of the posterior mediastinum and if some of the general signs are taken into account, other rare primary malignancies and metastases of the posterior and whole mediastinum.

As in neuroblastoma of other locations, the work-ups serve for diagnosis, staging, and biological characterization. In addition, chest x-rays, CT with i.v., and peroral contrast are necessary for delineation of the neuroblastoma, and in case of supposed involvement of the spinal canal, MRI with contrast.

Therapy, Prognosis

The therapeutic principles are similar to those of other sites of neuroblastoma with primary resection only in low stages followed by multiagent chemotherapy or chemotherapy followed second look resection if necessary #. In case of intraspinal extension, primary resection by laminotomy or laminectomy of the epidural part is followed shortly afterward by resection of the intrathoracic tumor.

For prognosis see Sect. 24.1.2.

8.3.2 Ganglioneuroma and Ganglioneuroblastoma

Occurrence, Pathology

The benign ganglioneuroma and the semimalignant ganglioneuroblastoma account for one third of all tumors of the mediastinum and are observed in contrast to neuroblastoma in older children. Whereas in ganglioneuroma tissue maturation is complete, ganglioneuroblastoma still contains islands of immature neural crest cells with the potential of malignancy #.

Clinical Significance

- The ganglioneuroma should be resected electively shortly after the diagnosis because it becomes very large with time that renders surgery difficult, especially if the cervicobra-chial plexus and large vessels are impinged.

Clinical Presentation

Ganglioneuroma are often *recognized incidentally by chest x-rays* performed for other reasons. *Ipsilateral chest, shoulder, and arm pain; heterochromia of the iris; and Horner's syndrome are relative characteristic signs* of ganglioneuroma although not specific. Depending on its location and size, the other symptoms and signs of mediastinal tumor may be observed and in case of extension to the spinal canal or neck, paraparesis, other neurological symptoms, or a visible or palpable neck mass.

Differential Diagnosis, Work-Ups

It includes all pathologies of the posterior mediastinum (and possibly of the neck) which lead to a slowly occurring displacement of the surrounding structures and more specifically with Horner's syndrome and chest, shoulder, and arm pain.

Chest x-rays in two plains demonstrate a roundish opacity extending from the mediastinum to the right or left upper or middle lung field what projects in the lateral x-ray in the posterior mediastinum. The probable diagnosis of ganglioneuroma is made more precisely by CT with contrast, and a neuroblastoma is excluded by 24-h urinalysis of catecholamines.

Ganglioneuroma with extension to the spinal canal or the neck needs delineation of the mass from the dura or the large vessels and important nerves by (angio) MRI of the spine and soft tissue.

Therapy, Prognosis

Ganglioneuroma is completely resected including possible foraminal extensions by posterolateral thoracotomy or thoracoscopically.

Preexisting Horner's syndrome persists after surgery and cannot be prevented at surgery. The ganglioneuroma should be examined histologically for possible immature parts within the tumor.

In so-called hourglass or dumbbell tumors with extension to the spinal canal, the latter should be removed first by laminectomy followed be excision of the main bulk of ganglioneuroma by thoracotomy. In thoracocervical ganglioneuroma,

excision of the intrathoracic part is followed by removal of the cervical part using a separate cervical incision. This demanding procedure needs careful dissection to avoid injuries to the nerves (cervicobrachial plexus, vagus, recurrent, and phrenic nerves) and large vessels and is time-consuming.

With complete resection and favorable histology, the prognosis of ganglioneuroma is excellent except for advanced cases with possible injury to the surrounding structures.

8.3.3   Neurogenic Tumors (Cranial and Peripheral Nerves)

Occurrence, Pathology

Schwannoma, neurinoma #, and neurofibroma occur much less frequently than the already quoted neuroblastoma and ganglioneuroma. They are observed either as an isolated mass or as multiple tumors, for instance, in **plexiform neurinoma of the upper thoracic aperture** or as neurofibromatosis.

8.3.4   Enteric and Neurenteric Cysts (Esophageal Duplication)

Occurrence, Surgical Pathology

Esophageal duplications are observed less frequently than bronchogenic cysts. They are lined by esophageal and/or gastric mucosa and belong to the duplications of the alimentary tract.

They develop probably from the notochord as by-product of detachment of the latter from the entoderm that explains the dorsal location of enteric cysts to the esophagus and the possibility of entering the spinal cord through a vertebral body defect. The **combined neurenteric cyst** is an intraspinal extension of parts of the enterogenic cyst. The **split notochord syndrome** belongs probably to the same embryological entity. Enterogenic cysts occur in the posterior mediastinum or neck, are separate from, have close connections to, and rarely enter into the esophagus. Sometimes they continue as a sinus or cord through the diaphragm, end blindly, or finish in the stomach or intestine below it.

Isolated intraspinal neurenteric cysts are rare malformations that are located in about 90 % in the intradural extramedullary compartment in front of the spinal cord, in 50 % in the cervical, and 50 % in thoracic or thoracolumbar spine and occur usually as single lesion. Possible complications are dissemination (e.g., after incomplete resection), infection, hemorrhage, and malignant degeneration.

They become symptomatic as spinal tumor in the second and third decade of life. If they present in childhood the mean age is 6.4 years, and children complain of localized back pain, develop myelopathic or radicular signs (focal weakness, radicular pain, and paresthesia), and rarely fever, meningism, paraplegia, and incontinence. Due to a waxing and waning course caused by fluctuation of cyst size or because the symptoms are overlooked or misinterpreted, some cysts are recognized only somewhere during childhood or even in adulthood.

In **neurenteric cyst of the back** also called **split notochord syndrome**, the remaining dorsal part of the former fistula between endoderm and ectoderm prolapses from the surface of the back skin as enteric mucosa. It may be combined with a myelomeningocele or meningocele.

Clinical Significance

- Enteric cysts increase in size and may compress the esophagus.
- The possible presence of gastric mucosa leads to ulceration wit pain, hemorrhage, or perforation.
- The rare combined or isolated neurenteric cyst may act as space-occupying mass or infectious process in the spinal canal.

Clinical Presentation

Some of the enteric cysts without or combined with a neurenteric cyst become clinically manifest *already in infancy by dysphagia, equivalents of pain, and symptoms and signs of complications such as hemorrhage or perforation* into the esophagus, mediastinum, or tracheobronchial tree and by *neurological signs of the thoracic spine*. Others are detected or supposed incidentally by *x-ray* (posterior mediastinal mass, thoracic spine abnormalities).

Chest and back pain combined with neurological signs and/or thoracic spine malformations are red flags of possible enteric cysts combined with a neurenteric cyst.

The clinical presentation of an isolated neurenteric cyst and neurenteric cyst of the back has been mentioned above.

The possibility of combined malformations should be taken into consideration in clinical presentation and work-ups. It concerns mainly minor to severe lower cervical and upper thoracic spine anomalies (anterior spina bifida, hemivertebrae, and butterfly vertebrae), additional alimentary tract duplications, other gastrointestinal, cardiac, urogenital malformations, myelomeningocele, and other anomalies.

Differential Diagnosis, Work-Ups

It includes all space-occupying or pain-triggering disorders of the (posterior) mediastinum and depending on the single signs, for example, of dysphagia, respiratory signs, etc., the varieties of possible pathologies.

Chest x-rays show a mass behind the heart silhouette and in front of the spine #. CT with i.v. and peroral contrast is diagnostic and demonstrates possible spine anomalies more precisely (present in 50 % of isolated neurenteric cysts).

It should be completed by MRI with contrast if an additional neurenteric cyst is supposed. The neurenteric cyst is depicted mostly as a nonenhancing lobulated homogenous mass without an associated mural nodule and is isodense on T1-weighted and hyperdense in T2-weighted images. Possibly present osseous anomalies are located in >80 at the level of the neurenteric cyst.

Therapy, Prognosis

In every case, elective complete resection is indicated by posterolateral thoracotomy or thoracoscopy #. In case of neurenteric cyst, it should be combined with total resection of the spinal part; in case of continuation to the abdomen, with laparotomy; and in case of notochord syndrome, with resection of the spinal and dorsal part.

Isolated neurenteric cysts can be removed by a dorsal access in spite of their ventral location.

Complete resection is necessary for permanent cure of enteric cyst, combined or isolated neurenteric cyst, and split notochord syndrome. Incomplete resection is the main cause of recurrences.

Webcodes

The following webcodes can be used on www. psurg.net for further images and data.

801 Chest x-ray in two plains,	813 Teratoma adultum, mediastinum
802 Tumor posterior mediastinum	814 Persistent thymic hyperplasia
803 Right Horner's syndrome, posterior mediastinal tumor	815 Thymoma
804 MRI and scintiscan	816 Right mediastinal tumor, suspected bronchogenic cyst
805 Neurogenic mediastinal tumor, PNET	817 Bronchogenic cyst at surgery
806 Lymph nodes, mediastinal Hodgkin's disease	818 Mediastinal neuroblastoma
807 Cystic lymphangioma mediastinum	819 Second look resection neuroblastoma
808 Chest x-rays, mediastinal teratoma	820 Mediastinal ganglioneuroblastoma
809 With thoracic deformity (upper pigeon breast)	821 Tumor thorax aperture, plexus neurinoma
810 Lateral chest x-ray, teeth in dermoid cyst	822 Neurinoma intercostal nerve
811 Sternotomy, dermoid cyst	823 Tomography, suspected enteric cyst
812 Dermoid cyst with teeth and sebum	824 Intraoperative enteric cyst, fibrous connection to esophagus

Bibliography

General: Textbooks, Anesthesia, Differential Diagnosis, Treatment

Anghelescu DL, Burgoyne LL, Liu T, Li CS, Pui CH, Hudson MM, Furman WL, Sandlund JT (2007) Clinical and diagnostic findings predict anesthetic complications in children presenting with malignant mediastinal masses. Paediatr Anaesth 17:1090–1098

Bölling T, Könemann S, Ernst I, Willich N (2008) Late effects of thoracic irradiation in children. Strahlenther Onkol 184:289–295

Cuendet A, Braun P (1982) Mediastinal tumoren. In: Bettex M et al (eds) Kinderchirur-gie, 2. Auflage, Thieme, Stuttgart

De Lorimier AA (1998) Respiratory problems related to the airway and lung. In: O'Neill JA Jr et al (eds) Pediatric surgery, vol 1, 5th edn. Mosby, St. Louis

Findik G, Gezer S, Sirmali M, Turut H, Aydogdu K, Tastepe I, Karaoglanoglu N, Kaya S (2008) Thoracotomies in children. Pediatr Surg Int 24:721–725

Hecker WC (1988) Neubildungen im bereich des thoray. In: Schulte FJ, Spranger J (eds) Neubildungen im bereich des thorax. Fischer, Stuttgart

Jaggers J, Balsara K (2004) Mediastinal masses in children. Semin Thorac Cardiovasc Surg 16:201–208

Philippart AI, Farmer DL (1998) Benign mediastinal cysts and tumors. In: O'Neill JA Jr et al (eds) Pediatric surgery, vol 1, 5th edn. Mosby, St. Louis

Saraswatula A, Mc Shane D, Tideswell D, Burke GA, Williams DM, Nicholson JC, Murray MJ (2009) Mediastinal masses masquerading as common respiratory conditions of childhood: a case series. Eur J Pediatr 168:1395–1399

Sharif K, Alton H, Clarke J, Desai M, Morland B, Parikh D (2006) Paediatric thoracic tumours presenting as empyema. Pediatr Surg Int 22:1009–1014

Tansel T, Onursal E, Dayloglu E, Basaran M, Sungur Z, Quamci E, Yilmazbayhan D, Eker R, Ertugrul T (2006) Childhood mediastinal masses in infants and children. Turk J Pediatr 48:8–12

Tsao K, St Peter SD, Sharp SW, Nair A, Andrews WS, Sharp RJ, Snyder CL, Ostlie DJ, Holcomb GW (2008) Current application of thoracoscopy in children. J Laparoendosc Adv Surg Tech A 18:131–135

Wright CD (2009) Mediastinal tumors and cysts in pediatric population. Thorac Surg Clin 19:47–61, vi

Section 8.1

Bayram AS, Gebitekin C, Bicer M (2007) Extrapulmonary sequestration mimicking mediastinal cyst: report of two identical cases. Tuberk Toraks 55:414–417

Bettschart RW, Bertschmann W, Bolliger CT (2008) Solide raumforderung im vorderen mediastinum (a solid tumour in the anterior mediastinum). Schweiz Med Forum 8:304–305

Blasimann B, Kuffer F, Bettex M (1977) Chirurgische Betrachtungen über die Thymushyperplasie (surgical consideration on hyperplasia of the thymus). Z Kinderchirurgie 21:214–230

De Backer A, Madern GC, Hakvoort-Cammel FG, Oosterhuis JW, Hazebroek FW (2006) Mediastinal germ cell tumors: clinical aspects and outcomes in 7 children. Eur J Pediatr Surg 16:318–322

De Backer A, Madern GC, Pieters R, Haentjens P, Hakvoort-Cammel FG, Oosterhuis JW, Hazebroek FW (2008) Influence of tumor site and histology on long-term survival in 193 children with extracranial germ cell tumors. Eur J Pediatr Surg 18:1–6

Gielda BT, Peng R, Coleman JL, Thomas CR, Cameron RB (2008) Treatment of early stage thymic tumors: surgery and radiation therapy. Curr Treat Options Oncol 9:258–268

Honda S, Morikawa T, Sasaki F, Okada T, Naito S, Itoh T, Kubota K, Todo S (2007) Cystic thymoma in a child: a rare case and review of the literature. Pediatr Surg Int 23:1015–1017

Hsueh C, Kuo TT, Tsang NM, Wu YC, Yang CP, Hung IJ (2006) Thymic lymphoepithelioma like carcinoma in children: clinicopathological features and molecular analysis. J Pediatr Hematol Oncol 28:785–790

Joshua BZ, Raveh E, Saute M, Schwarz M, Tobar A, Feinmesser R (2004) Familial thymic cyst. Int J Pediatr Otorhinolaryngol 68:573–579

Martino F, Avila LF, Encinas JL, Luis AL, Olivares P, Lassaletta L, Nistal M, Tovar JA (2006) Teratomas of the neck and mediastinum in children. Pediatr Surg Int 22:627–634

Rothstein DH, Voss SD, Isakoff M, Puder M (2005) Thymoma in a child: case report and review of the literature. Pediatr Surg Int 21:548–551

Salas Valverde S, Gamboa Y, Vega S, Barrantes M, Gonzales M, Zamora JB (2008) Diagnosis of anterior mediastinal mass lesions using the Chamberlain procedure in children. Pediatr Surg Int 24:935–937

Tomiyama N, Honda O, Tsubamoto M, Inoue A, Sumikawa H, Kuriyama K, Kusumoto M, Johkoh T, Nakamura H (2009) Anterior mediastinal tumors: diagnostic accuracy of CT and MRI. Eur J Radiol 69:280–288

Section 8.2

Bernasconi A, Yoo SJ, Golding F, Langer JC, Jaeggi ET (2007) Etiology and outcome of prenatally detected paracardial cystic lesions: a case series and review of the literature. Ultrasound Obstet Gynecol 29:388–394

Bluhm EC, Ronckers C, Hayashi RJ, Neglia JP, Mertens AC, Stovall M, Meadows AT, Mitby PA, Whitton JA, Hammond S, Barker JD, Donaldson SS, Robison LL, Inskip PD (2008) Cause-specific mortality and second cancer incidence after non-Hodgkin lymphoma: a report from the childhood cancer survivor study. Blood 111:4014–4021

Capra M, Hewitt M, Radford M, Hayward J, Weston CL, Machin D, Children's Cancer and Leukaemia Group (2007) Long-term outcome in children with Hodgkin's lymphoma: the United Kingdom Children's cancer study group HD82 trial. Eur J Cancer 43:1171–1179

Eldar AH, Futerman B, Abrahami G et al (2009) Burkitt lymphoma in children: the Israeli experience. J Pediatr Hematol Oncol 31:428–436

Karnak I, Alehan D, Ekinci S, Büyükpamukcu N (2007) Cardiac rhabdomyoma as an unusual mediastinal mass in a newborn. Pediatr Surg Int 23:811–814

Piedimonte G, Wolford ET, Fordham LA et al (1997) Mediastinal lymphadenopathy caused by mycobacterium avium-intracellulare complex in a child with normal immunity: successful treatment anti-mycobacterial drugs and laser bronchoscopy. Pediatr Pulmonol 24:287–291

Soor GS, Chakrabarti MO, Luk A, Abraham JR, Phillips K, Butany J (2010) Prenatal intrapericardial teratomas: diagnosis and management. Cardiovasc Pathol 19:e1–e4

Tang YJ, Tang JY, Pan C, Xue HL, Chen J, Shen SH, Dong L, Zhou M, Wang YP, Gu LJ, Jiang H, Ye QD (2009) Clinical characteristics and treatment outcome of 36 cases with non-Hodgkin's lymphoma arising from mediastinum in children. Zhonghua Er Ke Za Zhi 47:687–690

Venkateswaran RV, Barron DJ, Brawn WJ, Clarke JR, Desai M, Samuel M, Parikh DH (2005) A forgotten old disease: mediastinal tuberculous lymphadenitis in children. Eur J Cardiothorac Surg 27:401–404

Vogetseder A, Gengler C, Reineke T, Tinguely M (2011) Pädiatrische lymphom-diagnostik aktuelles aus der sicht der pathologen. Schweiz Med Forum 11:73–78

Von der Weid NX (2008) Adult life after surviving lymphoma in childhood. Support Care Cancer 16:339–345

Section 8.3

Alrabeeah A, Gillis DA, Giacomantonio M, Lau H (1988) Neurenteric cysts – a spectrum. J Pediatr Surg 23:752–754

Amra N, Amr SS (2009) Mediastinal lipoblastomatosis: report of a case with complex karyotype and review of the literature. Pediatr Dev Pathol 12:469–474

Bilik R, Ginzberg H, Superina RA (1995) Unconventional treatment of neuroenteric cyst in a newborn. J Pediatr Surg 30:115–117

Ebisu T, Odake G, Fujimoto M, Ueda S, Tsujii H, Morimoto M, Sawada T (1990) Neurenteric cysts with meningomyelocele or meningocele. Split notochord syndrome. Childs Nerv Syst 6:465–467

Häberle B, Hero B, Berthold F, von Schweinitz D (2002) Characteristics and outcome of thoracic neuroblastoma. Eur J Pediatr Surg 12:145–150

Kang CH, Kim YT, Jeon SH, Sung SW, Kim JH (2007) Surgical treatment of malignant mediastinal neurogenic tumors in children. Eur J Cardiothorac Surg 31:725–730

Kumar R, Jain R, Rao KM, Hussain N (2001) Intraspinal neurenteric cysts – report of three paediatric cases. Childs Nerv Syst 17:584–588

Rossi A, Cama A, Piatelli G, Ravegnani M, Biancheri R, Tortori-Donati P (2004) Spinal dysraphism: MR imaging rationale. J Neuroradiol 31:3–24

Savage JJ, Casey JN, McNeill IT, Sherman JH (2010) Neurenteric cysts of the spine. J Craniovertebr Junction Spine 1:58–63

Woo OH, Yong HS, Shin BK, Kim HK, Kang EY (2008) Wide spectrum of thoracic neurogenic tumours: a pictorial review of CT and pathological findings. Br J Radiol 81:668–676

Zhang KR, Jia HM, Pan EY, Wang LY (2006) Diagnosis and treatment of mediastinal enterogenous cysts in children. Chin Med Sci J 21:201–203

Respiratory Distress Syndrome of the Newborn and Young Infant

In the newborn and young infant, the leading symptoms and signs of the respiratory system are mainly those of a respiratory distress syndrome, whereas older infants and children present a large variety of different symptoms and signs or severity in clinical presentation.

This chapter deals with all pediatric surgical pathologies occurring in the neonatal and early infantile period which are relevant to differential diagnostic delineation and/or pediatric surgical treatment.

The following signs belong to the respiratory distress syndrome of the newborn and young infant of which at least two should be present for its diagnosis:

- Tachypnea (respiratory rate >60 breaths/min [up to 6 weeks of age] and >40 [up to 2 years of age])
- Cyanosis (under air condition)
- Nasal flaring
- Retractions and use of accessory muscles (suprasternal, intercostal, and costal margin retractions)
- Inspiratory and/or expiratory sounds (snoring, stridor, wheezing) #

The clinical presentation of older infants and children with disorders of the respiratory system reaches from noisy respiration to chest pain, abdominal symptoms (surgical abdomen), and cough or to peracute signs as quoted for respiratory syndrome of the newborn and young infant including dyspnea.

In Table 9.1 most of the pediatric surgical disorders of the newborn and young infant are listed that lead or may lead to respiratory

Table 9.1 Differential diagnosis of RDS of the newborn and young infant

Obstruction of the airways by disorders of head and neck or larynx and tracheobronchial tree
o Choanal atresia (CHARGE association)
• Congenital tumors of face, nasal or oral cavity and pharynx, or orbit
• Macroglossia
• Pierre Robin sequence
o Posterior laryngeal and laryngotracheoesophageal cleft
o Laryngeal disorders
o Tracheal atresia and stenosis
Obstruction of the airways by a valve mechanism
• Tracheobronchomalacia (airway malacia)
o Lobar emphysema
• Congenital cystic lung disorders, congenital cystic adenomatoid malformations
Obstruction of respiration by intrathoracic lung displacement
• Congenital diaphragmatic hernia
o Diaphragmatic hernia of morgagni
• Diaphragmatic eventration
o Chylothorax
o Mediastinal tumor
• Surgical abdomen
Obstruction of respiration by decreased pulmonary reserve
• Pulmonary hypoplasia
o Lung aplasia and agenesia, Post-pneumonectomy lung
o Anomalies of the thoracic cage
Obstruction of respiration by airway aspiration
• Esophageal atresia and gastroesophageal reflux
• Surgical abdomen, functional disorders of Suction and deglutination
Neurological disorders
o Arnold-Chiari II malformation, etc.

G.L. Kaiser, *Symptoms and Signs in Pediatric Surgery*, DOI 10.1007/978-3-642-31161-1_9, © Springer-Verlag Berlin Heidelberg 2012

distress syndrome. On that occasion, the causes of respiratory distress syndrome may be divided in six groups of pathologies for a clear overview. Embarrassment of respiration due to intrathoracic displacement or after aspiration is prominent numerically among the known causes of respiratory distress syndrome.

9.1 Obstruction of the Airways by Disorders of Head and Neck or Larynx and Tracheobronchial Tree

These disorders concern the nose and nasopharynx, mandibulofacial dysostoses and hypo- or retrognathia, oral cavity, larynx, and neck.

9.1.1 Choanal Atresia

Occurrence, Pathoanatomy
The osseous, fibrous, or mixed closure concerns the most posterior part of the nasal cavity between skull base and palatal bone #, either as uni- or bilateral anomaly with a prevalence of about 0.1‰ (Fig. 9.1).

Clinical Significance
- Bilateral choanal atresia is a life-threatening disorder leading to respiratory failure immediately after birth.
- About 25 % of uni- or bilateral forms are combined with a CHARGE association with a restricted prognostic outlook.

Clinical Presentation
Bilateral choanal atresia displays a *cyclic respiratory distress syndrome. The cyanotic newborn becomes rosy as he opens the mouth to cry and becomes again cyanotic as he closes the mouth.*

In case of unilateral choanal atresia, contralateral nasal breathing is possible. Therefore, the patient remains eupneic after birth. The diagnosis is suspected in the neonatal period or even later due to *difficult breastfeeding or increased discharge of watery or mucous fluid constantly on*

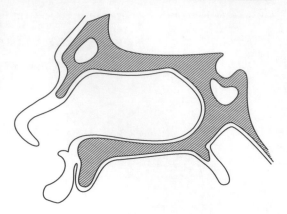

Fig. 9.1 Drawing of a sagittal section through the anterior basal fossa, nasal, and oral cavity of a newborn (the frontal and sphenoidal sinus is not yet developed in this age group but depicted for didactic reasons by M. Bettex). The lumen is closed by an osseous bridge between the hard palate and skull base in the most posterior part of the nasal cavity

the same side. Absent nasal flaring of the ipsilateral nostril may be seen by careful observation.

In a larger cohort of patients with uni- or bilateral choanal atresia, only one fourth has no additional malformations. Half have specific associated conditions such as cardiac malformations of which CHARGE syndrome is with altogether 25 % the most frequent.

CHARGE association is composed of ocular coloboma, heart anomaly, uni- or bilateral choanal atresia or stenosis, retardation of growth and development, genitourinary, and ear abnormalities. It is caused by a mutation in the CHD7 gene in chromosome 8 in two thirds. In the specific associated conditions, CHARGE syndrome, and in genitourinary abnormalities of the latter, a wide range of disorders may be observed. There is a clinical overlap of CHARGE association with **Treacher Collins syndrome** and other pathologies. Whereas in isolated choanal atresia, the incidence of unilateral is higher than in CHARGE syndrome, the inverse proportion is true for bilateral choanal atresia.

If radiological imaging and endocrinological tests are applied in addition to the clinical presentation, the most constant and important features for diagnosis of CHARGE syndrome are coloboma, choanal atresia or stenosis, absent semicircular canals, arhinencephaly, and rhombencephalic dysfunction (possible hypogonadism, growth hormone deficiency, and hypothyroidism). Possible hypocalcemia and cell-mediated or humoral immunodeficiency, concomitant disorders (such as otitis, upper and lower respiratory tract disorders, or feeding difficulties), and risks of postoperative air way events make CHARGE syndrome to a challenge for the involved multidisciplinary team and to a burden for the parents if the outcome is taken into consideration (only 50 % with satisfactory intellectual outcome at beginning school age).

Differential Diagnosis, Work-Ups
Immediately after birth, the differential diagnosis of bilateral choanal atresia includes all disorders which lead to a severe RDS, specifically the rare **congenital piriform aperture stenosis** with the same cyclical cyanosis. By careful observation of the newborn (after placement of an oropharyngeal airway), the suspicion arouses of a bilateral choanal atresia or stenosis by the cyclic RDS and absent nasal flaring.

The diagnosis may be substantiated by impossible cannulation of the nose with a catheter down to the pharynx. The diagnosis is confirmed by contrast instillation (with lateral plain x-ray in prone position of the head), by fiber-optic endoscopy, or by CT with thin slices. Further work-ups concern possible CHARGE association and other specific associated conditions.

Treatment, Prognosis
In bilateral choanal atresia or stenosis, surgery is indicated and performed as soon as possible. Restrictions exist in severe associated malformations and especially in CHARGE syndrome: Informed consent for treatment or not is only possible if all important malformations and their possible outcome are known and communicated. Surgery for unilateral choanal atresia is performed beyond the neonatal period and at the time of diagnosis and if other severe conditions are already treated.

Transpalatal repair and transnasal resections are the two main procedures. At present, there is no dominant approach although trends are directed toward the use of highly advanced endoscopic approaches. Postoperative stenting

is a matter of discussion. In transnasal resection, skull base damage with CSF leaks and fatal hemorrhage has been observed (0.4 %). In transpalatal repair, velar insufficiency, cross-bite, and arch deformities may be observed.

Long-term follow-ups by a multidisciplinary team are necessary for all patients with choanal atresia and even more for those with CHARGE syndrome including clinical evaluation (misted-up mirror), rhinometry, nasal endoscopy, and ear, speech, and orthodontic evaluation.

In transpalatal repair, permanent perfect choanal permeability is achieved in 90 % at 7 years of age and half of the patients required for it a complementary procedure. In transnasal resection, the early success rate is about 90 %.

9.1.2   Congenital Tumors of Face, Nasal or Oral Cavity and Pharynx, or Orbit

Occurrence, Pathology
Congenital tumors of the quoted regions are rare. The large ones may lead to feeding difficulties and/or obstruction of the upper air ways and include mainly germ cell tumors and congenital epulis.

Clinical Significance
- The often large tumors are disfiguring and may be life-threatening.
- If small, different relatively rare differential diagnoses must be considered.

Clinical Presentation
The usually histologically benign (mature) **teratomas** arise from the neck, face, oral cavity, nasopharynx, and oropharynx and account for about 5 % of all germ cell tumors. Facial, oral, and pharyngeal forms protruding through the mouth may cover the nares. **Epignathus** is a descriptive term of an oropharyngeal tumor protruding through the mouth and corresponds to a teratoma. Its site of attachment is the skull base of the nasopharynx (and rarely the palate or alveolar ridge), it involves the hard palate and sphenoid, and it leads to maxillary deformity. It may be

associated with other malformations such as cleft palate, bifid tongue or nose, duplication of pituitary gland, and intracranial extension has been reported.

Congenital granular cell tumor (**congenital epulis** or Neumann's tumor) originates from the gum of the *anterior* maxillary or mandibular *alveolar ridge*. Its immunohistochemical profile is different from the adult granular cell tumor. *The pedunculated or sessile, pink colored single or rarely multiple mass with a smooth or lobulated surface and a size from a few millimeters to several centimeters* (giant epulis) *is observed mostly in female newborns*. It may impair fetal deglutition and lead to polyhydramnios.

Differential Diagnosis, Work-Ups

It includes orofacial or cervicofacial vascular malformations, (cystic) lymphangioma #, hemangioma, nasoethmoid or sphenoid meningoencephalocele, ranula, dermoid cyst #, ectopic thyroid and glioma, thyroglossal duct cyst, neurofibromatosis, embryonic congenital rhabdomyosarcoma, and giant epulis.

Myoblastoma (derived from Schwann cells, occurring at any age, widespread distribution with possible recurrence and malignant degeneration), leiomyomatous hamartoma, Epstein's pearls (cystic remnants of odontogenic epithelium), sequestration of tooth buds, melanotic neuroectodermal tumor, and beyond the neonatal period or infancy, adult form of granular cell tumor (with different sites), granuloma, aneurysmatic bone cyst, fibroma, ameloblastic fibrosis, rhabdomyoma, and lymphoma are more **specific differential diagnoses of congenital epulis**. The preferred age of clinical presentation and the site of origin may be a useful tool for differentiation.

Sequestration of tooth buds is observed in neonates with cleft lip palate close to the cleft or in infants or small children due to maxillary osteomyelitis. Removal of the complete tooth bud(s) in the former situation has no consequence for permanent dentition.

Germ cell and congenital granular cell tumors are occasionally recognized by prenatal ultrasound if they are large and/or protruding. It makes birth planning possible and intrauterine or intrapartal removal of very large masses.

Postpartal work-ups include ultrasound, CT, and MRI depending on the tumor size. MRI is useful for characterization of the mass (in congenital epulis, the main part is isodense and combined with a contrast enhancing, hyperintense rim in T2-weighted images) and delineation of its extension. CT is indicated in epignathus to exclude intracranial extension.

Therapy, Prognosis

In germ cell tumor as well as in congenital granular cell tumor, complete excision by oral approach should be performed as soon as possible with throughout histopathological work-up (with search for immature components in epignathus). In epignathus, maxillary deformity needs orthodontic treatment and intracranial extension an additional access. For congenital epulis, covering of the remaining alveolar bone with gingivo-periosteal flaps is recommended to avoid a permanent notch in the alveolar ridge.

Permanent recovery follows usually the complete removal of teratomas and congenital epulis.

9.1.3 Macroglossia

Occurrence, Pathology

The prevalence is 2 in 1,000 schoolchildren. The tongue is either absolutely too large or in relation to a small oral cavity. Generalized hypertrophy and symmetrically or asymmetrically increased size due to numerous disorders are two principal pathoanatomical presentations. The following pathologies may be combined with macroglossia:

- **Down syndrome (trisomy 21)**, mental retardation, hypothyreosis (cretinism)
- Craniofacial dysostoses
- **Beckwith-Wiedemann syndrome** (present in about 10 % of omphalocele)
- Idiopathic macroglossia
- **Hemangioma, lymphangioma**, neurofibromatosis (symmetric/asymmetric, hemimacroglossia)
- Glycogenoses and mucopolysaccharidoses
- Large, localized masses

Clinical Significance

- Macroglossia may draw attention to specific disorders.
- It is a possible cause of functional or cosmetic impairment.

Clinical Presentation

In absolute or relative macroglossia, *a part of the tongue protrudes permanently through the mouth, occludes it, and is accompanied by drooling #*. Careful inspection of tongue and oral cavity may detect specific findings of some of the quoted disorders, for example, in diffuse lymphangioma, the symmetrically enlarged tongue reveals small vesicles like fish eggs and is rough on palpation #.

In severe forms of macroglossia, *the tongue touches the mouth corners, occupies the whole oral cavity, and is able to reach nearly the chin if actively sticked out.*

Macroglossia may lead to numerous early and late complications such as upper airway obstruction including obstructive sleep apnea (by closure of the mouth or posterior displacement [glossoptosis]), feeding difficulties (by impaired suction, deglutition, or chewing), speech disorders, prognathism or open bite, psychological consequences, and inadvertent injury by the teeth or glossitis.

Differential Diagnosis, Work-Ups

Based on the already quoted differential diagnoses, work-ups may be useful to recognize the pathology in the individual case. With history and local as well as general clinical examination, diagnosis is often possible or at least the suspected pathologies for work-ups by radiological imaging and/or laboratory tests.

Therapy, Prognosis

Indications of reduction surgery are mainly upper airway obstruction (e.g., obstructive sleep apnea in trisomy 21), feeding difficulties, repeated injury to the tongue, and cosmesis. Usually, reduction surgery is performed beyond the neonatal period and mostly in toddlers. It must consider a uniform, global reduction and the site of a possible cause, and retain mobility and sensation (hypoglossal nerve, lingual neurovascular bundle, sensitivity of taste).

Anterior wedge or keyhole reduction or combinations of both are the main procedures that are often performed by cold techniques including laser. Submucosal minimally invasive lingual excision is another option albeit expensive. The absorbable sutures should retain their tensile strength for 3 weeks.

Due to the possible postoperative swelling of the tongue during the first 3 days, supervision in the ICU with primary or secondary intubation may be necessary.

Whereas tongue protrusion and impairment of respiration or feeding difficulties are resolved by surgery, long-term results concerning speech and orthodontics remain open for larger cohorts of patients of the main three groups of pathologies.

9.1.4   Pierre Robin Sequence (Triad of Pierre Robin)

Occurrence, Pathology

The prevalence is 1 in 14,000 newborns. Micro- and retrognathia is the central finding of Pierre Robin sequence, whereas the often encountered cleft palate and glossoptosis are secondary events. The triad of Pierre Robin is either an **isolated clinical entity** (in about two thirds of the cases), a feature of a known syndrome, or combined with other malformations. **Syndromic Pierre Robin sequence** is observed in about one third. Stickler, bilateral facial microsomia, velocardiofacial, and Treacher Collins are the four most common syndromes.

Clinical Significance

- Pierre Robin syndrome is either isolated (isolated PRS) or a feature of a known syndrome (syndromic PRS), or combined with complex or simple malformations with different impact on clinical presentation and prognosis.
- Upper airway obstruction is nearly always present albeit to a different degree. Feeding difficulties are mainly due to the upper airway obstruction and amplified by possible pharyngeal and gastroesophageal dysfunction.
- If the respiratory problems are not recognized and treated, fatal outcome is possible with intellectual impairment or death (2 % and more).

Clinical Presentation

Today, prenatal diagnosis is possible by ultrasound in the middle of pregnancy. Retro-/micrognathia and glossoptosis are defined in the fetal profile (low frontal nasomental angle [the normal angles are not dependent on gestational age]).

In general, *the clinical presentation* of functional impairment such as respiratory and feeding difficulties is *heterogenous*. It is increased in intrauterine disorders such as fetal alcohol syndrome, premature or small for date neonates, and syndromic forms (familial and gestational history).

RDS, episodes of life-threatening choking, apnea, cyanosis, and other less severe or subtle manifestations of upper airway obstructions occur immediately after birth # or during the following weeks; they may be increased by neuromuscular pharyngeal and esophagogastric dysfunction (gastroesophageal reflux in less than one third up to >80 %) and by laryngotracheal abnormalities. *The respiratory problems occur mainly in supine position and are relieved by prone position.*

Hypo- and retrognathia is best seen in the profile of the face #, and inspection of the mouth yields a tongue that touches the palate and is dislocated in the oropharynx. Often breastfeeding is impossible and feeding with the bottle is difficult.

Feeding difficulties (observed in about 50 %) with failure to thrive, acute and chronic hypoxemia, carbon dioxide retention, and cor pulmonale with heart insufficiency are the consequences and may lead to mental retardation or death.

Clinically, a positive correlation exists between degree of hypo- and retrognathia or between type of Pierre Robin sequence and severity of respiratory difficulties.

Obstructive sleep apnea is possible before and after treatment of respiratory and feeding difficulties.

Differential Diagnosis, Work-Ups

It includes all surgical disorders with respiratory and feeding difficulties in the neonate and young infant, especially with RDS and episodic respiratory crises. **Congenital mandibular retro- and hypoplasia** is a frequent finding. It occurs mainly in oculoauriculovertebral spectrum, mandibulofacial dysostosis, and other syndromes. Pierre Robin sequence and **nonsyndromic mandibular hypoplasia** only amount to somewhat >10 and 5 %. The latter disorder has almost the same functional impairments as Pierre Robin sequence and is usually combined with other orofacial anomalies.

The work-ups include indispensably an early and comprehensive history and clinical evaluation, genetic consultation, and based on it, definition of the type of Pierre Robin sequence and throughout assessment of the upper airways and functional disorders by nasal fiber-optic endoscopy, radiological imaging, laboratory tests, and consultations by different specialists.

At the level of the oropharynx, 4 types of upper air way obstruction may be encountered by nasal fiber-optic endoscopy: In the most frequent type 1 (three fourths of the cases), the displaced tongue touches the wall of the oropharynx. In type 2, the displaced tongue compresses the soft palate against the posterior pharyngeal wall (about 10 %). In types 3 and 4 (about 10 %), the oropharynx closes either by medial movements of the lateral walls or concentric contractions. Other sites of obstruction such as laryngeal or tracheal must be recognized as well.

Treatment, Prognosis

The main topic is alleviation of upper airway obstruction and initiation of oral feeding as soon as possible. The therapeutic options are prone position treatment #, nasopharyngeal intubation, distraction osteogenesis, and tracheostomy.

An algorithm is usually recommended which is based on clinical follow-up including pulse oximetry without/with typifying the oropharyngeal obstruction and stepwise introduction of the least morbid procedure. For instance, prone position treatment after exclusion of a laryngotracheal anomaly and if not successful tongue-lip adhesion (that is indicated in isolated tongue-base airway obstruction) that is followed by mandibular distraction osteogenesis (significant increase of posterior distance from pharyngeal wall to the tongue base and hypopharyngeal airway volume) or tracheostomy if not successful. Or prone position treatment or nasopharyngeal intubation from the beginning (a method that can be applied by informed parents) or the latter if prone position treatment failed (both suitable for type 1 and 2). If not successful, glossopexy without or with tracheostomy; the latter is usually necessary in types 3 and 4.

Feeding by nasogastric tube or gastrostomy should be accompanied by different techniques of oral feeding because sucking and deglutition are necessary for the maturation of neuromuscular pharyngeal and esophagogastric dysfunction and mandibular position and growth.

The cleft palate is closed after alleviation of respiratory and feeding difficulties. Nevertheless, obstructive sleep apnea is possible afterward.

Before schoolage, the significant sagittal midface deficit of Pierre Robin syndrome is not resolved. In simple PRS, cognitive development is within the reference range of healthy children though they are performing significantly poorer but self concept and emotional and behavioral problems are not different.

9.1.5 Posterior Laryngeal and Laryngotracheoesophageal Cleft

Occurrence, Pathology
The laryngeal clefts are rare malformations with a prevalence of 1: 10,000–20,000 live births.

The posterior cleft concerns the larynx (type I) or the larynx and parts of the trachea and esophagus (type II), extends from the larynx to the carina (type III), or to one or both main stem bronchi (type IV). In addition, there exists a functional typification.

Clinical Significance
• Depending on the type, different clinical presentations are observed.
• If laryngeal clefts are not considered in the differential diagnosis of respiratory difficulties and voice disorders, the diagnosis is missed or delayed with worsening prognosis.

Clinical Presentation
In almost all **type II to IV clefts**, *an RDS and/or stridor* is observed which is *increased by feeding attempts. Feeding leads to coughing, cyanotic, or choking attacks, and repeated aspirations followed by recurrent respiratory infection and chronic pneumopathy*. Rarely, subglottic obstruction by inspired redundant mucosa increases the symptomatology or leads to manifestation of less severe clefts, or ventilation through an endotracheal tube gets impossible in the course of severe clefts with the need of emergent use of a laryngeal mask airway.

In **type I and minor types II**, a *history of recurrent respiratory tract infections and aspiration with thin liquids are the most common presentations*. On the other hand, some patients may be asymptomatic or present only subtle signs and remain undiagnosed.

In addition to the already mentioned signs, some *vocal impairment* such as hoarseness, weak cry, or aphonia is observed almost in all types.

Differential Diagnosis, Work-Ups
It includes all disorders of the neonate and young infant with RDS and stridor, and more specifically, disorders with choking attacks after or without feeding trials (with swallowing the wrong way) such as H-type tracheoesophageal fistula or Arnold-Chiari malformation type II (differential diagnosis of regurgitation, dysphagia, vomiting, and voice impairment).

For work-ups, rigid airway endoscopy (which spreads the laryngeal cleft apart) is the cornerstone tool. CT with reconstruction or MRI may be alternative methods. In suspected type I and minor type 2 clefts, modified barium swallow and functional fiberoptic endoscopic evaluation of swallow (with pathognomonic laryngeal penetration in a posterior to anterior direction) may enable the difficult diagnosis together with rigid airway endoscopy.

Treatment, Prognosis
In type I and smaller type II clefts, a trial of medical therapy may be useful, whereas all large type

II and the severe types III and IV need surgical reconstruction if they are not associated with a major comorbidity.

In type I, surgery is necessary if the conservative approach has failed, aspiration with feeding is clinically apparent, or other factors are encountered. In addition to the anterior translaryngeal approach with reconstruction of esophagus and larynx, and tracheostomy, endoscopic repair has been reported with good results and without the need of postoperative intubation or tracheostomy.

In large type II and the severe types, surgery must be individualized according to the specific findings. Prior reconstruction, respiration, and feeding must be maintained. The anterior extrathoracic or combined extra- and intrathoracic approach without or with ECMO and without or with interposition graft is confronted by many difficulties such as separation of trachea from the esophagus, postoperative exposure to gastroesophageal reflux due to microgastria, and nasopharyngeal feeding tube (possible need of early gastric division and gastrostomy), fistulization, and need for a continuous positive air pressure ventilation (tracheomalacia).

Whereas the prognosis of type I and minor type II clefts is good, the complication rate, revision quote, and fatal outcome amount to about 50, 25 and 10 % for a cohort of cleft I–III patients. In contrast, spontaneous and postoperative deaths occur in more than one third in type IV clefts. Therefore, especially the severe types need exclusion of major associated pathologies and fully informed parental consent.

9.1.6 Laryngeal Disorders, Tracheal Atresia and Stenosis

9.1.6.1 Laryngeal Disorders
Occurrence, Pathoanatomy
Congenital or acquired vocal cord paralysis and subglottic stenosis, and subglottic hemangioma occur less frequently than laryngomalacia. **Vocal cord paralysis** is more frequently unilateral than bilateral. It is caused by CNS malformations such as Chiari I and II malformation and possibly

reversible. Disorders along the recurrent laryngeal nerve must also be evaluated as possible causes of unilateral forms. The subglottic airway has a diameter of <3.5 mm in **congenital subglottic stenosis**. Long-term intubation, a too large tube used in elective interventions, and forceful bronchoscopy are possible causes of **acquired subglottic stenosis**. **Subglottic hemangioma** is observed in the posterolateral part and half of the children display cutaneous hemangiomas as well.

Clinical Significance
- Tracheotomy is indicated in the majority of patients with bilateral vocal cord paralysis in contrast to congenital subglottic stenosis or hemangioma in which only few of the children need tracheotomy

Clinical Presentation
Bilateral vocal cord paralysis leads *after birth to an acute high-pitched inspiratory stridor combined with normal crying* in contrast to the unilateral form with a *weak cry and amelioration after positioning of the child on the involved side.*

Patients with **congenital subglottic stenosis** become symptomatic mostly in the first months of life and *display recurrent signs of respiratory distress in upper respiratory tract infections.* **Hemangioma of the subglottis** leads during the growth of hemangioma in the first months of life to *inspiratory or biphasic stridor that increases at crying.*

Differential Diagnosis, Work-Ups
In addition to the quoted three disorders, laryngo- and tracheobronchomalacia must be considered in the differential diagnosis because the symptomatology is similar.

Direct laryngoscopy is indicated for confirmation of the specific disorder.

Treatment, Prognosis
Bilateral vocal cord paralysis is treated with temporary tracheotomy because spontaneous recovery is possible. Congenital or acquired subglottic stenosis needs in severe forms cricoid split or

endoscopic repair. Severe hemangiomas are treated with steroids or steroids combined with laser therapy.

Prognosis depends on the specific disorder and its severity, and the possibility of permanent relief or spontaneous healing.

9.1.6.2 Tracheal Atresia and Stenosis
Occurrence, Pathoanatomy
Both are rare malformations or acquired disorders. **Tracheal atresia** encompasses at least nine different forms in which a varying length of the trachea is not developed and variable communications of the residual tracheobronchial tree with the esophagus exist or no connection at all. In the most frequently observed forms, the carina joins the esophagus or the two stem bronchi communicate with it separately. Less frequent forms have no connection with the esophagus but a gap between the distal tracheobronchial tree and the proximal trachea or the larynx. In **tracheal stenosis**, the narrowing of lumen is short, segmental, or includes the whole trachea. In more than half of the patients, more than 50 % of the trachea is involved. Segmental stenoses are caused by complete tracheal cartilage rings, and several additional anomalies may accompany tracheal stenosis such as similar involvement of the bronchi, tracheal bronchus, and left pulmonary artery sling.

Clinical Significance
- Congenital subglottic stenosis, tracheal atresia, and stenosis may be suspected by prenatal ultrasound and MRI.
- The majority of tracheal atresia is not amenable to reconstructive surgery with long-term survival because substitute for long-segment tracheal atresia is not available.
- On the other hand, reconstructive surgery with long-term survival is possible for the majority of tracheal stenoses.

Clinical Presentation
The patients with **tracheal atresia** in which communication exists between the residual trachea and esophagus are able to breathe through the esophagus but are *cyanotic and dyspneic*. Those without communication *cannot breathe at all*. In the past, almost all patients died within 24 h due to respiratory insufficiency and/or associated severe cardiovascular malformation. Patient with **tracheal stenosis** are symptomatic from birth or *develop episodic cyanosis, in- and expiratory stridor, and wheezing in the first few months of life. Respiratory tract infection or mucous plugs lead to life-threatening RDS and possible respiratory arrest.*

Differential Diagnosis, Work-Ups
The differential diagnosis includes laryngeal disorders, severe tracheobronchomalacia, and the majority of lesions that lead to RDS in neonates and young infants.

In **tracheal atresia**, suspected diagnosis is confirmed by attempts to intubate the neonate combined with fiber-optic bronchoscopy and contrast application in the esophagus. **Esophageal stenosis** is confirmed by chest x-ray in two plains (outlining the proximal trachea by air accumulation in front of the stenosis and overinflation of the lungs) or ultrasound, and specifically by tracheobronchoscopy with a thin endoscope (site and length of the stenosis and the trachea). Echocardiogram is performed for exclusion of cardiovascular malformation. In addition, 3D reconstruction of the trachea is possible by CT or MRI.

Treatment, Prognosis
Long-term survival in **tracheal atresia** is possible if the anomaly is suspected by prenatal ultrasound and MRI, and tracheostomy is performed as EXIT (ex utero intrapartum treatment) procedure at birth in atresia of short distance that is followed later by primary anastomosis or in case of short-distance, esophageal component of the airway, after initial intubation which is followed by staged reconstructions.

In **tracheal stenosis**, treatment options depend on the site and the length of the stenosis: subglottic stenosis or stenosis of intrathoracic trachea above the carina vs. tracheal stenosis between them and short vs. segmental stenosis. It includes resection followed by primary anastomosis in short and short-segmental stenoses (e.g., 3–7 complete tracheal cartilage rings), slide tracheoplasty [=transverse incision of the trachea followed by superior anterior and inferior posterior longitudinal incision and overlapping anastomosis] without or with resection of maximum stenotic part in long-segmental stenoses (e.g., ≥ 8 complete rings), anterior incision and interposition of autologous cartilage in laryngotracheal (subglottic) stenosis, and resection in tracheal stenosis above the carina followed by longitudinal incision of the left stem bronchus and anastomosis. Tracheoplasty by anterior longitudinal incision and closure of the enlarged trachea by a graft sutured to the edges is also an alternative method for long-segment stenoses.

In contrast to the worse outcome of tracheal atresia, long-term survival is possible for the majority of tracheal stenoses. Possible postoperative formation of granulation tissue needs special consideration.

9.2 Obstruction of the Airways by Disorders with Valve Mechanism

9.2.1 Tracheobronchomalacia (Airway Malacia)

Occurrence, Pathology, Types

The incidence of primary airway malacia is as least 1 in 2,100 children. Tracheobronchomalacia is characterized by deficiency of the cartilage rings and hypotonia of the wall that leads to collapse with in- (extrathoracic) and expiration (intrathoracic) and consequent upper and/or lower airway obstruction.

Airway malacia is either localized (associated with esophageal atresia or H-type of tracheoesophageal fistula, vascular ring anomaly, or mediastinal tumor) or extending over a variable distance as in primary tracheomalacia, bronchomalacia, or the least frequent tracheobronchomalacia. It may be combined with laryngomalacia and is observed in connective tissue disorders such as achondroplasia.

Depending on the institution, more than two thirds or up to 85 % are primary types of airway malacia and nearly one third or 10–15 % secondary types such as the already quoted disorders, those after long-term high-pressure ventilatory support, or repair of severe laryngotracheal clefts.

Clinical Significance

- In the newborn, airway malacia may lead to RDS or extubation failure after surgery.
- Later in life, especially primary tracheobronchomalacia may be difficult to recognize because the clinical findings show overlap with those of common pulmonary diseases.

Clinical Presentation

The clinical manifestation and its course are heterogeneous, and respiratory difficulties due to airway obstruction are scattered from mild to severe.

In newborns and young infants, *RDS is in the foreground that is intensified during feeding* (with additional compression of the trachea between aorta and full distal esophagus), *by stress or pain, and forced respiration. Feeding difficulties in infants may be secondary due to airway malacia.*

Later in life, *brassy cough, expiratory secretory noise (wheeze), and stridor are observed, again increased by eating and drinking as well as recurrent lower respiratory tract infections. The last-mentioned, impaired exercise tolerance, atypical asthma, or asthma that is irreversible or resistant to medicaments, and localized radiological changes due to air-trapping are typical indications of possible airway malacia.* The difficult clinical diagnosis is emphasized by the observation that primary airway malacia is expected by experienced pediatric endoscopists in only 50 %.

In severe types of tracheobronchomalacia, *apneic ("dying") spells or the need of immediate intubation is encountered.*

Auscultation yields the described expiratory secretory noises or wheeze over the trachea and/ or both or one central lung field(s) and intermittently present between infections.

Differential Diagnosis, Work-Ups

The differential diagnosis includes all disorders with RDS of the newborn and young infant and later in life, the common lower respiratory tract, and pulmonic pathologies such as asthma.

Because the clinical diagnosis of airway malacia is difficult, chest x-rays in two plains should be performed in every case for differential diagnostic reasons. Chest fluoroscopy in lateral direction has been performed with video display in former times that demonstrated the air-filled trachea and main stem bronchi disappearing in expiration.

Today, rigid or fiberoptic bronchoscopy is used for diagnosis of airway malacia. It shows the characteristic airway collapse in in- or expiration, the extension of the malacia, and possibly abnormal cartilaginous rings.

Treatment, Prognosis

Therapy of airway malacia is not evidence-based. Spontaneous and resolution after surgical or endoscopic treatment is observed in most of the cases.

Therefore, conservative treatment is indicated in mild and noninvasive ventilation in moderate cases. For severe cases with episodic apnea, severe RDS, significant recurrent lower respiratory tract infections (>3 pneumonias per year), and failure to wean off ventilation, aortopexy, tracheostomy, or stent placement is available. Each procedure has its own indications and drawbacks. Aortopexy (and possibly pulmonary artery truncopexy) is indicated in tracheomalacia secondary to esophageal atresia or vascular ring anomalies and possibly in primary airway malacia. Tracheal patency should be verified by intraoperative tracheoscopy. It may lead to paracardial effusion. Some vascular ring anomalies with short-segment malacia may be treated by tracheal segment resection and other procedures. In addition to the well-known drawbacks of tracheostomy, possibly an extra-long tube becomes necessary or continuous positive airway breathing. Placement of one or several stents is the last therapeutic option because in spite of its effectiveness, it is associated with possible malposition and stent-related morbidity and mortality.

Prognosis

Except for some of the severe cases with fatal outcome (<5 %), most airway malacias gradually become asymptomatic within 1–2 years. Nevertheless, probably lifelong preposition to limitation of vigorous exercise and negative respiratory illness profiles persist.

9.2.2   Lobar Emphysema

Occurrence, Pathology

Congenital lobar emphysema is a rare disorder. Overexpansion of one or two pulmonic lobe(s) or segment(s) is caused by several groups of disorders with different pathophysiological mechanisms. Intrinsic or extrinsic bronchial obstruction by cartilage ring anomalies, vascular malformations (combined with postpartal arrest of alveolar development) or abnormal lung structures with increased number of alveoli (polyalveolar lobe) are the three most frequent encountered pathologies that are likewise responsible for the type of clinical presentation.

Left upper, right middle, or right upper lobe is in order of their citation the most frequently involved part of the lung #. If two lobes are affected mostly, the right middle and left upper lobe are overexpanded.

Beyond the neonatal period, acquired pathologies may lead to segmental or lobar emphysema such as a mucous plug, lymphadenopathy, or foreign body.

Clinical Significance

- Lobar emphysema may lead to life-threatening respiratory distress syndrome in the first days after birth, be mistaken as pneumothorax, and needs urgent or emergency surgery.

Clinical Presentation

The clinical presentation is heterogeneous. *Most of the patients develop within a few days after birth a more or less progressive RDS or become symptomatic after a few months or later by tachypnea, dyspnea, cyanosis, cough, wheezing, and hoarseness.* The development of pneumothorax or pneumonia is never excluded. About one fifth up to one third displays only minor symptoms or is or becomes even asymptomatic.

The involved thoracic side exhibits hyperresonance on percussion in its upper or middle field and diminished breath sounds on auscultation.

Differential Diagnosis, Work-Ups

Mistakes arise more likely from the radiological than from the clinical findings. The differential diagnosis includes mainly pneumothorax (with erroneous insertion of an intercostal drain) and pneumonia (the latter due to initial accumulation of lung fluid). But congenital cystic lung disorders and acquired lung cysts, congenital diaphragmatic hernia, atelectasis with compensatory emphysema, foreign body aspiration, and unilobar congenital lymphangiectasis should be considered as well.

The chest x-ray in two planes exhibits an increased anteroposterior diameter and flattened diaphragm, hyperlucidity of a localized zone in the upper and/or middle field combined with compression of the adjacent lung parts, and possible atelectasis #. In severe cases, mediastinal shift and herniation of parts of the overinflated lobe to the contralateral side is observed.

CT (and vascular MRI) defines the lobar emphysema, its site, and makes possible to differentiate it from other pathologies (and to describe suspected vascular malformations). Echocardiography is recommended for exclusion of possible cardiovascular anomalies which occur in up to 20 %. Blood gas analyses and perfusion scintigraphy are useful for specific questioning.

Therapy, Prognosis
In symptomatic cases, surgery is indicated. Depending on the severity and development of clinical presentation, emergency or elective lobectomy should be performed.

An initial tube thoracostomy may be necessary in extreme clinical presentations. Video-assisted thoracoscopic lobectomy (VATS) is a safe and efficacious alternative except for the need possible conversion into open lobectomy, especially after pneumonia.

In asymptomatic cases or if only a minor symptomatology is present, an observational strategy is possible on condition that no mediastinal shift is present, that long-term follow-up is maintained, and that informed consent of the parents is achieved.

In operated cases, clinically no respiratory embarrassment is observed on long-term follow-up. X-ray exhibits some hyperlucency or normal findings of the ipsilateral lung. The same applies probably for nonoperated patients if the

lobar emphysema becomes not symptomatic later. On the other hand, diminished hyperlucency can be observed in such patients.

9.2.3 Congenital Cystic Lung Disorders, Cystic Adenomatoid Malformation

Occurrence, Pathology
Among the congenital cystic lung disorders, **congenital cystic adenomatoid malformation (CCAM)** is the most frequently encountered form. It consists of cystic parts intermingled with solid elements and appears either cystic or solid depending on the predominance of one part. Although three types have been described, only the macrocystic type with few large cysts and normal alveolar tissue in between and the microcystic type with multiple cysts of less than 1 cm diameter and mixed with alveolar-like structures are of clinical significance.

The less frequent **single or multiple lung cyst(s)** # may be related to the macrocystic type of cystic adenomatoid malformation. Depending on the construction of their walls, bronchiolar or alveolar lung cysts can be differentiated, and on the location of the obstruction to air exchange, the increasing cyst(s) include(s) only multiple acini or acini and bronchioli in its final wall. For multiple cysts involving one lung, the term honeycomb lung has been used.

The described lung cyst(s) are mainly observed in the lower lung lobes, whereas the cystic adenomatoid malformation occurs in about 45 % in the left upper or lower lobe; in one third, in the right upper or lower lobe; and in the remaining, in more than one lobe or bilaterally.

Clinical Significance
- Cystic adenomatoid malformation is the most frequent type of clinically defined congenital lung cysts. It is prenatally recognizable and may be associated with considerable pre- and postnatal morbidity and mortality.
- Some lung cysts become symptomatic by pre- or postnatally effective valve mechanisms if communication exists to the bronchial tree.

Clinical Presentation

The **natural history** of cystic adenomatoid malformation during the second half of pregnancy depends on whether the cyst(s) increase(s) in size (in about one fifth), to which dimension, or if they remain stable. They should be followed by serial ultrasound. Pulmonary hypoplasia, polyhydramnios, and hydrops (in about 10 %, rarely with spontaneous resolution) are the possible sequels of very large and increasing cysts. Such varieties are associated with a significant pre- and postnatal morbidity and mortality. On the other hand, some cysts may decrease in size or even disappear. Thoracoamniotic shunting and fetal pulmonic resection are examples of fetal surgery in large cysts with mediastinal shift and/or hydrops with significant increase of survival rates. After prenatal diagnosis, CT evaluation is necessary in all CCAM (even if they are decreasing in size or disappearing) in the neonatal period, and the question arises, if asymptomatic cases should be operated prophylactically. Defined management plans are very important in pre- and postnatal counseling of the anxious parents.

About three fifths of the surviving newborns with cystic adenomatoid malformation *develop respiratory difficulties such as RDS in the first month of life*. The remaining become symptomatic in the first half of infancy, during childhood, and during adulthood (late-onset CCAM) or remain asymptomatic.

Multiple and single-lung cysts become symptomatic as they achieve a critical size with compression of the ipsilateral parts of the lung and possible mediastinal shift. It occurs usually later than in cystic adenomatoid malformation and earlier if the cysts are multiple than single.

Patients with gross **lung hypoplasia** caused by congenital pulmonary cystic disorders develop pulmonary hypertension and need artificial ventilation or even ECMO to overcome the respiratory insufficiency in the neonatal period.

Congenital pulmonary cystic disorders carry **a risk of infection, malignant degeneration** (rhabdomyosarcoma, bronchoalveolar carcinoma, pleuropulmonary blastoma), or **other complications** if not removed completely.

Differential Diagnosis, Work-Ups

It includes all congenital cystic lung disorders including pulmonary sequestration, bronchogenic cyst, and congenital lobar emphysema which are together with CCAM the 4 most common congenital cystic lung disorders if prenatally the ultrasound finding "hyperechoic lung lesion" is included. They share common histological characteristics such as abnormalities of the bronchial tree and occurrence of CCAM in sequestration and lobar emphysema. Later in life, CT differentiation between intrapulmonary bronchogenic cyst and CCAM may be impossible.

Both forms of congenital diaphragmatic hernia, pneumothorax, acquired lung cystics, for example, pneumatocele after staphylococci pneumonia, complicated purulent pleuropneumonia, isolated lung abscess, and parasitoses also must be considered in the differential diagnosis.

In small children, a seemingly benign cystic lung disorder may correspond to an early stage of **pleuropulmonary blastoma** that develops to a sarcoma within a few years. A combination of several possibly benign or malignant tumors and hamartomas, and multifocal or bilateral lung cysts in the involved patient or young relatives are red flags of a possible cystic pleuropulmonary blastoma and deserve early surgery for histological evaluation. Gross surgical excision has a good prognosis in contrast to the delayed treatment of sarcoma.

Chest x-rays in two plains and Doppler ultrasound (verification of a possible systemic circulation of the malformation) are useful for a preliminary diagnosis ##. CT demonstrates the precise expansion of the congenital pulmonary cystic disorder for planning of surgery or the presence of other differential diagnostically important disorders #.

Therapy, Prognosis

In symptomatic cases surgery is indicated. It includes mostly resection of the involved lobe(s) or segment(s) and may be performed by transthoracic open resection or by video-assisted thoracoscopic surgery (VATS). The latter procedure can be applied electively in prophylactic surgery of asymptomatic cases.

The prophylactic treatment of asymptomatic cases of CCAM and other congenital cystic lung disorders is discussed controversially. If prophylactic resection is performed in the first half of infancy, the following inherent complications are considered: recurrent bronchopneumonias, spontaneous pneumothorax, (massive) hemoptysis, malignancies (pleuropulmonary blastoma, brochoalveolar carcinoma, rhabdomyosarcoma), unnecessary treatments and hospitalizations (without and with loss of information about the underlying disorder), and technical difficulties by early occuring inflammations in spite of missing signs that leads to an increased conversion rate in VATS.

Solitary cysts can be removed by a lung tissue saving enucleation. It should be combined with closure of the draining bronchiolus and if necessary with endorrhaphy of the remaining cavity. Postoperative histological work-up is necessary in all cystic lung disorders.

Prognosis is good if there is no substantial lung hypoplasia. Respiratory signs such as tachypnea or cyanosis may be present already in the quiet child and/or on physical activity of severe hypoplasia. Nonoperated cases need long-term follow-ups as well as operated ones. Surgery has a minimal morbidity and nearly zero mortality. Morbidity includes intraoperative major bleeding in case of former pneumonia, postoperative pneumothorax due to bronchopulmonary fistulas with the possible need of operative closure, and recurrence due to incomplete resection of CCAM (about 5 %), for example, by atypical resection. VATS has conversion rate of less than 5 %.

9.3 Obstruction of Respiration by Intrathoracic Lung Displacement

9.3.1 Congenital Diaphragmatic Hernia

Occurrence, Pathology, Types and Forms
The congenital diaphragmatic hernia has a prevalence of 1 in 3,000 newborns. The congenital defect of the diaphragm leads to a permanent

or intermittent intrauterine (or postpartal) displacement of abdominal viscera in the thorax that includes most or parts of the intestine, the stomach, and the spleen on the left side and parts of the liver and intestinal tract on the right side.

The term "congenital diaphragmatic hernia" (Bochdalek's type) is used in the literature for the most frequently observed type IV with a posterolateral triangular defect of about 2 cm by 4 cm # although other types and another form with different locations and defect sizes occur.

In type I according to Vos et al., the residual diaphragm includes only its medial aspect and possibly a small rim on the lateral thoracic wall. Types II and III are eccentric and roundish defects (without or with a hernia sack) half-way between the anterior and posterior lateral chest wall. The rare diaphragmatic hernia of Morgagni concerns a uni- or bilateral defect at the anteromedial angle of the diaphragm # and Fig. 9.2.

Four fifths of congenital diaphragmatic hernia of the Bochdalek's type is left-sided and one fifth right-sided, and 10–15 % is combined with a hernia sack.

Up to 60 % of congenital diaphragmatic hernias have associated anomalies of which the nonchromosomal syndromes and nonsyndromic multiple anomalies are with 40 % the most frequent group followed by chromosomal aberrations with 30 %. Listed in order of frequency, cardiovascular malformations occur in one fourth followed by urogenital, musculoskeletal, and CNS anomalies.

Clinical Significance
- About one third of the patients with Bochdalek's hernia are stillbirths or die immediately after birth and never reach a tertiary center. This so-called hidden mortality is probably higher if the determination of pregnancy after prenatal diagnosis in the developed countries is considered.
- The surviving individuals are an important cause of severe RDS of the newborn.
- Instead of emergency surgery of former times, respiratory and cardiovascular resuscitation, medical treatment, and prognostication are the primary steps.

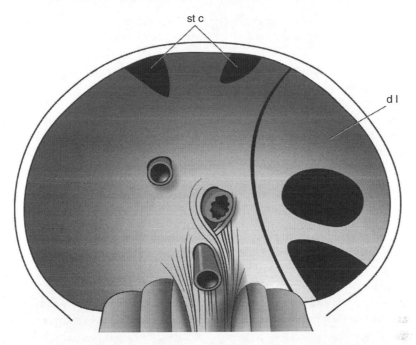

st c

d l

Fig. 9.2 Congenital diaphragmatic hernias. The diagrammatic drawing of the abdominal surface of the diaphragm shows in the middle the physiological apertures of esophagus, aorta, and inferior cava vein. On the left side of the patient, the three different types of dorsolateral diaphragmatic hernia are depicted (*dl*): The common triangular lumbocostal type, the type with an open pleuroperitoneal channel without and with hernia sack, and the less frequent type with open pleuroperitoneal foramen in which the defect encompasses nearly the whole left diaphragm. The term Bochdalek's hernia is used either for all dorsolateral diaphragmatic hernias or only for the lumbocostal type. In the front, the uni- or bilateral sternocostal hernia (*stc*) or Morgagni hernia is depicted

- In a significant proportion of the surviving patients, pulmonary hypoplasia and increased pulmonary artery pressure (with persistent fetal-type of circulation) display a demanding challenge for the intensive care medicine.
- Dependent on the criteria applied for the indication of surgery, the percentage of surviving patients with chronic lung disease is different.

Clinical Presentation

Prenatal diagnosis is possible somewhat before the 20th week of gestation in up to 90 %. It is based on the ultrasound finding of a fluid-filled stomach and/or intestinal loops at the same sectorial level as the heart. The diagnosis is missed in case of sporadic or late herniation of viscera, effacement of the herniation site by parts of the liver, or misinterpretation of the findings as congenital cystic lung or other disorders. The search for associated malformations is mandatory and should be accompanied by amniocentesis for karyotypization. Except for severe malformations such as cardiovascular or CNS anomalies, no safe prognostic findings for a poor outcome are available. Fetal tracheal occlusion therapy against severe lung hypoplasia is a matter of discussion.

Some patients develop a severe RDS immediately after birth and the majority within the next 24 h. A sunken belly contrasts with a unilaterally distended thorax #. Absent breath sounds on the involved side and lateralization of the heart sounds to the contralateral side may be recognized on auscultation.

Ten to twenty percent of the neonates have only mild respiratory signs or are even asymptomatic. *A part of them develops between the second week of life and adolescence at a median age of 2–3 years recurrent unspecific respiratory and/ or gastrointestinal signs or less frequently unexpected signs of surgical abdomen (due to incarceration of stomach or intestine) or RDS. The same applies to adulthood. The presence of* a hernia sack in some of them is not an exclusive explication for the delayed manifestation #.

Work-Ups, Differential Diagnosis

Chest x-ray in two plains is usually sufficient in the newborn for the diagnosis of congenital diaphragmatic hernia except for clinical and radiological findings in which one of the several differential diagnoses is possible or for older children. In such cases, CT and possibly antero- or retrograde contrast studies of the gastrointestinal tract should be performed.

The involved thoracic cavity is filled with multiple circular shadows with a central luminescence or air-fluid levels, and the mediastinum is shifted to the contralateral side #. In right-sided diaphragmatic hernia, the findings may be less distinct with effacement of the diaphragm and a parenchymatous area in the lower lung field.

The differential diagnosis includes all pathologies with RDS of the newborn and later in life, disorders with recurrent vague respiratory and/or gastrointestinal symptoms or acute respiratory signs or signs of a surgical abdomen.

If the radiological findings are included, congenital cystic lung disorders (and here especially the cystic adenomatoid malformation with similar circular shadows but with less regular arrangement and mixed with streaky shadows), eventration of the diaphragm, Morgagni diaphragmatic hernia, pneumothorax, lung lymphangiectasis, and acquired disorders such as multiple pneumatoceles or lower lobe pneumonia must be considered.

Treatment, Prognosis

It includes **resuscitation** (with nasogastric tube, intubation and conventional mechanical ventilation, and arterial and venous access for pre- and postductal blood gas analyses), respiratory and cardiovascular **stabilization**, and simultaneous **work-up examinations** (as quoted above and completed by echocardiogram, ultrasound, and other examinations for possible associated malformations) and **prognostication** (results of blood gas analyses, other examinations, and clinical findings in relation to the applied therapeutic measures).

High-frequency ventilation, NO or other drugs, or ECMO (extracorporeal membrane oxygenation) is applied if complete saturation of the preductal blood with oxygen and ventilation of PCO2 to less than 50 Torr is impossible. Surgery is only performed after a few to several days if control over the increased pulmonary artery pressure is achieved.

Surgery is mostly performed by an abdominal subcostal approach on the left and by a transthoracic approach on the right side. After gentle reduction of the viscera from the thorax # (reduction may be complicated in abnormal drainage of the hepatic vein or gross herniation of the liver with involvement of the pericardium), the whole intestine is inspected for malformations and pressure marks from the edges of the diaphragmatic defect with possible postoperative ileus. The defect is closed by interrupted nonabsorbable stitches (in case of hernia sac, after resection) or by a prosthetic patch or a reconstructive technique using adjacent tissue. To avoid a possible abdominal compartment syndrome, the abdominal wall is stretched, the meconium is expressed from the intestine, and all layers of the incision are only closed if easily possible. Otherwise, only the skin is closed or an interposed prosthetic siphon is used that is followed by a regular abdominal wall closure as soon as possible.

Prognosis depends on the following factors: severe associated anomalies, severity of lung hypoplasia and reversibility of increased pulmonary artery hypertension, and complications due to and during medical treatment (such as hemorrhages by ECMO or intestinal complications) and due to surgery (such as abdominal compartment syndrome or recurrence of diaphragmatic defect).

The reported survival rates are not uniform, and long-term results about the quality of life not yet available for the quoted treatment strategy in a large number of patients. Although a normal daily life is reported in most of the children, some of the following restrictions may be imposed on some individuals of older cohorts: Developmental delay and abnormalities of cognitive skills, nutritional and respiratory problems related to the frequently observed gastroesophageal reflux, mild restrictive small airway disorder and diminished physical performance, and thoracic asymmetries and scoliosis. Although lung functions achieve normal levels during childhood, some overinflation and diminished pulmonary blood flow remains throughout life.

9.3.2   Diaphragmatic Hernia of Morgagni

Occurrence, Pathology
Morgagni hernia occurs in about 5 % of all congenital diaphragmatic hernias. The defect of the sternocostal angle of the diaphragm is observed more frequently on the right side (Morgagni hernia) than on the left side (Larrey hernia), and at least one third is bilateral (Larrey-Morgagni hernia) and rarely with one single defect and sac. Frequently associated anomalies are encountered such as congenital heart disease, intestinal malrotation, and chromosomal aberrations (Down syndrome).

Clinical Significance
- Although Morgagni hernia is observed only rarely and diagnosis is difficult, prompt recognition is mandatory due to the inherent gastrointestinal complications.
- Often unexpectedly, bilaterality is recognized by radiological imaging or surgery.

Clinical Presentation
Infrequently, Morgagni hernia is recognized already prenatally by progressive herniation of viscera such as liver herniation in the pericardium and/or leads to RDS of the newborn.
In the majority of cases, Morgagni hernia manifests with subacute or chronic unspecific respiratory symptoms (recurrent chest infections) or is recognized incidentally either by chest x-ray or on the occasion of abdominal trauma or surgery at a mean age of 1–2 years (two thirds are younger than 1 year) from early infancy to school-age. *In about 15 %, acute presentation is observed mainly as surgical abdomen with unilateral tenderness of the epigastrium* after entrance of parts of the gastrointestinal tract, omentum, or liver in the hernia sac with possible obstruction or incarceration.

Few cases remain asymptomatic till adulthood and are detected incidentally or manifest with chronic recurrent vague gastrointestinal or respiratory complaints and occasionally as a surgical abdomen.

Work-Ups, Differential Diagnosis
Morgagni hernia may be suspected or recognized by chest x-ray in two plains by the findings of either a solid paracardial and anterior mass # or (an) air-fluid level(s). Diagnostics are CT or antero- or retrograde contrast studies of the gastrointestinal tract (if gastrointestinal parts have entered the hernia sac). For recognition of asymptomatic cases and search for bilaterality pneumoperitoneum has been used in the past. Today, CT or diagnostic laparoscopy is the main tool.

The differential diagnoses depend on the often unspecific clinical and radiological presentation, for example, anterior mediastinal tumor or hiatus hernia. In acute situations, lower lobe pneumonia or other causes of surgical abdomen are mostly considered.

Therapy
Surgery is indicated in symptomatic and asymptomatic patients (incidental finding, asymptomatic contralateral side). Except for cases with acute surgical abdomen, open transabdominal or transthoracic # and laparoscopic approach are suitable procedures. After reposition of the possible content, the hernia sac is resected and the defect is closed by nonabsorbable sutures or if large by a prosthetic patch. The transthoracic approach may be useful in case of intrathoracic adhesions of hernia sac or adhesions within the sac. In laparoscopic surgery, the sac is left behind after reduction of the content and inclusion of it in the stitches without or with a patch.

The prognosis is good although recurrences are not excluded.

9.3.3   Diaphragmatic Eventration

Occurrence, Pathology

Diaphragmatic eventration is a unilateral or less frequently bilateral elevation of the diaphragm due to flaccid muscle fibers. Congenital deficiency of the diaphragm and generalized neuromuscular diseases or acquired phrenic nerve paralysis after birth injury or following cardiac and thoracic surgery belong to the main large groups of diaphragmatic eventration. The degree of functional loss and capacity for recovery are different from case to case.

Clinical Significance

- Unilateral eventration leads to displacement of the ipsilateral lung and mediastinum; it is less well tolerated by neonates and infants than by older patients.
- Acquired bilateral eventrations need mechanical ventilatory support.
- Persistent asymptomatic eventration may be associated with troublesome recurrent or acute life-threatening gastric volvulus.

Clinical Presentation

Depending on the age and the degree of diaphragmatic involvement, *the symptomatology varies from respirator dependency and RDS to tachypnea, wheezing, recurrent bronchopneumonia, and failure to thrive*. For instance, even bilateral forms of congenital diaphragmatic eventration may remain undetected until adolescence.

Persistent eventrations may lead to *recurrent vomiting, dysphagia, and epigastric pain or surgical abdomen* due to recurrent or life-threatening **gastric volvulus** that is mostly associated with diaphragmatic anomalies.

In severe forms, ventilation and perfusion of the ipsilateral lung may be impaired in spite of absent symptoms.

Acquired diaphragmatic eventration must be considered in a newborn with RDS after a difficult birth with (in three fourths of all phrenic nerve palsies) or without **Erb's palsy** and/or clavicular fracture, or in children following heart or thoracic tumor surgery. The reported incidence of phrenic nerve palsy after **heart surgery** is 1.5 %

(up to 10 %), occurs mainly after previous cardiac surgery, and two fifths need diaphragmatic plication mostly at the age of less than 2 years.

Work-Ups, Differential Diagnosis

The leading radiological sign is elevation of the diaphragm in pa and lateral chest x-rays #, and diagnosis is confirmed by the sniff test by demonstration of paradox motions of the diaphragm on fluoroscopy. Differentiation between congenital eventration and paralyzed diaphragm is possible by evaluation of the shape or curvature of the diaphragm in the lateral chest x-ray. Ultrasound or CT is an additional examination to avoid fluoroscopy.

The differential diagnosis includes mainly congenital diaphragmatic hernia with a hernia sac and elevation due to lung hypo- or aplasia and disorders with reduction of the lung volume. Occasionally, newborns with RDS and pneumothorax develop temporary elevation of the diaphragm after chest tube insertion.

Therapy, Prognosis

In general, plication of the diaphragm # is indicated in persistently symptomatic children, in asymptomatic children with proven functional impairment of the ipsilateral lung, or as prevention from gastric volvulus. In children of less than 2 years of age with respirator dependency or RDS, surgery is indicated if there is no recovery of the phrenic nerve paresis after 1 month. The reported incidence of children who need plication is two thirds for congenital eventration and phrenic nerve paresis after birth injury and as quoted above less after cardiac surgery.

Surgery is performed by a transthoracic or alternatively, by an abdominal incision (more frequently on the left than on the right side). The former approach permits recognition of the point of entrance of the phrenic nerve, evaluation of a suspected diaphragmatic hernia with a sac, and an easier repair of a central eventration. The latter is useful if plication is combined with gastropexy.

After folding of the diaphragm in a frontal or sagittal plane, the base of the plica is sutured to the diaphragm with nonabsorbable stitches, and the plica is either sutured to the ribs or to the diaphragm avoiding the nonvisible main branches of the phrenic nerve. To avoid recurrences, the chosen plica should permit a tight reconstruction of the diaphragm.

If thoracoscopic plication is performed, lack of space may be a problem despite of insufflation into the pleural cavity.

A dramatic resolution of the symptomatology can be observed in most patients, and discontinuation of mechanical respiration is reported within a mean time of 3 days. In more than 90 %, a normal position of the diaphragm is achieved with almost immobility and without paradoxical motion. Preexisting gastroesophageal reflux is not resolved by plication.

9.3.4   Chylothorax

Occurrence, Pathology, Causes
Chylothorax is a relatively rare disorder that has attracted increased attention due to the frequency of cardiothoracic surgery and intensive care measures and progress in its treatment.

A lesion of the thoracic duct leads to escape of chyle in the thoracic cavity and specifically in the pleural space with pulmonary compression.

In neonates, birth injury, malformation of the thoracic duct, mediastinal lymphangioma or lymphangiomatosis of the adjacent bones, and spontaneous chylothorax must be considered as possible causes. Cardiothoracic surgery, superior vena cava thrombosis (e.g., after central venous catheter), rupture of the thoracic duct as a result of a violent bout of coughing or stretching maneuvers in sports, and malignancies become more important causes later in life.

Clinical Significance
- Chylothorax leads to a severe RDS in at least half of the involved neonates and young infants and possible respirator dependency. The remaining and older children develop less severe respiratory symptoms.
- In the long-term course, malnutrition and immune incompetence develop due to the enormous loss of fat, protein, and T cell lymphocytes.

Clinical Presentation
RDS or cyanosis, tachy- or dyspnea, and possible failure to thrive is the typical symptomatology.

The pleural effusion may be present already prenatally, is more frequently uni- than bilateral, and is recognizable by dullness on percussion, decreased breathing sounds, and diminished respiratory motion of the involved hemithorax. A right-sided effusion points to a leak of the thoracic duct in its lower part and a left-sided to a leak in its uppermost part. The chyle becomes only milky after beginning of oral nutrition. Before and pre- or postnatally, the chyle is clear or light yellow.

Work-Ups, Differential Diagnosis
Chest x-ray in two plains yields mostly a unilateral opaque hemithorax with contralateral mediastinal shift. After commencement of oral nutrition, the relatively radiolucent effusion demonstrates distinctly the lateral border of the ipsilateral compressed lung. Additional examinations are performed for evaluation of the suspected cause and/or nutritional and immunological state (e.g., possible lymphopenia).

The differential diagnosis includes other disorders of RDS (e.g., congenital diaphragmatic hernia) or less severe respiratory symptomatology and other types of pleural effusion. It also depends on the suspected cause of chylothorax and its clinical presentation.

Treatment, Prognosis
It includes mechanical respiration if needed, repeated thoracocenteses or better thoracotomy tube drainage (with quantification of the removed chyle), and total parenteral nutrition (instead of the less effective oral medium-chain triglyceride nutrition).

Depending on the age of the patient and the supposed cause of chylothorax, the medical treatment is continued for 4 weeks (e.g., in neonates) or less time and if not effective, completed by a pleuroperitoneal shunt with the need of regular postoperative pumping. The former transthoracic closure of the leak (by duct ligation below and above the leak) is today replaced by either shunting (with a success rate in three fourths) or video-assisted thoracoscopic procedure. This minimally invasive treatment cannot only better demonstrate the site of the leak but also allows closure of the duct at an earlier stage of chylothorax.

Prognosis depends on the cause of chylothorax. Most chylothoraces of the newborn disappear within 1–2 to 7–8 weeks with medical treatment and additional 1–3 months of shunting.

9.3.5 Mediastinal Tumor

Mediastinal tumor may be an important cause of obstruction of respiration by intrathoracic lung displacement. The reader is referred to the Chap. 8.

9.3.6 Surgical Abdomen

In general, every child with a surgical abdomen and specifically, every newborn and young infant with such a condition may display a very prominent belly in such a way that a disproportion between the size of the abdominal and the thoracic cavity results. In such cases, a secondary RDS develops due to the extreme elevation and immobilization of the diaphragm. If only a supradiaphragmatic cause of RDS is considered, the surgical abdomen may be missed. For the surgical abdomen, the reader is referred to Chap. 14.

9.4 Obstruction of Respiration by Decreased Pulmonary Reserve (Parenchymal Deficit)

9.4.1 Pulmonary Hypoplasia

Pathology, Causes
Several intrauterine disorders lead to a bi- or unilateral lung hypoplasia with consequent parenchymal deficit. The lung(s) remain(s) small and differentiation is permanently or transitorily delayed for various degrees.

Oligohydramnios in obstructive uropathies such as urethral valves or bilateral ureteropelvic junction obstruction, continuous loss of amniotic fluid, dysplasias of the thoracic cage, pleural effusions, congenital cystic lung disorders, diaphragmatic hernia #, and diaphragmatic eventration are possible causes of uni- or bilateral lung hypoplasia. Compression of one or both lung(s) is considered as the common pathophysiological mechanism of hypoplasia.

Pulmonary artery agenesis is combined with hypoplasia of the ipsilateral lung and occurs more frequently together with cardiac anomalies. **Unilateral lobar hypoplasia** is a rare example of a primary type of hypoplasia.

Clinical Significance
- Hypoplasia may lead to lethal respiratory insufficiency or to RDS shortly after birth and to exertional dyspnea later in life.
- For the pediatric surgeon, uni- and bilateral lung hypoplasia has prognostic implications such as indication of early surgery of the underlying disorder and final outcome and is an appeal for research (irreversibility of hypoplasia vs. possible delayed maturation).

Clinical Presentation
Postnatal death due to respiratory insufficiency, RDS with or without ventilator dependency, and respiratory signs due to recurrent bronchopulmonary infections and exercise stress on follow-up are the symptoms and signs and depend on the cause of hypoplasia, its degree, and extension,

Work-Ups, Differential Diagnosis
The clinical diagnosis of lung hypoplasia is possible by combination of a specific diagnosis (e.g., congenital diaphragmatic hernia) with possibly treatment-resistant signs of respiratory insufficiency. It may be supported by radiological signs on chest x-ray and CT or pulmonary functional tests. For instance, absent re-expansion of the ipsilateral lung after repair of diaphragmatic hernia points to hypoplasia. Final confirmation of hypoplasia needs histological work-up.

The differential diagnosis includes other causes of RDS in the neonate and young infant and respiratory signs in older children.

Treatment, Prognosis
Treatment options concern secondary and associated disorders of hypoplasia such as medication of recurrent respiratory tract infections and amelioration of increased vascular tone in persistent chronic pulmonary artery hypertension.

Prognosis depends on the degree of hypoplasia and the supposed possibility of delayed maturation. As long as the different disorders with pulmonary hypoplasia are not categorized and not followed prospectively with reliable parameters, precise outcome statements about lung hypoplasia are impossible.

9.4.2   Lung Aplasia and Agenesis, Post-Pneumonectomy Lung

Pathology
Single-lung patients have either a congenital aplasia (with carina and blindly ending stem bronchus), congenital agenesis of the lung (without any bronchial remnants), or had a pneumonectomy for different causes in the past.

Clinical Significance
- Single-lung patients have significant morbidity and mortality risks.
- Morbidity arises in congenital and acquired types from possible airway obstruction and decreased pulmonary reserve, and in addition from associated anomalies in congenital and from the underlying pathology in acquired types.

Clinical Presentation
Today, aplasia and agenesis may be suspected by prenatal ultrasound, and *a substantial part of them exhibits an RDS in the newborn period and recurrent respiratory infections and exertional dyspnea later in life.*

Chronic and acute respiratory insufficiency is possibly at any time due to airway obstruction in congenital and acquired single-lung patients

and in the latter by mediastinal shift of the contralateral lung with kinking of the tracheobronchial tree.

Work-Ups, Differential Diagnosis
In addition to prenatal ultrasound and possible MRI, after birth chest x-rays, CT, and in case of clinical manifestation, tracheobronchoscopy are the main diagnostic tools.

Prior or after birth and on follow-up, the differential diagnosis includes all disorders with similar findings and signs as lung aplasia or agenesis (e.g., foreign body aspiration in case of congenital unilateral lobar hypoplasia).

Therapy, Prognosis
Treatment is similar to lung hypoplasia. Surgery may become necessary in airway obstruction, in acquired types by implantation of an expander on the ipsilateral side.

Deaths result in acquired single-lung patients from recurrence of the underlying disease and in congenital aplasia from different causes in about half of the cases.

9.4.3   Anomalies of the Thoracic Cage

Generalized thoracic cage anomalies in the context of different syndromes with a too small thoracic cavity and deformed chest wall lead to respiratory failure or RDS in the newborn and cause in case of survival permanent reduction of lung function (due to lung hypoplasia and abnormal respiratory mechanism).

9.5   Obstruction of Respiration by Airway Aspiration

The following disorders are classic examples to demonstrate how a secondary RDS may come in the foreground of the clinical presentation if aspiration occurs into the laryngotracheobronchial tree as result of the primary symptomatology **"regurgitation or vomiting."**

9.5.1 Esophageal Atresia and Gastroesophageal Reflux

The leading sign of both are regurgitation and vomiting. As result of combined aspiration into the respiratory tract, laryngitis, tracheobronchitis, and bronchopneumonia develop. RDS or other signs of the respiratory tract involvement are now predominant.

In every case of RDS of the newborn or young infant, the individual cause of respiratory obstruction must be considered preferentially including secondary RDS due to aspiration. The same applies to the surgical abdomen or disorders of sucking and swallowing.

Webcodes

The following webcodes can be used on www. psurg.net for further images and data.

901 RDS young infant	914 x-ray chest, right cystic adenomatoidmalformation
902 Choanal atresia	915 CT, right cystic adenomatoid malformation
903 Cervicofacial cystic lymphangioma	916 Classic diaphragmatic hernia
904 Tongue teratoma	917 Types of congenital diaphragmatic hernias
905 Macroglossia (hemangioma)	918 RDS, diaphragmatic hernia
906 Cystic lymphohemangioma mouth	919 Diaphragmatic hernia with hernia sack
907 RDS Pierre Robin syndrome	920 Chest x-ray, diaphragmatic hernia
908 Retrognathia (Pierre Robin sequence)	921 Operative reduction diaphragmatic hernia
909 Prone position, Pierre Robin syndrome	922 Chest x-ray, Morgagni hernia
910 Lobar emphysema	923 Left (Morgagni) diaphragmatic hernia
911 X-ray chest, right upper lobe emphysema	924 Right phrenic nerve paralysis
912 Multilocular lung cyst	925 Plication for diaphragmatic eventration
913 Chest x-ray, lung cyst	926 Hypoplastic left lung

Bibliography

General: Textbooks, Differential Diagnosis, Radiological Imaging, Fetal Treatment, Surgery

Berrocal T, Madrid C, Novo S, Gutiérrez J, Arjonilla A, Gomez-Leon N (2004a) Congenital anomalies of the tracheobronchial tree, lung, and mediastinum: embryology, radiology and pathology. Radiographics 24(1): e17

Coley BD (2011) Chest sonography in children: current indications, techniques, and imaging findings. Radiol Clin North Am 49:825–846

Corbett HJ, Mann KS, Mitra I, Jesudason EC, Losty PD, Clarke RW (2007) Tracheostomy – a 10-year experience from a UK pediatric surgical center. J Pediatr Surg 42:1251–1254

Daniel SJ (2006) The upper airway: congenital malformations. Paediatr Respir Rev 7(Suppl 1):S260–S263

Holinger LD (1999) Histopathology of congenital subglottic stenosis. Ann Otol Rhinol Laryngol 108: 101–111

Huddleston CB (2006) Pediatric lung transplantation. Semin Pediatr Surg 15:199–207

Lee EY, Dorkin H, Vargas SO (2011) Congenital pulmonary malformations in pediatric patients: review and update on etiology, classification, and imaging findings. Radiol Clin North Am 49:921–948

Ley-Zaporozhan J, Ley S, Sommerburg O, Komm N, Müller FM, Schenk JP (2009) Clinical application of MRI in children for the assessment of pulmonary disease. Rofo 181:419–432

Shanmugam G, MacArthur K, Pollock JC (2005) Congenital lung malformations – antenatal and postnatal evaluation and management. Eur J Cardiothorac Surg 27:45–52

Wagner W, Harrison MR (2002) Fetal operations in the head and neck area: current state. Head Neck 24: 482–490

Weinberger M, Abu-Hasan M (2007) Pseudo-asthma: when cough, wheezing, and dyspnea are not asthma. Pediatrics 120:855–864

Section 9.1.1

Burrow TA, Saal HM, de Alarcon A, Martin LJ, Cotton RT, Hopkin RJ (2009) Characterization of congenital anomalies in individuals with choanal atresia. Arch Otolaryngol Head Neck Surg 135:543–547

Dave A (2002) Absent nasal flaring in a newborn with bilateral choanal stenosis. Pediatrics 109:989–990

Dobbelsteyn C, Peacocke SD, Blake K, Crist W, Rashid M (2008) Feeding difficulties in children with

CHARGE syndrome: prevalence, risk factors, and prognosis. Dysphagia 23:127–135

Durmaz A, Tosun F, Yldrm N, Sahan M, Kvrakdal C, Gerek M (2008) Transnasal endoscopic repair of choanal atresia: results of 13 cases and meta-analysis. J Craniofac Surg 19:1270–1274

Hengerer AS, Brickman TM, Jeyakumar A (2008) Choanal atresia: embryologic analysis and evolution of treatment, a 30-year experience. Laryngoscope 118: 862–866

Osovsky M, Aizer-Danon A, Horev G, Sirota L (2007) Congenital pyriform aperture stenosis. Pediatr Radiol 37:97–99

Ramsden JD, Campisi P, Forte V (2009) Choanal atresia and choanal stenosis. Otolaryngol Clin North Am 42: 339–352

Samadi DS, Shah UK, Handler SD (2003) Choanal atresia: a twenty-year review of medical comorbidities and surgical outcomes. Laryngoscope 113:254–258

Sanlaville D, Verloes A (2007) CHARGE syndrome: an update. Eur J Hum Genet 15:389–399

Schraff SA, Vijayasekaran S, Meinzen-Derr J, Myer CM (2006) Management of choanal atresia in CHARGE association patients: a retrospective review. Int J Pediatr Otorhinolaryngol 70:1291–1297

Triglia JM, Nicollas R, Roman S, Paris J (2003) Choanal atresia: therapeutic management and results in a series of 58 children. Rev Laryngol Otol Rhinol (Bord) 124: 65–69

Section 9.1.2

Cohen RL (1984) Clinical perspectives on premature tooth eruption and cyst formation in neonates. Pediatr Dermatol 1:301–303

Green LK, Mawn LA (2002) Orbital cellulitis secondary to tooth bud abscess in a neonate. J Pediatr Ophthalmol Strabismus 39:358–361

Izadi K, Smith M, Askari M, Hackam D, Hameed AA, Bradley JP (2003) A patient with an epignathus: management of a large oropharyngeal teratoma in a newborn. J Craniofac Surg 14:468–472

Kujan O, Clark S, Sloan P (2007) Leiomyomatous hamartoma presenting as a con-genital epulis. Br J Oral Maxillofac Surg 45:228–230

Kumar Dutta H (2009) Jaw and gum tumours in children. Pediatr Surg Int 25:781–784

Kumar B, Sharma SB (2008) Neonatal oral tumors: congenital epulis and epignathus. J Pediatr Surg 43: e9–e11

Küpers AM, Andriessen P, van Kempen MJ, van der Tol IG, Baart JA, Dumans AG, van der Waal I (2009) Congenital epulis of the jaw: a series of five cases and review of literature. Pediatr Surg Int 25:207–210

Mueller DT, Callanan VP (2007) Congenital malformations of the oral cavity. Otolaryngol Clin North Am 40:141–160, vii

Narasimhan K, Arneja JS, Rabah R (2007) Treatment of congenital epulis (granular cell tumor) with excision and gingivoperiosteoplasty. Can J Plast Surg 15: 215–218

Reinshagen K, Wessel LM, Roth H, Waag KL (2002) Congenital epulis: a rare diagnosis in paediatric surgery. Eur J Pediatr Surg 12:124–126

Silva GCC, Vieira TC, Vieira JC, Martins CR, Silva EC (2007) Congenital granular cell tumor (congenital epulis): a lesion of multidisciplinary interest. Med Oral Patol Oral Cir Bucal 12:E428–E430

Vandenhaute B, Leteurtre E, Lecompte-Houcke M, Pellerin P, Nuyts JP, Chisset JM, Soto-Ares G (2000) Epignathus teratoma: report of three cases with a review of the literature. Cleft Palate Craniofac J 37:83–91

Section 9.1.3

Bloom DC, Perkins JA, Manning SC (2009) Management of lymphatic malformations and macroglossia: results of a national treatment survey. Int J Pediatr Otorhinolaryngol 73:1114–1118

Guimaraes CV, Donnelly LF, Shott SR, Amin RS, Kalra M (2008) Relative rather than absolute macroglossia in patients with Down syndrome: implications for treatment of obstructive sleep apnea. Pediatr Radiol 38: 1062–1067

Jian XC (2005) Surgical management of lymphangiomatous or lymphangiohemangiomatous macroglossia. J Oral Maxillofac Surg 63:15–19

Matsune K, Miyoshi K, Kosaki R, Ohashi H, Maeda T (2006) Taste after reduction of the tongue in Beckwith-Wiedemann syndrome. Br J Oral Maxillofac Surg 44: 49–51

Maturo SC, Mair EA (2006a) Submucosal minimally invasive lingual excision: an effective, novel surgery for pediatric tongue base reduction. Ann Otol Rhinol Laryngol 115:624–630

Ugar-Cankal D, Denizci S, Hocaoglu T (2005) Prevalence of tongue lesions among Turkish schoolchildren. Saudi Med J 26:1962–1967

Section 9.1.4

Bijnen CL, Don Griot PJ, Mulder WJ, Haumann TJ, Van Hagen AJ (2009) Tongue-lip adhesion in the treatment of Pierre Robin sequence. J Craniofac Surg 20:315–320

Bravo G, Ysunza A, Arrieta J, Pamplona MC (2006) Videonasopharyngoscopy is useful for identifying

children with Pierre Robin sequence and severe
obstructive sleep apnea. Int J Pediatr Otorhinolaryngol
69:27–33

De Buys Roessingh AS, Herzog G, Cherpillod J, Trichet-
Zbinden C, Hohlfeld J (2008) Speech prognosis and
need for pharyngeal flap for non syndromic vs syndromic Pierre Robin sequence. J Pediatr Surg
43:668–674

Drescher FD, Jotzo M, Goelz R, Meyer TD, Bacher M,
Poets CF (2008) Cognitive and psychosocial develop-
ment of children with Pierre Robin sequence. Acta
Paediatr 97:653–656

Evans AK, Rahbar R, Rogers GF, Mulliken JB, Volk MS
(2006) Robin sequence: a retrospective review of 115
patients. Int J Pediatr Otorhinolaryngol 70:973–980

Kirschner RE, Low DW, Randall P, Bartlett SP, McDonald-
McGinn DM, Schultz PJ, Zackai EH, LaRossa D
(2003) Surgical airway management in Pierre Robin
sequence: is there a role for tongue-Lip adhesion?
Cleft Palate Craniofaci J 40:13–18

Marques IZ, de Sousa TV, Carneiro AF, Barbieri MA,
Bettiol H, Gutierrez MR (2001) Clinical experience
with infants with Robin sequence: a prospective study.
Cleft Palate Craniofac J 38:171–178

Marques IL, Monteiro LC, de Souza L, Bettiol H, Sassaki
CH, de Assumpcao CR (2009) Gastroesophageal
reflux in severe cases of Robin sequence treated with
nasopharyngeal intubation. Cleft Palate Craniofac J
46:448–453

Meyer AC, Lidsky ME, Sampson DE, Lander TA, Liu M,
Sidman JD (2008) Airway interventions in children
with Pierre Robin sequence. Otolaryngol Head Neck
Surg 138:782–787

Mondini CC, Marques IL, Fontes CM, Thomé S (2009)
Nasopharyngeal intubation in Robin sequence: technique and management. Cleft Palate Craniofac J
46:258–261

Nassar E, Marques IL, Trindade AS Jr, Bettiol H (2006)
Feeding-facilitating techniques for nursing infant with
Robin sequence. Cleft Palate Craniofac J 43:55–60

Palit G, Jacquemyn Y, Kerremans M (2008) An objective
measurement to diagnose micrognathia on prenatal
ultrasound. Clin Exp Obstet Gynecol 35:121–123

Roy S, Munson PD, Zhao L, Holinger LD, Patel PK
(2009) CT analysis after distraction osteogenesis in
Pierre Robin sequence. Laryngoscope 119:380–386

Singh DJ, Bartlett SP (2005) Congenital mandibular hypoplasia: analysis and classification. J Craniofac Surg
16:291–300

Smith MC, Senders CW (2006) Prognosis of airway
obstruction and feeding difficulty in the Robin
sequence. Int J Pediatr Otorhinolaryngol 70:319–324

Section 9.1.5

Chien W, Ashland J, Haver K, Hardy SC, Curren P,
Hartnick GJ (2006) Type 1 laryngeal cleft: establishing a functional diagnostic and management algorithm. Int J Pediatr Otorhinolaryngol 70:2073–2079

Delahunty JE, Cherry J (1969) Congenital laryngeal cleft.
Ann Otolaryngol 78:96–106

Denahoe PK, Gee PE (1984) Complete laryngotracheoesophageal cleft: management and repair. J Pediatr Surg
19:143–148

Kawaguchi AL, Donahoe PK, Ryan DP (2005)
Management and long-term follow-up of patients with
types III and IV laryngotracheoesophageal clefts. J
Pediatr Surg 40:158–164

Mathur NN, Peek GJ, Bailey CM, Elliott MJ (2006)
Strategies for managing type IV laryngotracheoesophageal clefts at Great Ormond Street Hospital
for Children. Int J Pediatr Otorhinolaryngol 70:
1901–1910

Maturo SI, Mair EA (2006b) Submucosal minimally invasive lingual excision: an effective, novel surgery for
pediatric tongue base reduction. Ann Otol Rhinol
Laryngol 115:624–630

Nassar E, Marques IL, Trindade AS Jr, Bettiol H (2006)
Feeding-facilitating techniques for nursing infant with
Robin sequence. Cleft Palate Craniofac J 43:55–60

Printzlau A, Andersen M (2004) Pierre robin sequence in
Denmark: a retrospective population-based epidemiological study. Cleft Palate Craniofac J 41:47–52

Rahbar R, Chen JL, Rosen RL, Lowry KC, Simon DM,
Perez JA, Buonomo C, Ferrari LR, Katz ES (2009)
Endoscopic repair of laryngeal cleft type I and type II:
when and why? Laryngoscope 119:1797–1802

Section 9.1.6

Backer CL, Kelle AM, Mavroudis C, Rigsby CK, Kaushal
S, Holinger LD (2009) Tracheal reconstruction in children with unilateral lung agenesis or severe hypoplasia. Ann Thorac Surg 88:624–630; discussion
630–631

Cotton RT, Willging JP (1998) Otolaryngological disorders. In: O'Neill JA Jr et al (eds) Pediatric surgery, vol 1,
5th edn. Mosby, St. Louis

De Lorimier AA (1998) Respiratory problems related to
the airway and lung. In: O'Neill JA Jr et al (eds)
Pediatric surgery, vol 1, 5th edn. Mosby, St. Louis

Filler RM, Forte W (1998) Lesions of the larynx and trachea. In: O'Neill JA Jr et al (eds) Pediatric surgery, vol 1,
5th edn. Mosby, St. Louis

Heyer CM, Nuesslein TG, Jung D, Peters SA, Lemburg
SP, Rieger CH, Nicolas V (2007) Tracheobronchial
anomalies and stenoses: detection with low-dose multidetector CT with virtual tracheobronchoscopy – comparison with flexible tracheobronchoscopy. Radiology
242:542–549

Lupi M, Bonetti LR, Trani N, Maccio L, Maiorana A
(2009) Congenital tracheal atresia in newborns: case
report and review of the literature. Pathologica
101:235–239

Schweizer P, Berger S, Petersen M, Kischner HJ, Schweizer M (2005) Tracheal surgery in children. Eur J Pediatr Surg 15:236–242

Section 9.2.1

Anton-Pacheco JL, Cabezali D, Tejedor R, Lopez M, Luna C, Comas JV, deMiguel E (2008) The role of airway stenting in pediatric tracheobronchial obstruction. Eur J Cardiothorac Surg 33:1069–1075

Boogaard R, Huijsmans SH, Pijnenburg MW, Tiddens HA, deJongste JC, Merkus PJ (2005) Tracheomalacia and bronchomalacia in children: incidence and patients characteristics. Chest 128:3391–3397; comment in: Chest 2006; 130:304; republished in Ned Tijdschr Geneeskd 2006; 16; 150: 2037–2042

Corbally MT, Spitz L, Kiely E, Brereton RJ, Drake DP (1993) Aortopexy for tracheomalacia in oesopgageal anomalies. Eur J Pediatr Surg 3:264–266

De Lorimier AA (1998) Respiratory problems related to the airway and lung. In: O'Neill JA Jr et al (eds) Pediatric surgery, vol 1, 5th edn. Mosby, St. Louis

Fayon M, Donato L (2010) Tracheomalacia (TM) or bronchomalacia (BM) in children: conservative or invasive therapy? Arch Pediatr 17:97–104

Finder JD (1997) Primary bronchomalacia in infants and children. J Pediatr 130:59–66

Kamata S, Usui N, Sawai T, Nose K, Kitayama Y, Okuyama H, Okada A (2000) Pexis of the great vessels for patients with tracheobronchomalacia in infancy. J Pediatr Surg 35:454–457

Masters IB, Chang AB, Patterson L, Wainwright C, Buntain H, Dean BW, Francis PW (2002) Series of laryngomalacia, tracheomalacia, and bronchomalacia disorders and their associations with other conditions in children. Pediatr Pulmonol 34:189–195

Masters IB, Zimmerman PV, Pandeya N, Petsky HL, Wilson SB, Chang AB (2008) Quantified tracheobronchomalacia disorders and their clinical profiles in children. Chest 133:461–467

Valerie EP, Durrant AC, Forte V, Wales P, Chait P, Kim PC (2005) A decade of using intraluminal tracheal/bronchial stents in the management of tracheomalacia and/or bronchomalacia: is it better than aortopexy? J Pediatr Surg 40:904–907; discussion 907

Section 9.2.2

Bush A (2009) Prenatal presentation and postnatal management of congenital thoracic malformations. Early Hum Dev 85:679–684

Chapdelaine J, Beaunoyer M, St-Vil D, Oligny LL, Garel L, Bütter A, Di Lorenzo M (2004) Unilobar congenital pulmonary lymphangiectasis mimicking congenital lobar emphysema: an underestimated presentation? J Pediatr Surg 39:677–680

Dogan R, Dogan OF, Yilmaz M, Demircin M, Passoglu M, Kiper N, Ozcelik U, Boke E (2004) Surgical management of infants with congenital lobar emphysema and concomitant congenital heart disease. Heart Surg Forum 7:E644–E649

Mani H, Suarez E, Stocker JT (2004) The morphological spectrum of infantile lobar emphysema: a study of 33 cases. Paediatr Respir Rev 5(Suppl A):S313–S320

Ozcelik U, Göcmen A, Kiper N, Dogru D, Dilber E, Yalcin EG (2003) Congenital lobar emphysema: evaluation and long-term follow-up of thirty cases at a single center. Pediatr Pulmonol 35:384–391

Section 9.2.3

Berrocal T, Madrid C, Novo S, Gutiérrez J, Arjonilla A, Gomez-Leon N (2004b) Congenital anomalies of the tracheobronchial tree, lung, and mediastinum: embryology, radiology and pathology. Radiographics 23(1):e17

Conforti A, Aloi I, Trucchi A, Morini F, Nahom A, Inserra A, Bagolan P (2009) Asymptomatic congenital cystic adenomatoid malformation of the lung: is it time to operate? J Thorac Cardiovasc Surg 138:826–830

Gardikis S, Didilis V, Polychronidis A, Mikroulis D, Sivridis E, Bougioukas G, Simopoulos C (2002) Spontaneous pneumothorax resulting from congenital cystic adenomatoid malformation in a pre-term infant: case report and literature review. Eur J Pediatr Surg 12:195–198

Lima M, Gargano T, Ruggeri T, Manuele R, Gentili A, Pilu G, Tani G, Salfi N (2008) Clinical spectrum and management of congenital pulmonary cystic lesions. Pediatr Med Chir 30:79–88

Nicolai T (2009) Management of the upper airway and congenital cystic lung diseases in neonates. Semin Fetal Neonatal Med 14:56–60

Papagiannopoulos K, Hughes S, Nicholson AG, Goldstraw P (2002) Cystic lung lesions in the pediatric and adult population: surgical experience at the Brompton Hospital. Ann Thorac Surg 73:1594–1598

Pelizzo G, Barbi E, Codrich D, Lembo MA, Zennaro F, Bussani R, Schleef J (2009) Chronic inflammation in congenital cystic adenomatoid malformation. An underestimated risk factor? J Pediatr Surg 44: 616–619

Priest JR, Williams GM, Hill DA, Dehner LP, Jaffé A (2009) Pulmonary cysts in early childhood and the risk of malignancy. Pediatr Pulmonol 44:14–30

Rothenberg SS (2008) First decade's experience with thoracoscopic lobectomy in infants and children. J Pediatr Surg 43:40–44; discussion 45

Stanton M, Njere I, Ade-Ajayi N, Patel S, Davenport M (2009) Systematic review and meta-analysis of postnatal management of congenital cystic lung lesions. J Pediatr Surg 44:1027–1033

Tran H, Fink MA, Crameri J, Culliane F (2008) Congenital cystic adenomatoid malformation: monitoring the antenatal and short-term neonatal outcome. Aust N Z J Obstet Gynaecol 48:462–466

Truitt AK, Carr SR, Cassese J, Kurkchubasche AG, Tracy TF Jr, Luks FI (2006) Perinatal management of congenital cystic lung lesions in the age of minimally invasive surgery. J Pediatr Surg 41:893–896

Tsai AY, Liechty KW, Hedrick HL, Bebbington M, Wilson RD, Johnson MP, Howell LJ, Flake AW, Adzick NS (2008) Outcomes after postnatal resection of prenatally diagnosed asymptomatic cystic lung lesions. J Pediatr Surg 43:513–517

Van Heurn LW, Harrison MR (2003) Fetal surgery: for selected patients. The experience of the Fetal Treatment Center in San Francisco. Ned Tijdschr Geneeskd 147:900–904

Wilson JM, Colin AA, Reid LM, Kozakewich HP (2006) Bronchial atresia is common to extralobular sequestration, intralobular sequestration, congenital cystic adenomatoid malformation, and lobar emphysema. Pediatr Dev Pathol 9:361–373

Wong A, Vieten D, Singh S, Harvey JG, Holland AJ (2009) Long-term outcome of asymptomatic patients with congenital cystic adenomatoid malformation. Pediatr Surg Int 25:479–485

Section 9.3.1

Cho SD, Krishnaswami S, Mckee JC, Zallen G, Silen ML, Bliss DW (2009) Analysis of 29 consecutive thoracoscopic repairs of congenital diaphragmatic hernia in neonates compared to historical controls. J Pediatr Surg 44:80–86; discussion 86

Cigdem MK, Onen A, Otcu S, Okur H (2007) Late presentation of bochdalek-type congenital diaphragmatic hernia in children: a 23-year experience at a single center. Surg Today 37:642–645

Clugston RD, Greer JJ (2007) Diaphragm development and congenital diaphragmatic hernia. Semin Pediatr Surg 16:94–100

Harrison MR, Adzick NS, Estes JM, Howell LJ (1994) A prospective study of the outcome for fetuses with diaphragmatic hernia. JAMA 271:382–384

Harrison MR, Keller RL, Hawgood SB et al (2003) A randomized trial of fetal endoscopic tracheal occlusion for severe fetal congenital diaphragmatic hernia. N Engl J Med 349:1916–1924

Karimova A, Brown K, Ridout D, Beierlein W, Cassidy J, Smith J, Pandya H, Firmin R, Liddell M, Davis C, Goldman A (2009) Neonatal extracorporeal membrane oxygenation: practice patterns and predictors of outcome in the UK. Arch Dis Child Fetal Neonatal Ed 94:F129–F132

Khwaja MS, al-Arfaj AL, Dawoodu AH (1989) Congenital right-sided diaphragmatic hernia: a heterogeneous lesion. J R Coll Surg Edinb 34:219–222

Koivusalo AI, Pakarinen MP, Lindahl HG, Rintala RJ (2008) The cumulative incidence of significant gastroesophageal reflux in patients with congenital diaphragmatic hernia – a systematic clinical, pH-metric, and endoscopic follow-up study. J Pediatr Surg 43: 279–282

Lin AE, Pober BR, Adatia I (2007) Congenital diaphragmatic hernia and associated cardiovascular malformations: type, frequency, and impact on management. Am J Med Genet C Semin Med Genet 145C(2):201–216

Mah VK, Zamakhshary M, Mah DY, Cameron B, Bass J, Bohn D, Scott L, Himidan S, Walker M, Kim PC (2009) Absolute vs relative improvements in congenital diaphragmatic hernia survival: what happened to "hidden mortality". J Pediatr Surg 44:877–882

Mann C, Baenziger O (2007) Management of newborns with congenital diaphragmatic hernia. Schweiz Med Forum 7:438–439

Mettauer N, Agrawal S, Pierce C, Ashworth M, Petros A (2009) Outcome of children with pulmonary lymphangiectasis. Pediatr Pulmonol 44:351–357

Newman KD, Anderson KD, Van Meurs K, Parson S, Loe W, Short B (1990) Extracorporeal membrane oxygenation and congenital diaphragmatic hernia: should any infant be excluded? J Pediatr Surg 25:1048–1053

Peetsold MG, Heij HA, Kneepkens CM, Nagelkerke AF, Huisman J, Gemke RJ (2009a) The long-term follow-up of patients with congenital diaphragmatic hernia: a broad spectrum of morbidity. Pediatr Surg Int 25:1–17

Peetsold MG, Heij HA, Nagelkerke AF, Ijsselstijn H, Tibboel D, Quanjer PH, Gemke RJ (2009b) Pulmonary function and exercise capacity in survivors of congenital diaphragmatic hernia. Eur Respir J 34: 1140–1147

Riedlinger WF, Vargas SO, Jennings RW, Estroff JA, Barnewolt CE, Lillehei CW, Shah SR, Wishnew J, Barsness K, Gaines BA, Potoka DA, Gittes GK, Kane TD (2009) Minimally invasive congenital diaphragmatic hernia repair: a 7-year review of one institutional's experience. Surg Endosc 23:1265–1271

Stolar CJH, Dillon PW (1998) Congenital diaphragmatic hernia and eventration. In: O'Neill JA Jr et al (eds) Pediatric surgery, vol 1, 5th edn. Mosby, St. Louis

Stoll C, Alembik Y, Dott B, Roth MP (2008) Associated malformations in cases with congenital diaphragmatic hernia. Genet Couns 19:331–339

Section 9.3.2

Al-Salem AH (2007) Congenital hernia of Morgagni in infants and children. J Pediatr Surg 42:1539–1543

Al-Salem AH (2010) Bilateral congenital Morgagni-Larrey's hernia. World J Pediatr 6:76–80

Antinolo G, De Agustin JC, Losada A, Marenco ML, Garcia-Diaz L, Morcillo J (2010) Diagnosis and management of fetal intrapericardial Morgagni diaphragmatic hernia with massive paracardial effusion. J Pediatr Surg 45:424–426

Iso Y, Sawada T, Rokkaku K, Furihata T, Shimoda M, Kita J et al (2006) A case of symptomatic Morgangni's hernia and a review of Morgangni's hernia in Japan (263 reported cases). Hernia 10:521–524

Loong TPF, Kocher HM (2005) Clinical presentation and operative repair of hernia of Morgagni. Postgrad Med J 81:41–44

Mallick MS, Alqahtani A (2009) Laparoscopic-assisted repair of Morgagni hernia in children. J Pediatr Surg 44:1621–1624

Yilmaz M, Isik B, Coban S, Sogutlu G, Ara C, Kirimlioglu V, Yilmaz S, Kayaalp C (2007) Transabdominal approach in the surgical management of Morgagni hernia. Surg Today 37:9–13

Section 9.3.3

De Vries TS, Koens BL, Vos A (1998) Surgical treatment of diaphragmatic eventration caused by phrenic nerve injury in the newborn. J Pediatr Surg 33:602–605

Hines MH (2003) Video-assisted diaphragm plication in children. Ann Thorac Surg 76:234–246

Jawad AJ, al-Sammarai AY, al-Rabeeah A (1991) Eventration of the diaphragm in children. J R Coll Surg Edinb 36:222–224

Kizilcan F, Tanyel FC, Hicsönmez A, Büyüpamukcu N (1993) The long-term results of diaphragmatic plication. J Pediatr Surg 28:42–44

McIntyre RC Jr, Bensard DD, Karrer FM, Hall RJ, Lilly JR (1994) The pediatric diaphragm in acute gastric volvulus. J Am Coll Surg 178:234–238

Tiryaki T, Livanelioglu XY, Atayurt H (2006) Eventration of diaphragm. Asian J Surg 29:8–10

Tönz M, von Segesser LK, Mihaljevic T, Arbenz U, Stauffer UG, Turina MI (1996) Clinical implications of phrenic nerve injury after pediatric cardiac surgery. J Pediatr Surg 31:1265–1267

Tsugawa C, Kimura K, Nishijima E, Muraji T, Yamaguchi M (1997) Diaphragmatic eventration in children: is conservative treatment justified? J Pediatr Surg 32:1643–1644

Verney PT, Grosselin MV, Primack SL, Kraemer AC (2007) Differentiating diaphragmatic paralysis and eventration. Acad Radiol 14:420–425

Section 9.3.4

Engum SA, Rescorla FJ, West KW, Scherer LR 3rd, Grosfeld JL (1999) The use of pleuroperitoneal shunts in the management of persistent chylothorax in infants. J Pediatr Surg 34:286–290

Tommasoni N, Mognato G, Gambla PG (2002) Congenital and acquired chylothorax. Pediatr Med Chir 24:21–28

Section 9.4

Furia S, Biban P, Benedetti M, Terzi A, Soffiati M, Calabro F (2009) Postpneumonectomy-like syndrome in an infant with right lung agenesis and left main bronchus hypoplasia. Ann Thorac Surg 87:e43–e45

Krivchenya DU, Rudenko EO, Lysak SV, Dubrovin AG, Khursin VN, Krivchenya TD (2007) Lung aplasia: anatomy, history, diagnosis and surgical management. Eur J Pediatr Surg 17:244–250

Langer M, Chiu PP, Kim PC (2009) Congenital and acquired single-lung patients: long-term follow-up reveals high mortality risk. J Pediatr Surg 44:100–105

The disorders of respiratory organs in infants and older children with pediatric surgical significance may be arranged in six categories as follows:

- Malformations or acquired disorders with similar presentation that become apparent in the neonatal period as well as later in childhood
- Malformations or acquired disorders with similar presentation that become apparent usually beyond the neonatal period or early infancy
- Thoracic injuries and foreign body aspiration and ingestion
- Complications of inflammatory lung diseases
- Parasitic diseases of the lung
- Neoplastic diseases of the lungs and respiratory tract

In Tables 10.1, 10.2, and 10.3, the relevant pathologies are arranged according to the described categories and quoted individually. The pathologies of the first, second, and third categories are supplemented by the most important presenting signs or by the circumstances of their occurrence. Many of the pathologies of the first category and some of the second category have been described in Chap. 9. The remaining disorders are described in detail in Chap. 10.

10.1 Malformations and Acquired Disorders with Similar Presentation in the Newborn or Later in Childhood

The reader is referred to Table 10.1 and Chap. 9.

10.2 Malformations and Acquired Disorders with Clinical Manifestation After the Neonatal Period

The individual pathologies are listed in Table 10.2, and the last four disorders are described in detail in Sect. 10.2. For visualization, see also Fig. 10.1.

10.2.1 Pulmonary Sequestration

Occurrence, Pathoanatomy

The prevalence of pulmonary sequestration is similar to bronchogenic cyst and congenital cystic lung disorders if prenatal ultrasound screening is performed and combined with postnatal work-up examinations.

Pulmonary sequestration is a combination of bronchopulmonary dysplasia with systemic arterial blood supply (with one or several branches from the supra- or infradiaphragmatic aorta, celiac trunk, or intercostal arteries) and venous outflow to the lung veins or azygos, hemiazygos, or portal vein.

Sequestration occurs either as intra- or extralobular type. The **intralobular sequestration** is mostly observed within the posterobasal or medial segment of the left lower lobe, and the **extralobular type** mostly close to the left lower lobe or infradiaphragmatically in the neighborhood of the left adrenal gland. In about one fifth, the sequestration is aerated either by a primary

Table 10.1 Malformations and acquired disorders with similar presentation in the newborn or later in childhood

Hem-/lymphangioma/vascular malformations	Dyspnea, dysphagia
Macroglossia #	Large tongue, hypersalivation
Tracheobronchomalacia	Wheezing respiration
Lobar emphysema (congenital/acquired) Congenital cystic lung disorders ### (Congenital/acquired [CCAM, pneumatocele])	} Symptoms and signs of respiratory organs
Congenital diaphragmatic hernia Bochdalek/ Diaphragmatic hernia of Morgagni #	Incidental finding, signs of respiratory organs, of gastrointestinal tract or heart
Diaphragmatic eventration	Recurrent respiratory tract infections, difficult food intake
Chylothorax (after thoracic surgery, trauma, or in neoplastic disease)	Signs of respiratory organs
Mediastinal tumor	} Possible dyspnea
Surgical abdomen	Combined with abdominal signs
Gastroesophageal reflux	Recurrent respiratory tract infections
Arnold-Chiari malformation	Apneic spells and cyanotic attacks, dysphagia, lower cranial nerve deficit

Table 10.2 Malformations and acquired disorders with clinical manifestation after the neonatal period

o Unilateral choanal atresia	Unilateral rhinorrhea
o Lung aplasia, agenesis, and post-pneumonectomy lung	Prenatal ultrasound, RDS and unexpected respiratory insufficiency/infection, exertional dyspnea
• Lung sequestration:	Prenatal ultrasound, postnatal work-up
Intralobular	Recurrent pneumonia at the same site
Extralobular	Accidental finding at surgery
• Bronchiectasis	After complicated pneumonia, foreign body aspiration, in cystic fibrosis,
Acquired/congenital	Primary ciliary dyskinesia
	Permanent cough, in schoolchildren
	Purulent expectorations
• Spontaneous pneumothorax	Chronic disease at </> 10 years of age (asthma, cystic fibrosis) sudden chest pain, shortness of breathing in teenagers
o Pneumomediastinum	Neck crepitation (emesis, asthma)

connection to the tracheobronchial tree or by secondary communication with the adjacent normal lung tissue.

In **communicating pulmonary sequestration** (communicating bronchopulmonary foregut malformation), the anomaly communicates through a fibrous cord or an open bronchus with the esophagus or stomach.

Clinical Significance
- Extralobular sequestration is associated with other anomalies in up to 40 %, congenital diaphragmatic hernia or eventration, congenital heart disease, and chest wall deformities belong to the more frequent.

- Both types may be combined with bronchogenic cyst, cystic adenomatoid malformation, enteric duplication, esophageal atresia, and with the other type of sequestration.
- Intralobular sequestration leads to recurrent bronchopneumonia.
- Both types may present as inferior posterior mediastinal tumor.

Clinical Presentation
Today, mainly supradiaphragmatic pulmonary sequestrations are suspected by prenatal ultrasound. In former times, sequestrations have been recognized somewhere between infancy and adulthood.

Clinically, intralobular sequestration presents mostly beyond the neonatal period as recurrent bronchopneumonia at the same site in the left *lower lobe and possibly as abscess and rarely with hemoptysis or "expectorations" tingled with blood.* In case of major systemic blood supply without or with arteriovenous fistula, *heart insufficiency* may be the first clinical manifestation.

Supradiaphragmatic pulmonary sequestration may present by chance as *mediastinal tumor on chest x-rays* performed for other reason, and *extralobular sequestrations are recognized in the course of or at surgery of the above quoted associated anomalies* and at thoracic or abdominal work-ups or surgical procedures performed for other reasons.

Differential Diagnosis, Work-Ups

The clinical and radiological differential diagnosis includes all disorders with symptoms and signs of the respiratory organs especially those with recurrent bronchopneumonia, hemoptysis, posterior mediastinal tumor, atelectasis, or cystic lung disorders.

Instead of former selective angiography, bronchography, and contrast swallow, plain chest x-rays and CT combined with intravascular contrast are used – the latter for differentiation of pulmonary sequestration from other pathologies, typification, and precise description of the vascular supply and outflow.

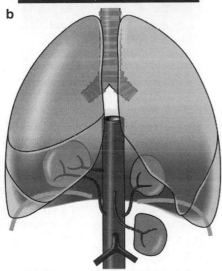

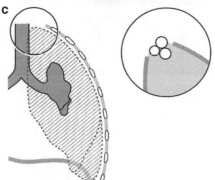

Fig. 10.1 Drawings of the three main pathologies that are observed usually beyond the neonatal period and early infancy: bronchiectasis, lung sequestration, and spontaneous pneumothorax. (**a**) Demonstrates cylindric bronchiectases of the basal segments of the left lower lobe that have been visualized by bronchography. (**b**) Displays different types of pulmonary sequestration: An intralobar sequestration is visible on the right and an extralobar sequestration on the left side of the patient above the diaphragm. The former is a part of lung, and the latter corresponds to an accessory lung lobe that is located mostly adjacent to the left lower lobe but may also be encountered below the diaphragm as illustrated in the drawing. The source of the systemic blood supply concerns one or several arteries directly from the supra- or infradiaphragmatic aorta, celiac, or intercostal artery. (**c**) Shows spontaneous pneumothorax on the left side that is often caused by blebs (bullae) in adolescence. Recurrent pneumothorax in cystic fibrosis is a typical example of the symptomatic type in childhood

For communicating pulmonary sequestration, the knowledge of the possible pathoanatomy and additional upper gastrointestinal contrast study are useful.

Treatment, Prognosis

Surgery is indicated in all supradiaphragmatic pulmonary sequestrations because of their already happened or forthcoming complications, in symptomatic infradiaphragmatic extralobular sequestrations or if they are encountered by chance at abdominal surgery.

Resection is stepwise performed: (1) careful ligation and division of the feeding arteries (e.g., within the inferior pulmonary ligament or along the aorta), (2) ligature and division of the outflowing veins, and (3) removal of the sequestration by lobectomy, segmentectomy, or atypical resection depending on the findings of the adjacent lung tissue and the type of sequestration (the sequestration consists of tissue similar to liver and is possibly intermingled with aerated cavities).

Prognosis is good if resection is performed in time except for severe cardiovascular compromise by the sequestration or ipsilateral lung hypoplasia in large sequestration.

10.2.2 Bronchiectasis

Occurrence, Pathology

Bronchiectasis is defined as cylindric or saccular dilatation of bronchi combined with recurrent purulent infections. In contrast to the developing countries where bronchiectasis is still one of the most common causes of lung resection in children, its prevalence is decreasing in the developed countries.

Bronchiectasis occurs in nearly 50 % in the basal segments of the two lower lobes, in one third in the right middle lobe or lingula on the left side, and in one sixth in both upper lobes. In 25–30 % bilateral involvement is observed.

The most frequent causes of bronchiectasis are chronic shrinking bronchopneumonic infections such as common bacterial and viral pneumonias and specifically those in influenza, pertussis, measles, and tuberculosis. Due to vaccinations and proper antibiotics, these causes are diminishing in the western hemisphere; therefore, congenital diseases such as cystic fibrosis, primary ciliary dyskinesia including Kartagener syndrome, Williams-Campbell syndrome (with deficit of the cartilaginous rings), and immunodeficiencies or delayed diagnosis of aspiration of foreign bodies are now numerically the main causes of bronchiectasis in this part of the world.

Clinical Significance

- Depending on the cause and extension of bronchiectasis, this disorder may become a limiting factor of survival or lead to irreparable destruction of lung tissue.
- In developing countries, surgery is still an important part of treatment with up to one fourth patients with lung resections in noncystic fibrosis bronchiectasis.
- In the latter situation, appropriate indications and technical skills are needed.

Clinical Presentation

Bronchiectasis develops after an acute or chronic disorder that explains a relatively silent period of different length. For instance, clinical manifestation of bronchiectasis in 2–3 % beyond 1 month in missed diagnosis of foreign body aspiration, in up to one fifth after a much longer period, or a delayed diagnosis of postpneumonic bronchiectasis at a mean age of beginning primary school.

Permanent or intermittent chronic cough and possible expectorations are the main signs. The purulent expectorations that may be tingled with blood or display a foetid smell are swallowed by small children but *may be gained by postural drainage.*

Tachypnea, exertional dyspnea, cyanosis, failure to thrive, clubbed fingers, and gross hemoptysis belong to the signs of advanced and extended bronchiectasis.

Differential Diagnosis, Work-Ups

The differential diagnosis includes all disorders with chronic cough and purulent expectorations. If these signs occur in the course of causative disorders, bronchiectasis must be excluded by appropriate work-ups. On the other hand, former foreign body aspiration must be considered in localized bronchiectasis of unusual site.

The work-ups include chest x-rays in two plains and high-resolution CT. The latter has replaced bronchography.

In addition, bronchoscopy, ventilation-perfusion scintiscan, and pulmonic function tests are applied. Bronchoscopy visualizes the involved bronchi with the possibility of biopsy, permits lavage and recovery of secretion for Gram stain and culture, and recognizes a possible foreign body.

Treatment, Prognosis

Treatment is primarily medical with appropriate antibiotics and physiotherapy with postural drainage of the secretions.

The indications of surgery must consider the course of bronchiectasis over a distinct period with radiological imaging, the severity of the clinical signs, and the cause of bronchiectasis. Resection is particularly indicated:

- In resistance to medical therapy.
- In localized bronchiectasis with irreparable damage and functional loss of the involved lung part.
- If complete resection of the involved lung parts is possible with sufficient functional reserve and if the underlying disorder does not lead to recurrence of the not yet involved parts.
- In cystic fibrosis, individualized indications are necessary, for instance, resection of a localized area with advanced bronchiectasis in relation to the findings in the residual lung.

Lobectomy (in two thirds or half of the children), pneumonectomy, lobectomy and segmentectomy, and segment resection arranged in order of their frequency and second resection on the contralateral side or completion pneumonectomy (in 7 or 14 %) are the expenditures of surgery in two recent studies with three fourths or >90 %

complete resections. In the larger study, the mortality was 0 %, the morbidity 13 %, and three fourths had a perfect outcome and only 3 % had no change.

For resections, specifically for lobectomy, video-assisted thoracoscopic resection is a possible alternative although difficulties of dissection of the hilum due to previous infections may necessitate conversion.

10.2.3   Spontaneous Pneumothorax

Occurrence, Causes, Pathology

Spontaneous pneumothorax occurs in 0.12 ‰ of the general population and less frequently in children. Depending on the cause of spontaneous pneumothorax, it may be observed throughout childhood or almost exclusively in teenagers as in primary spontaneous pneumothorax.

It is observed either due to an underlying generalized disorder such as cystic fibrosis or asthma, or a localized congenital malformation ## or acquired disease of the lung such as congenital cystic adenomatoid malformation or pneumatocele.

The term "**primary or idiopathic spontaneous pneumothorax**" refers to a disorder in which superficial blebs or bullae of the lung can be recognized only in a part of the children in spite of an equal clinical presentation. Familiality has been reported. The expected 1–6 blebs or bullae are mostly confined to the lung apices and less frequently to the lower parts of the lung and have radiologically a diameter of 2.5–45.0 mm. If blebs are present on one side, blebs on the contralateral side may occur in more than three fourths.

Clinical Significance

- The unexpected sudden onset of respiratory signs frightens parents and involved teenagers.
- Possible recurrences or involvements of the other side are troublesome.
- Spontaneous pneumothorax and spontaneous pneumomediastinum are related to each other.

Clinical Presentation

Sudden onset of cough, shortness of breathing, and chest pain is the clinical presentation. *Hyperresonance to percussion with decreased breathing sound* is the local finding. *In teenagers without a generalized disorder, primary spontaneous pneumothorax is the most likely cause.*

Bilateral primary spontaneous pneumothorax occurs in <10 %. The terms "first episode, persistent, and recurrent pneumothorax" mean first clinical manifestation of pneumothorax, the air leak lasts for more than 5 days, and the air leak occurs on the same side 7 days or more after initial resolution.

Differential Diagnosis, Work-Ups

It includes other disorders with sudden onset of shortness of breathing, dyspnea, and chest pain, and more specifically, isolated thoracic injury with pneumothorax and **primary or secondary spontaneous pneumomediastinum**. The latter disorder is observed in emesis, asthma flare-ups, and less frequently without recognizable cause. It may be combined with pleural effusion or pneumothorax. In addition to the symptomatology quoted above, *discomfort of the neck, expiratory wheezing, and neck crepitation due to subcutaneous air* may be present. Plain chest x-ray including the neck in two plains is performed, and if negative, CT is necessary for diagnosis. Pulmonary function tests are recommended to exclude asthma that has not been recognized up to now.

For spontaneous pneumothorax, chest x-ray is diagnostic. CT and diagnostic thoracoscopy are performed for detection of possible blebs or bullae of the same or contralateral side (CT yields no false-positive findings, but recognizes only a part of the blebs. So-called apical lines occur in normal and pathological CT and are probably a normal variant).

Treatment, Prognosis

Treatment must consider the cause of spontaneous pneumothorax.

In **idiopathic spontaneous pneumothorax**, primary tube thoracostomy is recommended with secondary VATS in case of recurrence. This is in spite of the superior outcome of VATS in

comparison with chest tube drainage due to the increased morbidity and costs of primary versus secondary VATS.

VATS (or open thoracotomy) includes blebectomy or wedge resection combined with mechanical pleurodesis and can be performed as prophylactic procedure of the contralateral side.

In **cystic fibrosis**, 1 in 167 patients experiences pneumothorax each year, mostly older patients are involved with advanced lung disease, and there is an increased morbidity and mortality after pneumothorax. Because neither chemical pleurodesis nor the quoted procedures have been assessed by randomized controlled trials so far, it is impossible to tell which is superior. On the other hand, it is suggested that pleurodesis renders lung transplantation impossible. If a surgical procedure is chosen, there is a greater risk of intra- and postoperative complications.

Prognosis depends on the cause of spontaneous pneumothorax and the possibility to treat the cause. For instance in localized lung anomalies and disorders, there is a minimal recurrence rate after some type of lung resection in CCAM or ligature of the bronchiolus and endorrhaphy in pneumatocele. The same may be true after proper treatment of asthma. On the other hand, the recurrence rate of primary spontaneous pneumothorax amounts to 23–42 % after tube thoracostomy and to 0–13 % after VATS; the recurrence rate is much higher if involvement of the contralateral side is also considered as recurrence. Absence of contralateral blebs does not mean that pneumothorax is excluded later.

10.3   Thoracic Injuries

10.3.1 General Remarks

Occurrence, Causes

Depending on the cause, two thirds or more of thoracic traumas are multisystemic organ injuries, for instance, in child abuse or falls of infants and toddlers or in motor vehicle accidents of schoolchildren as pedestrians or cyclists. Thoracic injury is with about 5 % of all accidents grouped according to the involved region after head injury, and abdominal trauma the **third most frequent of the trunk** and has after head injury **the second**

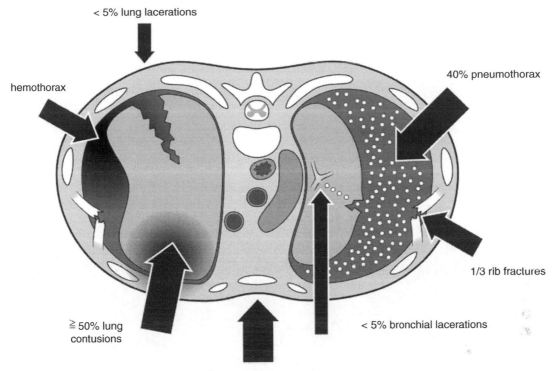

< 5% lung lacerations

hemothorax

40% pneumothorax

1/3 rib fractures

≧ 50% lung contusions

< 5% bronchial lacerations

≧ 50% combined injuries

Fig. 10.2 Types of thoracic injuries in a large number of consecutive children with trauma to the chest. About two thirds of the involved children have additional extrathoracic injuries, and the thoracic injuries are combined in half of the patients. The most frequent single injuries are lung contusion, hemothorax, and/or pneumothorax. Rib fractures are observed less frequently and the most severe thoracic injuries lung or bronchial laceration amount each to <5 %

rank in mortality (<10 %) that is mainly due to a combination with head or abdominal trauma. In >85 %, the thoracic injury is **blunt** and in <15 % a **penetrating trauma**. The quoted figures may be different depending on the catchment area of a country and the state of development.

Birth trauma, child abuse, falls (from a height or ground level), impalement injuries, motor vehicle accident as occupant, pedestrian, or cyclist, sports, stab injuries (knife or gunshot injuries) are the preferred **causes** of thoracic injury and arranged in order of increasing age.

The younger the child, the more the typical **pattern of childhood thoracic injury** is observed with lung contusion and pneumo- and/or hemothorax as the most frequent single injuries in contrast to adulthood with rib fracture(s) as the most common single thoracic injury.

More than 50 % of chest injuries are combined intrathoracic lesions. In blunt thoracic trauma,

trauma to the lung, mostly lung contusion is observed in >50 % and pneumo- and/or hemothorax in nearly 40 %, whereas rib fractures are observed only in about one third as shown in Fig. 10.2. The relevant thoracic injuries are listed in Table 10.3 and supplemented by the most important presenting signs.

Severe thoracic injury that occurs in <5 % of trauma to the chest may be defined as follows: pediatric trauma score ≤4, presence of multiple significant thoracic injuries or a multisystemic organ injury, cardiovascular and respiratory instability at presentation or on follow-up, and need for mechanical ventilation.

In general, chest x-ray and ultrasound with Doppler belong to the **first-line work-ups** of thoracic injury. In the conscious pediatric patient, selective use of individual component of a full trauma series is safe if adequate clinical examination can be performed. On the other hand, single

Table 10.3 Relevant thoracic injuries and their most important presenting signs

Combined thoracic injury	History of trauma including child abuse
	≥ two thirds multisystemic organ injuries
	≥50 % combined thoracic injuries
	Second rank in mortality
	>85 % blunt, <15 % penetrating injuries
Lung contusion, hematoma	>50 % no specific clinical signs
	Diagnosis by chest x-ray
Pneumothorax	40 %
Simple	Possibly tachy- and dyspnea
	Hyperresonance, ↓ breathing sounds
Open	Sucking chest wall sound
Tension	Severe tachy- and dyspnea, cyanosis, distended neck veins. Lung collapse in spite of tube thoracostomy
Hemothorax	Possibly combined with pneumothorax
	Dullness, ↓ breathing sounds
	Possibly hemodynamic instability and anemia
Lung laceration	Imminent shock, respiratory impairment
Less common in children with blunt trauma	Injury of major blood vessel
Rib fractures	One third
	Localized pain or crepitation. Avoidance of respiratory motion
	Notice differential diagnosis
Lung laceration	Often pneumo- and hemothorax together
Injury tracheobronchial tree	Signs of tension pneumothorax, imminent shock, possibly hemoptysis, s.c. emphysema, inability to speak
Air embolism	Severe deterioration, frothy blood sample from arterial line
Small tracheal tear	Neck pain, s.c. emphysema, torticollis
Cardiovascular injuries	Less common in children in blunt trauma
Cardiac injuries	
Heart contusion	Possibly arrhythmia, arterial hypotonia
Heart rupture	Tachycardia, arterial hypotonia, peripheral vasoconstriction, jugular vein distension
	Resistance to fluid resuscitation
	Cardiosonogram, needle catheterization
Commotio cordis	Sports, unexpected sudden collapse
	Ventricular fibrillation
Aortic rupture	Severe trauma, widening mediastinum on chest x-ray

contrast- or spiral multidetector-CT is indicated in severe thoracic or significant multisystemic organ injuries including penetrating torso trauma.

The **therapeutic requirements** of thoracic injury are in >1/3 tube thoracostomy, in <10 % mechanical ventilation, and in <5 % thoracotomy. Except for some specific, mainly diagnostic indications (e.g., evaluation of suspected diaphragmatic injury), VATS has not yet attained a major acceptance in severe thoracic trauma.

Possible **sequels of thoracic injury** are pneumonitis, pleural empyema, lung abscess, bronchiectasis, pleural membranous peel, and traumatic pulmonary pseudocyst (posttraumatic pneumatocele).

Initial management and work-ups of **penetrating thoracic injuries** do not differ from that of blunt chest trauma except for the greater chance of associated abdominal trauma (especially in wounds below the nipples), cardiovascular injuries (e.g., wounds near the heart), and gross lesions of the airways and esophagus.

If plain chest and abdominal x-rays are performed, the entry and exit wounds should be marked. Echocardiography and torso CT combined with angiography are the most informative work-ups.

Urgent surgery is indicated in shock (massive bleeding), gross air leak, and heart tamponade, and the site of access depends on the results of work-ups and suspected injuries. Occasionally, a subxiphoid pericardial window may be useful if echocardiography is not available.

10.3.2 Lung Contusion and Hematoma

Occurrence
Lung contusion and hematoma are the most frequent single type of thoracic injury in children. It is observed even after focal low or moderate trauma to the chest.

Clinical Presentation
Lung contusion and hematoma have no specific clinical features. Although a history of thoracic injury and contusional marks, abrasions, or lacerations of the chest wall may point to the possibility of lung contusion and although its possible complications "pleural effusion, pneumo- and/or hemathorax, and pneumonitis" can draw attention to an underlying lung contusion, *the diagnosis is only possible by radiological imaging at first presentation.*

Nevertheless, careful clinical examination should be performed initially for primary survey including cardiorespiratory repercussions, injury severity score, possible multisystemic organ injury, and possible combined thoracic injuries.

Work-Ups
Plain chest x-ray and measurement of oxygen saturation are the first line examinations. Because contusion that are not visible on chest x-ray have no clinical significance, CT should only be performed in selected cases, for example, in multisystemic organ injury, in severe thoracic trauma, or suspected specific thoracic injuries.

Treatment
Depending on the severity of lung contusion and the presence or possibility of combined thoracic injuries or multisystemic organ injury, the child is monitored on the ICU with continuous measurement of the arterial oxygen saturation and laboratory, and radiological follow-ups of the thoracic and other injuries and treatment by analgetics, blood transfusions if necessary, physiotherapy, and antibiotics.

The combined injuries and already quoted complications may become apparent within 1–2 days or several days later and need additional measures such as chest tube insertion. Lung contusion as isolated chest injury does not need frequently mechanical ventilation.

Prognosis
Complete resolution occurs in the majority of lung contusions without sequels. Severe contusions may need ventilation from the beginning or with progressive manifestation of respiratory signs. Pneumonia, lung abscess, or pneumatocele(s) develop rarely. Pneumatoceles need follow-ups until radiological disappearance due to their inherent complications.

10.3.3 Pneumothorax

Pathology, Pathophysiology
The air in the pleural space stems from an injury of the lung parenchyma, chest wall, tracheobronchial tree, or esophagus. In **simple pneumothorax**, the air leak is not large. The usually large and continuous air leak of **tension pneumothorax** cannot escape because of the effect of a one-way valve, the pressure in the pleural space exceeds that of the atmosphere, and pushes the collapsed lung with the mediastinum to the contralateral side. In **open pneumothorax,** there is a communication to the outside by a penetrating chest wall injury.

Clinical Presentation
The clinical signs and findings progress in severity from simple to open and to tension pneumothorax.

In **simple pneumothorax**, *the child is tachy- and possibly dyspneic. On the other hand, pneu- mothorax may be symptomless especially in case of small mantle pneumothorax that emphasizes the necessity of routine plain chest x-ray in all children with thoracic injury.*

Clinical examination yields possibly external signs of thoracic injury such as contusional marks or localized pain and crepitation in case of rib fractures. *Percussion of the involved hemithorax is hyperresonant, and the breath sounds are diminished on auscultation in comparison with the contralateral side.*

In **open pneumothorax**, the penetrating injury presents often as *sucking chest wall wound.* It is life-threatening and should be immediately closed by an occlusive dressing that changes the open in a closed simple pneumothorax.

In **tension pneumothorax**, *severe dyspnea develops with tachycardia and tachypnea. In addi- tion to the local findings of simple pneumothorax, the neck veins are distended, cyanosis develops, and the trachea is displaced to the contralateral side.* This life-threatening condition needs imme- diate catheter needle insertion through the second intercostal space in the midclavicular line.

Work-Ups

First-line examination is chest x-ray which shows all degrees of pneumothorax although a clinically important pneumothorax may be recognized by ultrasound.

Pneumomediastinum in blunt trauma as addi- tional finding needs not further evaluation if the patient has an isolated type of thoracic injury and is asymptomatic. Additional examinations are necessary in tension and possibly in open pneumothorax.

Treatment, Prognosis

All children with simple pneumothorax need chest tube insertion and connection to an under- water seal with a pump of low suction force, except for small mantle pneumothorax without hemothorax. The tube is inserted parallel to the chest wall in the fifth intercostal space in the anterior axillary line; its size depends on the age of the child and whether the pneumothorax is combined with hemothorax or not.

Open pneumothorax needs after preliminary wound dressing chest tube insertion followed by debridement and closure of the wound.

In tension pneumothorax, the preliminary catheter needle insertion should be followed by chest tube insertion, emergency work-up, and surgery for the underlying gross lung laceration or injury of the tracheobronchial tree as source of the major air leak.

Prognosis of traumatic simple pneumothorax is usually good with spontaneous closure of the air leak of the lung within several days. In open and tension pneumothorax, prognosis depends on prompt preliminary measures and the severity of the underlying cause.

10.3.4 Hemothorax

Pathology

Hemothorax results mostly from injury to the lung and much less frequently from injury of the chest wall arteries (intercostal or internal mam- mary artery) or from major vessels of the medi- astinum. The latter conditions occur more frequently in penetrating thoracic injury; they lead to gross, continuous, and life-threatening hemorrhage and result in progressive shock. Occasionally, hemothorax results from percuta- neous insertion of central venous catheter, a chest tube placement, or other interventions.

Clinical Significance

- Pneumo- and hemothorax may be a sign of another major and life-threatening thoracic injury such as injury to the tracheobronchial tree, lung laceration, or injury of large vessels of the mediastinum, especially if the lung remains collapsed after chest tube insertion, if hemodynamic instability is initially present, or shock is developing

Clinical Signs

In addition to a history of an appropriate trauma and recognizable signs of chest wall injury, signs of imminent shock and respiratory impairment may be present. The involved hemithorax displays dullness on percussion and decreased breath sounds on auscultation if the hemothorax is large enough. In combination with pneumothorax, the corresponding local findings may dominate or be mixed with those of hemothorax.

Work-Ups

Plain chest x-ray shows peripheral or complete opacity of the involved hemithorax combined with signs of the frequently combined lung contusion or an air-fluid level if combined with pneumothorax. The severity of lung contusion determined by chest x-ray may correlate with impairment of oxygenation, CO_2 exchange, and need and duration of mechanical ventilation. Simultaneously, blood examinations and testing are necessary.

CT or CT angiography is indicated in major hemothorax and suspicion of major combined thoracic injury. If CT angiography in blunt thoracic trauma is indeterminate, conventional angiography is unnecessary because it is unlikely that it displays aortic or intrathoracic great vessel injury.

Therapy, Prognosis

After initial resuscitation of airways, respiration, and blood volume loss, chest tube placement is necessary with measurement and follow-up of the attained blood.

Intervention with blood stanching and repair of the involved vessels may be indicated if the initial loss is more than one fifth of the estimated blood volume, if hemorrhage continues by more than 1–2 ml/kg body weight/h, or if the pleural space cannot be drained from blood and clots and/or the emergency work-ups have shown the site of hemorrhage. Intrapleural fibrinolysis beyond 1 week after trauma may be an alternative to surgery in unresolved hemothoraces because of failure of chest drainage; it is reported to have a low morbidity, for example, bleeding complications.

In common hemothorax due to lung contusion, the hemorrhage stops usually within 1–2 days and does not leave sequels if prompt and complete evacuation has been performed. If large amounts of blood and clots are left behind, sanguineous effusions and later membranous peels may develop with the inherent morbidity similar to empyema. Rarely, posttraumatic empyema and lung abscess may develop 1–2 weeks

after hemothorax and lung contusion. In massive hemothorax, the prognosis depends on the initial measures and the underlying cause.

10.3.5 Rib Fractures

Clinical Significance

Although rib fractures are observed less frequently in children than in adults, they have a distinct clinical significance:

- Rib fractures may be an indication of a severe thoracic injury and necessitate together with other findings further work-ups.
- Fracture of the first rib may be combined with **thoracic outlet syndrome** and Horner's syndrome.

Relative mydriasis of the contralateral pupil may be interpreted as a sign of head injury. Diagnosis of **Horner's syndrome** is possible with 0.5 % apraclonidine drops and recovery after trauma is partially possible.

- A fractured accessory rib may lead to **neurogenic thoracic outlet syndrome** with delayed neurological impairment of the ipsilateral arm.
- Rib fractures in infants and toddlers point to a possible **battered child syndrome.**
- In the rare **flail chest** with multiple fractures in a row (<2.2 %), respiration of involved hemithorax may become inefficient due to paradoxical movements and associated lung contusion that needs supervision or mechanical ventilation in the ICU.

Clinical Presentation

Spontaneous localized chest pain combined with anxious avoidance of normal ventilatory movements of the involved hemithorax, localized pain, and possible crepitation on palpation belong to the characteristic symptomatology.

Work-Ups, Differential Diagnosis

Rib fractures are usually recognized by the routine chest x-ray although acute rib fractures may be missed. In equivocal findings, ultrasound may be used as an adjunct in acute trauma and CT for precision of the extent of trauma to the chest wall in suspected nonaccidental thoracic injury.

The differential diagnosis includes:

- Midposterior rib fractures may be related to birth trauma (high birth weight, shoulder dystocia, associated homolateral clavicular fracture).
- Neonatal rib fractures occur in metabolic bone disease (e.g., hypocalciuric hypercalcemia, absence of significant traumatic events).
- Anterior rib fractures may be observed after cardiopulmonary resuscitation (>0.3 %) and lateral rib fractures after physiotherapy for bronchiolitis and pneumonia (1 ‰).
- Rib fractures in **nonaccidental trauma.**

The latter concern the posterior part or the transition zone of the ribs to the cartilage and display varying stages of healing. Rib fractures in extremely low birth weight preterm infants who are rehospitalized within a few weeks after discharge because respiratory disorder may be caused by nonaccidental trauma.

Treatment
It includes regular medication of analgetics, rest, and if necessary physiotherapy for 1–2 weeks.

10.3.6 Lung Laceration and/or Injuries to the Tracheobronchial Tree

Occurrence, Causes
Although both injuries occur in less than 5 % of all types of chest wall and lung trauma, they belong together with cardiovascular injuries to the possibly fatal injuries.

Lung lacerations are caused either by penetrating injuries or by broken ribs, whereas tears of the membranous trachea or partial or complete transections of the main and more distal bronchi occur mostly in blunt thoracic trauma. Complications after endotracheal intubation or endoscopy must be considered as well as possible causes of tracheobronchial lesion.

Clinical Significance
- Lung laceration may lead to fatal air embolism.
- Both types of thoracic injury must be supposed in the differential diagnosis in case of large and continuous pneumothorax in spite of tube thoracotomy and possibly combined with hemothorax.

Clinical Presentation
Pulmonic laceration must be considered *in every case of pneumothorax especially if combined with hemothorax and if the lung remains collapsed, or deterioration occurs in spite of primary measures such as pleural drainage, blood volume replacement, and intubation with ventilation with positive pressure.*

Severe deterioration and more specifically frothy blood samples from an arterial line are indications of complicating **air embolism** from the lacerated site.

Injury to the tracheobronchial tree leads rapidly to tension pneumothorax that is characterized by *dyspnea and cyanosis, possible hemoptysis, and palpable subcutaneous emphysema of chest wall and neck. Difficult breathing, inability to speak, and a bruise on the neck point specifically to a tracheal lesion. Failure of re-expansion of the lung after pleural drainage is a further indication of such an injury.*

In unrecognized cases, spontaneous healing of a partial transection occurs rarely with subsequent atelectasis, recurrent respiratory infections, and localized bronchiectasis due to bronchial stricture. Rarely an acquired tracheoesophageal fistula has been observed.

Small tears of the membranous trachea occur probably more frequently than overt injury to the tracheobronchial tree. Trivial neck trauma or spontaneous occurrence, for example, after heavy coughing is reported by some children or parents. *Neck pain, torticollis, and transient subcutaneous emphysema of the neck* are the main complaints and findings. Recovery occurs without major measures within a few days.

Work-Ups, Differential Diagnosis
In suspected laceration, radiological imaging has first priority, whereas in supposed injury of the tracheobronchial tree, bronchoscopy describes precisely the site and type of laceration or transection.

Plain chest x-ray shows pneumothorax with a collapsed lung, tracheal deviation, and possible pneumomediastinum, high-resolution CT of the site of laceration or transection of lung, trachea, or bronchi. The occasionally observed "fallen lung" sign displays a collapsed lung with a position that is dependent on the gravity; the lung is attached only to the vessels of the hilum.

The precise site and extension of the wall defect or the exposure of cartilage is visible by a rigid ventilating bronchoscope performed in general anesthesia or by a flexible bronchoscope in an only slightly sedated child (unstable child or supposed trauma to the cervical spine).

The differential diagnosis in advanced tension pneumothorax or air embolism is **pericardial tamponade**.

Treatment, Prognosis
If either of the disorders is confirmed immediately, posterolateral thoracotomy is performed for debridement, repair of the lung laceration (possibly with some type of lung resection), or tracheal laceration or bronchial dissection.

Air embolism needs emergency thoracotomy, clamping of the pulmonic hilus, aspiration of air from the heart, and revision of the lung laceration.

Prognosis is for both disorders, good if prompt surgery can be performed. If a more distal bronchial lesion is not recognized, delayed bronchostenosis will occur with distal atelectasis, recurrent respiratory infection, and bronchiectasis.

10.4 Cardiovascular Injuries

Occurrence, Causes
In contrast to chest wall and lung injuries, significant trauma to the heart and aorta is less common in children than in adults if only the blunt motor vehicle accidents are considered. But if blunt injuries in competitive sports and penetrating trauma are included, the proportion of childhood cardiovascular injuries is also much larger.

10.4.1 Cardiac Injuries

Types, Clinical Significance
In **heart contusion**, structural changes of different dimensions may be observed from localized types without functional impairment and bleeding up to myocardial aneurysm or rupture. **Rupture** may concern the myocardium, valves, septa, coronary arteries (including dissection and thrombosis), or pericardium.

Commotio cordis, **impingement** of left coronary artery with abnormal origin, and **dissection** of coronary, vertebral, or internal carotid arteries are typical examples of injuries in contact sports:
- Commotio cordis may lead to death due to ventricular fibrillation already in teenagers.
- Heart contusion must be considered in multisystemic organ and thoracic injuries.
- Rupture of the myocardium leads to heart tamponade that needs immediate recognition and treatment.
- Most of the other quoted injuries require prompt diagnosis and elective surgery.

Clinical Presentation
In relevant **commotio cordis**, *unexpected, sudden collapse* is observed. Innocent-appearing blows to the chest wall especially to the precordium or to the neck by projectiles or body contact in competitive sports such as karate, football, hockey, rugby, baseball, and lacrosse ball lead to cardiac death in the sports field or intimal tear and dissection (with subsequent thrombosis or hemorrhage) of the coronary, vertebral, or internal carotid artery. The collapse due to ventricular fibrillation is mostly observed in teenagers (mean age 14 years) and mostly followed by ineffective resuscitation, whereas the latter injuries occur less frequently and lead to posttraumatic chest pain because of myocardial infarction or to fatal outcome due to intracranial hemorrhage.

Arrhythmia or arterial hypotonia belong to the signs of significant **heart contusion** *although contusion may be observed with unexpected, sudden collapse or more often without any clinical signs.* In **rupture of heart**, the cardiac tamponade leads to *tachycardia, arterial hypotonia, and peripheral vasoconstriction. The combination of arterial hypotonia resistant to fluid resuscitation and jugular vein distension in trauma patient should draw the attention to a possible heart tamponade* because pulsus paradoxus and decreased heart sound are less reliable signs.

In **rupture of valves, septa, or pericardium**, *a new cardiac murmur, signs of heart insufficiency, and electrocardiographic abnormalities* may be observed.

Work-Ups, Differential Diagnosis

Heart contusion may be confirmed by 12-lead electrocardiography, echocardiography, scintiscan, and heart enzymes. If the latter belongs to a battery of blood examinations in multisystemic organ or thoracic injuries, further work-up is only necessary in case of positive results or clinical manifestation.

Rupture of the heart is confirmed if possible by echocardiography or immediate diagnostic and therapeutic needle catheterization of the pericardium. The other injuries need echocardiography and/or heart catheterism.

In case of sudden collapse or recurrent syncope and chest pain, or cardiovascular compromise on follow-up, the already quoted types of cardiovascular injuries must be considered.

The most important differential diagnosis of **cardiac tamponade** is **tension pneumothorax** in which local and chest x-ray findings are characteristic, **heart contusion**, **commotio cordis**, and intima tear or **anomalies of the coronary artery**. Abnormal origin of the left coronary artery from the contralateral coronary sinus with impingement between aorta and pulmonary artery is an example of coronary artery anomaly. **The anomaly** is best visualized by 3D-MR angiography or coronary angiography and treated by surgical repositioning.

Treatment, Prognosis

Commotio cordis with collapse needs immediate heart resuscitation, and heart tamponade prompts needle catheterization followed by surgical repair. In heart contusion, monitoring in the ICU is necessary, and most of the other injuries need elective surgery after rapid and precise work-up.

Most of the injuries are curable with good result including heart tamponade, whereas immediate resuscitation of commotio cordis is possible in only 15 %. The prognosis of the quoted arterial ruptures, dissections, and thromboses are equivocal.

Commotio cordis and blows to the neck should be prevented by effective protective devices of the chest and neck.

10.4.2 Rupture of the Aorta and Its Branches

Occurrence, Types

Aortic rupture is less frequently observed in children than in adults. It concerns either the proximal or the distal arch and in the former location at specific sites.

Clinical Significance

- Aortic rupture is mostly fatal.
- Less than 10 % survive the acute stage of injury due to containment of the blood by the adventitia and pleura.

Clinical Findings

Aortic rupture can only be considered in severe trauma and suspected if chest x-ray shows widened mediastinum (mediastinum/chest ratio >0.25).

Work-Ups, Differential Diagnosis

Transesophageal ultrasound may be a more reliable screening test than chest x-ray.

Aortic rupture must be confirmed by CT or MRI angiography or by aortography. The differential diagnosis includes other causes of a widened mediastinum.

Treatment

If the diagnosis of aortic rupture is confirmed, elective repair is indicated after surgery of major bleeding sources, for example, due to blunt abdominal trauma or head injury and stabilization of the child. Possible complications are intracranial hypertension, heart or renal insufficiency, and spinal cord injury.

10.5   Foreign Body Aspiration

Occurrence, Pathology, Types of Foreign Body
Foreign body aspiration occurs mainly in preschool children although all ages may be involved from 2 months on to adolescence.

Aspiration takes place during eating, playing, or other daily activities if normal deglutition is suddenly interrupted by a strong inspiration and if medical including anesthesiological or dental, and other activities are carried out.

Foreign bodies and solid parts of the food or body are then aspirated, and their **site** depends partly on the body position at the moment of aspiration. Although it is more likely to enter the right bronchial tree, preference of the right side is less marked in children than in adults because of the variation in the position of the carina in relation to the middle of the trachea. Aspiration occurs in an overwhelming number of children in the tracheobronchial tree. Nevertheless, foreign bodies may be encountered either in the larynx or pharynx in nearly one fourth.

The **effects** on the laryngotracheobronchial tree depend on the size, shape, composition (plant and animal parts or synthetic, metallic, and mineral objects), initial and final site of foreign body, and age of the patient.

Some of **the most frequently aspirated foreign bodies** are peanuts, other nuts, and berries and seeds, fish, and chicken bones as examples of plant and animal foreign bodies that may contain bacteria and/or swell up. In addition, plastic and metallic parts of playthings or of utensils of daily activity, for example, button batteries or coins, in addition, pen caps, scarf pins, piercing tools, thumb tacks, or darting pins in teenagers.

Depending on the size, shape, and possible swelling of the foreign body and the reaction of the bronchial wall, incomplete or complete **obstruction of the involved bronchus** occurs leading either to **emphysema or atelectasis** of the distal part of the lung that is combined with retention of secretion. **Recurrent purulent bronchitis, pneumonia, lung abscess, and bronchiectasis or bronchial stenosis** are the inevitable sequels.

On the other hand, some unrecognized foreign bodies have only minimal effect and remain therefore clinically silent.

Clinical Significance
- Aspirated foreign bodies require immediate endoscopic removal.
- In developing countries with delayed referral, aspirated foreign body must be always considered as a cause of recurrent bronchitis and pneumonia at the same site as well as lung abscess and localized bronchiectasis.
- Large and irregularly shaped foreign bodies get stuck in the larynx and lead by a bolus effect to death or remain there and are mistaken as recurrent laryngitis. In North America, hot dog aspiration is the most frequently event associated with fatal outcome.

Clinical Presentation
The natural history of foreign body aspiration can be divided into *three stages*. The **acute** or initial stage concerns the clinical presentation of aspiration and the subsequent period of several to 24–48 h. The subacute, **intermediate**, or latent stage may be clinically silent in some but not all of the children and lasts for a variable time of weeks to months. The **chronic** or late stage becomes manifest by recurrent bronchitis and persistent pneumonia, lung abscess, or bronchiectasis.

Initial stage: *The chocking episode may include sensation of suffocation with tickling in the throat, cyanosis, dyspnea, and coughing-fits and is observed in three fourths of the children. It is followed by attacks of coughing or wheezing.* **Intermediate stage**: *Often obvious signs are missing*, or the signs of initial stage are replaced by chronic and permanent cough or wheezing. **Late stage**: *In addition to signs of recurrent bronchitis and pneumonia, signs of lung abscess and bronchiectasis including purulent sputum and hemoptysis may be observed.*

The physical findings include *localized hyperresonance to percussion and localized diminished breath sounds and possible wheezing.*

Complications of foreign body occur in more than 10 %. Perforation of the airways with possible migration in the surrounding tissue belongs to the early complications. Pneumomediastinum, pneumothorax, and neck crepitation are possible sequels.

Work-Ups, Differential Diagnosis

Chest x-ray is not very helpful in the acute stage except for pathological findings such as radiopaque foreign bodies and localized overdistension of the lung. After the acute stage, the incidence of pathological findings increases with overdistension, atelectasis, and permanent pneumonia as the most frequent.

CT and especially in the 3D application has a higher sensitivity and specificity. But radiation exposure must be considered in children, and false-positive findings are possible. Diagnostic bronchoscopy is therapeutic at the same time. But it may be unnecessary due to potentially negative findings (in 5 % up to 1/4–1/3) and is not without risks (airway edema and bleeding, hypoxia, laryngospasm, and pneumothorax with the need of temporary mechanical ventilation).

The differential diagnosis of the acute stage includes many other causes of chocking episodes and coughing-fits – in the subacute stage, those of persistent cough and wheezing, for example, asthma and in the late stage, those of the complicating disorders, for example, permanent pneumonia. In case of baby wipe aspiration, **child abuse** may be the underlying cause, and beyond the acute stage, tuberculous hilar and mediastinal lymphadenitis is an important differential diagnosis of foreign body aspiration beyond the acute stage.

Treatment, Prognosis

A history of foreign body aspiration with description of the observed chocking episode, coughing-fits, or missing of a part of playthings combined with unexpected onset of coughing attacks is the key for the diagnosis of foreign body aspiration and sufficient for immediate work-up including endoscopy. Out of the pathological findings, unilateral diminished breath sounds and overdistension on the chest x-ray are the most sensitive and specific independent findings of referral before or after 2 weeks since aspiration.

Endoscopies with a rigid or flexible bronchoscope are complementary tools. The former method is more successful in removal of foreign bodies, and the latter is minimally invasive and superior in diagnosis and location. Therefore, endoscopic removal of foreign bodies should be performed rather with a rigid than a flexible bronchoscope. Delay of the bronchoscopy to the next available daytime operating list does not lead to any adverse outcome if the patient is stable.

Regular prevention campaigns are absolutely necessary. They may reduce the incidence of foreign body aspiration and of delayed referrals.

Prognosis depends on the time between aspiration and diagnosis. In the acute stage, bronchoscopic removal of an aspirated foreign body is possible in <95 % with complete recovery.

In some developed countries, only half of the children are referred to a tertiary center within 24 h of aspiration, and still 5 % at a median time 3 months in developing countries. Organic foreign bodies and a delay of 1 month or more are risk factors of the development of bronchiectasis. At a median time of 3 months after aspiration, one half of the children displays complete recovery of their symptomatology after removal of the foreign body, one fourth has chronic respiratory problems, and nearly one fourth will develop or has developed bronchiectasis.

10.6 Complications of Inflammatory Disorders of the Lung

The treatment of inflammatory diseases of the lung is medical. Exceptions are residual focuses of active infection not accessible by or resistant to antibiotics, complications and irreparable sequels of the inflammatory diseases, and differential diagnostic indications. Loculated pleural empyema, chronic lung abscess, fungal cavities, and echinococcal cyst(s) are such **focuses**; pyopneumothorax and expanding pneumothorax are possible **complications**; and membranous pleural peel, localized bronchiectasis, and destroyed lung parts are **irreparable sequels** or possibly infected congenital cystic disorders of the lung and malignancies are **differential diagnostic indication** that all need surgical intervention.

10.6.1 Pleural Empyema

Occurrence, Pathoanatomy

Between the 1990s and the first decade of the twenty-first century, a distinct increase of complicated pneumonia (= pneumonia combined with empyema or abscess) and empyema has been observed in the developed countries, for example, an increase of hospitalizations because of complicated pneumonias by a factor of 1.4, 2.6, 3, and 7.7 in the USA (5.5 with complicated pneumonia in 100,000 children in 2006), Australia, Belgium, and France (complicated pneumonias with 92 % empyemas in 11.7 % of admitted pneumonias). References about empyema in newborns and preterm infants are rare.

Pleural empyema is observed mostly in the course of pneumonia and less frequently in children after penetrating chest injury, surgical procedures, or intrathoracic perforation of the esophagus or bronchial tree.

In at least 40 % of community-acquired pneumonias, an accompanying pleural effusion is observed (**stage 1**). In case of complicated pneumonia, the effusion is followed by accumulation of large amounts of fibrinopurulent fluid (= pleural empyema, **stage 2**) that becomes often loculated within a few days by fibrinoid deposits. **Stage 3** with organization of the deposits by fibrous tissue with development of a thick fibrous pleural peel and encasement of the underlying lung is reached in 10–14 days from the beginning of pneumonia. Spontaneous complete normalization is unlikely in advanced stage 2 and in stage 3 pleural effusion.

Streptococcus pneumoniae is an uncommon but important cause of hemolytic-uremic syndrome in combination with complicated pneumonia.

Clinical Significance
- Pleural empyema as the most frequent and prominent feature of complicated pneumonia

leads to considerable morbidity and may result in death not only in developing countries.
- Appropriate antibiotic treatment combined with early chest tube placement or early video-assisted thoracoscopic treatment (VATS) avoids further progression of empyema and secondary surgery.

Clinical Presentation

The history of a preceding influenza-like symptomatology, skin or soft tissue infection, or gastroenteritis in infants with transient amelioration and secondary deterioration are possible risk factors. In the course of community-acquired pneumonia, the development of an empyema must always be considered especially in case of longer symptomatology before hospitalization and/or of medication of anti-inflammatory drugs and inappropriate antibiotics.

Tachy- and dyspnea, pyrexia, and hypoxia and their severity characterize children who need hospitalization for pneumonia. If these signs persist in spite of appropriate antibiotics or if there is only a partial or superficial amelioration in combination with the risk factors quoted above, empyema must be excluded by follow-ups of the local clinical findings, radiological imaging, and laboratory tests.

In addition to dullness to percussion and diminished breath sounds on auscultation, the possibly changing local findings are the following: *The involved hemithorax becomes smaller with narrow intercostal spaces and flattening of the contours combined with thoracic scoliosis. These findings as well as homolateral decreased respiratory movements become permanent in the third stage of empyema.*

Differential Diagnosis, Work-Ups

It includes other causes of empyema than the postpneumonic type such as infected congenital malformations of the lung (e.g., CCAM), mediastinitis, parasitosis (such as thoracic amebiasis) and malignancies of the thoracic cage, pleura, or lungs.

As in every inflammatory disorder, leukocytes and neutrophil counts, C-reactive protein, and erythrocyte sedimentation rate can be used for follow-up in the acute period. Pleural empyema is diagnosed by a combination of plain chest x-rays and ultrasound (US). It must be confirmed by US-guided aspiration of the pleural effusion with Gram stain, culture, and if needed with cell count and differentiation (>10,000 white blood cells/microL = empyema).

CT with small slices and MRI (contrast enhancement for differentiation between active inflammation and noninflammatory changes) are only necessary for differential diagnosis and long-term follow-up (bronchiectasis, destroyed lung). The same is true for Xenon 133 perfusion-ventilation scintiscan. In general, imaging techniques alone cannot accurately stage empyema, guide decisions regarding surgical versus medical management, and predict outcome.

Chest X-Rays: **Empyema** may be recognizable as peripheral or diffuse opacity. Circumscript clearings with air-fluid level at the site of effusion correspond to a pyopneumothorax or to aerobes, and thin-walled cyst-like clearings within the lung parenchyma to pneumatoceles. In lateral decubitus views, empyema does not change its position like the simple parapneumonic effusion. Indirect signs of **pleural peel** are reduction of the size of the involved hemithorax, narrow intercostal spaces, and thoracic scoliosis concave to the involved side. Direct signs are a constricted lung with a thick-walled rim at its periphery.

Ultrasound is useful for estimation of the quantity of effusion, for detection of free flow or loculation of pleural fluid, of anecho- or echogenicity of the content, and as guide for subsequent aspiration. Loculation and echogenicity need chest tube or VATS.

Cultures from pleural fluid or tissue are often negative due to antibiotics prior fluid sampling and low sensitivity. Molecular (including direct molecular typing of culture-negative samples) and antigen detection-based techniques are important adjuncts of epidemiology, etiology, and appropriate treatment of empyemas. *Streptococcus pneumoniae* real-time fluorescence polymerase chain reaction is an example.

Treatment, Prognosis

Presumably, some serotypes of pneumococci are still the most frequently encountered bacteria in spite of vaccination followed by *Streptococcus pneumoniae*, *Streptococcus pyogenes*, *Staphylococcus aureus*, *Haemophilus influenzae*, and anaerobic bacteria (*Pseudomonas aeruginosa*, *Klebsiella*). *Staphylococcus aureus* plays still a specific role in severe necrotizing pneumonia of small children. Recent reports describe strains with different toxin expressing genes (e.g., the Panton-Valentine leukocidin **(PVL)-positive** *Staphylococcus aureus* with particular virulence and potential lethality including bilateral multilobular infiltrates, pneumatocele, recurrent pneumothorax, pleural empyema, lung abscess, diaphragmatic paresis, and Horner's syndrome).

It is important to know that the current epidemiology does not apply completely to the developing countries and that it may change unpredictably.

Treatment of pleural empyema is antibiotic medication either combined with early (= in the first few days of hospitalization or in less than 10–14 days after commencement of complicated pneumonia) chest tube placement and instillation of fibrinolytics or with early video-assisted thoracoscopic surgery (=VATS) including debridement, decortication, and chest tube placement under endoscopic control. In large bronchopleural fistula(s), VATS is contraindicated.

From a surgical point of view, it is hardly imaginable that chest tube placement and fibrinolytics are effective in loculated empyema. Unfortunately, still an insufficient number of appropriately performed studies exist to answer the question if VATS is superior to nonoperative treatment in all respects that include **treatment failures** (up to 7 % in VATS) such as recurrences and conversions to thoracotomy; **intraoperative morbidity** (up to 6 % in VATS) such as lung tearing, air leaks, or chest wall infection; and **length of hospitalization** (median time 7 days for VATS), **duration of tube thoracostomy** (median time 4 days for VATS), and **antibiotic therapy**. Nevertheless, it is important to involve the pediatric or thoracic surgeon early in the case management.

In chronic cases of complicated pneumonia (<5 %), thoracotomy or VATS is indicated for decortication of the trapped lung and possible resection of destroyed lung parts without/with bronchopleural fistula, lung abscess, or localized bronchiectasis.

Prognosis is much better with the treatment options quoted above than with antibiotics alone. In contrast to the late outcome in the 1970s after complicated pneumonia with diminished mobility and asymmetry of the involved hemithorax or thoracic scoliosis in one third, recurrent respiratory infections, and radiological signs of membranous peel in one fourth, the early and intermediated outcome of early VATS displays for the majority of children neither chest wall restrictions nor chronic lung disease with complete recovery in at least 91 %.

10.6.2 Lung Abscess

Occurrence, Causes, Pathology

Lung abscess is quoted as a rare disease. It is observed in 0.9 % of hospitalized and in 8 % of complicated pneumonias. The proportion of primary to secondary lung abscess with an underlying disease is different in the available studies.

The possible causes of lung abscess are the following:

- Lung aspiration (gastroesophageal reflux and other disorders of vomiting, deglutition, dysphagia, and regurgitation; aspiration during anesthesia, inhalation of toxic substances [e.g., turpentine oil, kerosene], and missed aspirated foreign bodies)
- Complicated pneumonia
- Septicemia, especially in congenital or acquired immunodeficiency [e.g., medicamentous] and/or triggered by manipulations, instrumentations, or operations [e.g., Port-A-Cath implantation and punctures], and following gastrointestinal infections [e.g., Salmonellae or Yersinia enterocolitica]. Bilateral and multiple abscesses may occur specifically in septicemia.

The site of abscess depends in lung aspiration on the present posture. In acute abscess, a fluid- and air-filled cavity develops in the area of infiltration due to suppuration followed by necrosis and communication to the bronchial tree. The wall is irregular and thin. In chronic lung abscess, the cavity is roundish with a thick wall.

Clinical Significance

- Lung abscess has considerable morbidity with increased length of hospitalization, and even death is possible mainly due to the underlying disease.

Clinical Presentation

In **primary lung abscess**, *the following symptomatology dominates arranged in order of occurrence: Cough and purulent, possibly foetid sputum (not in infants and toddlers), chest pain and hemoptysis, weight loss, fever, chills, and night sweats.*

Early recognition of **secondary lung abscess** *needs a high grade of suspicion. The already existing clinical presentation becomes protracted and undergoes a significant deterioration combined with some of the already quoted symptoms.*

Work-Ups, Differential Diagnosis

The chest x-ray in two planes demonstrates in the acute phase an irregular, thin-walled lucency in the center of a lung infiltration. In the lateral decubitus view of the involved hemithorax, an air-fluid level may be visible in this cavity. The chronic abscess is characterized by a round lucency combined with an air-fluid level and a peripheral, thick, and regular opacity corresponding to the thick membrane of the abscess.

CT is superior to plain x-rays by its larger sensitivity and specificity for recognition of abscess and descriptions of its characteristics.

For appropriate antibiotic treatment, Gram stain and culture of the abscess content is essential that is recovered by bronchoscopy, ultrasound-guided, or CT-guided percutaneous catheterization of the abscess cavity. The predominant germs are often mixed and include oropharyngeal anaerobic pathogens (in aspiration, pepto-streptococcus), streptococcal species, *Staphylococcus aureus*, *Klebsiella pneumonia*, *Pseudomonas aeruginosa*, *Proteus mirabilis*, and *Aspergillus*.

If Gram stain and culture are negative, serological methods and molecular techniques must be considered.

C-reactive protein, ESR, and blood white cell count and differentiation are useful adjuncts for diagnosis, differential diagnosis, and mainly for follow-up.

The differential diagnosis includes bronchiectasis, pyopneumothorax, infected pneumatocele, complicated hydatid cyst, and infected congenital cystic lung disorders.

Therapy, Prognosis

The first-line treatment is i.v. antibiotics and if available percutaneous catheter drainage. Open pneumonostomy may be performed in case of continuous progression of lung abscess despite medical therapy or large amounts of purulent secretion in infants and toddlers. In chronic abscess, some type of lung resection is indicated since an infected congenital cystic malformation or a missed foreign body may be the cause of resistance to medical therapy. VATS is used alternatively for catheter drainage especially if combined pleura empyema needs debridement or for lung resection.

Eighty to ninety percent of all lung abscesses are definitely curable by medical treatment. Prognosis is less favorable if a severe underlying disease exists, bilateral or multiple abscesses are present, the abscess is progressive and involves larger parts of the lung, and if complete and safe resection is not possible in chronic abscess.

10.6.3 Pneumatocele

Occurrence, Pathoanatomy, Pathophysiology

Pneumatocele is an acquired disorder and occurs either as single or multiple lesion in up to 5 % of motor vehicle-related blunt thoracic injury, in up to 8 % of hospitalized children with pneumonia, and in 20 up to >40 % of complicated pneumonia #. Although all ages are involved, the preferred age is less than 3 years.

Pneumatocele is a thin-walled cyst of the lung parenchyma that contains air. The wall is lined by acinous and bronchiolar epithelium, and the air stems from feeding bronchioli or surrounding normal acini.

In **tension pneumatocele**, a considerable increase of the pneumatocele (up >50 % of the hemithorax) is observed due to a check-valve mechanism and potential effect of mechanical ventilation with compression of the adjacent lung. Tension and superficial pneumatocele may lead to **pneumothorax**.

The suggested pathogenesis of pneumatocele depends on the known causes. For instance, a bursting lesion of the parenchyma in blunt thoracic injury or a necrotizing process in complicated pneumonia. The causes include primary or secondary **complicated pneumonia** (mainly in staphylococcal or pneumococcal pneumonia or less frequently in other types of necrotizing or chronic pneumonias such as tuberculosis or pneumocystis carinii pneumonia), **blunt thoracic injury**, and potentially **high pressure ventilation**.

Clinical Significance

- The individual pneumatoceles develop pathoanatomically and clinically an unpredictable course.
- Pneumatoceles are prone to complications.
- They may lead to intractable cardiorespiratory insufficiency and death.

Clinical Presentation

Pneumatoceles are *either accidental findings on the first chest x-rays* of complicated pneumonias or *become manifest in the course of complicated pneumonias because of complications that lead to a sudden cardiorespiratory compromise.*

The **complications of pneumatocele** are tension pneumatocele, pneumothorax, persistent bronchopleural fistula, or infected pneumatocele. They occur in the first to second or less frequently in the third to fourth week of complicated pneumonia or in the first days of thoracic injury, and later in infected pneumatocele. For estimation of the period in which a clinical manifestation of pneumatocele can be expected, the knowledge of the **natural history of pneu-matoceles is useful**: About two thirds disappear radiologically within 2 months, about one fifth gradually decrease in size and disappear within a mean time of 6.1 months, and 10–15 % develop life-threatening tension pneumatocele, involve more than 50 % of the hemithorax, or display no reduction in size.

Work-Ups, Differential Diagnosis
Work-up examinations are serial chest x-rays in two plains and before intervention, CT.

The differential diagnosis includes congenital cystic disorders of the lung, lung abscess (that might be difficult in case of infected pneumatocele), and pneumothorax.

Treatment, Prognosis
Treatment is expectative except for complications. Pneumothorax needs tube thoracostomy. Surgery is indicated in persistent bronchopulmonary fistula, infected pneumatocele, and unsuccessful catheter drainage. It consists of atypical or segmental resection, or lobectomy.

In tension pneumatocele, very large, and persistent pneumatocele, ultra- or CT-guided catheter drainage may be performed or alternatively surgery with closure of the draining bronchiolus and so-called endorrhaphy ## or with some type of lung resection. The persistence of moderate- to large-sized pneumatoceles beyond 2 months is a relative indication for intervention because they need follow-ups of 6–12 months and are prone to complications.

If pneumatoceles spontaneously disappear radiologically or after intervention, permanent cure can be expected.

10.7 Lung Parasitosis

10.7.1 Pulmonary Cystic Echinococcosis (Pulmonary Hydatid Cyst)

Occurrence, Forms, Pathoanatomy
Hydatid disease is a significant health problem in endemic areas especially in the Mediterranean or developing countries all over the world.

In three fourths of the patients, larvae of the tape worm *Echinococcus granulosus* are responsible for which the dog is the important final and man only an occasional intermediate host. Transmission occurs mainly by direct contact (e.g., sheepdogs), contaminated water, and not washed foodstuffs such as mushrooms, berries, etc. Up to ¼ of the echinococcoses are caused by the larvae of *Echinococcus multilocularis*, a tapeworm which occurs in many countries in strictly limited areas with the fox and wolf as final host. The so-called alveolar form of echinococcosis resembles histologically and clinically a malignant tumor.

In about 90 %, one organ is involved by mostly one and occasionally by two and more cysts (mean number of cysts per patient 1.8). After the liver with 60 % (often in the upper dome), the lung is with 30 % (often in the right lower lobe) the second most frequently involved part, and in about 10 %, other organs are the site of a cyst. In 6 % up to 25 % liver echinococcosis includes the lung as well.

Clinical Significance
• Cystic echinococcosis is increasingly observed in developed countries because of migration.
• Alveolar echinococcosis has a particularly long incubation of 10–15 years and leads to misinterpretation of the clinical presentation due to a loss of information about the exposition.

Clinical Presentation
In large studies, *the mean age at diagnosis of cystic echinococcosis is 10 years (SD ±3–4 years). It is recognized either due the incidental characteristic finding on chest x-ray performed for other reasons or because of clinical manifestation (in up to 40 %).*

The latter is mainly observed in giant, multiorgan, and complicated forms of hydatid cysts (in more than 10 %). Lung compression leads to *recurrent bronchopneumonia, atelectasis, bronchiectasis, and cyst perforation to bronchopneumonia, lung abscess, and hydropneumothorax with the corresponding clinical presentation (e.g., dyspnea and pneumothorax with collapsed lung* and prolonged massive air leak). *In general, chest pain, cough, vomiting, and (massive or life-threatening) hemoptysis* belong to the most often quoted and typical signs and symptoms of hydatid cyst.

Work-Ups, Differential Diagnosis

Chest x-ray in two planes shows a spherical, homogeneous, and opaque mass with projection to the lung. For recognition of cyst rupture ("air-bubble" sign is a sensitive indication), preoperative work-up, and postoperative follow-up, CT should be performed. Ultrasound is reliable tool for community-based screening for cystic echinococcosis. The diagnosis is confirmed by ELISA, serum indirect hemagglutination titers, and DNA analysis.

Differential diagnosis includes lung abscess, congenital cystic disorders without and with infection, and primary or metastatic lung tumor.

Treatment, Prognosis

Treatment is surgical and should be performed whenever possible as parenchyma-saving procedure.

It includes cyst enucleation after injection of a scolicidal agent and sutures of localized air leaks in the remaining cavity that is left open. Lung resections such as lobectomy are necessary in giant and complicated cysts. The former procedure is possible in >80 %, whereas resections become necessary in 10–20 % of children. The role of pre-, peri-, and postoperative treatment with mebendazole is controversial. It may be indicated in giant, complicated, and multiple or multiorgan echinococcosis or in intraoperative rupture. The role of VATS is not completely elucidated.

The prognosis is excellent in case of single cyst in which uneventful cyst enucleation has been performed. In all other cases, recurrences are possible.

10.8   Lung and Pleural Tumors

10.8.1 Lung Tumors

Occurrence, Pathoanatomy

Lung and pleural neoplasms are relatively rare in children. At least three fourths of lung tumors are metastatic, and the remainder are primary lung tumors with more malignant than benign forms.

The most common primary malignant tumors are bronchial adenoma followed by pulmonary blastoma and bronchogenic carcinoma. Sarcomas and other malignancies occur less frequently. Pulmonary capillary hemangiomatosis and pulmonary epitheloid hemangioendothelioma are examples of rare malignant lung tumors. Plasma cell granuloma (inflammatory myoblastic tumor, fibroxanthoma, and [fibro] histiocytoma are synonyms) and hamartoma belong to the most common primary benign tumors. Calcifying fibrous pseudotumor is an example of a rare benign tumor.

Clinical Significance

- Bronchial adenoma is often not considered in the differential diagnosis of signs caused by partial bronchial obstruction and leads to a delayed diagnosis.
- The other malignant lung tumors manifest themselves often in a far advanced stage because the clinical setting is with few exceptions unspecific and a pulmonic malignancy is not considered in the differential diagnosis. A high index of suspicion in children with recurrent or persistent respiratory sign is therefore necessary.
- Congenital cystic lung malformations should be removed at diagnosis because malignant lung tumors are observed later in life in up to 10 %.
- A pulmonic malignancy may be hidden behind a purulent pleuropneumonia.

Clinical Presentation

Bronchial adenoma is primarily an endobronchial lesion, displays occasionally malignant behavior, and manifests as carcinoid tumor (≥80 %), mucoepidermoid, or adenoid cystic carcinoma. Recurrences are observed in <5 %, metastases in >5 %, and locally invasive growth may occur especially as submucous spread in adenoid cystic carcinoma.

The endobronchial site and growth leads to partial bronchial obstruction with *cough, possible inspiratory wheezing, hemoptysis, recurrent bronchopneumonia, and localized bronchiectasis. Interpretation of the symptomatology as asthma explains a delayed diagnosis of several months to years.*

Bronchogenic carcinoma, pulmonary blastoma, fibrosarcoma, and rhabdomyosarcoma *have several features in common*: advanced tumor stage at diagnosis with possible metastatic disease (e.g., 20 % in pulmonary blastoma), possible occurrence together with nontreated congenital cystic lung disorder, chest pain and signs of respiratory restriction in addition to the already quoted signs, and thoracic mass in chest x-ray, localized lung collapse, or consolidation.

In **bronchogenic carcinoma**, an undifferentiated or adenocarcinoma is mostly encountered, **pulmonary blastoma** is localized in the periphery of the lungs and manifests usually in infants and toddlers below 4 years of age, and **rhabdomyosarcoma** originates from the bronchial wall or from congenital cystic anomalies.

The peripheral or pleural site of **pleuropulmonary blastoma** (PPB) explains possible pleural involvement with signs of pleurisy, pleural effusion, or (tension) pneumothorax. Onset in the area of a previously diagnosed cystic lung disorder, for example, lung cyst is observed as well in pleuropulmonary blastoma as in the other malignancies. The three histological types "cystic type, cystic and solid type, and solid type" can be suspected by CT. The early form of PPB (type I) is clinically and radiographically indistinguishable from benign congenital lung cysts. Not all type I PPB progress probably to types II and II. Great vessel, cardiac extension, and tumor embolism are observed in <5 % of type II and III PPB.

Less than one third of PPB has a familial predisposition or belongs to a heritable syndrome (lung cysts, cystic nephroma, childhood cancer, stromal sex-cord ovarian tumors, seminomas or dysgerminomas, intestinal polyps, thyroid hyperplasias, and hamartomas in members of the same family).

Pleuropulmonary blastoma must be considered:

- Age of <4 years
- Pleural involvement (pleurisy, pleural effusion, pneumothorax)

- Cystic lung disorders and bilateral and multifocal cysts
- Familial syndrome

Plasma cell granuloma is a slowly growing **benign primary lung tumor** which may be observed after pneumonia, displays local invasive growth and lymphadenopathy, and rarely recurs after resection. The less frequent **hamartoma** becomes symptomatic because of the large size and coarse calcifications like popcorn are visible on chest x-ray in some of them. *Fever, unspecific respiratory signs or signs of intrathoracic mass effect, or asymptomatic mass on chest x-ray* lead to their diagnosis. Differentiation from a malignant lung tumor is often impossible by radiological imaging.

Differential Diagnosis, Work-Ups

It includes disorders with localized partial bronchial obstruction of which foreign body aspiration and peribronchial lymphadenopathies belong to the most common. Disorders with hemoptysis, purulent expectoration, and recurrent bronchopneumonia must be considered as well.

Bronchoscopy with sampling of secretions and washouts and chest x-ray in two plains, CT, and MRI belong to the main work-ups. Endoscopic biopsy and excision of bronchial adenoma should be performed only in selected cases due to the risk of hemorrhage and recurrence. CT delineates possible localized bronchiectases and excludes other malignant tumors than bronchial adenoma. Cytologic and bacteriological examination of the secretions and possible pleural effusion, determination of inflammatory blood signs, and percutaneous or thoracoscopic biopsies belong also to the work-ups. Additional radiological imaging is necessary depending on the suspected type of malignancy, for instance, bone scan, brain imagery (most common site of metastasis), and abdominal ultrasound in type II and III of pulmonary blastoma.

Treatment, Prognosis

At first, surgery permits often differentiation of benign from malignant tumor by examination of frozen section. Sleeve segmental bronchial resection is occasionally possible in bronchial adenoma. Often conservative resection techniques which consider complete resection of the involved bronchus (e.g., in cylindromas with submucosal growth), removal of the involved lymphatics, and localized bronchiectasis are often superior to sleeve segmental bronchial resection. The other malignant tumors need depending on the type, stage, and location of the neoplasm extensive pulmonary resection including possible lobectomy or pneumonectomy and multimodal treatment.

Prognosis is favorable in the majority of childhood bronchial adenomas with permanent cure. Prognosis of the other malignant tumors depends on the respectability and type of the primary tumor and presence of a metastatic disease.

Resection cures the cystic type of pleuropulmonary blastoma in 85–90 %, and only 45–60 % is cured by surgery and chemotherapy in the cystic-solid or solid types.

Treatment of metastatic lung disease by resection is an option in osteogenic sarcomas, some types of soft tissue sarcomas, and adrenocortical carcinoma; less in nephroblastoma and Ewing's sarcoma; and rarely in neuroblastoma, thyroid cancer, and rhabdomyosarcoma. Prerequisites are cure of the primary lesion, exclusion of other organ involvement by metastases, and insufficient response of the metastases to chemotherapy. ###

Resection of metastases includes wedge resection, segment resection, or lobectomy which is performed by bilateral muscle-sparing thoracotomy or sternotomy. Favorable conditions are complete resection of all lung metastases including those only identified by palpation, metachronous metastases, and absent involvement of the pleura. For instance, a 5-year event-free survival of 36 % is observed in high-grade osteosarcoma of the extremities with localized disease who later relapsed with lung metastasis.

10.8.2 Pleural Tumors

Occurrence, Pathoanatomy

Pleural tumors are mostly lung or chest wall tumors with pleural involvement. Ewing's sarcoma of the rib (with pleural effusion in up to two thirds at first clinical presentation) and pleuropul-

monary blastoma (with possible pleural effusion or pneumothorax) are characteristic examples. Sarcomatoid and desmoplastic mesothelioma, solitary fibrous or desmoid tumor, and benign mesothelioma belong to the primary pleural tumors.

Clinical Presentation

The spectrum of clinical presentation extends from *localized or diffuse chest pain to tachy- and dyspnea depending on the type and amount of pleural effusion.*

Differential Diagnosis, Work-Ups, and Treatment

It includes the more common parapneumonic and tuberculous pleural effusions. The work-ups are the same as for lung or chest wall tumors. Thoracocentesis and diagnostic thoracoscopy are specific tools.

Treatment encompasses the primary tumor such as rib and soft tissue resection and chemotherapy in Ewing's sarcoma and possibly decortication in gross involvement of the pleural space by a primary or secondary tumor.

Webcodes

The following webcodes can be used on www.psurg.net for further images and data.

1001 Macroglossia, hemangioma	1008 Pneumatoceles after Staphylococcuspneumonia and
1002 Solitary lung cyst	1009 At surgery the involved lung with
1003 Spontaneous pneumothorax with	1010 Feeding bronchiolus of pneumatoceles
1004 Diagnosis of CCAM in infancy	1011 Metastasis left lung lobe, after
1005 Bochdalek's hernia, manifestation in infancy	1012 Treated nephroblastoma and
1006 Clinical presentation, subcutaneous emphysema in	1013 After cytostatic treatment
1007 Spontaneous bilateral pneumothorax and -mediastinum	

Bibliography

General: Transfusion Related Lung Injury, Thoracoscopy, Lung Transplantation

Sanchez R, Toy P (2005) Transfusion related acute lung injury: a pediatric perspective. Pediatr Blood Cancer 45:248–255

Speich R, Nicod LP, Aubert JD, Spiliopoulos A, Wellinger J, Robert JH, Stocker R, Zalunardo M, Gasche-Soccal P, Boehler A, Weder W (2004) Ten years of lung transplantation in Switzerland: results of the Swiss lung transplant registry. Swiss Med Wkly 134: 18–23

Tsao K, St Peter SD, Sharp SW, Nair A, Andrews WS, Sharp RJ, Snyder CL, Ostlie DJ, Holcomb GW (2008) Current application of thoracoscopy in children. J Laparoendosc Adv Surg Tech A 18: 131–135

Section 10.1

Gokhale J, Selbst SM (2009) Chest pain and chest wall deformity. Pediatr Clin North Am 56:49–65, x

Selbst SM, Ruddy RM, Clark BJ, Henretig FM, Santulli T Jr (1988) Pediatric chest pain: a prospective study. Pediatrics 82:319–323

Section 10.2.1: Pulmonary Sequestration

Gezer S, Tastepe I, Sirmali M, Findik G, Türüt H, Kaya S, Karaoglanoglu N, Cetin G (2007) Pulmonary sequestration: a single-institutional series composed of 27cases. J Thorac Cardiovasc Surg 133:955–959

Kang M, Khandelwal N, Ojili V, Rao KL, Rana SS (2006) Multidetector CT angiography in pulmonary sequestration. J Comput Assist Tomogr 30:926–932

Morikawa N, Kuroda T, Honna T, Kitano Y, Fuchimoto Y, Terawaki K, Kawasaki K, Koinuma G, Matsuoka K, Saeki M (2005) Congenital bronchial atresia in infants and children. J Pediatr Surg 40:1822–1826

Section 10.2.2: Bronchiectasis

Banjar HH (2007) Clinical profile of Saudi children with bronchiectasis. Indian J Pediatr 74:149–152

Karadag B, Karakoc F, Ersu R, Kut A, Bakac S, Dagli E (2005) Non-cystic-fibrosis bronchiectasis in children: a persisting problem in developing countries. Respiration 72:233–238, Comment in: Respiration (2005) 72:225–226

Otgün I, Karnak I, Tanyel FC, Senocak ME, Büyükpamukcu N (2004) Surgical treatment of bronchiectasis in children. J Pediatr Surg 39:1532–1536

Sirmali M, Karasu S, Türüt H, Gezer S, Kaya S, Tastepe I, Karaoglanoglu N (2007) Surgical management of bronchiectasis in childhood. Eur J CardiothoracSurg31: 120–123

Tsao PC, Lin CY (2002) Clinical spectrum of bronchiectasis in children. Acta Paediatr Taiwan 43: 271–275

Section 10.2.3: Spontaneous Pneumothorax

Amin R, Noone PG, Ratjen F (2009) Chemical pleurodesis versus surgical intervention for persistent and recurrent pneumothoraces in cystic fibrosis. Cochrane Database Syst Rev. (2):CD007481

Bialas RC, Weiner TM, Phillips JD (2008) Video-assisted thoracic surgery for primary spontaneous pneumothorax in children: is there an optimal technique? J Pediatr Surg 43:2151–2155

Caceres M, Ali SZ, Braud R, Weiman D, Garrett HE Jr (2008) Spontaneous pneumomediastinum: a comparative study and review of the literature. Ann Thorac Surg 86:862–866

Chambers A, Scarci M (2009) In patients with first-episode primary spontaneous pneumothorax is video-assisted thoracoscopy superior to tube thoracostomy alone in terms of time to resolution of pneumothorax and incidence of recurrence? Interact Cardiovasc Thorac Surg 9:1003–1008

Chiu CY, Wong KS, Yao TC, Huang JL (2005) Asthmatic versus non-asthmatic spontaneous pneumomediastinum in children. Asian Pac J Allergy Immunol 23: 19–22

de Lorimier AA (1998) Respiratory problems related to the airway and lung. In: O'Neill JA Jr et al (eds) Pediatric surgery, vol 1, 5th edn. Mosby, St. Louis

de Perrot M, Deléaval J, Robert J, Spiliopoulos A (2000) Spontaneous hemopneumothorax – results of conservative treatment. Swiss Surg 6:62–64

Even L, Heno N, Talmon Y, Samet E, Zonis Z, Kugelman A (2005) Diagnostic evaluation of foreign body aspiration in children: a prospective study. J Pediatr Surg 40:1122–1127

Guimaraes CV, Donnelly LF, Warner BW (2007) CT findings for blebs and bullae in children with spontaneous pneumothorax and comparison with findings in normal age-matched controls. Pediatr Radiol 37: 879–884

Nathan N, Guilbert J, Larroquet M, Lenoir M, Clement A, Epaud R (2010) Efficacy of blebs detection for preventive surgery in children's idiopathic spontaneous pneumothorax. World J Surg 34:185–189

Poenaru D, Yazbeck S, Murphy S (1994) Primary spontaneous pneumothorax in children. J Pediatr Surg 29: 1183–1185

Reynolds M (1998) Disorders of the thoracic cavity and pleura and infections of the lung, pleura, and mediastinum. In: O'Neill JA Jr et al (ed) Pediatric surgery, vol 1, 5th edn. Mosby, St. Louis

Robinson PD, Cooper P, Ranganathan SC (2009) Evidence-based management of paediatric primary spontaneous pneumothorax. Paediatr Respir Rev 10: 110–117; quiz 117

Sections 10.3.1–10.3.6: Thoracic Injuries

Cheli M, Alberti D, Adriana T, Zaranko E, Colusso M, Arnoldi R, Codazzi D, Locatelli G (2009) Successful bleeding control by a combined conventional surgical approach and video-assisted surgery: a case report. Ann Thorac Cardiovasc Surg 15:253–256

Cullen ML (2001) Pulmonary and respiratory complications of pediatric trauma. Respir Care Clin N Am 7:59–77

Frommelt PC, Frommelt MA (2004) Congenital coronary artery anomalies. Pediatr Clin North Am 51:1273–1288

Maguire S, Mann M, John N, Ellaway B, Sibert JR, Kemp AM, Welsh Child Protection Systematic Review Group (2006) Does cardiopulmonary resuscitation cause rib fractures in children? A systematic review. Child Abuse Negl 30:739–751

Nakayama DK, Ramenofsky ML, Rowe MI (1989) Chest injuries in childhood. Ann Surg 210:770–775

Neal MD, Sippey M, Gaines BA, Hackam DJ (2009) Presence of pneumomediastinum after blunt trauma in children: what does it really mean? J Pediatr Surg 44:1322–1327

Ramirez RM, Cureton EL, Ereso AQ, Kwan RO, Dozier KC, Sadjadi J, Bullard MK, Liu TH, Victorino GP (2009) Single-contrast computed tomography for the triage of patients with penetrating torso trauma. J Trauma 67:583–588

Rodgers BM, McGahren ED III (1998) Laryngoscopy, bronchoscopy, and thoracoscopy. In: O'Neill JA Jr et al (eds) Pediatric surgery, vol 1, 5th edn. Mosby, St. Louis

Roux P, Fisher RM (1992) Chest injuries in children: an analysis of 100 cases of blunt chest trauma from motor vehicle accidents. J Pediatr Surg 27:551–555

Samarasekera SP, Mikocka-Walus A, Butt W, Cameron P (2009) Epidemiology of major paediatric chest trauma. J Paediatr Child Health 45:676–680

Tsitouridis I, Tsinoglou K, Tsandiridis C, Papastergiou C, Bintoudi A (2007) Traumatic pulmonary pseudocysts: CT findings. J Thorac Imaging 22:247–251

Wesson DE (1998) Thoracic injuries. In: O'Neill JA Jr et al (eds) Pediatric surgery, vol 1, 5th edn. Mosby, St. Louis

Wylie J, Morrison GC, Nalk K, Kotylak TB, Fraser DD, Kornecki A (2009) Lung contusion in children – early computed tomography versus radiography. Pediatr Crit Care Med 10:643–647

Section 10.4: Cardiovascular Injuries

Allison ND, Anderson CM, Shah SK, Lally KP, Hayes-Jordan A, Tsao KJ, Andrassy RJ, Cox CS Jr (2009) Outcomes of truncal vascular injuries in children. J Pediatr Surg 44:1958–1964

Bajor G, Bijata W, Szczeklik M, Bohosiewicz J, Bochenek A, Daab M (2005) Traumatic rupture of the aorta in adolescence – description of two cases. Eur J Pediatr Surg 15:287–291

Grapow MTR, Lampert FM, Handschin R, Bremerich J, Eckstein F, Carrel T (2009) Rezidivierende Synkope und Thoraxschmerz bei einem jugendlichen Fussballspie-ler. Schweiz Med Forum 9:695–697

Link MS, Bir C, Dau N, Madias C, Estes NAM 3rd, Maron BJ (2008) Commentary protecting our children from the consequences of chest blows on the playing field: a time for science over marketing. Pediatrics 122:437–439

Maron BJ, Gohman TE, Kyle SB et al (2002) Clinical profile and spectrum of commotio cordis. JAMA 287: 1142–1146

Vasudevan AR, Kabinoff GS, Keltz TN et al (2003) Blunt chest trauma producing acute myocardial infarction in a rugby player. Lancet 362:370

Section 10.5: Foreign Body Aspiration

Bhat KV, Hedge JS, Nagalotimath US, Patil GC (2010) Evaluation of computed tomography virtual bronchoscopy in paediatric tracheobronchial foreign body aspiration. J Laryngol Otol 29:1–5

Cohen S, Avital A, Godfrey S, Gross M, Kerem E, Springer C (2009) Suspected foreign body inhalation in children: what are the indications for bronchoscopy? J Pediatr 155:276–280, Comment in: J Pediatr (2010) 156:690–691; author reply 691

de Sousa ST, Ribeiro VS, de Menezes Filho JM, dos Santos AM, Barbieri MA, de Figueiredo Neto JA (2009) Foreign body aspiration in children and adolescents: experience of a Brazilian referral center. J Bras Pneumol 35:653–659

Girardi G, Contador AM, Castro-Rodriguez JA (2004) Two new radiological findings to improve the diagnosis of bronchial foreign-body aspiration in children. Pediatr Pulmonol 38:261–264

Göktas O, Snidero S, Jahnke V, Passali D, Gregori D (2010) Foreign body aspiration in children: field report of a German hospital. Pediatr Int 52:100–103

Karakoc F, Cakir E, Ersu R, Uyan ZS, Colak B, Karadag B, Kiyan G, Dagli T, Dagli E (2007) Late diagnosis of foreign body aspiration in children with chronic respiratory symptoms. Int J Pediatr Otorhinolaryngol 71:241–246

Krugman SD, Lantz PE, Sinal S, De Jong AR, Coffman K (2007) Forced suffocation of infants with baby wipes: a previously undescribed form of child abuse. Child Abuse Negl 31:615–621

Li Y, Wu W, Yang X, Li J (2009) Treatment of 38 cases of foreign body aspiration in children causing life-threatening complications. Int J Pediatr Otorhinolaryngol 73:1624–1629

Ludemann JP, Riding KH (2007) Choking on pins, needles and a blowdart: aspiration of sharp, metallic foreign bodies secondary to careless behaviour in seven adolescents. Int J Pediatr Otorhinolaryngol 71: 307–310

Mani N, Soma M, Massey S, Albert D, Bailey CM (2009) Removal of inhaled foreign bodies – middle of the night or the next morning? Int J Pediatr Otorhinolaryngol 73:1058–1089, Comment in: Int J Pediatr Otorhinolaryngol (2010) 74:104; author reply 104–105

Riess KP, Cogbill TH, Patel NY, Lambert PJ, Mathiason MA (2007) Tracheal rupture in a child with blunt chest injury. J Trauma 63:1021–1025

Roh JL, Lee JH (2006) Spontaneous tracheal rupture after severe coughing in a 7-year-old boy. Pediatrics 118: e224 e227

Roux P, Fisher RM (1992) Chest injuries in children: an analysis of 100 cases of blunt chest trauma from motor vehicle accidents. J Pediatr Surg 27:551–555

Sammer M, Wang E, Blackmore CC, Burdick TR, Hollingworth W (2007) Indeterminate CT angiography in blunt thoracic trauma: is CT angiography enough? AJR Am J Roentgenol 189: 603–608

Saquib Mallick M, Rauf Khan A, Al-Bassam A (2005) Late presentation of tracheobronchial foreign body aspiration in children. J Trop Pediatr 51:145–148

Schimpl G, Schneider U (1996) Traumatic pneumatoceles in an infant: case report and review of the literature. Eur J Pediatr Surg 6:104–106

Shin SM, Kim WS, Cheon JE, Jung BJ, Kim IO, Yeon KM (2009) CT in children with suspected residual foreign body in airway after bronchoscopy. AJR Am J Roentgenol 192:1744–1751

Shlizerman L, Mazzawi S, Rakover Y, Ashkenazi D (2010) Foreign body aspiration in children: the effects of delayed diagnosis. Am J Otolaryngol 31: 320–324

Shubha AM, Das K (2009) Tracheobronchial foreign bodies in infants. Int J Pediatr Otorhinolaryngol 73: 1385–1389

Sirmali M, Türüt H, Kisacik E, Findik G, Kaya S, Tastepe I (2005) The relationship between time of admittance and complications in paediatric tracheobronchial foreign body aspiration. Acta Chir Belg 105:631–634

Tomaske M, Gerber AC, Stocker S, Weiss M (2006) Tracheobronchial foreign body aspiration in childrenz – diagnostic value of symptoms and signs. Swiss Med Wkly 136:533–538

Tovar JA (2008) The lung and pediatric trauma. Semin Pediatr Surg 17:53–59

Weissberg D, Weissberg-Kasav D (2008) Foreign bodies in pleura and chest wall. Ann Thorac Surg 86: 958–961

Section 10.6.1: Pleural Empyema

Avansino JR, Goldman B, Sawin RS, Flum DR (2005) Primary operative versus nonoperative therapy for pediatric empyema: a meta-analysis. Pediatrics 115:1652–1659, Comment in: Pediatrics (2006) 117:1462–1463 and 117:261–262

Bishay M, Short M, Shah K, Nagraj S, Arul S, Parikh D, Jawaheer G (2009) Efficacy of video-assisted thoracoscopic surgery in managing childhood empyema; a large single center study. J Pediatr Surg 44:337–342

Calder A, Owens CM (2009) Imaging of parapneumonic pleural effusions and empyema in children. Pediatr Radiol 39:527–537

Carey JA, Hamilton JR, Spencer DA, Gould K, Hasan A (1998) Empyema thoracis: a role for open thoracotomy and decortication. Arch Dis Child 79:510–513

Gustafson RA, Murray GF, Warden HE, Hill RC (1990) Role of lung decortication in symptomatic empyemas in children. Ann Thorac Surg 49:940–946, discussion 946–947

Kokoska ER, Chen MK, Committee New Technology (2009) Position paper on video-assisted thoracoscopic surgery as treatment of pediatric empyema. J Pediatr Surg 44:289–293

Li ST, Tancredi DJ (2010) Empyema hospitalizations increased in US children despite pneumococcal conjugate vaccine. Pediatrics 125:26–33

Roberts JE, Bezack BJ, Winger DI, Pollack S, Shah RA, Cataletto M, Katz DS, Montoya-Iraheta C, Schroeder SA, Quintos-Alagheband ML (2008) Association between parapneumonic effusion and pericardial effusion in a pediatric cohort. Pediatrics 122:e1231–e1235

Shamsuzzaman SM, Hashiguchi Y (2002) Thoracic amebiasis. Clin Chest Med 23:479–492

Sharif K, Alton H, Clarke J, Desai M, Morland B, Parikh D (2006) Paediatric thoracic tumours presenting as empyema. Pediatr Surg Int 22:1009–1014

St Peter SD, Tsao K, Spilde TL, Keckler SJ, Harrison C, Jackson MA, Sharp SW, Andrews WS, Rivard DC, Doug C, Morello FP, Frank P, Holcomb GW 3rd, Ostlie DJ (2009) Thoracoscopic decortication vs tube thoracostomy with fibrinolysis for empyema in children: a prospective, randomized trial. J Pediatr Surg 44:106–111; discussion 111

Tönz M, Ris HB, Casaulta C, Kaiser G (2000) Is there a place for thoracoscopic debridement in the treatment of empyema in children. Eur J Pediatr Surg 10:88–91

Sections 10.6.2–10.6.3: Lung Abscess and Pneumatocele

Al-Saleh S, Grasemann H, Cox P (2008) Necrotizing pneumonia complicated by early and late pneumatoceles. Can Respir J 15:129–132

Ayed AK, Al-Rowayeh A (2005) Lung resection in children for infectious pulmonary diseases. Pediatr Surg Int 21:604–608

Caksen H, Oztürk MK, Uzüm K, Yüksel S, Ustünbas HB (2000) Pulmonary complications in patients with staphylococcal sepsis. Pediatr Int 42:268–271

Chan PC, Huang LM, Wu PS, Chang PY, Yang TT, Lu CY, Lee PI, Chen JM, Lee CY, Chang LY (2005) Clinical management and outcome of childhood lung abscess: a 16-year experience. J Microbiol Immunol Infect 38:183–188

Cowles RA, Lelli JL Jr, Takayasu J, Coran AG (2002) Lung resection in infants and children with pulmonary infections refractory to medical therapy. J Pediatr Surg 37:643–647

Imamoglu M, Cay A, Kosucu P, Ozedmir O, Cobanoglu U, Orhan F, Akyol A, Sarihan H (2005) Pneumatoceles in postpneumonic empyema: an algorithmic approach. J Pediatr Surg 40:1111–1117

Jetley NK, El-Wahed Hussein MR, Softha AL (2009) Air filled, inflammatory, lung pseudo-cyst: etiopathogenesis and management. Indian J Pediatr 76:324–326

Joosten KF, Hazelzet JA, Tiddens HA, Hazebroek FW, Dzoljic-Danilovic G, Neijens HJ, de Groot R (1995) Staphylococcal pneumonia in childhood: will early surgical intervention lower mortality? Pediatr Pulmonol 20:83–88

Kunyoshi V, Cataneo DC, Cataneo AJ (2006) Complicated pneumonias with empyema and/or pneumatocele in children. Pediatr Surg Int 22:186–190

Nagasawa KK, Johnson SM (2010) Thoracoscopic treatment of pediatric lung abscesses. J Pediatr Surg 45:574–578

Puligandla PS, Laberge JM (2008) Respiratory infections: pneumonia, lung abscess, and empyema. Semin Pediatr Surg 17:42–52

Reynolds M (1998) Disorders of the thoracic cavity and pleura and infections of the lung, pleura, and mediastinum. In: O'Neill JA Jr et al (ed) Pediatric surgery, vol 1, 5th edn. Mosby, St. Louis

Thomas B, Pugalenthi A, Chilvers M (2009) Pleuropulmonary complications of PVL-positive *Staphylococcus aureus* infection in children. Acta Paediatr 98: 1372–1375

Section 10.7: Lung Parasitosis

Aghajanzadeh M, Safarpoor F, Amani H, Alavi A (2008) One-stage procedures for lung and liver hydatid cysts. Asian Cardiovasc Thorac Ann 16:392–395

Chopdat N, Menezes CN, John MA, Mahomed N, Grobusch MP (2007) A gardener who coughed up blood. Lancet 370:1520

Darwish B (2006) Clinical and radiological manifestations of 206 patients with pulmonary hydatidosis over a ten-year period. Prim Care Respir J 15:246–251

Demirbilek S, Sander S, Atayurt HF, Aydin G (2001) Hydatid disease of the liver in childhood: the success of medical therapy and surgical alternatives. Pediatr Surg Int 17:373–377

Dincer SI, Demir A, Sayar A, Gunluoglu MZ, Kara HV, Gurses A (2006) Surgical treatment of pulmonary hydatid disease: a comparison of children and adults. J Pediatr Surg 41:1230–1236

Djuricic SM, Grebeldinger S, Kafka DI, Djan I, Vukadin M, Vasiljevicz ZV (2010) Cystic echinococcosis in children – the seventeen-year experience of two large medical centers in Serbia. Parasitol Int 59:257–261

Gavidia CM, Gonzales AE, Zhang W, McManus DP, Lopera L, Ninaquispe B, Garcia HH, Rodriguez S, Verastegui M, Calderon C, Pan WK, Gilman RH (2008) Diagnosis of cystic echinococcosis, central Peruvian highlands. Emerg Infect Dis 14:260–266

Kilimcioglu AA, Ozkol M, Bayindir P, Girginkardesler N, Ostan I, Ok UZ (2006) The value of ultrasonography alone in screening surveys of cystic echinococcosis in children in turkey. Parasitol Int 55:273–275

Mishra PK, Agrawal A, Joshi M, Sanghvi B, Gupta R, Parelkar SV (2010) Minimal access surgery for multiorgan hydatid cysts. Afr J Paediatr Surg 7:40–42

Olmez D, Babayigit A, Arslan H, Uzuner N, Ozturk Y, Karaman O, Cakmakci H (2008) Multiorgan involvement in a pediatric patient with hydatid disease. J Trop Pediatr 54:417–419

Reynolds M (1998) Disorders of the thoracic cavity and pleura and infections of the lung, pleura, and mediastinum. In: O'Neill JA Jr et al (ed) Pediatric surgery, vol 1, 5th edn. Mosby, St. Louis

Tuncözgür B, Isik AF, Nacak I, Akar E, Elbeyli L (2007) Dilemma on the treatment of haemoptysis: an analysis of 249 patients. Acta Chir Belg 107:302–306

Ulkü R, Eren N, Cakir O, Balci A, Onat S (2004) Extrapulmonary intrathoracic hydatid cysts. Can J Surg 47:95–98

Zeyrek D, Savas R, Gulen F, Demir E, Tanac R (2008) "Air-bubble" signs in the CT diagnosis of perforated pulmonary hydatid cyst: three case reports. Minerva Pediatr 60:361–364

Section 10.8: Lung and Pleural Tumors

Bagan P, Hassan M, Le Pimpec Barthes F, Peyrard S, Souilamas R, Danel C, Riquet M (2006) Prognostic factors and surgical indications of pulmonary epithelioid hemangioepithelioma: a review of the literature. Ann Thorac Surg 82:2010–2013

Bartyik K, Bede O, Tiszlavicz L, Onozo B, Virag I, Turi S (2004) Pulmonary capillary haemangiomatosis in children and adolescents: report of a new case and review of the literature. Eur J Pediatr 163: 731–737

Briccoli A, Rocca M, Salone M, Guzzardella GA, Balladelli A, Bacci G (2010) High grade osteosarcoma of the extremities metastatic to the lung: long-term results in 323 patients treated combining surgery and chemotherapy, 1985–2005. Surg Oncol 19:193–199

Dishop MK, Kuruvilla S (2008) Primary and metastatic lung tumors in the pediatric population: a review and 25-year experience at a large children's hospital. Arch Pathol Lab Med 132:1079–1103

Dommange-Romero F, Collardeau-Frachon S, Hameury F (2010) Child pleuropulmonary blastoma. Bull Cancer 97:1047–1052

Harting MT, Blakely ML (2006) Management of osteosarcoma pulmonary metastases. Semin Pediatr Surg 15:25–29

Hill DA, Jarzembowski JA, Priest JR, Williams G, Schoettler P, Dehner LP (2008) Type I pleuropulmonary blastoma: pathology and biology study of 51 cases from the international pleuropulmonary blastoma registry. Am J Surg Pathol 32:282–295

Hullo E, Cotta L, Rabeyrin M, Larroquet M, Plantaz D (2011) Bronchial carcinoid tumors in children. Bull Cancer 98:709–715

Kayton ML (2006) Pulmonary metastasectomy in pediatric patients. Thorac Surg Clin 16:167–183, vi

Kovach SJ, Fischer AC, Katzman PJ, Salloum RM, Ettinghausen SE, Madeb R, Koniaris LG (2006) Inflammatory myofibroblastic tumors. J Surg Oncol 94:385–391

Naik-Mathuria BJ, Cotton RT, Fitch ME, Popek EJ, Brandt ML (2008) Thoracoscopic excision of an intrathoracic mesothelial cyst in a child. J Laparoendosc Adv Surg Tech A 18:317–320

Newman B (2011) Thoracic neoplasms in children. Radiol Clin North Am 49:633–664, v

Priest JR, Andic D, Arbuckle S, Gonzalez-Gomez I, Hill DA, Williams G (2011) Great vessel/cardiac extension and tumor embolism in pleuropulmonary blastoma: a report from the International Pleuropulmonary Blastoma Registry. Pediatr Blood Cancer 56:604–609

Shochat S (1998) Tumors of the lung. In: O'Neill JA Jr et al (eds) Pediatric surgery, vol 1, 5th edn. Mosby, St. Louis

Soyer T, Ciftci AO, Gücer S, Orhan D, Senocak ME (2004) Calcifying fibrous pseudotumor of the lung: a previously unreported entity. J Pediatr Surg 39:1729–1730

Tagge EP, Mulvihill D, Chandler JC, Richardson M, Uflacker R, Othersen HD (1996) Childhood pleuropulmonary blastoma: caution against nonoperative management of congenital lung cysts. J Pediatr Surg 31:187–189; discussion 190

Temeck BK, Wexler LH, Steinberg SM, McClure LL, Horowitz M, Pass HI (1995) Metastasectomy for sarcomatous pediatric histologies: results and prognostic factors. Ann Thorac Surg 59:1385–1389; discussion 1390

Travis WD (2010) Sarcomatoid neoplasms of the lung and pleura. Arch Pathol Lab Med 134:1645–1658

Utine GE, Ozcelik U, Kiper N, Dogru D, Yalcn E, Cobanoglu N, Pekcan S, Kara A, Cengiz AB, Ceyhan M, Secmeer G, Göcmen A (2009) Pediatric pleural effusions: etiological evaluation in 492 patients over 29 years. Turk J Pediatr 51:214–219

Warmann SW, Fuchs J (2009) Principles of oncological surgery for lung metastases in paediatric solid tumours. Zentralbl Chir 134:537–541

Weldon CB, Shamberger RC (2008) Pediatric pulmonary tumors: primary and metastastic. Semin Pediatr Surg 17:17–29

This chapter concerns the most frequent and important congenital deformities of the thoracic wall. They are not always recognized at birth because no attention is paid to it or they only emerge distinctly during growth.

Chest wall deformities can be divided in five groups as listed in Table 11.1 according to their clinical and numerical significance.

11.1 Funnel Chest

11.1.1 Occurrence, Pathology, Associated Anomalies

The prevalence of pectus excavatum is 1 in 100 teenagers, and three thirds to 80 % are boys.

The sternum and the adjacent cartilaginous parts of several rib pairs are inverted similar to funnel #. Funnel chest may be combined with other malformations such as scoliosis or heart failure. It may be a part of a syndrome such as Marfan,

Table 11.1 Differential diagnosis of chest wall deformities

- Funnel chest (pectus excavatum)
- Protrusion deformity (pectus carinatum, pigeon breast)
- Poland's syndrome
- o Sternal defects including ectopia cordis
- o Other chest wall deformities: Shield-shaped thorax in Turner's syndrome or chest wall deformities with or without systemic skeletal pathologies

Noonan, and Poland's syndrome. Familiality is present in up to two thirds of patients.

11.1.2 Clinical Significance

- In small children, the parents may be worried about the deformity. For teenagers, funnel chest may be a psychological problem.
- Young people may be handicapped in competitive sports.
- Important associated syndromes such as **Marfan syndrome** # should be recognized early.
- Combined disorders and postural abnormalities of the spine should be treated early to avoid permanent impairment.
- Corrective surgery is easier to perform in children.

11.1.3 Natural History, Clinical Presentation

Although the majority of cases with funnel chest is recognizable already in small children or even in newborns if looked for, the deformity may increase during growth and become therefore more visible. On the other hand, the degree of deformity remains stable in most children, and amelioration takes place only in a few.

The **symptoms and signs** depend on the age. In small children, anorexia and failure to thrive, motionless, stridor, and dysphagia have been observed in single patients. In schoolchildren, *psychological problems* are in the foreground: Disorders of self-esteem combined with pathological behavior are sometimes triggered by the reaction of the schoolfellows, for example, avoidance of swimming pools.

In teenagers, *reduced tolerance to exercise*, for instance, in cycling, swimming, or competitive sports, is added to possible psychological problems.

In up to two thirds of all schoolchildren, *minor cardiovascular and respiratory symptoms* are described such as chest pain, shortness of breathing, palpitations, and crampedness, or *major signs such as reduced endurance fitness* (=reduced physical work capacity) with tachypnea, tachycardia, and shortage of breath on exertion.

Severe functional restrictions are occasionally observed in young adult, especially while working in a sitting position.

The **local findings** display a large variability of degree and type of the individual deformity. The assignment of the patients to either asthenic (with a characteristic posture) or muscular constitution, the differentiation between four types of funnel chest, and measurements of the thoracic cage are trials to objectively define the individual type of funnel chest and its degree of deformity.

The four **types of pectus excavatum** are as follows if shape and depth of the funnel are considered:

- Symmetric ## (Fig. 11.1).
- Asymmetric shallow type: The funnel is shallow like a saucer and up to 17 cm broad, and the rib bows are only slightly everted #.
- Symmetric #.
- Asymmetric deep type ##: The funnel is small and up to 7 cm deep (it touches nearly the anterior thoracic spine), and the rib bows are distinctly everted (Fig. 11.2).

The asymmetric deep type and the asymmetric and symmetric shallow types are the most frequently observed forms. In such cases, the

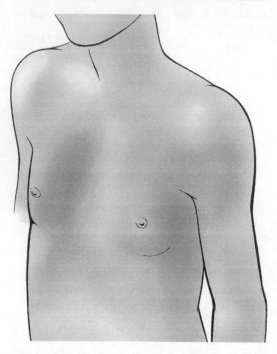

Fig. 11.1 Drawings of the main types of funnel chest. The symmetrical sternal depression is broad and has a shape like a mould or small hollow

external sternal surface is turned to the right side and forms the border of the left-sided funnel; the corresponding adjacent rib pairs are more prominent on the left than on the right side #. At surgery, 51 % of pectus excavatum are asymmetric.

Associated S-shaped scoliosis of the thoracic and lumbar spine (in >10 % of the cases) and postural kyphosis of the thoracic spine are possible disorders of the spine. The latter is often combined with an asthenic constitution.

The **clinical skills** include determination of the **external sternovertebral distance** and other distances. *A calliper measures the distance between the deepest point of the funnel and the opposite spine.* The obtained value is compared with normal values for age and sex: In body length of 55, 105, or 155 cm, values of 8, 12, and 14 cm or less are pathological. In addition, photos of the chest in ap and semioblique projections are taken.

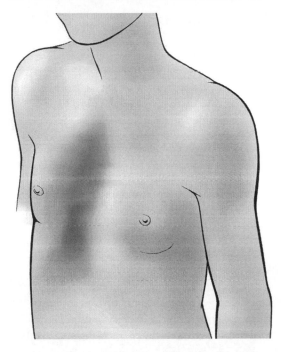

Fig. 11.2 Drawings of the main types of funnel chest. The depression of the sternum and adjacent ribs is deep, narrow, and asymmetrical

The degree of malposition of the spine and possible associated anomalies must be measured or recorded precisely.

11.1.4 Work-Ups, Differential Diagnosis

Chest x-rays in two planes are useful for measurement of the internal sternovertebral distance ##, for description of the heart silhouette, and for recognition of spine or thoracic anomalies.

For the **internal sternovertebral diameter**, the distance between the deepest point of the marked funnel to the opposite anterior spine surface is measured. In body length of 55, 105, and 155 cm, values of <5, 7, and 8 cm or less are pathological.

The heart silhouette is either displaced to the left side combined with abnormal configuration and prominent right hilus, or less frequently widened with equal distribution of both sides.

Because findings that affect the decision to perform surgery can be obtained by chest x-rays, 3D CT with larger radiation risks and medical costs should only be performed in specific indications. It shows precisely the type of deformity and the Haller index, and new indexes for better definition of asymmetry and depression may be calculated.

The **Haller index** can be calculated on an appropriate single CT image by dividing the narrowest central diameter into the cross-sectional diameter of the chest. Values of the pectus index > 3.25 belong to a distinct funnel chest, whereas indices <3.25 belong to a normal chest or only a minimal depression. The pectus index is not age-dependent and corresponds to the same index achieved by chest x-rays in two planes. It seems inadequate to quantify the postoperative change in shape.

(Doppler) Echocardiography is useful in suspected heart failure or Marfan syndrome (possible dilatation of the aortic root), to exclude mitral prolapse (in 15 %, not influenced by surgery), and as part of **exercise tests**. **Static and dynamic lung function tests** are applied for recognition of a possible restrictive disorder and associated asthma that needs preoperative treatment.

The **differential diagnosis** includes **combined pectus excavatum and pigeon breast** (in <5 % of funnel chests with surgery, see also Fig. 11.4), Marfan syndrome, other collagenoses, and **postoperative chest deformities (funnel chest)** #.

11.1.5 Treatment, Prognosis

Treatment is exclusively surgical and the **indications** are symptomatic and/or progressive funnel chests: Physical symptoms and signs with relevant impairment or relevance to the patient, for example, exertional dyspnea and reduced endurance fitness and/or severe psychosocial impairment.

Whereas physical impairment has a correlation to the degree of funnel chest, for instance, documented by a low sternovertebral distance, the psychosocial impairment is unrelated to the severity of funnel chest.

A **decision in favor of or against surgery** only should be taken if the following topics are evaluated and discussed with patient and parents:

- Severity of the individual funnel chest and patient suffering from it
- Informed consent about the possible natural history (possible deterioration of the physical signs in some young adults, possible impact on survival)
- Informed consent about the available surgical procedures including advantages and disadvantages, complications, and outcomes
- Possible necessity of pre- and postoperative physiotherapy: Maintenance of a normal posture and strength of trunk muscles and/or asthma medication

Available are **the minimally invasive Nuss** or **the open reconstructive Ravitch technique** and other surgical procedures (including magnetic mini-mover procedure in the future). If the repair has failed with one method, some recommend the alternative approach for reoperation.

The original indication of **Nuss procedure** was symmetric funnel chest in schoolchildren. The sternum is raised by a retrosternal bar which has been placed under thoracoscopic guidance and turned. Nuss technique has undergone a serious learning curve since its introduction in 1998 due to failure in asymmetric and severe types, or after former cardiovascular surgery, displacement of the bar, and complications such as injury to heart and aorta, or pneumothorax and pleural, and pericardial effusions. Introduction of two bars, use of stabilizers, short subxyphoid approach, and incisions along the cartilaginous ribs are examples of modified techniques to overcome the quoted drawbacks ##.

The modified **Ravitch technique** requires minimal costal cartilage resection and sternal osteotomy, and most of the patients receive a temporary sternal support strut. Sternochondroplasty is specifically useful for asymmetric funnel chests. Main disadvantages are chest wall reactions to the resection, possibly diminished flexibility and elasticity of the chest wall, and a visible scar ##.

11.1.6 Prognosis

Untreated funnel chest does mostly not improve with time and can affect survival.

After surgery, normalization is reported to a large extent for the Nuss procedure and the Ravitch technique. After Nuss operation, the sternovertebral distance increases during the first year after surgery by a mean value of 33.8 mm and decreases after bar removal by 8.6 mm. The mean Haller index decreases from a preoperative value of 5.97 ± 3.31 to a postoperative value of 3.08 ± 0.64 after bar removal regardless of age and severity, and between the latter value and the value of a control cohort, no significant difference is reported. Unfortunately, normalization concerns only the mean value, and the application of 1SD shows that already several patients of two thirds of the study group have pathological values. Therefore, a complete normalization is not achieved in all.

Static and dynamic lung function test is pathological in some patients with funnel chest, and slight to moderate restrictive lung disorder can be observed. The results of the postoperative permanent recovery are controversially reported. On the other hand, preoperative reduced endurance fitness in some of the patients objectively recorded by exercise testing can be improved by surgery which is attributed to amelioration of cardiac function. Yet, a generally valid statement is still impossible because there is considerable overlap of the results of some patients with funnel chest and those of age-matched normal children.

In general, surgical repair leads significantly to improvement of self-consciousness and body image. Chronic chest pain after any surgery may be observed occasionally; in Nuss procedure, it may be related to the bar or stabilizer.

The survey of the first 20 years' data on Nuss procedure quotes no mortality and 15.4 % complications of which bar-related adverse advents and pneumothorax have been the most frequent. In other studies, the recent complication quote was 3.8 %, and the recurrence rate was 1.6 %; the long-term results were excellent in almost all patients.

If surgery is performed before 10 years of age, recurrences have been observed during the growth spurt. In addition to preoperative information of the parents and long-term follow-ups, delayed removal of the bar is an option.

Metal allergy is observed in <5 %, is often misdiagnosed as infection, and needs removal or replacement by a titanium bar. Patients with a history of atopy should be tested for metal allergy before insertion of a metallic bar. Rarely, reactive pectus carinatum does occur.

In Nuss procedure, the deformity is forcibly corrected that leads to concentrated stress to the thoracic cage in children recognized later by costal cartilaginous changes on ultrasound.

In Ravitch technique, very good or excellent results are reported in 94 % (–98 %) with a mean follow-up time of 7.6 years. There were no deaths and complications in 2.6 % such as pleural or pericardial effusion, hematoma or seroma, dislodged sternal strut, and localized infection. The recurrence rate was 8 % (–0.9 %) and 2 % needed resection of localized cartilage protrusion.

In addition, asphyxiating thoracic dystrophy and reactive pectus carinatum has been reported as rare complications of Ravitch technique occurring several years after or within a year of original correction. Whereas the former condition can be improved by sternal split with rib craft placement, the latter needs pectus carinatum repair after puberty or in case of Nuss technique early bar removal. In Ravitch technique, sustained bone and cartilage changes are recognizable years after surgery by shortening of the regenerated costal cartilages and clubbing of the ends of the osseous ribs.

11.2   Pectus Carinatum (Protrusion Deformity of the Chest, Pigeon Breast)

11.2.1   Occurrence, Surgical Pathology

Pigeon breast is observed in 1 of 1,000 teenagers and mostly in boys. Familiality is present in up to a fourth (Fig. 11.3).

In pectus carinatum, the body of the sternum and adjacent costal cartilages are protruded mostly symmetrically or less frequently asymmetrically only on one side. It is associated with a bi- or unilateral groove of the lateral ribs. The rare superior type of pigeon breast or protrusion deformity of the manubrium is combined with a relative impression of the sternal body.

Except for scoliosis and infrequent congenital heart failure, pigeon breast is usually not associated with other malformations. In congenital heart failure or mediastinal tumor, localized protrusion may be present.

11.2.2   Clinical Significance

• Pectus carinatum is mainly an aesthetic and psychological problem of teenagers that is often underestimated.

11.2.3   Clinical Presentation

All protrusion deformities are recognizable by careful inspection from different angles of view. In addition, it should be looked for constitution and spinal abnormalities.

The sternal body is together with the adjacent costal cartilages protruding ##. The degree of protrusion can be expressed by measurement of

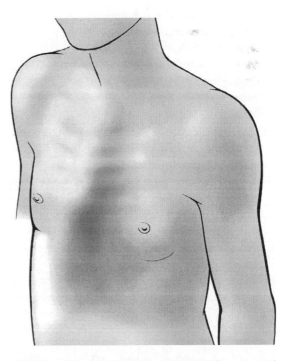

Fig. 11.3 Drawing of pectus carinatum. Sternum and adjacent ribs protrude symmetrically (pigeon breast)

the external sternovertebral distance. In asymmetric pigeon breast, the protruding cartilages of one side lead together with a posterior torsion of sternum on the contralateral side to a keel-like deformity #. In the rare superior type, the protruded manubrium describes a comma-like transition to the relatively depressed sternal body if looked from the side.

11.2.4 Work-Ups, Differential Diagnosis

Except for asymmetric and combined types of pigeon breast, chest x-rays in two planes together with photos from the front and both sides are sufficient for documentation of the individual case. CT with possible 3D reconstruction is useful in complex types of pigeon breast. Other work-ups including cardiovascular and respiratory functional tests are only necessary in suspected heart failure or in specific questioning.

The differential diagnosis includes protrusion deformities due to congenital mediastinal tumor or heart failure, pectus carinatum combined with funnel chest, reactive pectus carinatum after surgery of funnel chest or thoracic surgery, and **postoperative chest deformity (pectus carinatum)** #.

In **combined pectus carinatum**, the proximal part of sternal body is protruding, whereas the distal part is depressed. The sternum is S-shaped in the sagittal plane and is rotated with its posterior part to the depressed side (Fig. 11.4).

Reactive pectus carinatum develops within the first year after Nuss or Ravitch procedure for funnel chest. It can be corrected by early bar removal or by postpubertal repair.

11.2.5 Treatment, Prognosis

In symmetric pigeon breast of the sternal body, dynamic compression combined with physical exercises is indicated. Bracing needs long-term adherence and supervision of the patient and parents, especially during the growth spurt and until the end of growth.

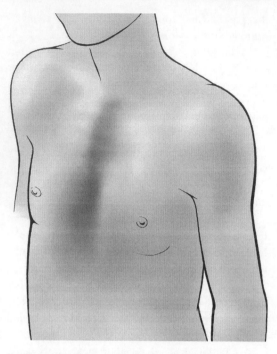

Fig. 11.4 The drawing displays a combination of pectus carinatum (*middle part of the sternum*) and funnel chest (*lower part of the sternum*)

In case of an asymmetric or combined funnel chest, or a very rigid pigeon breast, surgery is superior to bracing. The modified sternochondroplasty must consider the abnormal position of the protruding sternum in all three planes.

Prognosis is excellent if the appropriate treatment option is chosen and proper performed with minor morbidity, for example, skin reactions in bracing or surgical morbidity.

11.3 Poland's Syndrome

11.3.1 Occurrence, Pathology

Poland's syndrome is a rare and sporadic combination of mostly unilateral aplasia or hypoplasia of the sternocostal portion of the major pectoralis muscle with at least another of the known associated malformations. Associated anomalies are present in variable combinations and include anomalies of the homolateral thoracic cage and its soft tissues, hand, and arm of different degrees. Poland's syndrome is observed more frequently on the right side, and if the left side is involved, dextrocardia may be encountered. Later in life, association with various malignancies, for example, breast carcinoma, occurs rarely.

11.3.2 Clinical Significance

- The single or multiple associated unilateral anomalies should attract the attention to the possibility of Poland's syndrome because aplasia or hypoplasia of the major pectoralis muscle is often not recognized at first glance.
- Severe hand and/or chest wall anomalies may lead to functional and/or aesthetic impairment.

11.3.3 Clinical Presentation

Aplasia or hypoplasia of the sternocostal portion of the major pectoralis muscle and possibly of other chest and trunk muscles *is recognized by loss of the anterior axillary fold combined with a transverse skin fold, an infraclavicular depression, and deficit and abnormal contour of the breast #.*

The most frequently occurring **hand and arm anomalies** # consist of *cutaneous syndactyly, brachydactyly with fingers of equal length,* carpal bone anomalies, smaller hand and shorter arm in comparison to the contralateral side, and more mutilating anomalies. **Malformations of the breast** occur in two thirds of patients and vary from absence of breast or nipple to hypoplasia of one or both. The aesthetically most disturbing forms are *absent breast in a developing girl* or *hypoplastic nipple in adolescent boy with cranial displacement.*

Malformations of the chest wall occur in less than 50 % of the patients: hypoplasia or aplasia of one or several ribs. The latter is combined with depression of the adjacent ribs, rotation of the sternum to the involved side, and possible lung hernia. The funnel chest-like depression of ribs is combined with a depression and rotation of sternum, and protrusion deformity of the contralateral side (combined funnel chest with pigeon breast). *The frequency of hypoplasia, depression deformity, and aplasia of the ribs corresponds to the quoted order.*

In addition, the subcutaneous fat and hair of chest wall including axilla may be thin and sparse.

11.3.4 Work-Ups, Differential Diagnosis

In addition to the precise clinical description including measurement of arm and hand, palpation of the breast, and appropriate photo documentation, chest x-rays, CT, and MRI may be useful for evaluation of the thoracic cage and chest wall soft tissues. In developed patients, mammography and hand x-ray may be added, and at any age ultrasound as preliminary examination. To avoid unnecessary radiological imaging, it is useful to perform them as far as they are needed for forthcoming surgery.

The differential diagnosis includes differentiation from all possible associated anomalies. The hallmark of Poland's syndrome is always the major pectoralis muscle hypoplasia or aplasia of one side that is recognized be clinical comparison with the contralateral side or confirmed by ultrasound. Specific conditions include anterior thoracic hypoplasia and unilateral accentuated thelarche.

11.3.5 Treatment, Prognosis

Early reconstruction of the chest wall is necessary in aplasia of the ribs with lung hernia and can be performed by autologous rib transplantation and synthetic patch. Syndactyly or depression deformities of the ribs (chest wall deformities) should be corrected in preschool or in school age by a modified Fonkalsrud procedure, whereas reconstructive surgery of breast and chest wall soft tissue is best performed at the end of development and growth by (endoscopically assisted) autologous latissimus dorsi flap (the muscles are rarely hypoplastic), autologous fat tissue transfer, contralateral breast resection and/or silicone implant insertion.

11.3.6 Prognosis

It depends on the degree of severity of Poland's syndrome (grades I to III according to Foucras et al.). The possibilities and growing experience of reconstructive surgery for the individual anomalies play an important role as well.

11.4 Sternal Defects

The complex of different sternal defects occurs much less frequently than pigeon breast. Today, prenatal ultrasound diagnosis is possible.

11.4.1 Cleft Sternum

11.4.1.1 Pathology
The sternal midline defect is more frequently partial than total and concerns mostly the upper part in the partial type. The osseous defect is covered by normal skin. The heart is normal in its location, morphology, and investment.

11.4.1.2 Clinical Significance
- The underlying heart is not protected by a firm chest wall, and the paradoxical respiratory motions of the soft tissue mantle hinder an effective mechanics of respiration.

11.4.1.3 Clinical Presentation
A dent is visible and palpable in the midline of the sternum corresponding to the sternal defect. In addition, paradoxical respiratory movements can be observed of the soft tissue overlying the defect and the anteroinferior part of the neck with depression on inspiration and swelling on expiration, and especially on crying.

11.4.1.4 Work-Ups, Differential Diagnosis
The former are chest x-ray into planes and 3D CT with specific reference to the sternum. The latter includes tumors of neck and mediastinum, for example, cystic lymphangioma and postoperative sternal cleft.

11.4.1.5 Treatment, Prognosis
Closure of the defect should be performed in the first trimenon for correction of the quoted pathophysiological mechanisms and a greater flexibility and elasticity of the sternal halves and costal cartilages.

After blunt dissection of the endothoracic fascia from the sternal halves and possible wedge excision at the lower sternal end, the two sternal parts are sutured together with nonabsorbable threads.

Prognosis is favorable. Older children need additional mobilization of the cartilaginous costal arch.

11.4.2 Ectopia Cordis

11.4.2.1 Pathology
In ectopia cordis, the often malformed heart is displaced through a soft tissue and sternal defect in front of the thorax, in an abdominal or cervical direction by an anterior diaphragmatic and lower sternal defect or upper sternal defect with fusion between mouth region and apex of the heart.

11.4.2.2 Clinical Significance
- In contrast to the inoperable cervical ectopia cordis, surgery is possible in the thoracoabdominal and thoracic ectopia cordis.

11.4.2.3 Clinical Presentation
Thoracic ectopia cordis is easily recognized by the protrusion of the anteriorly directed heart through a skin and sternal defect #.

In the thoracoabdominal ectopia cordis, a subcostal abdominal wall defect is observed at first glance that is often composed of an omphalocele in its lower part and a part of the heart combined with a lower sternal defect and covered by a thin membrane.

11.4.2.4 Work-Ups, Differential Diagnosis

It includes ultrasound, thoracoabdominal CT, and echocardiography. Some types of simple omphalocele must be differentiated from thoracoabdominal ectopia cordis because the location of the heart is variable.

11.4.2.5 Treatment

Surgery must consider that there is not sufficient space available for the heart in the thoracic cage and congenital heart failure occurs frequently.

In a first step, the skin defect should be closed as early as possible. After evaluation for possible heart failure, surgery should be performed accordingly. Finally, the thoracic and/or abdominal defect is reconstructed.

Prognosis concerning survival and quality of life is better in thoracoabdominal than in thoracic ectopia cordis. It depends largely on the individual type of malformation and the possibilities of reconstructive surgery.

Webcodes

The following webcodes can be used on www. psurg.net for further images and data.

1101 Funnel chest	1113 Step of Nuss procedure,
1102 Funnel chest in Marfan syndrome	1114 After reduction of funnel chest
1103 Shallow symmetrical type,	1115 Step in Ravitch technique and
1104 Better visible from an oblique view	1116 After removal of stitches
1105 Shallow asymmetrical type	1117 Protrusion deformity, frontal and
1106 Deep symmetrical type	1118 Lateral view
1107 Deep asymmetrical type,	1119 Postoperative protrusion deformity (laparoschisis)
1108 Better visible from an oblique view	1120 Hypoplasia major pectoralis muscle
1109 Close-up view, deep asymmetrical type	1121 Poland's syndrome, arm and hand anomaly
1110 Pa chest x-ray, heart silhouette	1122 Ectopia cordis

1111 Lateral chest x-ray, internal sternovertebral diameter	1123 Asymmetrical pigeon breast
1112 Postoperative funnel chest	

Bibliography

Sections 11.1–11.2 General

Carrel T, Schnyder A, Zurmühle P, Matyas G, Velasco R, Körner F, Ammann K (2003) Das Marfan-Syndrom. Schweiz Med Forum 46:1096–1107

De Paepe A, Devereux RB, Dietz HC, Henekam RC, Pyeritz RE (1996) Revised diagnostic criteria for the Marfan syndrome. Am J Med Genet 62: 417–426

Fokin AA, Steuerwald NM, Ahrens WA, Allen KE (2009) Anatomical, histological, and genetic characteristics of congenital chest wall deformities. Semin Thorac Cardiovasc Surg 21:44–57

Haller JA Jr, Kramer SS, Lietman SA (1987) Use of CT scans in selection of patients for pectus excavatum surgery: a preliminary report. J Pediatr Surg 22: 904–906

Kelly RE Jr (2008) Pectus excavatum: historical background, clinical picture, preoperative evaluation and criteria for operation. Semin Pediatr Surg 17: 181–193

Kelly RE Jr, Lawson ML, Paidas CN, Hruban RH (2005) Pectus excavatum in a 112-year autopsy series: anatomic findings and the effect on survival. J Pediatr Surg 40:1275–1278

Ravitch MM (1986) The chest wall. In: Welch KJ et al (eds) Pediatric surgery, vol I, 4th edn. Mosby, St. Louis

Rowland T, Moriarty K, Banever G (2005) Effect of pectus excavatum deformity on cardiorespiratory fitness in adolescent boys. Arch Pediatr Adolesc Med 159:1069–1073

Shamberger RC (1998) Congenital chest wall deformities. In: O'Neill JA Jr et al (eds) Pediatric surgery, vol I, 5th edn. Mosby, St. Louis

Stucki HR (1972) Bestimmung des sagitallen Thoraxdurchmessers bei Kindern. Z Kinderchir 11: 21–31

Section 11.1.1 Surgery

Antonoff MB, Saltzman DA, Hess DJ, Acton RD (2010) Retrospective review of reoperative pectus excavatum repairs. J Pediatr Surg 45:200–205

Bouchard S, Hong AR, Gilchrist BF, Kuenzler KA (2009) Catastrophic cardiac injuries encountered during the minimally invasive repair of pectus excavatum. Semin Pediatr Surg 18:66–72

Castellani C, Schaalamon J, Saxena AK, Hoellwarth ME (2008) Early complications of the Nuss procedure for pectus excavatum: a prospective study. Pediatr Surg Int 24:659–666

Castellani C, Saxena AK, Zebedin D, Hoelwarth ME (2009) Pleural and pericardial morbidity after minimal access repair of pectus excavatum. Langenbecks Arch Surg 394:717–721

Felts E, Jouve JL, Blondel B, Launay F, Lacroix F, Bollini G (2009) Child pectus excavatum: correction by minimally invasive surgery. Orthop Traumatol Surg Res 95:190–195

Fonkalsrud EW (2009) 912 Open pectus excavatum repairs: changing trends, lessons learned: one surgeon's experience. World J Surg 33:180–190

Fonkalsrud EW, Mendoza J, Finn PJ, Cooper CB (2006) Recent experience with open repair of pectus excavatum with minimal cartilage resection. Arch Surg 141:823–829

Harrison MR, Curran PF, Jamshidi R, Christensen D, Bratton DJ, Fechter R, Hirose S (2010) Magnetic mini-mover procedure for pectus excavatum II: initial findings of a food and drug administration-sponsored trial. J Pediatr Surg 45:185–191

Hosie S, Sitkiewicz T, Petersen C, Göbel P, Schaarschmidt K, Till H, Noatnick M, Winiker H, Hagl C, Schmedding A, Waag K-L (2002) Minimally invasive repair of pectus excavatum – the Nuss procedure. A European multicentre experience. Eur J Pediatr Surg 12:235–238

Kilda A, Lukosevicius S, Barauskas V, Jankauskaite Z, Basevicius A (2009) Radiological changes after Nuss operation for pectus excavatum. Medicina (Kaunas) 45:699–705

Nuss D, Kelly RE Jr (2008) Minimally invasive surgical correction of chest wall deformities in children (Nuss procedure). Adv Pediatr 55:395–410

Nuss D, Croitoru DP, Kelly RE Jr, Goretsky MJ, Nuss KJ, Gustin ST (2002) Review and discussion of the complications of minimally invasive pectus excavatum repair. Eur J Pediatr Surg 12:230–238

Palmer B, Yedlin S, Kim S (2007) Decreased risk of complications with bilateral thoracoscopy and left-to-right mediastinal dissection during minimally invasive repair of pectus excavatum. Eur J Pediatr Surg 17:81–83

Protopapas AD, Athanasiou T (2008) Peri-operative data on the Nuss procedure in children with pectus excavatum: independent survey of the first 20 years' data. J Cardiothorac Surg 3:40, Review

Rushing GD, Goretsky MJ, Gustin T, Morales M, Kelly RE Jr, Nuss D (2007) When it is not an infection: metal allergy after the Nuss procedure for repair of pectus excavatum. J Pediatr Surg 42:93–97

Swanson JW, Colombani PM (2008) Reactive pectus carinatum in patients treated for pectus excavatum. J Pediatr Surg 43:1468–1473

Section 11.1.2 Long-Term Outcome

Al-Assiri A, Kravarusic D, Wong V, Dicken B, Milbrandt K, Sigalet DL (2009) Operative innovation to the "Nuss" procedure for pectus excavatum. Operative and functional effects. J Pediatr Surg 44:888–892

Kelly RE Jr, Crash TF, Shamberger RC, Mitchell KK, Mellins RB, Lawson ML, Oldham K, Azizkhan RG, Hebra AV, Nuss D, Goretsky MJ, Sharp RJ, Holcomb GW III, Shim WK, Megison SM, Moss RL, Fecteau AH, Colombani PM, Bagley T, Quinn A, Moskowitz AB (2009) Surgical repair of pectus excavatum markedly improves body image and perceived ability for physical activity: multi-center study. Pediatrics 122:1218–1222

Kubiak R, Habelt S, Hammer J, Häcker FM, Mayr J, Bielek J (2007) Pulmonary function following completion of minimally invasive repair for pectus excavatum (MIRPE). Eur J Pediatr Surg 17:255–260

Lam MW, Klassen AF, Montgomery CJ, LeBlanc JG, Skarsgard ED (2008) Quality-of-life outcomes after surgical correction of pectus excavatum: a comparison of the Ravitch and Nuss procedures. J Pediatr Surg 43:819–825

Section 11.3

Bock K, Hadji P, Schulz KD, Wagner U, Duda FV (2004) Differential diagnosis of Poland-syndrome versus unilateral accentuated thelarche. Ultraschall Med 25:377–382

Delay E, Sinna R, Chekaroua K, Delaporte T, Garson S, Tousson G (2010) Lipomodeling of Poland's syndrome: a new treatment of the thoracic deformity. Aesthet Surg J 34:218–225

Ireland DCR, Takayama N, Flatt AE (1976) Poland's syndrome: a review of forty-three cases. J Bone Joint Surg Am 58A:52–58

Ribeiro RC, Saltz R, Mangles MG, Koch H (2009) Clinical and radiographic Poland syndrome classification: a proposal. Aesthet Surg J 29:494–504

Shamberger RC, Welch KJ, Upton J III (1989) Surgical treatment of thoracic deformity in Poland's syndrome. J Pediatr Surg 24:760–765; discussion 766

Spear SL, Pelletiere CV, Lee ES, Grotting JC (2004) Anterior thoracic hypoplasia: a separate entity from Poland syndrome. Plast Reconstr Surg 113:69–77; discussion 78–79

Urschel HC Jr (2009) Poland syndrome. Semin Thorac Cardiovasc Surg 21:89–94

Section 11.4

Luthra S, Dhaliwal RS, Singh H (2007) Sternal cleft – a natural absurdity or surgical opportunity. J Pediatr Surg 42:582–584

Tumors, Tumor-Like Masses, Nipple Discharge, and Anomalies of the Breast

12

These presenting signs concern exclusively the breast. A surview of the many and diverse disorders of congenital or acquired origin is listed in Tables 12.1 and 12.2.

Spontaneous pain, tenderness, and firm swelling of the breast are observed mainly in acquired disorders and may be recorded in a cyclic fashion as in 25 % of female teenagers with **premenstrual syndrome** and sometimes already before menarche. The observation of diverse symptoms 7 days before beginning of menstruation is probably underreported; only just one of ten young women is symptomless. Unilateral or bilateral nipple pain may be observed as transient phenomenon in the second stage of breast development.

12.1 Congenital Pathologies

12.1.1 Hypoplasia and Aplasia of Breast and/or of Nipple (Micromastia, Amastia, and/or Athelia)

Occurrence
They occur as part of a Poland's syndrome or as isolated unilateral or bilateral disorder.

Clinical Significance
• Micromastia, amastia, and/or athelia bothers already school children and their mothers, particularly if they are unilateral or become overt during pubertal development

Table 12.1 Differential diagnosis of congenital breast tumors and anomalies including nipple discharge

o Unilateral and bilateral breast and/or nipple hypoplsia or aplasia (micromastia, amastia, and/or athelia)

● Gross enlargement of the breast in newborns

o Inversion, hypertrophy, or multiplication of the nipple(s)

Table 12.2 Acquired disorders of breast including nipple discharge and diffuse and localized enlargement of the breast including tumors

o Acquired and secondary hypoplasia and aplasia of the breast

o Discharge from the nipple

● Mastitis

● Diffuse enlargement of the breast(s)

  o Precocious thelarche

  o Precocious puberty

  o Precocious pseudopuberty

  o Macromastia

    ● Gynecomastia

● Localized enlargement of the breast, tumors of the breast

Clinical Presentation
An absent or hypoplastic is nipple and areola is already recognizable in early childhood whereas hypoplasia and aplasia of the breast of one and to a lesser degree of both sides can be suspected during pubertal development (at latest by 14 years of age) and diagnosed almost certainly at the end of growth (e.g., by 17 years if the size of the breast(s) does not change anymore within 6 months). *Sizes of less than one to two fifth of the measured contralateral breast correspond to hypoplasia of one side. A history of neonatal breast enlargement excludes congenital breast aplasia.*

G.L. Kaiser, *Symptoms and Signs in Pediatric Surgery*,
DOI 10.1007/978-3-642-31161-1_12, © Springer-Verlag Berlin Heidelberg 2012

Work-Ups, Differential Diagnosis

They include clinical examination of the whole body including for signs of puberty; inspection, palpation, and measurement of breast size; measurement of body length; weight; and percentiles, photographs, and radiological imaging for bone age.

In girls, the differential diagnosis includes **several variations** and disorders:

1. During puberty, the development of one breast may differ from that of the other breast with equalization in size and shape at the end of growth #. Hence, small differences in size and shape belong to the general right-left asymmetry of the whole body.

2. The absent growth of the breasts is part of a delayed sexual development that is often a familial variation. Nevertheless, some breast development should be present at the age of 14 years at latest.

3. The mammary gland and the mammilla remain infantile in spite of normal maturation of the other signs of puberty.

In addition, Turner syndrome, testicular feminization, and other **chromosomal aberrations or disorders of sex development** (premenarcheal, virilizing congenital adrenal cortical hyperplasia = CAH) must be considered in bilateral hypoplasia or aplasia. Finally, **acquired and secondary types of unilateral and bilateral hypoplasia and aplasia** of the breast belong to the possible differential diagnoses. The latter diagnoses may be supported by a history of injury to the breast or ovaries, by local findings such as scars after surgery, or by primary amenorrhea and absent secondary sex characteristics. In addition, **delayed puberty** (no signs of pubertal development up to the thirteenth year in girls and up to the fourteenth years of age in boys) must be considered in which a constitutional cause, a severe chronic disease, and rarely an endocrinological disorder is encountered (primary, secondary, and tertiary gonadal insufficiency, e.g., Turner syndrome in girls, Klinefelter's syndrome, or congenital or acquired testicular insufficiency).

In unilateral hypoplasia, a reliable diagnosis may be possible by comparison with the other breast. On the other hand, differentiation between true hypoplasia is difficult in bilateral forms because of a continuous transition from a normal to a pathological size, especially since the imagination of the young women is different.

Treatment, Prognosis

Breast augmentation should not be performed before the clinically confirmed end of growth and development. It is indicated in bilateral aplasia or unilateral aplasia and hypoplasia, whereas bilateral hypoplastic forms are a matter of discussion and dependent on the mental distress.

12.1.2 Diffuse Enlargement of the Breast in the Newborn

Occurrence

Congenital breast enlargement that is observed in almost all neonates born at term starts in the late fetal life and reaches a maximum size of about 14 mm 2–3 weeks after birth. It occurs less frequently in premature infants.

Clinical Significance

- The large variability of enlargement of the neonatal breast bud and its different course may arouse the suspicion of a tumor especially in the large and persistent variety if a physiological phenomenon is not considered. Carcinoma of the breast has been observed only rarely in infancy.

Clinical Presentation

At birth, slight enlargement of the breast is visible and palpable with a mean size of about 8 mm diameter although the breast may be larger # and reach several centimeters in the following few weeks in some. Initially, a watery or milky excretion may be observed. The involution to the original size at birth or less may take several months #. Unilateral or bilateral atresia of the breast is excluded if a physiological breast enlargement has been observed in the neonatal period.

Work-Ups, Differential Diagnosis

Work-ups are only necessary if unusual local findings lead to discussion about the origin of enlargement and secretion.

Sometimes, the initial stage of mastitis of the newborn or a developing hemangioma of the breast must be considered. Short-term observations, inflammatory laboratory signs, and ultrasound are the tools for differential diagnosis.

Treatment, Prognosis

Treatment is not necessary. Expression of the breast bud should be avoided. Except for puberty or pregnancy and breastfeeding, enlargement and/or secretion beyond late infancy is pathological.

Prognosis is excellent and no correlation exists between size of neonatal enlargement and chance of development of neonatal mastitis.

12.1.3 Inversion, Hypertrophy, and Multiplication of the Nipple(s)

Pathology, Clinical Significance

The nipple is either turned upside down or effaced because the whole areola forms a bulbous, large, and soft projection or is multiplied into two or more nipples.
- All three congenital anomalies may cause mental stress, but only inversion may have functional consequences leading to subareolar abscess and difficulties in breastfeeding.

Therapy

Reconstructive surgery may become necessary after puberty.

12.2 Acquired Pathologies

12.2.1 Acquired and Secondary Hypoplasia and Aplasia of the Breast

Causes

Several injuries to the chest wall and breast may lead to acquired hypoplasia or aplasia of the breast:
- Burns including chemical or electrical injuries and child abuse
- Blunt and penetrating thoracic injuries (motor vehicle accident, sports, stab and gunshot injuries, bites)

- Inflammatory or neoplastic disorders, for example, purulent mastitis of the neonate or hemangioma of chest wall and breast
- Sequels of surgery or radiation, for example, chest tube thoracostomy in recurrent pneumothorax of the preterm infant or biopsy of the breast bud

The secondary hypoplasia or aplasia of the breast is due to endogenous estrogen deficit after primary or secondary functional loss of the ovaries or because of absent reactivity of the breast to hormonal stimulation.

Clinical Significance
- Surgeons and all interventional therapists should be aware of possible injury to the breast if the thoracic cavity and chest wall or the lower abdomen is involved at any age of childhood ##.

12.2.2 Nipple Discharge

Occurrence, Clinical Significance

It occurs as presenting symptom in at least 7 % of adult surgical breast pathologies and in 10–15 % of benign and <5 % of malignant tumors in childhood.

Clinical Significance
- Except for discharge in combination with neonatal breast enlargement and milky secretion in pregnancy and after birth, any secretion from the breast is pathological.
- Discharge from the nipple is like a palpable mass of the breast not specific for a single pathology because it may be observed in many disorders although less often than a palpable mass.

Clinical Presentation

Breast secretion is milky, multicolored and sticky, purulent, clear (watery), yellow (serous), pink (serosanguineous), and bloody (sanguineous with red or brownish color). It has been observed by the child or mother or has led to discoloration of the underwear or nightclothes. Secretion may be gathered on consultation by compression of the breast.

Depending on the cause of abnormal secretion, several local findings of the breast, mammilla, or overlying or adjacent skin may be present.

Work-Ups, Differential Diagnosis

A precise history may disclose some of the possible causes such as medication with tranquilizers or contraceptives, or indications of possible endocrinological disorders, for example, hypothyroidism or pituitary tumor if the galactorrhea is not associated with pregnancy. Dependent on the suspected disorder, ultrasound including Doppler (vascularization), mammography, MRI, US-guided FNA cytology or core needle biopsy, galactography, ductoscopy, and surgical biopsy are the next steps.

In ultrasound, the examiner should be well acquainted with the specific findings and variations of breast development and of the expected specific pathologies.

The differential diagnosis includes:

- Medicamentous or endocrinological causes
- Subareolar abscess or purulent mastitis
- Cystic ductal hyperplasia (mammary duct ectasia)
- Intraductal papilloma or papillomatosis
- The other benign or malignant tumors of the breast

Of the quoted seven types of discharge, the last four are significant for benign and malignant tumors. The most likely cause of bloody nipple discharge is mammary duct ectasia especially in small children although other causes such as mastitis, fibrocystic disease, and even gynecomastia are observed.

The **subareolar abscess** occurs in lacteal duct obstruction. The abscess is evacuated insufficiently by secondary periareolar sinus tract(s). The small mass beneath the areola may fluctuate on palpation.

In **cystic ductal hyperplasia (mammary duct ectasia)**, a small, nontender, and soft mass near the areola may be palpated.

Treatment, Prognosis

Treatment is mostly successful if the appropriate measures are taken. They include in subareolar abscess combined excision of the sinus tract(s), abscess, and corresponding major duct and in cystic ductal hyperplasia, primarily a conservative approach.

12.2.3 Mastitis

Occurrence, Causes

In contrast to the mastitis of toddlers and schoolchildren that is observed sporadically, several cohorts with neonatal mastitis have been described for evaluation of the common characteristics.

Physiological breast enlargement of the newborn is not the cause of mastitis of neonates. The abscess is mainly caused by staphylococci but, Gram-negative and mixed germs are also observed. Only a small percentage has a positive blood culture.

In schoolchildren with a developing breast, sports without or with necrosis of the fatty tissue, injuries to the chest wall with abrasions, or tight underwear and sweating may lead to mastitis. Breastfeeding adolescents may obtain mastitis like women after birth.

Clinical Significance

- Purulent mastitis or its inappropriate treatment is a possible cause of acquired unilateral hypoplasia or aplasia of the breast.

Clinical Presentation

Mastitis occurs uniformly in female and male newborns without any preference of one side during the first 2 weeks after birth #.

Two thirds of mastites with abscess present either in the second or third postnatal week. The phlegmonous infection of the breast bud includes the overlying and adjacent skin and leads to an inflammatory enlargement of the breast. *In three fourths, systemic signs of infection are absent and the body temperature does not exceed 38 °C. The breast becomes swollen, red, and warm with palpable periareolar fluctuation #.*

In schoolchildren, a history as mentioned before may be ascertained in some. *The patients complain of discomfort, tension, or a vague pain in the breast. Initially, the overlaying and adjacent skin is faintly reddened #.*

Differential Diagnosis, Work-Ups

It includes **chronic subareolar abscess, cellulitis of the chest wall, infection after trauma to the chest wall,** and **chest wall tumors with inflammatory signs of the skin**. Rarely obese teenagers complain of a tender swelling of one breast. On clinical examination, a hard and painful cord is subcutaneously palpable that corresponds to a thrombophlebitis of the thoraco-epigastric, lateral thoracic, and superior epigastric veins and is called **Mondor disease**.

Leukocyte count and shift and C-reactive protein are necessary as well as Gram stain and culture of the pus obtained by fine needle aspiration or incision. Depending on the severity of the general and local findings, blood cultures should be performed especially in neonates.

Treatment, Prognosis

Antibiotic treatment should be started immediately corresponding to the expected germs to avoid abscess. Abscess needs prompt incision and drainage by a semicircular periareolar incision close to the mammilla.

Prognosis depends on the stage of mastitis at the beginning of treatment. Specifically in newborns, advanced mastitis with gross abscess may lead to breast hypoplasia or aplasia and to septicemia with osteomyelitis.

12.2.4 Diffuse Enlargement of the Breast

Clinical Significance

- Diffuse enlargement of one or both breasts may cause anxiety to the parents and involved child or psychological disturbances if it occurs before puberty in both sexes or at puberty in girls in excess or in boys in general.

Types

Precocious thelarche, precocious puberty, iso- or heterosexual precocious pseudopuberty, macromastia (virginal hypertrophy), and **gynecomastia** of the boy are the main types of diffuse breast enlargement.

Clinical Presentation

Unilateral or bilateral **precocious thelarche** (in girls, at <8 and in boys, at <9 years) *is mainly observed in the first 3 years of life and in girls* although boys may also be involved. *The breast buds have a palpable and/or visible size of the hazelnut # to the plum or even of the developed breast.* Normalization occurs within a year or the breast enlargement persists until the onset of puberty. *Areola, nipple, and primary and secondary sexual characteristics remain infantile.*

Benign pubic hair of infancy and premature onset of menses are other types of isolated manifestation of one single pubertal sign. In a population of children referred for evaluation of precocious puberty, 80 % belong to such variations of normal sex development. The change from 8 to 7 years of age for white girls and to six for black girls at which signs of puberty are considered precocious according to the PROS guidelines is controversial because serious pathologies may be missed due to late referrals.

Precocious puberty: *Development of all sexual characteristics occurs before 8 years in girls and 9 years in boys. The latter are less frequently involved; the order of development is the same as in normal puberty*. The possible causes are different from those of precocious pseudopuberty. It is observed in 1:5–10,000 children and much more frequently in girls ## than in boys.

Precocious pseudopuberty: *The sexual characteristic may occur as single signs, do not follow the normal order of development, and manifests as isosexual and/or heterosexual form #.*

In **virginal hypertrophy**, *one or both breasts increase to a grotesque size and pendulous shape that leads to fatigue, chest pain, backache, and premenstrual mastalgia, abnormal posture, intertrigo, rarely to thoracic outlet compression syndrome, and psychological disorders.*

Gynecomastia: A *palpable and/or visible enlargement of one or both breasts at puberty occurs in up to 70 % of all boys. The breasts look in some of the patients like those of a girl at puberty # although the increase in size is for the majority of involved boys less than in the pubertal girl #.* Often spontaneous resolution is observed in 1–2 years. About 10 % persist with no resolution within 3 years. However, the exorbitant size of one or both breasts and/or the delay in involution causes emotional distress and/or raises carcinophobia in the mother.

Work-Ups, Differential Diagnosis

Peak height velocity, radiological imaging (ultrasound, CT, and MRI), and hormonal evaluation (examinations should be performed before manual examination of the breast and include estradiol, testosterone, LH/FSH prior and after LRH stimulation) belong to the work-ups depending on the suspected disorder as quoted above and for differential diagnosis.

Precocious thelarche, virginal hypertrophy, and gynecomastia are in the majority of cases clinical diagnoses. In precocious thelarche, the quoted differential diagnoses may be excluded by a normal abdominal ultrasound and estradiol level.

In contrast to a positive LRH stimulation in precocious puberty, the test is negative in precocious pseudopuberty. In unilateral gynecomastia, the demonstration of normal breast tissue by ultrasound excludes a tumor as cause of macromastia.

In **precocious thelarche**, precocious puberty and pseudopuberty, an estradiol-producing tumor of the ovary, testis, or adrenal gland must be excluded. In addition, precocious thelarche may be the beginning of precocious puberty. Occasionally, fat may simulate precocious thelarche that is best confirmed by ultrasound.

In **precocious puberty**, CNS disorders (such as hydrocephalus, malformations, neurofibromatosis, trauma, infection, or tumor), late-onset CAH, hypothyroidism, acanthosis nigricans (altogether 10–15 %), and an idiopathic form must be considered, and in **precocious pseudopuberty**, hormonally active tumors of the ovary (arrhenoblastoma) or testis, McCune-Albright syndrome, CAH, virilizing adrenal gland tumor, and ectopic tumors with LH-FSH formation must be excluded.

In **virginal hypertrophy**, tuberous breast hypertrophy, hypertrophy of the nipple(s), or normal but large breasts are the main differential diagnoses.

In **gynecomastia**, the most frequent differential diagnosis is **pseudogynecomastia** in which breast enlargement is simulated by obesity. The clinical examination yields a prepubertal obese boy with an infantile breast bud and penis without any signs of puberty #.

Rarely Klinefelter's syndrome, disorder of testosteron synthesis, other DSD, feminizing tumor, medication of drugs such as estradiol or antiepileptics or severe diseases such as leukemia or disorders with hepatic or renal insufficiency are the **cause of gynecomastia.**

If only **one breast is diffusely enlarged** in one of the already quoted disorders, a variation of normal development in girls or a large breast tumor in both sexes must be considered in the differential diagnosis.

Treatment, Prognosis

Premature thelarche needs no treatment except for reassurance of the parents and regular clinical follow-ups.

Virginal hypertrophy should be treated by reduction mammoplasty as soon as growth is finished by the seventeenth year of life.

In boys with gynecomastia, the role of estrogen receptor inhibitors is not yet established by prospective, randomized clinical trials. Subcutaneous mastectomy should be considered if the size of the enlarged breast bud is ≥5 cm in diameter and/or persists beyond 1–2 years and/or if the boy exhibits severe psychological impairment.

In virginal hypertrophy, the prognosis is excellent if the appropriate measures are taken.

Treatment and prognosis of the other disorders depend on their causes.

12.2.5 Localized Masses of the Breast

Occurrence, Pathology

Tumors and tumor-like masses of the breast are rare in children and somewhat more frequently at puberty and in adolescence. Up to three fourths are fibroadenomas followed by diffuse mastopathies (about 10 %). Intraductal papilloma, cysts, and chronic subareolar abscess are observed each in 5 %. Only 1 % concerns malignant tumors such as metastatic disease (rhabdomyosarcoma, leukemia, lymphoma, and neuroblastoma) and breast carcinoma. Only ≥8 % of all patients with breast carcinoma are younger than 20 years. A palpable mass and/or nipple discharge and/or some breast discomfort is the main symptom and sign.

Clinical Significance

- In breast tumors of children, always the suspicion of malignancy arises and often mutilating diagnostic and therapeutic interventions are taken although a malignant tumor is rare in this age group.

Clinical Skills

Inspection should be performed in a sitting position without and with raised arms. The breasts are **palpated** in a supine and in a sitting position with the finger tips in a circular manner from the outer margins of the breast to the center and from one quadrant to the next, and again after crossing one arm over the contralateral shoulder. Palpation is repeated with the palmar surface of the hand(s) for each breast and simultaneously for both breasts. Masses of at least ≥1 cm can be identified by an appropriate technique of palpation.

Afterward, the axilla and supraclavicular region are palpated for lymph nodes. For specific indications, **breast size and development is measured** with a centimeter tape. The distances between the inner and outer and upper and lower margin of each breast are multiplied and used as objective measure of breast size.

Clinical Presentation

Fibroadenoma is the most frequently observed tumor that develops around puberty and has a peak incidence in the late 20s to early 30s and earlier in blacks. *Its size is usually 2–3 cm at first consultation. However, large masses may be encountered simulating a diffuse enlargement of one breast #. Approximately two thirds occur in the lateral quadrants of the breast.* Due to the fast growth and possible development of a second tumor at an average time of 3.3 years (several months to 15 years), the suspicion of a malignant tumor arises. The latter observation is attributed to serial presentations of multicentric lesions in the same and/or contralateral breast, and true malignant degeneration has been observed rarely.

Solitary or multiple **cysts** are often associated with **fibrocystic disease**.

Papillary duct hyperplasia consists of intraductal sclerosing papilloma, papilloma, or papillomatosis. The median age at diagnosis is 17 years with one fourth less than 15 years old. Mostly females are involved. *A palpable nodule below the areola and hemorrhagic nipple discharge are the main signs.* Recurrences are observed in 16 % at a median interval of 3 years (median age at last follow-up 28 years), but there is no predisposition to breast carcinoma or another malignancy before the fourth decade.

The rare **phyllodes tumor** (cystosarcoma phyllodes of Müller) of the breast is *initially a small mass that may rapidly increase in size and then give the impression of a malignancy or inflammation because of skin distension with discoloration and venous dilatation.* Nevertheless, the tumor is mostly benign and *large, mobile, multilobulated, and firm with possibly cystic areas on palpation.*

Other benign tumors include lipoma, fibrolipoma, cystic and other types of lymphangioma #, hemangioma, and lymphangioma. The latter tumors become manifest already in early infancy #.

Most **malignancies** in children are metastases of rhabdomyosarcoma, leukemia, lymphoma, and neuroblastoma. **Breast carcinoma** and other malignancies may occur at any age of childhood though rarely and somewhat more frequently in adolescence. A palpable mass and much less frequently a watery, bloody, pink, or yellow nipple discharge are the usual findings.

Work-Ups, Differential Diagnosis

Work-ups include regular observation for a short time, ultrasound and mammography, cyst aspiration with cytological examination, and biopsy or excision with histological examination.

The differential diagnosis of hemorrhagic unilateral or bilateral **nipple discharge** is **mammary duct ectasia** (cystic ductal hyperplasia) that is already observed in neonates, infants, and older children, is the most common cause of bloody discharge in this age group, and is a matter of psychic stress to parents and physicians. The sanguineous discharge may last several months but is often self-limited. Diagnosis is possible by ultrasound that shows dilated mammary ducts. Expectant approach is indicated except for persistent or increasing secretion of one breast and/or signs of inflammation, combination with a palpable tumor, or equivocal ultrasound findings that need further work-ups and possible segmental resection including the involved duct or excision of the mass.

In addition, **discharge from an areolar gland** must be considered in which the secretion is not from the nipple but from somewhere in the areola.

The differential diagnosis of a solitary cyst includes a **galactocele** that is observed in newborns and small children because of occlusion of a duct. The roundish and painless cyst is usually small but can reach five and more centimeters.

The differential diagnosis of a **palpable nodule** must consider development variations such as a small, flat, button-like mass beneath the nipple in the second stage, a plaque-like mould of the areola in the fourth stage of puberty, and granularity at the end of breast development and somewhat larger nodules around menstrual bleeding. These variations disappear with time.

Treatment, Prognosis

In **persistent cysts**, aspiration with cytological examination is indicated and followed by excision if aspiration fails, the cyst recurs, or equivocal findings are encountered by cytological examination. Papillary duct hyperplasia with persistent nipple discharge needs segmental resection combined with the excision of the involved duct(s).

Masses that persist, become larger, or are suspicious of a neoplasm need excision often with a rim of healthy tissue outside the capsule # and including the duct in papillomas. Treatment of breast carcinoma follows the principles of adult surgery. If breast surgery is performed for biopsy or excision, circumareolar incisions along the skin lines, sharp dissection, and subcuticular sutures should be used.

The prognosis is excellent with permanent cure in most of the cysts and tumors with a few exceptions. Nipple discharge in cystic ductal hyperplasia or galactocele may disap-

pear spontaneously after aspiration. Some disorders need lifelong follow-up, (e.g., papillary duct hyperplasia) and all adolescents should be instructed for self-examination.

Webcodes

The following webcodes can be used on www.psurg.net for further images and data.

1201 Different breast development in the girl	1212 Precocious puberty, 5-year old girl (hydrocephalus)
1202 Diffuse breast enlargement, newborn	1213 Pseudoprecocious puberty, development breast in
1203 Persistent diffuse breast enlargement, infancy	1214 Hormonally active testicular tumor
1204 Acquired left breast hypoplasia after	1215 Extreme bilateral gynecomastia
1205 Chest wall hemangioma	1216 Right gynecomastia
1206 Right mastitis, newborn	1217 Pseudogynecomastia
1207 Left mastitis with abscess, newborn	1218 Large fibroadenoma right breast
1208 Right mastitis in a developing girl	1219 Pigmented nevus left areola
1209 Premature thelarche, 5-year old girl	1220 Cutaneous and subcutaneous hemangioma left breast
1210 Precocious puberty, 1-year old girl with	1221 Large fibroadenoma
1211 Pubic hair and clitoris hypertrophy	

Bibliography

General: Textbooks, Related Disorders

Cleckner-Smith CS et al (1998) Premenstrual symptoms: prevalence and severity in an adolescent sample. J Adolesc Health 22:403

Hiersche H-D (1987) Jugendliche Mamma. In: Huber A, Hiersche H-D (eds) Praxis der Gynäkologie im Kindes- und Jugendalter, 2nd edn. Thieme, Stuttgart

Huffman JW, Caprano VJ, Dewhurst CJ (1981) The breast and its disorders in childhood and adolescence. In: Huffman JW et al (eds) The gynecology of childhood and adolescence. Saunders, Philadelphia

Seashore HJ (1998) Disorders of the breast. In: O'Neill JA Jr et al (eds) Pediatric surgery, vol I, 5th edn. Mosby, St. Louis

Section 12.1

Bach AD, Kneser U, Beier JP, Breuel C, Horch RE, Leffler M (2009) Aesthetic correction of tuberous breast deformity: lessons learned with single-stage procedure. Breast J 15:279–286

Faridi MM, Dewan P (2008) Successful breastfeeding with breast malformations. J Hum Lact 24:446–450

Grotto I, Browner-Elhanan K, Mimouni D et al (2001) Occurrence of supernumerary nipples in children with kidney and urinary tract malformations. Pediatr Dermatol 18:291–294

Ishida LH, Alves HR, Munhoz AM, Kaimoto C, Ishida LC, Saito FL, Gemperli R, Ferreira MC (2005) Athelia: case report and review of the literature. Br J Plast Surg 58:833–837; comment in: J Plast Reconstr Aesthet Surg 2006; 59:1006-1008

Leung W, Heaton JP, Morales A (1997) An uncommon urologic presentation of a supernumerary breast. Urology 5:122–124

Mandrekas AD, Zambacos GJ, Anastasopoulos A, Hapsas D, Lambrinaki N, Ioannidou-Mouzaka L (2003) Aesthetic reconstruction of the tuberous breast deformity. Plast Reconstr Surg 112:1099–1108; discussion 1109

Section 12.2.1

Sadove AM, van Aalst JA (2005) Congenital and acquired pediatric breast anomalies: a review of 20 years' experience. Plast Reconstr Surg 115:1039–1050

Versaci AD, Balkovich ME, Goldstein SA (1986) Breast reconstruction by tissue expansion for congenital and burn deformities. Ann Plast Surg 16:20–31

Section 12.2.2

Imamoglu M, Cay A, Reis A, Ozdemir O, Sapan L, Sarihan H (2006) Bloody nipple discharge in children: possible etiologies and selection of appropriate therapy. Pediatr Surg Int 22:158 163

Leis HP Jr (1989) Management of nipple discharge. World J Surg 13:736–744

Weiman E (2003) Clinical management of nipple discharge in neonates and children. J Paediatr Child Health 39: 155–156

Section 12.2.3

Rudoy RC, Nelson JD (1975) Breast abscess during the neonatal period. Am J Dis Child 129:1031–1034

Section 12.2.4

Chalumeau M, Hadjiathanasiou CG, Ng SM et al (2003) Selecting girls with precocious puberty for brain imaging: validation of European evidence-based diagnosis rule. J Pediatr 143:445–450

Gabra HO, Morabito A, Bianchi A, Bowen J (2004) Gynaecomastia in the adolescent: a surgically relevant condition. Eur J Pediatr Surg 14:3–6

Kaplowitz P (2004) Extensive personal experience: clinical characteristics of 104 children referred for evaluation of precocious puberty. J Clin Endocrinol Metab 89:3644 3650

Kaplowitz PB, Oberfield SE (1999) Re-examination of the age limit for defining when puberty is precocious in girls in the Unites States: implications for evaluation and treatment. Drug and Therapeutics and Executive Committees of the Lawson-Wilkins Pediatric Endocrinology Society. Pediatrics 104:936–941

Lawrence SE, Faught KA, Vethamuthu J et al (2004) Beneficial effects of Raloxifene and Tamoxifen in the treatment of pubertal gynecomastia. J Pediatr 145:71–76

Midyett LK, Moore WV, Jacobson JD (2003) Are pubertal changes in girls before age 8 benign? Pediatrics 111:47–51

Stolecke H (1987) Klinische und endokrinologische Merkmale der weiblichen Puber-tät. In: Stolecke H, Terrhun V (eds) Pädiatrische gynäkologie. Springer, Berlin

Section 12.2.5

Bock K, Duda VF, Hadji P, Ramaswamy A, Schulz-Wendtland R, Klose KJ, Wagner U (2005) Pathological breast conditions in childhood and adolescence: evaluation by sonographic diagnosis. J Ultrasound Med 24:1347–1354; quiz 1356-1357

Chung EM, Cube R, Hall GJ, Gonzales C, Stocker JT, Glassman LM (2009) From the archives of the AFIP: breast masses in children and adolescents: radiologic-pathologic correlation. Radiographics 29:907–931

Cox EM, Siegel DM (1997) Mondor disease: an unusual consideration in a young woman with a breast mass. J Adolesc Health 21:183–185

Garcia CJ, Espinoza A, Dinamarca V, Navarro O, Daneman A, Garcia H, Cattani A (2000) Breast US in children and adolescents. Radiographics 20:1605–1612

Jones PG, Campell PE (1976) Tumors of infancy and childhood. Blackwell, London

Kenney LB, Yasui Y, Inskip PD, (Dana-Farber Cancer Inst, Boston) et al (2004) Breast cancer after childhood cancer: a report from the childhood cancer survivor study. Ann Intern Med 141:590–597

Martino A, Zamparelli M, Santinelli A, Cobellis G, Rossi L, Amici G (2001) Unusual clinical presentation of a rare case of phyllodes tumor of the breast in an adolescent girl. J Pediatr Surg 36:941–943

Nigro DM, Organ CH Jr (1976) Fibroadenoma of the female breast. Some epidemiologic surprises. Postgrad Med 59:113–117

Pacinda SJ, Ramzy I (1998) Fine-needle aspiration of breast masses: a review of its role in diagnosis and management in adolescent patients. J Adolesc Health 23:3–6

Pistolese CA, Tanga I, Cossu E, Perretta T, Yamgoue M, Bonanno E, Simonetti G (2009) A phyllodes tumor in a child. J Pediatr Adolesc Gynecol 22:e21

Wilson M, Cranor ML, Rosen PP (1993) Papillary duct hyperplasia of the breast in children and young women. Mod Pathol 6:570–574

Malformations, Neoplasms, and Other Disorders of the Chest Wall

13

The differential diagnosis of congenital and acquired tumors, tumor-like masses, and anomalies of the chest wall is listed in Table 13.1.

13.1 Congenital Pathologies

13.1.1 Polythelia, Polymastia

Pathology

Polythelia, polythelia areolaris, and polymastia arc abnormalities with one or more additional

Table 13.1 Congenital and acquired tumors and anomalies of the chest wall

Congenital pathologies
● Polythelia, polymastia
o Circumscribed anomalies of the ribs
Acquired pathologies: soft tissue tumors and tumor-like masses
● Pilomatricoma
● Fibromatosis
● Hemangiomas, lymphangiomas, vascular malformations, and lipomas
● Melanotic nevus including syndromic disorders and malignant melanoma
Acquired pathologies: tumors and tumor-like masses of the ribs
● Hereditary multiple exostoses
● Solitary osteochondroma and other benign tumors
● Ewing sarcoma and other malignant tumors
Acquired pathologies of the chest wall: inflammatory disorders
● Axillary lymphadenitis, inflammation of sudoriparous glands
o Cellulitis chest wall

nipple(s), areola(s), and breast bud(s) along the bilateral embryonic milk streak from the lateral third of the clavicle to the symphysis or outside of it.

Clinical Significance
- One or more additional nipples and/or areolas are a differential diagnosis of melanotic nevus and may be an esthetic problem.
- Breast bud without nipple and areola and particularly with a location outside of the milk streak simulates a growing soft tissue mass (soft tissue neoplasm, axillary sudoriparous abscess, or lymphadenopathy).

Clinical Presentation
One or more circumscribed pigmentations without or with a hardly recognizable nipple are encountered on the chest or abdominal wall above or below the normal breasts along the former milk streak # or outside of it. Less frequently, an additional breast bud is palpated underneath a supernumerary areola or without any external signs of a breast that is growing at puberty and changing in size after beginning of menstrual cycle.

Differential Diagnosis, Work-Ups
In supernumerary areola and/or nipple, a pigmented nevus or another skin tumor must be considered, and in polymastia, a subcutaneous soft tissue tumor.

Except for ectopic polymastia, the clinical diagnosis is mostly possibly by inspection and palpation. In ectopic polymastia, ultrasound shows the characteristics of breast gland tissue.

Treatment, Prognosis
Complete excision regarding esthetic principles confirms the clinical diagnosis, avoids possible complications of areolar and breast tissue, and reliefs the cosmetic problems with good results. Malignancies have been described in ectopic polymastia.

13.1.2 Circumscribed Anomalies of the Ribs

Pathology
In circumscribed anomalies of the thoracic cage, number, shape, spatial arrangement, and relation to each other of the involved ribs are abnormal. They belong to the group of anatomic variations that occur in chest CT in one third of the children and may be an additional feature of the major chest wall deformities such as funnel and pigeon breast.

Clinical Significance
- Circumscribed anomalies of the ribs may be mixed up with a tumor of the thoracic cage and is regarded as an esthetic problem by some parents and adolescents.

Clinical Presentation
The strictly circumscribed anomalies of the thoracic cage and disorder of the underlying ribs, for example, a paracostal subcutaneous nodule or prominent convexity of the anterior rib, or costal cartilage, are recognized by inspection and palpation of the deformity and the adjacent ribs.

Differential Diagnosis, Work-Ups
It includes consolidating rib fractures that have been acquired at or after birth by resuscitation, physiotherapy, battering, or trauma, chest wall deformity after thoracotomy or chest wall surgery, or a tumor of the thoracic cage.

Chest x-rays and CT with 3D reconstruction confirm the clinical diagnosis and describe precisely the deformity if reconstructive surgery is intended.

Treatment
Reconstructive surgery is rarely indicated.

13.2 Acquired Pathologies: Soft Tissue Tumors and Tumor-Like Masses

In general, soft tissue tumors display a wide histological variety and biological behavior, and the histological features of tumor dignity are not always identical with biological behavior especially in young children. This applies also to soft tissue tumors of the chest wall in which the thorax and trunk is the preferred site or that occur only occasionally there. Some of the soft tissue tumors are quoted here because they are often recognized early due to the exposed location, some belong to common and well-known disorders, some point to a systemic disease, and some are malignant and/or important for an appropriate treatment. Soft tissue tumors of the chest wall occur in 1:1,000,000 children.

13.2.1 Pilomatricoma (Pilomatrixoma, Calcifying Epithelioma of Malherbe)

Occurrence, Pathology
The pilomatricoma that is derived from matrix cells of hair follicles belongs to the most common tumors of the skin adnexa.

Clinical Presentation
Pilomatricoma occurs mostly in the head (scalp, face), neck, and upper extremity regions. *The slowly growing subcutaneous mass of several millimeter to 1 and more cm size is hard or firm, has an irregular contour, and is fixed to the skin with free mobility against the surrounding area on palpation, and the overlying skin is normal or may display a red to purple discoloration.* Multiple pilomatricomas occur in less than 5 %. Sometimes, a giant pilomatricoma may be observed and only anecdotally a malignant degeneration. In multiple pilomatricoma, a possible **Turner syndrome** should be considered.

Work-Ups, Differential Diagnosis

A clinical diagnosis is possible in more than three fourths, and additional examinations such as FNA (not conclusive if not all major components are in the aspirate), ultrasound (heterogeneous echotexture, internal echogenic foci in scattered-dot pattern, and a hypoechoic rim or a posterior shadowing are the typical features), CT, and MRI are only necessary in extraordinary cases because excision biopsy is performed anyway.

The number of differential diagnoses is large: dermoid cyst, sebaceous nevus, juvenile xanthogranuloma, viral tumors, pyogenic granuloma, foreign body reaction, fat necrosis, calcifying lymphoma.

Treatment, Prognosis

Complete excision including a spindle of the overlying skin and clear margins leads to permanent cure. Nevertheless, histologic work-up are indicated to confirm the diagnosis. Recurrences are due to incomplete resection.

13.2.2 Fibromatosis

Occurrence, Pathology

Most soft tissue tumors have a fibrous or vascular origin, and many of them are benign. One large group of soft tissue tumors is **fibromatosis** that belongs to the soft tissue tumors with fibroblastic or myofibroblastic origin.

Subgroups are **infantile (congenital) and aggressive fibromatosis (desmoid tumor)**, **juvenile angiofibroma** (occurring in the nasopharynx at puberty with epistaxis or bleeding from the mouth as leading symptom), **fibrous hamartoma** (occurring in the first 2 years of life in the upper extremity and axillary region with spontaneous regression), and localized fibroses of the extremities.

The malignant varieties are the **infantile and adult-type fibrosarcomas** that are usually put together to one group with other non-rhabdomyosarcoma soft tissue sarcomas. Synovial sarcoma, malignant peripheric neuroectodermal tumors (MPNET), and Askin's tumor (a thoracopulmonic small cell tumor of the second decade)

belong to the same group. They have a prevalence of <1–1.5 in 100,000 children below 15 years of age.

Clinical Significance

- Fibromatosis has a large variety of histology, discrepancy between histology and biology, and equivocal dignity. Therefore, experienced histological work-up is necessary, and primary mutilating resection is not indicated.

Clinical Presentation

The solitary node or less frequently multiple nodes of **infantile fibromatosis** are observed already in neonates or young infants (mean age <6 months). Head, neck, upper extremity, shoulder, and thigh are the mostly observed sites although they occur occasionally at the chest wall or trunk. The tumor is either subcutaneous or/and intramuscular or involves bones and visceral organs (e.g., gastrointestinal tract). Additional bone involvement corresponds to the multiple type and bone and visceral involvement to the generalized type of fibromatosis.

The initially growing mass is firm, well demarcated, but fixed on the underlying surface on palpation, and the skin may be red to blue. At surgery and follow-up, the tumor has no capsule and is locally aggressive.

In contrast, **aggressive fibromatosis** occurs in the second decade and concerns the musculoaponeuroses and is occasionally observed at the same place after former surgery. *Abdominal wall or similar involvement of chest wall, back, and thigh are typical regions of manifestation. The uni- or less frequently multilocal tumors are solid and painless on palpation.*

A possible association with **Gardner's syndrome** must always be considered. The autosomal dominant inherited disorder leads to desmoid tumors, familial adenomatous polyposis of the gastrointestinal tract, and osteomas.

Work-Ups, Differential Diagnosis

In addition to incisional biopsy for a precise diagnosis, some of the characteristics of the fibromatoses is recognizable by ultrasound and MRI or CT including possible skeleton and visceral involvement and differentiation from other soft tissue masses such as infantile or adult-type fibrosarcoma, **mesenchymal (fibrous) hamartoma**, hemangioma and lymphangioma, and vascular malformations, peripheral neurogenic tumors, lipomas, and lipoblastomas (-tosis), nodular fasciitis, and soft tissue sarcomas and **rhabdomyosarcoma**.

Mesenchymal hamartoma is a benign tumor at or shortly after birth and presents as an extrapleural mass that arises from the rib cage. The sometimes huge mass and a possible RDS may mimic a malignant tumor. Histology shows an admixture of hyaline cartilage resembling growth plate cartilage. Resection is followed by permanent cure.

Rhabdomyosarcoma is the most frequently encountered malignant soft tissue tumor of the chest wall. Immunochemically, muscle markers like desmin and myogenin are useful for differentiation from other malignant soft tissue tumors.

Treatment, Prognosis

Complete resection is recommended in symptomatic or equivocal tumors of infantile fibromatosis, or if the intestine or other visceral organs are involved. In adult-type fibromatosis, complete excision is necessary whenever possible to avoid local recurrences. In a not completely resectable cases and recurrences, chemotherapy, radiation, or other medicamentous treatments are necessary.

The local recurrence rate is low in infantile fibromatosis and high in adult-type fibromatosis. Generalized forms and all types of adult-type fibromatoses may lead to death.

13.2.3 Hemangiomas, Lymphangiomas, Vascular Malformations, and Lipomas

Clinical Significance
- Involvement of the breast bud by the lesion itself or because of its treatment may lead to acquired hypoplasia or aplasia of the breast that is especially of significance in girls.

- Extension to the thoracic cavity or into the muscles of the back, chest, and abdominal wall is a challenge to an appropriate treatment.
- Due to the exposition of the chest wall, these disorders have a great esthetic significance ###.

13.2.4 Melanotic Nevi

Occurrence
Melanotic nevi are frequently observed especially in areas exposed to the sun.

Clinical Significance
- Melanotic nevi and specifically disorders with hyperpigmentation are at risk for the development of malignant melanoma.
- Melanotic nevi may be a sign of systemic disorders, for example, neurofibromatosis.

Clinical Presentation
Acquired melanotic nevi have a size of less than 5 mm before puberty and well-defined borders. They increase in size up to 15 mm and number during childhood. Their risk of development of melanoma is increased at sites where they are exposed mechanically or to the sun, for example, at the sole of the foot.

Work-Ups, Differential Diagnosis
Work-ups are not necessary in common melanotic nevi except for measurement and photographic documentation of mechanically exposed types or types with unusual clinical presentation, and in the differential diagnostic significant disorders.

The differential diagnosis includes the following important disorders in order of increased risk of malignant melanoma or other malignancies:
- **Single dysplastic nevus**, **dysplastic nevus syndrome** (atypical nevus syndrome), and **FAMM syndrome** (familial atypical mole melanoma):

Dysplastic nevi have blurred borders; their size may be >5 mm before and >15 mm at puberty and also occur in regions not exposed to the sun. In contrast to dysplastic nevus syndrome with manifestation in small children, FAMM syndrome appears often around puberty

- **Xeroderma pigmentosum**:

It is a disorder with hypersensitivity to ultra-light violet light.

- **Giant congenital nevus** (giant congenital melanotic nevus, giant hairy nevus):

In the classic type, the largest diameter is >20 cm and the nevus is combined with hairy and dark parts, an irregular surface, and smaller satellite nevi #. The scalp and trunk are the main sites. Midline and scalp giant congenital nevus may be associated with CNS melanoma.

- **Cellular blue nevus and juvenile melanoma (Spitz nevus)** occur mostly in the head and neck region at any age of childhood. Their oncological dignity is different from that of malignant melanoma. The latter tumor presents as a small and pink mass with a smooth surface shaped like a dome. Both tumors may recur locally and lead to involvement of the regional lymph nodes.

- **Sebaceous nevus** (due to enlarged sebaceous glands) involves often the scalp and exhibits a hairless and orange zone with a morphology changing at puberty. In up to 15 %, skin carcinomas develop later.

- **Malignant melanoma** occurs occasionally as congenital tumor, in acquired melanotic nevus, and in the three first disorders of hyperpigmentation quoted above, or as malignant melanoma like in adulthood, and altogether more frequently in the second decade than before.

The history should include possible risk factors for development of malignant melanoma. Such risk factors are acquired melanotic nevus and the already quoted disorders with hyperpigmentation, mechanical and excessive sun exposition, fair hair and skin, and congenital and acquired immunodeficiency.

The incidence of **malignant melanoma** has steadily increased in Caucasians people in the last 50 years and is highest in Australia and lowest in Africa. The primary cutaneous malignant melanoma is divided into four clinical types. *Change of a melanotic nevus in size, color, and shape with irregular borders and ulceration as well as bleeding or itch are possible signs of malignant degeneration.* The most important tool for diagnosis is the ABCD role that includes possible asymmetry, types of border, color, and dynamic (regression or growth) or differential structure. The clinical diagnosis may be improved by epiluminescence microscopy and quantification.

Clinical diagnosis must be confirmed by excision biopsy including the whole pigmented nevus except for very large forms of face and extremities in which incisional biopsy is permitted. Histology enables confirmation of the clinical diagnosis and substaging of the primary tumor by evaluation of the prognostic important thickness of the melanoma according to Breslow (≤1 mm, >1–2 mm, >2–4 mm, and >4 mm). The TNM/AJCC classification differentiates five subtypes of primary tumor, three of involvement of the regional lymph nodes and three of distant metastases.

Treatment depends on the individual tumor stage including tumor thickness. The secondary therapeutic resection of the primary tumor should be performed within 1 month and includes a safety zone of 0.5, 1, or 2 cm of normally appearing skin depending on the tumor thickness and exceptionally a smaller rim and histological control of it. Tumor thickness of >1 mm needs additional sentinel lymph node biopsy (90 % of all lymph node metastases are micrometastases (diameter ≤ 2 mm) at the time of resection of the primary tumor). It is followed by complete resection of the regional lymph nodes in case of histological or clinically recognizable involvement and search for distant metastasis. The treatment of stages with involvement of the lymph nodes and distant metastases includes interferon alpha-2b, perfusion of involved extremities, single or multiagent chemotherapy, and surgical resection (e.g., single lung metastasis).

The follow-ups including times and methods depend on tumor thickness, time of diagnosis, and state after lymph node or distant organ involvement and the experience that 90 % of metastases occur in the first 5 years after primary excision. The 10-year survival is >80 % if the tumor thickness is <1 mm and <60 % if it is

>4 mm, 30 % if regional lymph nodes are involved, and <5 % in distant metastases. The outlook of children seems to be somewhat better.

- **Neurofibromatosis** is divided in two types that differ in frequency, genetics, and clinical presentation. **Neurofibromatosis 1** (Recklinghausen's disease) occurs in 1 of 3,000 births and has an autosomal dominant inheritance with spontaneous mutation in half of the cases (and therefore a negative family history). The presenting symptoms and signs are:
  - Café-au-lait spots (≥6 spots). The preferred site is the trunk #; the size is >5 mm before and >15 mm after the onset of puberty.
  - Neurinomas and neurofibromas (≥2) along the peripheral nerves or plexiform neurinoma (≥1).
  - Multiple small light-brown spots (freckling) in the axilla and groin.
  - Melanocytic hamartomas of the iris (Lisch nodules). Recognizable by slit-lamp examination.
  - Optic nerve glioma (reduction of visual acuity/precocious puberty) and other CNS tumors.
  - Kyphoscoliosis or pseudarthrosis of tibia/fibula.
  - Involved first-degree relative.

Treatment, Prognosis

The **common melanotic nevus** needs only excisional biopsy in case of mechanical exposition or if malignant melanoma is suspected. In contrast to single dysplastic nevus, **Spitz, cellular blue nevus,** and **sebaceous nevus** that should be excised because of the increased risk of malignant degeneration or equivocal dignity, in **the other disorders with hyperpigmentation,** excision is only possible in single efflorescences with increased risk or possible malignant degeneration. Nevertheless, lifelong follow-ups are necessary.

In **giant congenital nevus**, early complete resection is recommended for prophylactic and particularly esthetic reasons. Repeated full-thickness resections are needed after skin expansion.

For the quoted disorders, no common informations are available due to the diversity and small numbers of the different disorders and individual findings.

13.3 Acquired Pathologies: Tumors and Tumor-Like Masses of the Chest Wall and Ribs

Occurrence, Pathology

Chest wall tumors and specifically those of the ribs are rare. Arranged in order of their frequency, mainly metastatic and primary malignant tumors are observed followed by benign neoplasms and such that originate from the thoracic cavity.

Clinical Significance

- Rib tumors and tumor-like masses of the ribs may be observed earlier than other skeletal and soft tissue tumors because of their exposed location.

Clinical Presentation

Depending on the age, site, and in- or outward growth of the tumor, different symptoms can be recorded: *vague or localized chest or back pain, pain after minor trauma due to a pathological rib fracture, or pleuritic pain, persistent cough, and shortness of breathing.*

Incidental findings on chest x-rays performed for other reasons or as part of work-ups in malignant extrathoracic tumors are frequent occasions of recognition of a rib tumor.

A visible and/or palpable mass with continuation along the rib (s) that is hard or firm on palpation without/with inflammatory signs of the overlying skin is a typical local finding. In addition, dullness on percussion and diminished breathing sounds on auscultation point to a possible intrathoracic extension or pleural effusion.

Work-Ups, Differential Diagnosis

The former depend on the history, local findings, and data of general examination. If a metastatic or generalized tumor is suspected, specific urine, blood, and bone marrow examinations and scintiscan, for example, early and delayed bone scan, are necessary. The characteristics, extension, and precise origin of the rib tumor are demonstrated by chest x-ray, ultrasound, CT, and MRI. The final diagnosis is attained best by open surgical biopsy although FNA or trucut biopsy is less invasive.

The differential diagnosis includes the following pathologies:

- Metastatic and multifocal tumors such as neuroblastoma, histiocytosis X, leukemia, Ewing and osteosarcoma, and **hereditary multiple exostoses** or lymphangiomatosis of the ribs
- Primary malignant and benign tumors such as **Ewing sarcoma** # or rhabdomyosarcoma, and osteo- and chondrosarcoma, extranodal non-Hodgkin's lymphoma, giant cell tumor ##, and **solitary osteochondroma**, fibrous dysplasia, chondromas, aneurysmatic bone cyst #, eosinophilic granuloma, and mesenchymal hamartoma of the chest wall
- Tumors originating from the thoracic cavity such lung metastases, pleuropulmonary blastoma, mesothelioma, and neurofibromas of the intercostal nerves
- Inflammatory disorders such as osteomyelitis, chest wall cellulitis, actinomycosis

Hereditary multiple exostoses and solitary osteochondroma may lead to spontaneous hematothorax, pericardial effusion, and diaphragmatic rupture.

Ewing sarcoma is the most frequent primary malignant tumor and occurs in 10–15 % in the ribs. Localized or pleuritic pain, a visible and/or a palpable mass, and pleural effusion are the most frequent symptoms and signs. Clinically and radiologically, it may be mixed up more than the other rib and chest wall tumors with **rib osteomyelitis**, chest wall cellulitis, actinomycosis, and other disorders.

Osteomyelitis is observed in <1 % in the rib. It is mostly caused by staphylococci. **Chronic multifocal nonbacterial osteomyelitis** in which the ribs may be involved can also mimic a rib malignancy. It is observed in hypophosphatasia that leads to chronic hyperprostaglandinism in children and is recognized by elevated levels of pyroxidal-5'-phosphate and inorganic pyrophosphate in urine and serum.

Treatment, Prognosis

Benign tumors should be resected with a part of the rib and free margins except for osteochondromas with resection of the mass itself.

Some principles of treatment for Ewing sarcoma applies more or less to the other malig-

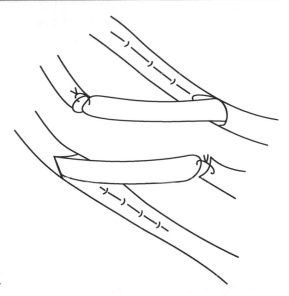

Fig. 13.1 Example of a simple chest wall reconstruction after resection of a single rib tumor. After resection of a piece of the involved rib together with the tumor, periosteum, and adjacent rim of bone and soft tissue, the next upper and lower ribs are used to cover the defect after degloving them from the periosteum along an appropriate distance. The periosteum is afterward closed with absorbable single sutures. The upper and lower cortical hemicircumference is incised at the exit site from the periosteum depending on the elasticity of the used ribs and the free ends of the corresponding ribs connected to the free edges of the resected rib and stabilized with absorbable miniplates. In small children, connection with nonabsorbable sutures is sufficient

nancies. The **primary Ewing sarcoma** should be considered as a systemic disease. Therefore after an incisional biopsy, multiagent chemotherapy is performed. The residual tumor is resected with wide tumor-free borders (but including at least one adjacent rib below and above is not a significant prognostic factor for survival). Depending on the dimensions of resection, chest wall reconstruction becomes necessary to avoid scoliosis, restrictive pulmonary disorder, sensation disorders, and motion-dependent pain. Their techniques must consider a growing chest wall and stability. A method of chest wall reconstruction is depicted in Fig. 13.1 that cannot be applied in every case.

Local recurrence of Ewing sarcoma is observed in about 20 % and is associated with fatal outcome.

13.4 Acquired Pathologies of the Chest Wall: Inflammatory Disorders

Occurrence, Pathoanatomy

Inflammatory disorders of the chest wall concern the soft tissues, ribs, and the axillary lymph nodes and sudoriparous glands of the axilla of which the latter are most frequently involved. Secondary infections of the soft tissues occur after scalds, burns, or abrasions and in chest wall tumors.

Clinical Significance

- In contrast to axillary lymphadenitis, infection and abscess of sudoriparous glands are only encountered at and after puberty.
- Hematogenic osteomyelitis of ribs is an important differential diagnosis of Ewing's sarcoma (and is mentioned in Sect. 13.3).
- Cellulitis of the chest wall soft tissues is a rare disorder in early infancy that involves progressively large areas and leads to skin necrosis ###.
- Local inflammatory signs may point to an infectious or neoplastic intrathoracic disorder that breaks through the chest wall.

Clinical Presentation

The local findings of the axillary lymphadenitis are identical with the more frequent adenitis of the neck. The responsible cause may be encountered in the draining area that includes shoulder, arm, and lateral chest wall. Chronic lymphadenitis after BCG vaccination is such an example. It leads to lengthy visible swelling of the axillary lymph nodes with possible fistulization ##.

Inflammation of the sudoriparous # glands is characterized by pain, redness, and induration and is observed in neglected body care or immunodeficiency. Formation of one or several abscesses leads to a palpable fluctuation.

Differential Diagnosis, Work-Ups

Clinical diagnosis is possible after a careful history and examination. **Actinomycosis** with its chronic soft tissue induration, redness, and possible fistulization is a possible differential diagnosis of bacterial cellulitis.

Radiological imaging with ultrasound, chest x-ray, or CT is indicated if a deep soft tissue abscess or rib or intrathoracic lesion is suspected. Abscess needs after punction or incision bacteriological examination including resistance screening and chronic lymphadenitis, specific serological examination.

Treatment, Prognosis

Acute lymphadenitis with abscess needs incision, drainage, and antibiotic treatment of the underlying cause. Chronic BCG lymphadenitis should be excised and not incised. In inflammation of the sudoriparous glands, antibiotics and possible abscess incision must be supplemented by hair cutting, regular skin disinfection, and abduction splint of the shoulder. Delayed healing is observed in BCG lymphadenitis and recurrence in sudoriparous gland inflammation if the adherence of the patient is not appropriate; en bloc resection must be considered in the latter disorder.

Webcodes

The following webcodes can be used on www.psurg.net for further images and data.

1301 Left polythelia	1309 Histology: giant cells
1302 Large cystic lymphangioma, newborn	1310 Aneurysmatic bone cyst, right sixth rib
1303 Cystic lymphangioma, infant	1311 Chest wall cellulitis,
1304 Bilateral lipomas	1312 Clinical course, and
1305 Giant congenital nevus	1313 Final stage
1306 Multiple pigmented nevi, neurofibromatosis	1314 Chronic lymphadenitis
1307 Ewing sarcoma, right sixth rib	1315 Chronic lymphadenitis, abscess
1308 Recurrent giant cell tumor, right fourth rib	1316 Sudoriparous gland, histology

Bibliography

Section 13.1

Donnelly LF, Frush DP, Foss JN, O'Hara SM, Bisset GS III (1999) Anterior chest wall: frequency of anatomic variations in children. Radiology 212:837–840

Merks JH, Smets AM, Van Rijn RR, Kobes J, Caron HN, Maas M, Hennekam RC (2005) Prevalence of rib anomalies in normal Caucasian children and childhood cancer patients. Eur J Med Genet 48:113–129

Section 13.2.1

Choo HJ, Lee SJ, Lee YH, Lee JH, Oh M, Kim MH, Lee EJ, Song JW, Kim SJ, Kim DW (2010) Pilomatricomas: the diagnostic value of ultrasound. Skeletal Radiol 39:243–250

Cigliano B, Baltogiannis N, De Marco M, Faviou E, Settimi A, Tilemis S, Soutis M, Papandreou E, D'Agostino S, Fabbro MA (2005) Pilomatricoma in childhood: a retrospective study from three European paediatric centres. Eur J Pediatr 164:673–677

Pirouzmanesh A, Reinisch JF, Gonzalez-Gomez I, Smith EM, Meara JG (2003) Pilomatrixoma: a review of 346 cases. Plast Reconstr Surg 112:1784–1789

Section 13.2.2

Andreou D, Tunn PU (2009) Sentinel node biopsy in soft tissue sarcoma. Recent Results Cancer Res 179:25–36

Baerg J, Murphy JJ, Magee JF (1999) Fibromatoses: clinical and pathological features suggestive of recurrence. J Pediatr Surg 34:1112–1114

Bedford CD, Sills JA, Sommelet-Olive D, Boman F, Beltramo F, Cornu G (1991) Juvenile hyaline fibromatosis: a report of two severe cases. J Pediatr 119:404–410

Coffin CM, Dehner LP (1990) Soft tissue tumors in the first year of life: a report of 190 cases. Pediatr Pathol 10:509–526

Coffin CM, Dehner LP (1991) Fibroblastic-myofibroblastic tumors in children and adolescents: a clinicopathological study of 108 examples in 103 patients. Pediatr Pathol 11:569–588

Corsi A, Boldrini R, Bosman C (1994) Congenital-infantile fibrosarcoma: a study of two cases and review of the literature. Tumori 80:392–400

Eich GF, Hoeffel JC, Tschäppeler H, Gassner I, Willi UV (1998) Fibrous tumours in children: imaging features of a heterogeneous group of disorders. Pediatr Radiol 28:500–509

Fetsch JF, Miettinen M, Laskin WB, Michal M, Enzinger FM (2000) A clinicopathological study of 45 pediatric soft tissue tumors with an admixture of adipose tissue and fibroblastic elements, and a proposal for classification as lipofibromatosis. Am J Surg Pathol 24:1491–1500

Hicks J, Mierau G (2004) The spectrum of pediatric fibroblastic and myofibroblastic tumors. Ultrastruct Pathol 28:265–281

Inwards CY, Unni KK, Beabout JW, Shives TC (1991) Solitary congenital fibromatosis (infantile myofibromatosis) of bone. Am J Surg Pathol 15:935–941

Patrick LE, O'Shea P, Simoneaux SF, Gay BB Jr, Atkinson GO (1996) Fibromatoses of childhood: the spectrum of radiographic findings. AJR Am J Roentgenol 166:163–169

Wehrli BM, Weiss SW, Yandow S, Coffin CM (2001) Gardner-associated fibromas (GAF) in young patients: a distinct fibrous lesion that identifies unsuspected Gardner syndrome and risk for fibromatosis. Am J Surg Pathol 25:645–651

Section 13.2.3

Harrer J, Hammon G, Wagner T, Bolkenius M (2001) Lipoblastoma and Lipoblastomatosis: a report of two cases and review of the literature. Eur J Pediatr Surg 11:342–349

Lucas A, Bettloch I, Planelles M, Martinez T, Perez-Crespo M, Mataix J, Belinchon I (2007) Non-melanocytic benign skin tumors in children. Am J Clin Dermatol 8:365–369

Price HN, Zaenglein AL (2007) Diagnosis and management of benign lumps and bumps in childhood. Curr Opin Pediatr 19:420–424

Section 13.2.4

Blum A, Rassner G, Garbe C (2003) Modified ABC-point list of dermoscopy: a simplified and highly accurate dermoscopic algorithm for the diagnosis of cutaneous melanocytic lesions. J Am Acad Dermatol 48:672–678

Dummer R, Meier S, Beyeler M, Hafner J, Burg G (2006) Die aktualisierten schweizerischen Richtlinien zur Behandlung des kutanen Melanoms-wo stehen wir heute? Schweiz Med Forum 6:196–201

Morton DL, Wen DR, Wong HJ, Economou JS, Cagle LA, Storm FK et al (1992) Technical details of intraoperative lymphatic mapping for early stage melanoma. Arch Surg 127:392–399

Thompson JF, Scolyer RA, Kefford RF (2005) Cutaneous melanoma review. Lancet 365:687–701

Tsao H, Atkins MB, Sober AJ (2004) Management of cutaneous melanoma. N Engl J Med 351:998–1012

Section 13.3 Differential Diagnosis

Kim S, Lee S, Arsenault DA, Strijbosch RA, Shamberger RC, Puder M (2008) Pediatric rib lesions: a 13-year experience. J Pediatr Surg 43:1781–1785

La Quaglia MP (2008) Chest wall tumors in childhood and adolescence. Semin Pediatr Surg 17:173–180

Soyer T, Karnak I, Ciftci AO, Senocak ME, Tanyel FC, Büyümamukcu N (2006) The result of surgical treatment of chest wall tumors in childhood. Pediatr Surg Int 22:135–139

Van den Berg H, van Rijn RR, Merks JH (2008) Management of tumors of the chest wall in childhood: a review. J Pediatr Hematol Oncol 30:214–221

Section 13.3 Benign Tumors

Ayadi-Kaddour A, Mlika M, Chaabouni S, Kilani T, Mezni F (2007) Mesenchymal hamartoma of the chest wall in an infant. Pathologica 99:440–442

Coffin CM, Dehner LP (1989) Peripheral neurogenic tumors of the soft tissues in children and adolescents: a clinicopathological study of 139 cases. Pediatr Pathol 4:387–407

Cowles RA, Rowe DH, Arkovitz MS (2005) Hereditary multiple exostoses of the ribs; an unusual cause of hemothorax and pericardial effusion. J Pediatr Surg 40:1197–1200

Dubois J, Chigot V, Grimard G, Isler M, Garel L (2003) Sclerotherapy in aneurysmal bone cyst in children: a review of 17 cases. Pediatr Radiol 33:365–372

Eugster EA, the McCune-Albright Study Group (2003) Tamoxifen treatment for Precocious Puberty in McCune-Albright syndrome: a multicenter trial. J Pediatr 143:60–66

Golla S, Wit J, Guschmann M, Lübbert E, Kerner T (2002) Rare mesenchymal lesions: hamartoma of the chest wall and juvenile active ossifying fibroma in siblings. J Pediatr Surg 37:E27

Groom KR, Murphey MD, Howard LM, Lonergan GJ, Rosado-De-Christenson ML, Torop AH (2002) Mesenchymal hamartoma of the chest wall: radiologic manifestations with emphasis on cross-sectional imaging and histopathological comparison. Radiology 222:205–211

Karabakhtsian R, Heller D, Hameed M, Bethel C (2005) Periosteal chondroma of the rib – report of a case and literature review. J Pediatr Surg 40:1505–1507

Leonhardt J, Schirg E, Schmidt H, Glüer S (2004) Imaging characteristics of childhood lipoblastoma. Rofo 176:972–975

Mentzel T, Kutzner H (2009) Dermatomyofibroma: clinicopathological and immunohistochemical analysis of 56 cases and reappraisal of a rare and district cutaneous neoplasm. Am J Dermatopathol 31:44–49

Pawel BR, Crobleholme TM (2006) Mesenchymal hamartoma of the chest wall. Pediatr Surg Int 22:398–400

Rakoto-Ratsimba HN, Rakotomena SD, Rakotoarivony ST, Randrianjafisamindra-kotroka N (2008) An uncommon rib tumor in a child: aneurysmal bone cyst. Arch Pediatr 15:1538–1540

Rosenberg AE, Nielsen GP, Fletcher CDM (2002) Aneurysmal bone cyst. In: Fletcher CDM et al (eds) Pathology and genetics: tumours of soft tissue and bone. WHO, IARC Press, Lyon

Tomita S, Thompson K, Carver T, Vazquez WD (2009) Nodular fasciitis: a sarcomatous impersonator. J Pediatr Surg 44:e17–e19

Section 13.3 Malignant Tumors

Abbas AE, Deschamps C, Cassivi SD, Nichols FC III, Allen MS, Schleck CD, Capany C, Raffoul W, Zambelli PY, Joseph JM (2009) Latissimus dorsi muscle-flap over Gore-Tex patch for coverage of large thoracic defects in pediatric Ewing sarcoma. Pediatr Blood Cancer 52:679–681

Chattopadhyay A, Nagendhar Y, Kumar V (2004) Osteosarcoma of the rib. Indian J Pediatr 71:543–544

Demir A, Gunluoglu MZ, Dagoglu N, Turna A, Dizdar Y, Kaynak K, Dilege S, Mandel NM, Yilmazbayhan D, Dincer SI, Gurses A (2009) Surgical treatment and prognosis of primitive neuroectodermal tumors of the thorax. J Thorac Oncol 4:185–192

Gladish GW, Sabloff BM, Munden RF, Truong MT, Erasmus JJ, Chasen MH (2002) Primary thoracic sarcomas. Radiographics 22:621–637

Hayes-Jordan A, Stoner JA, Anderson JR, Rodeberg D, Weiner G, Meyer WH, Haw-kins DS, Arndt CA, Paidas C; Children's Oncology Group (2008) The impact of surgical excision in chest wall rhabdomyosarcoma: a report from the Children's Oncology Group. J Pediatr Surg 43:831–836

Khong PL, Chan GC, Shek TW, Tam PK, Chan FL (2002) Imaging of peripheral PNET: common and uncommon locations. Clin Radiol 57:272–277

Meys KM, Heinen RC, van den Berg H, Aronson DC (2008) Recurrence of Ewing sarcomas of the chest wall. Pediatr Blood Cancer 51:765–767

Murphy F, Corbally MT (2007) The novel use of small intestine submucosal matrix for chest wall reconstruction following Ewing's tumour resection. Pediatr Surg Int 23:353–356

Mysorekar VV, Harish K, Kilara N, Subramanian M, Giridhar AG (2008) Embryonal rhabdomyosarcoma of the chest wall: a case report and review of the literature. Indian J Pathol Microbiol 51:274–276

Naffaa LN, Donnelly LF (2005) Imaging findings in pleuropulmonary blastoma. Pediatr Radiol 35:387–391

Orazi C, Inserra A, Schingo PM, De Sio L, Cutrera R, Boldrini R, Malena S (2007) Pleuropulmonary blastoma, a distinctive neoplasm of childhood: report of three cases. Pediatr Radiol 37:337–344

Pairolero PC (2004) Chest-wall desmoids tumors: results of surgical intervention. Ann Thorac Surg 78:1219–1223; discussion 1219-1223

Parasuraman S, Rao BN, Bodner S, Cain A, Pratt CB, Merchant TE, Pappo AS (1999) Clear cell sarcoma of soft tissues in children and young adults: the St. Jude Children's Research Hospital experience. Pediatr Hematol Oncol 16:539-544

Rastogi R, Garg R, Thulkar S, Bakhshi S, Gupta A (2008) Unusual thoracic CT manifestations of osteosarcoma: review of 16 cases. Pediatr Radiol 38:551–558

Shivastava R, Saha A, Mehera B, Batra P, Gagne NM (2007) Pleuropulmonary blastoma: transition from type I (cystic) to type III (solid). Singapore Med J 48: e190–e192

Taneli C, Genc A, Erikci V, Yüce G, Balik E (1998) Askin tumors in children: a report of four cases. Eur J Pediatr Surg 8:312–314

Waldhausen JH, Redding GJ, Song KM (2007) Vertical expandable prosthetic titanium rib for thoracic insufficiency syndrome: a new method to treat an old problem. J Pediatr Surg 42:76–80

Widhe B, Widhe T, Bauer HC (2007) Ewing sarcoma of the rib – initial symptoms and clinical features: tumor missed at the first visit in 21 of 16 patients. Acta Orthop 78:840–844

Section 13.4

Basa NR, Si M, Ndiforchu F (2004) Staphylococcal rib osteomyelitis in a pediatric patient. J Pediatr Surg 39:1576–1577

Girschick HJ, Mornet E, Beer M, Warmuth-Metz M, Schneider P (2007) Chronic multifocal non-bacterial osteomyelitis in hypophosphatasia mimicking malignancy. BMC Pediatr 7:3

Karagöz B, Köksal Y, Varan A, Haliloglu M, Ekinci S, Büyüpamukcu M (2006) An un-usual case of grass inflorescence aspiration presenting as chest wall tumour. Pediatr Radiol 36:434–436

Pinarli FG, Mutlu B, Celenk C, Yildiz L, Elli M, Dagdemir A, Acar S (2005) Pulmonary actinomycosis mimicking chest wall tumor in a child. Jpn J Infect Dis 58:247–249

Yeung VH, Wong QH, Chao NS, Leung MW, Kwok WK (2008) Thoracic action-mycosis in an adolescent mimicking chest wall tumor or pulmonary tuberculosis. Pediatr Surg Int 24:751–754

Part IV
Abdomen

Surgical Abdomen

14

14.1 Surgical Abdomen, General Remarks

"Surgical abdomen" is a clinical term that has been developed by surgeons but is described differently. According to Siewert, the term means a preliminary description of a clinical condition that is dictated by shortness of time and concerns at first a not exactly definable, painful, and imminent abdominal disorder up to the final diagnosis, and for which the indication of a surgical intervention seems urgent.

The following remarks are important to the referring physicians for psychological reasons and consider the distinctive features of surgical abdomen in children. In this age group, the examiner has to rely often on the history of the parent rather than on the child itself, and nearly exclusively on the clinical presentation.

The spectrum of possible disorders as well as their clinical presentation is quite different from that in adults. On the other hand, the number of symptoms and signs is relatively small in comparison to the possible pathologies: Their modification, combination, and order of occurrence are important

and admit together with other factors a preliminary differential diagnosis. The natural course of the disorder must be considered at the same time because the clinical presentation may differ from stage to stage.

In mnemotechnical respect, two divisions of the surgical abdomen are useful in children: in the first place, the age groups "newborns, toddlers, schoolchildren, and adolescents" due to age-specific pathologies and in second place, the grouping by pathoanatomical criteria as quoted in Table 14.1 (overview) and in Tables 14.2, 15.1, 15.2, and 15.3, Table 22.1, 23.1, and 24.1 for the subgroups.

The surgical abdomen is very frequent in children and has a great significance for physicians who care for children because failure to recognize and to denote it yields an enormous morbidity or even mortality.

In case of an unclear abdomen, the element of urgency does not apply for work-up and indication for surgery at the first glance. Nevertheless, there is a continuous transition from the acute abdomen to chronic abdominal pain that becomes a nuisance to parents and family doctor.

G.L. Kaiser, *Symptoms and Signs in Pediatric Surgery*,
DOI 10.1007/978-3-642-31161-1_14, © Springer-Verlag Berlin Heidelberg 2012

Table 14.1 Differential diagnosis of the surgical abdomen. Overview of the pathoanatomical subdivisions

Disorders with peritonitis

- Acute appendicitis
- o Meckel's diverticulitis
- o Cholecystitis, cholelithiasis
- o Pancreatitis
- Primary peritonitis
- o Omental infarction

Acute/chronic partial intestinal obstructions

- Ileus of the newborn
- o Spontaneous gastrointestinal perforation
- Incarcerated inguinal hernia
- Hypertrophic pyloric stenosis
- Intussusception
- Postoperative ileus due to adhesions
- Volvulus
- Constipation (acute decompensation, sigmoid volvulus)
- Hirschsprung's disease (ileus of the newborn, colon perforation, enterocolitis) and the corresponding findings
- Sickle cell disease, vasoocclusive events
- o Rare hernias
- o Intestinal duplications
- Inflammatory bowel diseases (Crohn's disease, ulcerative colitis)

Gastrointestinal hemorrhage

Leading symptoms hematemesis and lower intestinal bleeding

Abdominal tumor

Leading symptom intra- and retroperitoneal tumor including acute manifestations

Retroperitoneal disorders

- Nephrolithiasis

Disorders close to the abdomen and other pathologies

- Testicular torsion
- Premenstrual syndrome
- Acute stool and urinary retention
- Pneumonia, meningitis, and other disorders

14.2 Surgical Abdomen, Disorders with Peritonitis

The specific disorders with peritonitis that lead to a surgical abdomen are listed in Table 14.2:

Table 14.2 Surgical abdomen. Disorders with peritonitis

- Acute appendicitis
- o Stump appendicitis
- o Meckel's diverticulitis
- o Cholecystitis, cholelithiasis
- o Pancreatitis
- Primary and secondary peritonitis
- o Spontaneous bile duct perforation
- Ventriculoperitoneal shunt or peritoneal dialysis catheter infection
- o Abdominal yersiniosis
- o Infected urachal cyst
- Inflammatory bowel disease

14.2.1 Acute Appendicitis

Occurrence, Clinical Significance

Appendicitis is the most frequent cause of surgical abdomen in schoolchildren (2–4:1,000 children). Its clinical significance is as follows:

- Delayed recognition leads to a considerable morbidity and possible mortality, increases the public health costs significantly, and decreases the reputation of the referring physician.
- Perforated appendicitis is a major cause of postoperative obstruction due to adhesions in children and of primary sterility in women ##.

In children, timely diagnosis of appendicitis may be difficult. Therefore, a varying rate of perforated appendicitis is observed dependent on the medical experience. Delayed forms of appendicitis are even more difficult to be recognized. Therefore, acute or complicated appendicitis must be considered always in abdominal pain and/or inflammatory symptoms and signs.

Clinical Presentation

A relatively short history of 1–2 days with progressive abdominal pain is followed by inappetence, nausea, and vomiting. The vague abdominal discomfort or continuous epigastric pain moves in the right lower abdomen, becomes severe, has not been experienced before, and deprives the child from sleeping. Vibration and motion during the drive to the hospital are painful, and a history

Fig. 14.1 Diagrammatic drawing of the normal site of cecum and appendix in the lower abdomen and of their relation to two visible and palpable auxiliary lines in the right abdomen. The *first line* lies between the navel and the anterior upper iliac spine; the *second line* lies between the right and left spine. Mc Burney's point lies in the middle of the *first line* and corresponds to the base of the appendix. The point of Lanz lies between the right and middle third of the *second line* and corresponds to the tip of the appendix

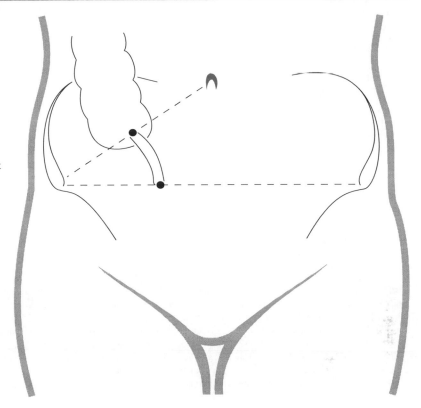

of complicated appendicitis can be ascertained in family members. Constipation (as coexisting or associated disorder) or less frequently loose stools interpreted as diarrhea with mucus or dysuria may be encountered.

This history does not necessarily apply to small children or to patients with a prodromal disease such as gastroenteritis or measles (appendicitis occurs prior the rush), in immunodeficiency, for example, due to oncological disease, or in case of already occurred perforation. On the other hand, dissimulation must always be considered in schoolchildren who are afraid of surgery or have something better to do.

Clinical Skills

Pain to coughing, motion as sitting up, or gentle percussion in the right lower abdomen, and palpation for tenderness and guarding (muscular defense, défense musculaire) at the Mc Burney's and Lanz point should be tested first in children

(Fig. 14.1), *and if at all, before the others tests quoted for adults. To perform them, gentle percussion and palpation with warm hands are necessary that start at a point where no pain is expected. Simultaneously, some involuntary reactions to pain should be observed such as acceleration of breathing, movements of the fingers, or facial expression.*

[Rovsing's sign (tenderness in the right lower abdomen released by retrograde palpation of the ascending colon), rebound tenderness in the right lower abdomen or released from the contralateral side (Blumberg's sign), and observation of rigidity of psoas muscle by right hip extension are mainly used in adults].

The already described local findings at the Mc Burney's point may be displaced in direction of the flank, to the bladder, left lower or right upper abdomen depending on the site of the involved appendix (retrocecally, in the pelvis #, left lower or right upper abdomen).

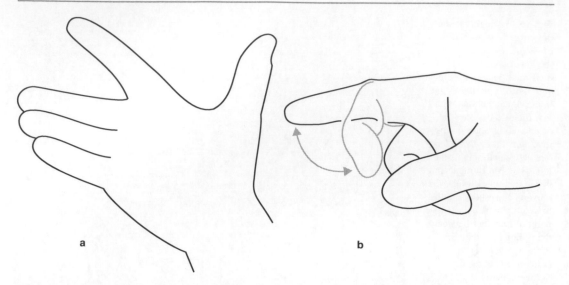

a   b

Fig. 14.2 Rectal examination: after pausing with the index finger introduced into the anus (the three ulnar fingers should be extended and deviated in an ulnar direction for introduction and examination) = **a** and calming, the child may be asked about pain in the Douglas' cul-de-sac. The *up and down* movements of the examining index finger = **b** can be demonstrated by simultaneous movements of the index finger of the other hand. Only after that, the rectal lumen and its environment are palpated. A differentiated rectal examination with the index finger is only useful in cooperative schoolchildren. In younger children, simple rectal examination is only indicated if specific findings should be excluded such as Douglas' abscess, torsion of the ovary, low intussusception or rectal polyp, pelvic tumor, or other pathologies. The rectal examination may be combined with a rectoabdominal examination in pelvic pathologies

Rectal examination is often excluded today although it makes still a sense if indicated and performed correctly. For instance, if an abscess of the Douglas' pouch or a lower abdominal mass in small children is expected. In cooperative school-children, localized pain, infiltration, or prominence of the ceiling may be recorded (Fig. 14.2).

Rarely appendicitis may be combined with priapism.

In advanced localized and specifically **generalized peritonitis**, the child *is quiet, has an increased heart rate, distinctly fever, missing respiratory movements of the abdominal wall, peristaltic silence on auscultation, and diffuse tenderness and guarding on palpation.*

Additional Examinations

They include measurement of body temperature, white blood cell count (WBC), differentiation, C-reactive protein (CRP), and erythrocyte sedimentation rate (ESR).

The **rectal temperature** is still the gold standard for determination of core body temperature although it is lower by a mean of 0.3 °C and lags behind by 1–2 h if the core body temperature changes rapidly. The widely used infrared tympanic thermometry differs by >0.3 °C in 1/4th–2/3rd and by >0.6 °C in one third of the children. Therefore, the formerly used axillorectal difference should not be used anymore.

Fever ≥38°, white blood cell count of >10,000/mm³, left shift (>11 % granulocytes), and increased C-reactive protein (>6) increase the sensitivity and specificity of clinical findings for acute and perforated appendicitis.

In general, timing at which the laboratory data have been drawn in relation to the onset of symptomatology plays an important role. Determination of ESR is only useful in and for follow-up after suspected complicated appendicitis.

The first-line radiological imaging is ultrasound (equivocal clinical findings, differential diagnostic delineation). CT is indicated in complicated appendicitis especially if a perityphlitis, another intra-abdominal abscess, or a tumor is suspected #.

Table 14.3 Differential diagnosis of acute appendicitis

- Gastroenteritis
- o Enterocolitis, e.g., E. coli (VTEC) leading to diarrhea
- Constipation, e.g., acute decompensation of constipation
- o Mesenteric lymphadenitis
- o Bilharziasis, enterocolitis includig appendicitis
- o Yersiniosis
- o Crohn's disease
- o Stump appendicitis
- o Carcinoid tumor
- *Primary or secondary peritonitis*
- o Benign abacterial peritonitis
- Urinary tract infections (infants, girls)
- Premenstrual syndrome and related disorders (teenagers)
- o Lobar pneumonia, diabetes mellitus, meningitis, etc.
- Testicular and hydatid torsion
- Ovarian mass and/or torsion

Differential Diagnosis

The differential diagnosis of acute appendicitis includes several pathologies as quoted in Table 14.3. Some of them are frequent (•) and others age-dependent, *surgical*, and/or less frequent (o). The differential diagnosis of **complicated appendicitis** includes abdominal tumor, intra-abdominal abscesses of nonappendical cause, primary peritonitis, and other causes of secondary peritonitis, ovarian torsion, and hematometrocolpos.

Yersiniosis is caused by specific serotypes of Yersinia enterocolitica or pseudotuberculosis and presents as acute or chronic enteritis with mucous and mushy stools without/with blood or watery stools.

In one fourth of the cases, a right lower abdominal symptomatology is present and mimics appendicitis although the appendix is mostly not involved at surgery. However, a considerable mesenteric lymphadenopathy and occasionally localized ileitis terminalis is present which resembles **Crohn's disease**. In the latter condition, the inflammatory signs (redness and swelling) are less distinctly limited and creeping fat sign is present. Because yersiniosis is self-limited, antibiotics are not necessary except for rare septicemia. Positive cultures of stool and mesenteric

lymph node tissue and a serum agglutinin titer of ≥1,160 are diagnostic.

Stump appendicitis is probably underreported. It occurs if an appendiceal remnant is left behind and occurs in inverted and not inverted appendiceal stump. With the introduction of laparoscopic appendectomy, stump appendicitis has initially increased. It presents with symptoms and signs of appendicitis, but the possibility of stump appendicitis is usually not considered because of prior surgery. Therefore, the reported number of perforations in stump appendicitis is very high. It is prevented by avoidance of a long appendiceal stump, and in laparoscopic appendectomy, ligature is recommended instead of the use of a surgical stapler. Also malignancies and hemorrhage do occur in appendiceal stump.

Carcinoid tumor is rarely suspected clinically because the majority of children presents with acute appendicitis (>70 %) with the tumor located at the tip of the appendix (tumor sizes < 0.5–1 cm) or less frequently with right lower peritonitis with tumor on the base of the appendix (tumor size ≥ 2 cm). Appendectomy in carcinoid tumors at the tip of the appendix is sufficient whereas larger tumors at the base need recognition at primary surgery and appropriate techniques: cecectomy if serosa and/or mesoappendix is involved without metastases, and ileocecal resection in infiltration beyond the cecum with local metastases, and if only incomplete gross resection has been performed at initial surgery. The prevalence of carcinoid tumor is 0.4 % in a large population of children and adults.

Treatment

The indication of surgery in suspected appendicitis relying on history, clinical findings, and laboratory results is questioned today due to the relatively high rates of unnecessary appendectomies and missed appendicitis. In the background of this trend, length and costs of hospitalization, possibility of ensuing, 100 % safety mania, and loss of clinical experience are hidden and lead to an overuse of imaging techniques.

One way to overcome this dilemma is **appendicitis scores**. They are based on statistically proofed clinical and laboratory findings and allow grouping in three categories: (1) children with obvious signs of appendicitis, (2) children with equivocal findings, and (3) children with minimal chance of appendicitis. Group 1 is submitted to appendectomy and group 3 discharged with surveillance by the family doctor. Short-term clinical examinations are performed (by evaluation of useful clusters of signs) or sonography in group 2, and in case of equivocal findings laparoscopic evaluation or CT. This procedure saves a lot of unnecessary examinations and, in case of CT, radiation and altogether costs. A 100 % security that a normal appendix is excluded and no appendicitis is missed is impossible in spite of the numerous quoted work-ups with often controversial results.

A lot of change is communicated in the literature regarding treatment of appendicitis:

(1) Antibiotic treatment with/without interval appendectomy versus immediate appendectomy in simple appendicitis, (2) antibiotic treatment with/without drainage and delayed appendectomy versus immediate appendectomy and evacuation of abscess in perforated appendicitis, and (3) laparoscopic appendectomy in every case of appendicitis versus selective open or minimally invasive surgery. It is possible that the experience of several generations of pediatric surgeons must be reinvented due to fatal outcomes in the near future if all the suggested therapeutic options are realized.

In case of obvious clinical and laboratory signs of appendicitis, open or minimally invasive appendectomy should be performed as soon as possible #. Laparoscopic appendicitis is specifically indicated in pubertal girls and obese children of any age with equivocal findings #.

In perforated appendicitis ###, appropriate triple antibiotics including metronidazole are started immediately followed by urgent appendectomy, lavage, and drainage either by open or minimally invasive surgery. The latter procedure has a somewhat higher rate of postoperative abscesses.

To avoid intra-abdominal or abdominal wall abscesses, perioperative single-shot antibiotics are indicated in phlegmonous or gangrenous appendicitis.

The appendix should be sent for histological examination even if it looks normal for exclusion of Enterobius vermicularis (pinworms, 0.2–42 % worldwide) and other zoonoses, carcinoid (0.4 %), neurogenic appendicopathy (53 % of normal appendices with presenting signs of appendicitis).

Prognosis

The prognosis is much more favorable after simple than after complicated appendicitis with ≤1.2 % **intra-abdominal** and **abdominal wall abscess** # in the former and 3.4–6.5 % in latter, with **early ileus or primary sterility in women** in the latter, and **intestinal obstruction due to postoperative adhesions** # 1.2 % in the former and 6.2 % in the latter.

In young children especially in infants, the occurrence of perforated appendicitis is very high (<3 years of age 60 %) in contrast to older children with rates of ≥15–20 %.

14.2.2 Meckel's Diverticulitis

Meckel's diverticulitis # is discussed in the Chap. 23.

14.2.3 Cholelithiasis, Cholecystitis

Occurrence

Gallstones are increasingly recognized in children and occur more frequently because of new therapeutic options in many fields of pediatrics. Their prevalence is probably more than 0.3 %, and in ultrasound performed for abdominal pain in children, gallstones are recognized in about 5 %.

Although the majority of gallbladders removed for gallstones yields histological signs of chronic inflammation, acute calculous and acalculous cystitis confirmed by ultrasound and inflammatory tests is much less frequent than cholelithiasis.

Clinical Significance

• In children, only about 50 % of gallstones are symptomatic, and the asymptomatic remain so in the majority of cases during childhood.

- Laparoscopic cholecystectomy or cholecystotomy in selected cases are established methods with low morbidity and relief of the symptomatology in >95 %.
- Although complicated cholecystitis is observed much less frequently in children, their possible occurrence must be considered in every case of surgical abdomen.

Causes and Predisposing Factors

The numerous causes and predisposing factors can be used to divide cholelithiasis into three groups:

1. Hematological cholelithiasis. In this group, the hemolytic disorders play a major role: sickle cell disease (45 % of children develop cholelithiasis), hereditary spherocytosis (≤ two thirds develop cholelithiasis), thalassemia major (≤45 % develop cholelithiasis in the first half of the second decade; mainly SS homozygous and Sb heterozygous types), and other types of hemolysis
2. Miscellaneous causes and predisposing factors:
- Obesity and pregnancy in adolescent girls including rapid loss of weight and familial cholelithiasis (2 % of obese pubertal children previously treated with diet develop stones)
- Severe generalized disorders such as leukemia or other malignancies, septicemia, organ transplantations, metabolic diseases (e.g., cystic fibrosis, hypothyreosis)
- Prematurity and associated treatment options
- Hepatobiliary disorders such as malformations (e.g., choledochal cyst, other anomalies of cystic, hepatic, and common duct, biliary dyskinesia), hepatitis and cirrhosis
- Total parenteral nutrition (TPN) and/or small intestine resections or disorders such as small bowel syndrome (even after bowel lengthening), necrotizing enterocolitis (NEC), Crohn's disease, ulcerative colitis
- Drugs like cyclosporine, ceftriaxone, and contraceptives
- Gallbladder parasitosis (**e.g., Dicrocoelium dendriticum** belongs to the Plathelminthes that enter the biliary tree and liver by the portal vein system)

3. Idiopathic cholelithiasis. None of the known etiopathological factors are present.

There is a wide variation in occurrence of the three groups and of the single pathologies the world over. For instance, hematological cholelithiasis is observed in <5 % up to 30 %.

In contrast to adults with more than three fourths of patients with cholesterol stones, this type is observed only in about one fifth (mostly in adolescent girls). About 50 % of the children have black pigmented bilirubinate (mainly after hemolysis, TPN, neonatal abdominal surgery) or less frequently calcium carbonate stones (mainly after neonatal intensive care or abdominal surgery).

Clinical Presentation

The triad right subcostal pain, nausea/vomiting, and intolerance to fatty foods may be encountered in the second decade.

In most children, recurrent chronic or acute abdominal pain is the main presenting symptom followed by nausea and vomiting, intolerance to fatty food, pain radiating to the ipsilateral shoulder or subscapular region, and attacks of pancreatitis in order of decreasing frequency. Often the pain is vague and poorly localized or may be assigned to the right upper abdominal quadrant and/or less frequently to the epigastrium, sometimes with sudden onset of crescendo- and decrescendo-type colic.

In case of abdominal pain, the history should be checked for the disorders quoted under the headline "causes and predisposing factor," and symptomless patients with such disorders should be checked for gallstones at intervals.

In acute abdominal pain without/with complicated cholelithiasis, the right upper quadrant is tender on percussion and pressure with possible guarding.

Complications of cholecystitis occur in about 10 % and include **acute cholecystitis, choledocholithiasis/cholangitis, and biliary pancreatitis** (each with similar incidence of <5 %). Clinically, inflammatory signs, jaundice, and abdominal pain of different location and character may be observed although the patients may be symptomless in choledocholithiasis and jaundice may be due to hemolysis.

Work-Ups, Differential Diagnosis

The main imaging procedure is ultrasound that has a sensitivity and specificity of gallstones of at least 95 %. Less reliable is the demonstration of infundibular, cystic duct and common hepatic and bile duct stones although dilatation is clearly recognizable.

In addition, biliary sludge that consists of thickened gall with sprinkled radiopaque bits of 1 mm size as possible precursors of gallstones, signs of acute cholecystitis or empyema, and hydrops of the gallbladder may be recognized.

Laboratory tests are performed for exclusion of complicated cholelithiasis and include inflammatory parameters, gammaglutamyl transferase, alkaline phosphatase, bilirubin, transaminases, and amylase.

If choledocholithiasis or biliary pancreatitis is suspected (the diagnosis may be difficult in children because of the unreliability of clinical signs and laboratory findings), endoscopic retrograde cholangiopancreatography (ECRP) or magnetic resonance cholangiopancreatic perfusion (MRCP) is available.

Although ECRP needs special experience in infants and may lead to pancreatitis (about 4 %), it is possible to remove choledochal stones. MRCP needs as the latter examination general anesthesia or at least sedation and the possibility to avoid breathing artifacts but yields high spatial resolution.

The differential diagnosis includes disorders of surgical abdomen and chronic recurrent abdominal pain, and, more specifically, **biliary dyskinesia**, **acalculous cystitis**, malformations of the biliary tree (e.g., juvenile type of choledochal cyst, obstruction and anomalous junction of cystic duct), gallbladder polyp and biliary parasitoses, pancreatitis, and gastric and duodenal ulcer. In case of **complicated cholelithiasis**, disorders with jaundice and/or peritonitis must be considered.

Biliary dyskinesia (diminished gallbladder contractility) has the same symptomatology as symptomatic gallstones although the occurrence of the single symptoms may be somewhat different. The diagnosis is established by a DISIDA (= 99 m-Tc di-isopropyl iminodiacetic acid)

scintiscan during cholecystokinin injection with a preoperative gallbladder ejection fraction of ≤35–40 %. After cholecystectomy, the relief or amelioration of symptoms is about 85 % and independent of the value of gallbladder ejection fraction.

Acalculous cholecystitis is often associated with severe illness such as septicemia (e.g., Haemophilus influenzae infection) and trauma including burns. In cohorts with childhood cholecystectomy, it is usually not quoted as major cause.

Treatment, Prognosis

Surgery is indicated in all symptomatic gallstones whereas this approach is controversial in asymptomatic gallstones because the majority remains symptomless during childhood, for instance, in sickle cell disease. On the other hand, increased complicated cholelithiasis has been observed in idiopathic gallstones of adolescents.

Laparoscopic cholecystectomy or in selected cases cholecystotomy needs before surgery exclusion or treatment of possible choledochal stones. It takes place by laboratory tests and ultrasound and if needed by ECRP to avoid intraoperative cholangiography and choledochal revision. During surgery, variations of the extrahepatic biliary and vascular system must be considered that occur in up to 20 %.

The prognosis in operated gallstones is good with >95 % relief of the symptomatology.

Although morbidity of laparoscopic cholecystectomy is low, biliary leak, major bleeding, lesions of the structures adjacent to the choledochus, and common duct stricture are not excluded.

In asymptomatic gallstones, the overall outcome during childhood is not known although some informations are available. Spontaneous resolution of bile sludge has been observed in two thirds of very young patients with Down syndrome and only in one fourth of the gallstones that occur in 9 % of this population. Ursodeoxycholic acid is not very effective in dissolution of gallstones, but it may have a benefit for the symptomatology of older and for prophylaxis in small children. Nevertheless, long-term follow-ups are necessary in all patients with asymptomatic gallstones.

14.2.4 Acute Pancreatitis

Occurrence

Acute, recurrent, and chronic pancreatitis is encountered in children as well although less frequently than in adults in whom alcohol abuse and cholelithiasis are the main causes.

Clinical Significance

- Pancreatitis must be considered in all children with acute and specifically with recurrent or chronic abdominal pain.
- The main causes are systemic infections, blunt abdominal trauma, disorders of the pancreaticobiliary duct system, and drugs.
- If acute pancreatitis is not recognized, specific treatment is withhold from the child, and complicated or chronic pancreatitis may develop.

Clinical Presentation

Although vague or delayed upper abdominal pain may be recorded in some children, *the classic pain is peracute, epigastric, severe, continuous, and possibly combined with nausea and vomiting, and/or radiation in the lower abdomen or waist.*

The abdomen may be distended and tender, and bowel sounds are absent on auscultation if paralytic ileus is present. In severe cases, periumbilical or flank ecchymoses may be recognizable.

Depending on the natural history, either interstitial-edematous or less frequently hemorrhagic-necrotizing pancreatitis occurs. The latter is less frequently observed in children than in adults (about 20 %). *In* **hemorrhagic-necrotizing pancreatitis** or **complications** such as infection and abscess, *fever, exsiccosis, shock, signs of the respiratory organs, and guarding of the distended and tender belly are present.*

The possible causes of pancreatitis are listed in Table 14.4.

Differential Diagnosis, Work-up Examinations

It includes disorders of surgical abdomen specifically those with intestinal perforation or obstruction, cholelithiasis, acalculous cystitis, gastroduodenal ulcer, and disorders of chronic recurrent abdominal pain.

Table 14.4 Causes of childhood pancreatitis

- Systemic infections such as mumps, other virus infections, or septicemia, burns, or multisystemic organ injury
- Trauma such as blunt abdominal trauma or abdominal pancreaticobiliary instrumentation
- Disorders of the pancreaticobiliary duct system such as choledochal cyst or cholelithiasis, and malunion, pancreas divisum, and stenosis of the ampulla of Vater
- Drugs such as antibiotics, antiepileptics, immunosuppressants
- Metabolic disorders such as cystic fibrosis and miscellaneous causes such as hereditary pancreatitis

The diagnosis of acute pancreatitis is possible by more than threefold elevated levels of serum amylase and/or lipase; normal values do not exclude acute pancreatitis; those that are only moderately elevated are not specific for pancreatitis because they may also be observed in secondary peritonitis and other disorders. On the other hand, enzyme determination immediately after the onset of the symptomatology or after several days may be normal or not conclusive.

Other laboratory examinations are performed for follow-up (prognostication, complications) or recognition of the cause of pancreatitis: hemoglobin, hematocrit, inflammatory parameters, LDH, glucose, calcium, creatinine, PO2, base deficit, and ALT/AST (threefold increase corresponds in 95 % to a biliary pancreatitis). For prognostication, either single tests such as CRP and creatinine increase, or PO2 and hemoglobin decrease, or scores composed of clinical and laboratory data as the Ranson Score may be used.

If plain chest and/or abdominal x-rays have been performed for other reasons, some hints of pancreatitis may be recognized such as left pleural effusion or mottling of the lung, and/or radiopaque stones, gas-filled right colon, or a single distended loop of small intestine.

Imaging techniques are only necessary in case of suspected hemorrhagic-necrotizing or complicated pancreatitis, or for evaluation of the cause of pancreatitis.

Treatment, Prognosis

Treatment is medical and supportive: analgetics, parenteral fluid replacement, nasogastric suction in case of vomiting and paralytic ileus, and enteral nutrition by a jejunal tube. Antibiotics are only indicated in case of hemorrhagic-necrotizing and complicated pancreatitis.

In the latter situations, ultrasound and i.v. contrast CT and in suspected pancreaticobiliary duct disorders ERCP or MRCP are necessary for further work-up. Supposed infection may be confirmed by fine needle aspiration (FNA) from the pancreas with Gram stain and cultures.

The **infected hemorrhagic-necrotizing pancreatitis** and **abscess** need surgical evacuation including necrosectomy, lavage and drainage, **choledocholithiasis** removal of the stones by ERCP, **choledochal cyst** or **stenosis of the papilla of Vater** Roux-en-Y hepaticojejunostomy and sphincteroplasty, respectively, and **pancreas divisum** or **malunion of the biliary and pancreatic duct** ductoplasty of the minor papilla or more extensive procedures.

The prognosis of acute pancreatitis is often uneventful. On the other hand, a mortality of ≤17 % exists due to multiorgan failure, hemorrhagic-necrotizing pancreatitis, or severe underlying disease and chronic pancreatitis.

After pancreatitis, development of pseudocysts or fistulas may be observed in 15 or <5 %. The transition to a chronic pancreatitis occurs mainly in missed anomalies of the pancreaticobiliary duct system, rare causes of pancreatitis, and cystic fibrosis.

14.2.5 Chronic Pancreatitis (Chronic Relapsing Pancreatitis)

Occurrence, Pathology

Chronic pancreatitis is less frequently observed in children than in adults. It is characterized by a progressive fibrosis, irreversible destruction of glandular tissue, and abnormalities of the duct system (stenoses and dilatations) of the pancreas. Chronic relapsing pancreatitis refers to the clinical stage in which recurrent episodes of abdominal pain are combined with varying degrees of pancreatic dysfunction.

Clinical Significance

- Episodes of abdominal pain may present as surgical abdomen and are not recognized as part of a chronic relapsing pancreatitis because additional signs such as weight loss and steatorrhea are only present in a far advanced stage.
- Depending on the cause of chronic relapsing pancreatitis, the progress of the disease may be stopped with preservation of pancreatic function if appropriate surgical treatment is and can be performed.

Clinical Presentation

The abdominal pain mostly located in the epigastrium and radiating in the back is usually the sole symptom because weight loss, steatorrhea, and diabetes occur only if up to 90% of the pancreas is distroyed. Such stools are voluminous, soft, and sticky.

The epigastric pain occurs early after a meal, may be combined with nausea and vomiting, and is observed intermittently (with intervals of several months to years) or in a later stage constantly with daily severe attacks.

The **causes** are the same as in acute pancreatitis. In addition, chronic inflammatory disorders such as Crohn's disease and ulcerative colitis or idiopathic chronic pancreatitis must be considered. Important causes are anomalies of the pancreaticobiliary duct system without or with annular pancreas or pancreas divisum (pancreas secretion is mainly [and possibly insufficiently] drained by the minor duct of Santorini).

Differential Diagnosis, Work-Ups

It includes the surgical abdomen and disorders with chronic relapsing abdominal pain, for instance, intermittent ureteropelvic junction obstruction.

Work-ups for pancreatic insufficiency are limited because steatorrhea (>7 g fat in the stool of 24 h) and secretin test need intubation of the papilla of Vater for determination of bicarbonate. The determination of elastase in the stool is less complicated for collection and yields somewhat earlier pathological results (<200 μg/g stool). Ultrasound, CT, ECRP, MRCP (with secretin test), and endosonography yield informations about possible causes of chronic pancreatitis, and endosonography demonstrates the ductal and parenchymal morphology.

Treatment, Prognosis

Treatment is medical and includes alleviation of pain, appropriate diet, and lipase replacement.

In ductal abnormalities with obstruction of pancreas secretion, sphincteroplasty of the major or minor duct and longitudinal pancreaticojejunostomy are surgical options with good results.

The prognosis depends on the cause and the stage of chronic pancreatitis, and the practicality of surgical options. In children, pancreatectomy, bouginage, or stenting for pain relief is usually not discussed.

14.2.6   Primary (Spontaneous) Peritonitis

Occurrence, Pathology

In primary peritonitis, the cause is not perforation of a hollow organ, for example, perforated appendicitis or an abscess of a parenchymatous organ, for example, **hepatic amebiasis** (= secondary peritonitis), but the bacterial infection occurs by hematogenous, lymphatic, or urogenital routes or as sequels of diagnostic and therapeutic interventions such as v-p shunt or peritoneal dialysis. Whereas primary peritonitis due to pneumo- or streptococci in relation to acute and perforated appendicitis occurs in <0.5 %, primary peritonitis due to predisposing diseases or abdominal foreign bodies is frequent.

Clinical Significance

- In case of acute abdominal pain and fever or a symptomatology of surgical abdomen specifically of peritonitis combined with specific causes and predisposing factors, the possibility of primary peritonitis should be considered and excluded.

Predisposing Factors and Causes

Nephrotic syndrome, chronic liver diseases with/ without hepatic insufficiency and formation of ascites, cystic fibrosis, abdominal lymphatic disorders, CAH, postsplenectomy syndrome, and long-term steroid administration are risks for primary peritonitis.

Causes are urogenital (e.g., jumps into the water, ascending vulvovaginitis, labial synechia, or sexual abuse), pneumonic (streptococci pneumoniae group A) infections, and inappropriate handling of abdominal implants in v-p shunt and peritoneal dialysis.

Depending on the predisposing factors and causes, different bacteria are in the fore:

In nephrotic syndrome, streptococcus pneumonia and Gram-negative germs are prominent. In chronic liver disease, mostly Gram-negative germs are encountered and less frequently Streptococci pneumonia and *Staphylococcus aureus*. In peritoneal dialysis, *Staphylococcus aureus* and epidermidis are the most frequent bacteria followed by other bacteria or fungi such as *Pseudomonas* species or *Candida*. In v-p shunt, *Staphylococcus epidermidis* is the most frequent bacterium although all well-known and some rare germs may be encountered. In primary peritonitis caused by an initial infection somewhere in the body, *Streptococcus pneumoniae*, gonococcus, group A and *β-hemolytic streptococci*, haemophilus influenzae, Gram-negative bacteria, *Salmonella*, *Serratia*, and *Yersinia enterocolitica* are observed.

Clinical Presentation

The leading symptoms are abdominal pain and/or fever possibly combined with nausea/ vomiting and diarrhea. In carriers of abdominal foreign bodies, they may be superimposed by signs of shunt malfunction and by a cloudy effluent dialysate or difficulties to perform dialysis.

Due to a paralytic ileus and fluid accumulation, *the abdomen is often distended and tender with diminished bowel sounds. Sometimes, diffuse or localized guarding or rebound tenderness may be recorded although the local findings are less impressive in comparison with secondary peritonitis and develop protractedly. If large amounts of exudate are present, shifting dullness to percussion and perceptible fluid wave is present.*

In case of an open processus vaginalis (inguinal or inguinoscrotal hernia), an inflammatory groin or scrotal swelling may point to the ongoing primary or secondary peritonitis.

Differential Diagnosis, Work-Ups
The differential diagnosis must consider secondary peritonitis, benign nonbacterial peritonitis, familial Mediterranean fever, and abdominal tuberculosis.

Examples of less known secondary peritonitis are **intestinal complications in children undergoing chemotherapy**, **intestinal perforation in S. typhi,** or **hepatic amebiasis**.

Benign nonbacterial peritonitis occurs mainly in toddlers and at the beginning of school age. It is observed in 2 of 100 children with appendicitis who complain of acute diffuse or localized pain in the right lower abdomen or periumbilical region. On clinical examination, diffuse or localized tenderness to palpation and guarding is present combined with diminished bowel sound. Surgery is performed with the indication of acute appendicitis or peritonitis and yields distinct hyperemia of the peritoneum including the serosa of the appendix and a moderate amount of mucous and viscous exudate all over the abdominal cavity. Recovery is uneventful without antibiotics.

Familial Mediterranean fever is an autosomal recessive inherited disorder that is observed in the Mediterranean population. It starts already in small children with episodic attacks of fever and abdominal pain resembling acute appendicitis that flare off after 1–2 days. The abdominal symptomatology is combined with monoarthralgia or oligarthralgia, an erysipelas-like exanthema, and possibly with chest pain. Pain is caused by sterile effusions. Before recognition of the disease, up to one fourth of the children have received appendectomy. Family history, characteristic episodes, and genetic examinations confirm the diagnosis. Unfortunately, abdominal attacks may occur in spite of colchicine treatment what may again lead to unnecessary surgical interventions. On the other hand, obstructive ileus due to inflammatory adhesions may occur in <5 %.

Abdominal tuberculosis includes infection of the peritoneum, abdominal lymph nodes, liver, spleen, pancreas, and the gastrointestinal tract. Most common are peritonitis and nodal disease. **Tuberculous peritonitis** is observed in endemic regions in <1 % of all tuberculosis cases, may occur more frequently in developed countries in relation to other tuberculosis cases because of migration, and is also observed in schoolchildren.

A history of night sweats, intermittent fever, and weight loss may be recorded that are followed by abdominal pain and distension. Occasionally fever, an abdominal tumor, or surgical abdomen may be suspected. Gross ascites may be observed in three fourths of the cases. The exudate has increased levels of protein and leukocytes with predominantly lymphocytes. Laparoscopy is most useful for diagnosis because it shows the characteristic thickening of the peritoneum and filiform adhesions; if combined with tissue biopsy for cultures, it yields the best chance for diagnosis of tuberculosis.

In addition to determination of the inflammatory blood parameters, **examination of the peritoneal fluid** should be performed that is recovered by paracentesis, diagnostic laparoscopy, effluent dialysate, or surgery. In infected v-p shunt, CSF recovered from the shunt reservoir is often diagnostic. The results of protein (serum-ascites-albumin gradient < 11 g/dl), leukocyte count and differentiation (with >500 Lc/mm^3 and mainly granulocytes), pH < 7.35, and lactate > 25 mg/dl are diagnostic for infectious peritonitis.

Gram stain and cultures should be performed in peritoneal exudate or biopsy, and depending on the individual case in blood, urine, fluor vaginalis, and respiratory tract.

Imaging techniques are used for exclusion of a secondary peritonitis and yield additional informations about the peritonitis. Plain abdominal and chest x-ray display: e.g., pneumoperitoneum and air-fluid levels in intestinal perforation or obstructive ileus or signs of pneumonia. Ultrasound shows: Demonstration of exudate and of its amount, site, and distribution or pseudocysts and compartmentalization of the peritoneal cavity.

Treatment, Prognosis
It is usually medical and includes immediate systemic antibiotics depending on the expected germs, nasogastric suction, and parenteral infusion.

Whereas dialysis catheters need only replacement if the system does not work properly or if infection cannot be eradicated, v-p shunt must be exteriorated in every case with replacement of the whole system after cure of CSF infection and peritonitis.

In the preantibiotic area, morbidity and mortality of primary peritonitis were considerable. Today, primary peritonitis due to predisposing disorders and medications, and abdominal interventions including implants, is the great majority that has a better prognosis. Nevertheless, fatal outcomes because of the causal disorder or septicemia still occur. In addition, long-term sequels must be considered such a loss of absorptive capacity of the peritoneum or obstructive ileus due to postinflammatory adhesions.

14.2.7 Omental Infarction

Occurrence, Pathoanatomy
Primary omental infarction is a rare disorder of schoolchildren and adults.

Clinical Significance
- It is a differential diagnosis of acute abdominal pain and acute appendicitis.

Clinical Presentation
Omental infarction leads to acute onset of abdominal pain which may be untractable and indistinguishable from acute appendicitis (≤ 50 %) or another localized inflammatory process. Localized abdominal tenderness and guarding is often observed.

Work-Ups
Confirmation of suspected omental infarction is possible by ultrasound, CT, or diagnostic laparoscopy.

Treatment, Prognosis
Laparoscopic or open surgery with resection of the involved omentum and elective appendectomy depends on the severity and duration of symptomatology and certainty of diagnosis. Conservative treatment is possible in selected cases with uneventful outcome so far.

Webcodes

The following webcodes can be used on www.psurg.net for further images and data.

1401 Perforated appendicitis with	1407 Perforated appendicitis, localized peritonitis
1402 Localized peritonitis	1408 Perforated appendicitis with
1403 Pelvic appendicitis	1409 Mucocele of the appendix
1404 CT, perityphlitic abscess	1410 Postoperative abdominal wall abscess
1405 Phlegmonous, retrocecal appendicitis	1411 Postoperative ileus due to adhesions
1406 Acute appendicitis, laparoscopicappendectomy	1412 Meckel's diverticulitis, diffuse peritonitis

Bibliography

Section 14.1: Thermometry, Abdominal Manifestations in Cystic Fibrosis

Chaudry G, Navarro OM, Levine DS, Oudjhane K (2006) Abdominal manifestations of cystic fibrosis in children. Pediatr Radiol 36:233–240

Craig JV, Lancaster GA, Taylor S et al (2002) Infrared ear thermometry compared with rectal thermometry in children: a systematic review. Lancet 360:603–609

Greenes DS, Fleisher GR (2004) When body temperature changes, does rectal temperature lag? J Pediatr 144:824–826

Mc Carthy VP, Mischler EH, Hubbard VS, Chernick MS, di Sant'Agnese PA (1984) Appendiceal abscess in cystic fibrosis: a diagnostic challenge. Gastroenterology 86:564–568

Section 14.2.1: Clinical Presentation and Work-Ups

Alaedeen DI, Cook M, Chwals WJ (2008) Appendiceal fecalith is associated with early perforation in pediatric patients. J Pediatr Surg 43:889–892

Ang A, Chong NK, Daneman A (2001) Pediatric appendicitis in "real-time": the value of sonography in diagnosis and treatment. Pediatr Emerg Care 17:334–340

Beltran MA, Almonacid J, Vicencio A, Gutierrrez J, Cruces KS, Cumsille MA (2007) Predictive value of white blood cell count and C-reactive protein in children with appendicitis. J Pediatr Surg 42:1208–1214, Comment in: J Pediatr Surg 2008 43:256; author reply 256-257

Bixby S, Lucey B, Soto J et al (2006) Perforated versus nonperforated acute appendicitis: accuracy of multidetector CT detection. Radiology 241:780–786

Bundy DG, Byerley JS, Liles EA et al (2007) Does this child have appendicitis? J Am Med Assoc 298:438–451

Chiang DT, Tan EI, Birks D (2008) 'To have…or not to have'. Should computed tomography and ultrasonography be implemented as a routine work-up for patients with suspected acute appendicitis in a regional hospital? Ann R Coll Surg Engl 90:17–21

Colvin JM, Bachur R, Kharbanda A (2007) The presentation of appendicitis in preadolescent children. Pediatr Emerg Care 23:849–855

Fishman SJ, Pelosi L, Klavon SL, O'Rourke EJ (2000) Perforated appendicitis: prospective outcome analysis for 150 children. J Pediatr Surg 35:923–926

Flum DR, Morris A, Koepsell T et al (2001) Has misdiagnosis of appendicitis de-creased over time? A population-based analysis. JAMA 286:1748–1753

Fraser ID, Aguayo P, Sharp SW, Snyder CL, Holcomb GW III, Ostlie DJ, St Peter SD (2010) Physiological predictors of postoperative abscess in children with perforated appendicitis: subset analysis from a prospective randomized trial. Surgery 147:729–732

Goldman RD, Carter S, Stephens D, Antoon R, Mounstephen W, Langer JC (2008) Prospective validation of the pediatric appendicitis score. J Pediatr 153:278–282

Jancelewicz T, Kim G, Miniati D (2008) Neonatal appendicitis: a new look at an old zebra. J Pediatr Surg 43:e1–e5

Lee SL, Ho HS (2006) Acute appendicitis: is there a difference between children and adults? Am Surg 72:409–413

Levine CD, Aizenstein O, Wachsberg RH (2004) Pitfalls in the CT diagnosis of appendicitis. Br J Radiol 77: 792–799

Molenaar JC (1997) The physical examination. Semin Pediatr Surg 6:62–64

Nance M, Adamson W, Hedrick H (2000) Appendicitis in the young child: a continuing diagnostic challenge. Pediatr Emerg Care 16:160–162

Paajanen H, Somppi E (1996) Early childhood appendicitis is still a difficult diagnosis. Acta Paediatr 85:459–462

Puig S, Staudenherz A, Felder-Puig R, Paya K (2008) Imaging of appendicitis in children and adolescents: useful or useless? A comparison of imaging techniques and a critical review of the current literature. Semin Roentgenol 43:22–28

Rappaport W, Peterson M, Stanton C (1989) Factors responsible for the high perforation rate seen in early childhood appendicitis. Am Surg 55:602–605

Samuel M (2002) Pediatric appendicitis score. J Pediatr Surg 37:877–881

Spitz L, Kimber C (1997) The history. Semin Pediatr Surg 6:58–61

Wang LT, Prentiss KA, Simon JZ, Doody DP, Ryan DP (2007) The use of white blood cell count and left shift in the diagnosis of appendicitis in children. Pediatr Emerg Care 23:69–76

Section 14.2.1: Treatment

Andersen BR, Kallehave FL, Andersen HK (2005) Antibiotics versus placebo for prevention of postoperative infection after appendectomy. Cochrane Database Syst Rev (3):CD001439

Henry MC, Moss RL (2005) Primary versus delayed wound closure in complicated appendicitis: an international systemic review and meta-analysis. Pediatr Surg Int 21:625–630

Kokoska ER, Minkes RK, Silen ML et al (2001) Effect of pediatric surgical practice on the treatment of children with appendicitis. Pediatrics 107:1298–1301

Martin LC, Puente I, Sosa JL et al (1995) Open versus laparoscopic appendectomy: a prospective randomized comparison. Ann Surg 222:256–262

Oldham KT (2004) Financial considerations in laparoscopic and open appendectomy. Arch Pediatr Adolesc Med 158:11–12

Samuel M, Hosie G, Holmes K (2002) Prospective evaluation of nonsurgical versus surgical management of appendiceal mass. J Pediatr Surg 37:882–886

Sauerland S, Lefering R, Neugebauer EA (2004) Laparoscopic versus open surgery for suspected appendicitis. Cochrane Database Syst Rev (4):CD001546

Solomkin JS, Mazuski JE, Bradley JS, Rodvolt KA, Goldstein EJ, Baron EJ, O'Neill PJ, Chow AW, Dellinger EP, Eachempati SR, Gorbach S, Hilfiker M, May AK, Nathens AB, Sawyer RG, Bartlett JG (2010) Diagnosis and management of complicated intra-abdominal infection in adults and children: guidelines by the Surgical Infection Society and the Infectious Diseases Society of America. Surg Infect (Larchmt) 11:79–109

Whyte C, Levin T, Harris BH (2008) Early decisions in perforated appendicitis in children: lessons from a study of nonoperative management. J Pediatr Surg 43:1459–1463

Section 14.2.1: Pathology

Güller U, Oertli D, Terracciano L, Harder F (2001) Neurogenic appendicopathy: a frequent, almost unknown disease picture. Evaluation of 816 appendices and review of the literature. Chirurg 72:684–689

Section 14.2.1: Differential Diagnosis

Anonymus (2006) Outbreaks of Escherichia coli O157. H7 associated with petting zoos. JAMA 295:378–380

Arca MJ, Gates RL, Groner JI, Hammond S, Caniano DA (2004) Clinical manifestations of appendiceal pinworms in children: an institutional experience and review of the literature. Pediatr Surg Int 20:372–375

Bettex M (1953) La péritonite bénigne abacteriénne de l'enfant. Helv Paediat Acta 8:166–173

Black RE et al (1978) Epidemic Yersinia Enterocolitica infection due to contaminated chocolate milk. N Engl J Med 298:76–79

Burnens AP (2001) Aktuelle Diagnostik von Verotoxin bildenden Escherichia coli. Bundesamt für Gesundheit, Epidemiology und Infektionskrankheiten. Bulletin 2:27–30

Centers for Disease Control and Prevention (CDC) (2005) Outbreaks of Escherichia coli O157:H7 associated with petting zoos – North Carolina, Florida, and Arizona, 2004 and 2005. MMWR Morb Mortal Wkly Rep. 23;54:1277–1280

Defechereux T, Coimbra C, De Roover A, Meurisse M, Honoré P (2006) Carcinoid tumor of the appendix: a consecutive series from 1237 appendectomies. World J Gastroenterol 12:6699–6701

Ein SH, Miller S, Rutka JT (2006) Appendicitis in the child with a ventriculoperitoneal shunt: a 30-year review. J Pediatr Surg 41:1255–1258

Gasmi M, Fitouri F, Sahli S, Jemai R, Hamzaoui M (2009) A stump appendicitis in a child: a case report. Ital J Pediatr 35:35

Grynspan D, Rabah R (2008) Adenoviral appendicitis presenting clinically as acute appendicitis. Pediatr Dev Pathol 11:138–141

Hassler H, von Dach B, Gössi U, Schwarz H (1986) Die Yersiniosis enterocolitica als Differentialdiagnose zur Appendicitis und zum Morbus Crohn. Helv Chir Acta 53:649–652

Kasifoglu T, Cansu DU, Korkmaz C (2009) Frequency of abdominal surgery in patients with familial Mediterranean fever. Intern Med 48:523–526

Liang MK, Lo HG, Marks JL (2006) Stump appendicitis: a comprehensive review of literature. Am Surg 72:162–166

Pelizzo G, La Riccia A, Bouvier R, Chappuis JP, Franchella A (2001) Carcinoid tumors of the appendix in children. Pediatr Surg Int 17:399–402

Sandler G, Soundappan SS, Cass D (2008) Appendicitis and low-flow priapism in children. J Pediatr Surg 43:2091–2095

Section 14.2.3

Boechat MC, Silva KS, Llerena JC Jr, Boechat PR (2007) Cholelithiasis and biliary sludge in Downs syndrome patients. Sao Paulo Med J 125:329–332

Chan S, Currie J, Malik AI, Mahomed AA (2008) Paediatric cholecystectomy: shifting goalposts in the laparoscopic era. Surg Endosc 22:1392–1395

Criblez D, Frey M (2001) Choledocholithiasis. Schweiz Med Forum 32(33):810–813

De Caluwe D, Akl U, Corbally M (2001) Cholecystectomy versus cholecystolithotomy for cholelithiasis: long-term outcome. J Pediatr Surg 36:1518–1521

Frey M, Criblez D (2001) Cholecystolithiasis. Schweiz Med Forum 32(33):805–809

Gumiero AP, Bellomo-Brandao MA, Costa-Pinto EA (2008) Gallstones in children with sickle cell disease followed up at a Brazilian hematology center. Arq Gastroenterol 45:313–318

Herzog D, Bouchard G (2008) High rate of complicated idiopathic gallstone disease in pediatric patients of a North American tertiary care center. World J Gastroenterol 14:1544–1548

Hofeldt M, Richmond B, Huffman K, Nestor J, Maxwell D (2008) Laparoscopic cholecystectomy for treatment of biliary dyskinesia is safe and effective in the pediatric population. Am Surg 74:1069–1072

Holcomb GW III, Pietsch JB (1998) Gallbladder disease and hepatic infections. In: O'Neill JA Jr et al (eds) Pediatric surgery, vol II, 5th edn. Mosby, St. Louis

Kaechele V, Wabitsch M, Thiere D, Kessler AL, Haenle MM, Mayer H, Kratzer W (2006) Prevalence of gallbladder stone disease in obese children and adolescents: influence of the degree of obesity, sex, and pubertal development. J Pediatr Gastroenterol Nutr 42:66–70

Klimek P, Kessler U, Schibli S, Berger S, Zachariou Z (2009) Gallensteine bei Kin-dern. Schweiz Med Forum 9:246–250

Kumar R, Nguyen K, Shun A (2000) Gallstones and common bile duct calculi in infancy and childhood. Aust N Z J Surg 70:188–191

Neuhaus P, Schmidt SC, Hintze RE, Adler A, Veltzke W, Raakow R, Langrehr JM, Bechstein WO (2000) Classification and treatment of bile duct injuries after laparoscopic cholecystectomy. Chirurg 71:166–173

Palasciano G, Portincasa P, Vinciguerra V, Velardi A, Tardi S, Baldassarre G et al (1989) Gallstone prevalence and gallbladder volume in children and adolescents: an epidemiological ultrasonographic survey and relationship to body mass index. Am J Gastroenterol 84:1378–1382

Reif S, Sloven DG, Lebenthal E (1991) Gallstones in children: characterization by age, etiology, and outcome. Am J Dis Child 145:105–108

Schweizer P, Lenz MP, Kirschner HJ (2000) Pathogenesis and symptomatology of cholelithiasis in childhood: a prospective study. Dig Surg 17:459–467

Soyer T, Turkmen F, Tatar N, Bozdogan O, Yagmurlu A, Cakmak M (2008) Rare gallbladder parasitosis mimicking cholelithiasis: dicrocoelium dendriticum. Eur J Pediatr Surg 18:280–281

St Peter SD, Keckler SJ, Nair A, Andrews WS, Sharp RJ, Snyder CL, Ostlie DJ, Holcomb GW (2008) Laparoscopic cholecystectomy in the pediatric population. J Laparoendosc Adv Surg Tech A 18:127–130

Talpur KA, Laghari AA, Yousfani SA, Malik AM, Memon AI, Khan SA (2010) Anatomical variations and congenital anomalies of the extra hepatic biliary system encountered during laparoscopy. J Pak Med Assoc 60:89 93

Teh SH, Pham TH, Lee A, Stavlo PL, Hanna AM, Moir C (2006) Pancreatic pseudocyst in children: the impact of management strategies on outcome. J Pediatr Surg 41:1889–1893

Tipnis NA, Werlin SL (2007) The use of magnetic resonance cholangiopancreatography in children. Curr Gastroenterol Rep 9:225–229

Vegting IL, Tabbers MM, Taminiau JA, Aronson DC, Benninga MA, Rauws EA (2009) Is endoscopic retrograde cholangiopancreatography valuable and safe in children of all ages? J Pediatr Gastroenterol Nutr 48:66–71

Vegunta RK, Raso M, Pollock J, Misra S, Wallace LJ, Torres A Jr, Pearl RH (2005) Biliary dyskinesia: the most common indicator for cholecystectomy in children. Surgery 138:726–731; discussion 731-733

Wesdorp I, Bosman D, de Graaff A et al (2000) Clinical presentation and predisposing factors of cholelithiasis and sludge in children. J Pediatr Gastroenterol Nutr 31:411–417

Yedlin ST, Dubois RS, Philippart AI (1984) Pancreas divisum: a cause of pancreatitis in childhood. J Pediatr Surg 19:793–794

Sections 14.2.4–14.2.5

Abou-Assi S, Craig K, O'Keefe SJ (2002) Hypocaloric jejunal feeding is better than total parenteral nutrition in acute pancreatitis: results of a randomized comparative study. Am J Gastroenterol 97:2255–2262

Bühler H, Bertschinger P (2004) Akute Pankreatitis: Diagnostik undTherapie. Schweiz Med Forum 4:43–48

Etemad B, Withcomb D (2001) Chronic pancreatitis: diagnosis, classification, and new genetic developments. Gastroenterology 120:682–707

Frossard JL, Nicolet T (2007) Chronische Pankreatitis und Pankreasinsuffizienz. Schweiz Med Forum 7:75–80

Gloor B, Wente MN, Müller CA, Worni M, Uhl W, Büchler MW (2000) Indikation zur chirurgischen Therapie und operative Technik bei akuter Pankreatitis. Swiss Surg 6:241–245. doi:10.1024/1023-9332.6.5.241

Inderbitzi R, Hohenberger W, Triller J (1989) Die operative Therapie der Pankreas-pseudozysten. Helv Chir Acta 53:699–701

Lee SP, Nicholls JF, Park HZ (1992) Biliary sludge as a cause of acute pancreatitis. N Engl J Med 326:589–593

Monkemuller K, Kahl S, Malfertheiner P (2004) Endoscopic therapy for chronic pancreatitis. Dig Dis 22:280–291

Rocca R, Castellino F, Daperno M, Masoero G, Sostegni R, Ercole E et al (2005) Therapeutic ERCP in paediatric patients. Dig Liver Dis 37:357–362

Schlosser W, Rau BM, Poch B, Beger HG (2005) Surgical treatment of pancreas divisum causing chronic pancreatitis: the outcome benefits of duodenum-preserving pancreatic head resection. J Gastrointest Surg 9:710–715

Sharma VK, Howden CW (1999) Metaanalysis of randomized controlled trials of endoscopic retrograde cholangiography and endoscopic sphincterotomy in the treatment of acute biliary pancreatitis. Am J Gastroenterol 94:3211–3214

Sharma VK, Howden CW (2001) Prophylactic antibiotic administration reduces sepsis and mortality in acute necrotizing pancreatitis: a meta-analysis. Pancreas 22:28–31

Shea J, Bishop M, Parker E, Gelrud A, Freedman S (2003) An enteral therapy containing medium-chain triglycerides and hydrolyzed peptides reduces postprandial pain associated with chronic pancreatitis. Pancreatology 3:36–40

Terui K, Yoshida H, Kouchi K, Hishiki T, Saito T, Mitsunaga T, Takenouchi A, Tsuyuguchi T, Yamaguchi T, Ohnuma N (2008) Endoscopic sphincterotomy is a useful preoperative management for refractory pancreatitis associated with pancreaticobiliary maljunction. J Pediatr Surg 43:495–499

Yadav D, Agarwal N, Pitchumoni CS (2002) A critical evaluation of laboratory tests in acute pancreatitis. Am J Gastroenterol 97:1309–1318

Yu ZL, Zhang LJ, Fu JZ, Li J, Zhang QY, Chen FL (2004) Anomalous pancreatico-biliary junction: imaging analysis and treatment principles. Hepatobiliary Pancreat Dis Int 3:136–139

Section 14.2.6

Lane JC, Warady BA, Feneberg R, Majkowski NL, Watson AR, Fischbach M, Kang HG, Bonzel KE, Simkova E, Stefanidis CJ, Klaus G, Alexander SR, Ekim M, Bilge I, Quinlan C, Cantwell M, Rees L (2010) Eosinophilic peritonitis in children on chronic peritoneal dialysis. Pediatr Nephrol 25:517–522

Schaefer F, International Pediatric Peritonitis Registry (2010) Relapsing peritonitis in children who undergo chronic peritoneal dialysis: a prospective study of the international pediatric peritonitis registry. Clin J Am Soc Nephrol 5:1041–1046

Tinsa F, Essaddam L, Fitouri Z, Brini I, Douira W, Ben Becher S, Boussetta K, Bousnina S (2010) Abdominal tuberculosis in children. J Pediatr Gastroenterol Nutr 50:634–638

Uncu N, Bülbül M, Yildiz N et al (2010) Primary peritonitis in children with nephrotic syndrome: results of a 5-year multicenter study. Eur J Pediatr 169:73–76

West KW (1998) Primary peritonitis. In: O'Neill JA Jr et al (eds) Pediatric surgery, vol II, 5th edn. Mosby, St. Louis

Section 14.2.6: Differential Diagnosis

Brook I (2004) Intra-abdominal, retroperitoneal, and visceral abscesses in children. Eur J Pediatr Surg 14: 265–273

Hata S, Pietsch J, Shankar S (2004) Intestinal complications in children undergoing chemotherapy for mediastinal non-Hodgkin's lymphoma. Pediatr Hematol Oncol 21:707–710

Muyembe-Tamfum JJ, Veyi J, Kaswa M, Lunguya O, Verhaegen J, Boelaert M (2009) An outbreak of peritonitis caused by multidrug-resistant Salmonella Typhi in Kinshasa, Democratic Republic of Congo. Travel Med Infect Dis 7:40–43

Rao S, Solaymani-Mohammadi S, Petri WA Jr, Parker SK (2009) Hepatic amebiasis: a reminder of the complications. Curr Opin Pediatr 21:145–149

Zorludemir U, Koca M, Olcay I, Yücesan S (1992) Neonatal peritonitis. Turk J Pediatr 34:157–166

Section 14.2.7

Houben CH, Powis M, Wright VM (2003) Segmental infarction of the omentum: a difficult diagnosis. Eur J Pediatr Surg 13:57–59

Nubi A, McBride W, Stringel G (2009) Primary omental infarct: conservative vs operative management in the era of ultrasound, computerized tomography, and laparoscopy. J Pediatr Surg 44:953–956

Rimon A, Daneman A, Gerstle JT, Ratnapalan S (2009) Omental infarction in children. J Pediatr 155:427–431.e1

Surgical Abdomen due to Intestinal Obstructions

15

The pathoanatomical subdivision of the surgical abdomen due to intestinal obstructions and other pathologies is quoted in Table 15.1.

15.1 Surgical Abdomen of the Newborn

15.1.1 Obstructive Ileus of the Newborn, General Remarks

Occurrence

Obstructive ileus is the most significant cause of surgical abdomen in the newborn.

Clinical Significance, Causes

- Prompt recognition of obstructive ileus of the newborn and its possible or probable cause is

crucial for outcome and successful parenteral and patient-related guidance

The main causes of neonatal obstructive ileus are listed in Table 15.2.

Clinical Presentation

At first, the clinical triad consisting of vomiting (or regurgitation), distended abdomen, and missing or abnormal passage of meconium or stool must be looked for.

With a precise observation of these signs and order of appearance, it is already possible to restrict the probable causes to a few disorders. Immediate bringing up of saliva or feeds correlates with regurgitation and probably with esophageal atresia. Bilious vomiting with increasing delay points to an obstruction of increasing distance from the papilla of Vater. Whereas only the upper belly is distended in upper intestinal obstruction, a global

Table 15.1 Acute/chronic partial intestinal obstruction in newborns and older children

• Ileus of the newborn	
• Incarcerated inguinal hernia	Swelling of the groin and umbilicus[a]
• Hypertrophic pyloric stenosis	Vomiting, regurgitation, and dysphagia[a]
• Intussusception	
• Postoperative ileus due to adhesions	
o Spontaneous gastrointestinal perforation	
o Rare abdominal wall, pelvic floor, and internal hernias	
o Sickle cell disease, abdominal vasoocclusive events	
o Massive colon dilatation due to fecal impaction	

[a]The leading sign is quoted for disorders that are not discussed in this chapter

Table 15.2 Main causes of neonatal obstructive ileus

• Esophageal atresia	Vomiting, regurgitation, and dysphagia[a]
• Intrinsic and extrinsic duodenal obstruction	
• Small intestine atresia and stenosis	
• Meconium ileus	
o Meconium peritonitis	
• Anomalies of intestinal rotation and fixation	
o Gastrointestinal duplications	
o Colonic atresia and stenosis	
• Hirschsprung's disease	Constipation[a]
• Anorectal malformations	

[a]The leading sign is quoted for disorders that are not discussed in this chapter

G.L. Kaiser, *Symptoms and Signs in Pediatric Surgery*, DOI 10.1007/978-3-642-31161-1_15, © Springer-Verlag Berlin Heidelberg 2012

distension is observed in intermediate or low intestinal obstruction #.

Regular passage of normal meconium is absent in complete duodenal and small intestinal obstruction, and meconium passage may be present in anomalies of rotation and fixation and occurs either delayed in Hirschsprung's disease or by an abnormal route (by a fistula or micturition) or not at all in anorectal malformations without an anus at the normal site or possible fistula.

Additional Examinations, Differential Diagnosis

The available radiological imaging can be reduced to plain abdominal X-ray in one or two plane(s) in hanging position and by contrast enema (except for specific formulation of question) and yield the following informations:

- Double-bubble air-fluid level in duodenal obstruction
- Few air-fluid levels in jejunal obstruction
- Many air-fluid levels in ileal obstruction #
- Ubiquitous (incl. pelvis) air-fluid levels of different sizes in Hirschsprung's disease with ileus and in some anorectal malformations
- Microcolon in ileal or colonic atresia
- Pathological position of colon in intestinal anomalies of rotation and fixation

The differential diagnosis is dealt with in the single disorders. In general, other causes of surgical abdomen of the neonate than obstructive ileus must be considered.

15.1.2 Intrinsic and Extrinsic Duodenal Obstruction

Occurrence, Pathoanatomy

Intrinsic duodenal obstruction is observed in ≥1:10,000 newborns. It is either complete or partial. The three types of **atresia** consist of a diaphragm or web (the site of the diaphragm is recognizable by the transition of a dilated proximal to a narrow distal duodenum), of two blind duodenal ends connected by a fibrous cord or separated by a defect including a gap of the mesentery (Fig. 15.1).

In **type 1**, the origin of the web may be several centimeters apart from the site of duodenal caliber difference. At surgery, this @@@windsock anomaly and its origin can be recognized by an indentation of duodenal wall if a gastric tube is advanced against the bottom of the web. Duodenal atresia occurs in about 85 % distal to the ampulla of Vater and in 15 % proximal to it.

In **duodenal stenosis**, there is either narrowing of a duodenal part, or the already described membrane or web has an opening, or an external compression of the duodenum is present. The T-shaped duodenal stenosis associated with the ampulla of Vater in its middle needs special attention and is an example of possible pancreaticobiliary duct anomalies encountered in intrinsic duodenal atresia.

Annular pancreas is often combined with intrinsic complete or partial obstruction of the duodenum although occasionally external compression or no compression at all may be observed. In addition, **disorders of intestinal rotation and fixation, ectopic pancreas tissue, gastrointestinal duplication, or preduodenal portal vein** may lead to extrinsic duodenal obstruction.

Clinical Significance

- Duodenal atresia or stenosis belongs to the most common intestinal obstructions of the newborn, can be relieved mostly by a standardized procedure, and has a favorable outcome in the large majority of cases.

Clinical Presentation

Duodenal obstruction is an example of high intestinal obstructions that leads to polyhydramnios and induces the search for specific signs on prenatal ultrasound. Depending on the view, a dilated, fluid-filled stomach and proximal duodenum is demonstrated.

Except for some cases of duodenal stenosis, *vomiting of bile-stained material or copious, bilious gastric aspirate in the first hours after birth is the most frequent leading sign that may be colorless in case of atresia proximal to the papilla of Vater.* Often the sunken belly is more striking than some epigastric distension. Stool evacuation is often abnormal with delay beyond 24 h and little dry or no meconium feces.

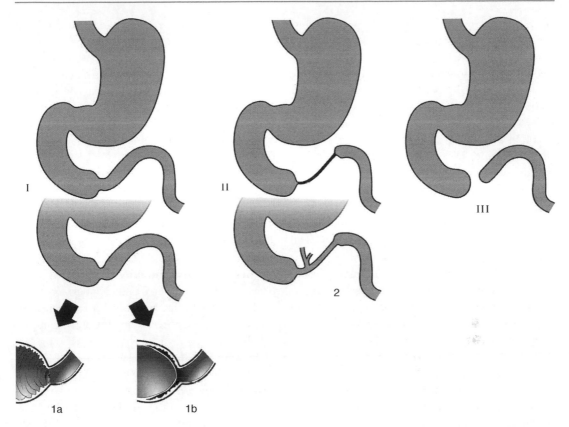

Fig. 15.1 Types of duodenal atresia and stenosis. *I*: The proximal part of duodenum is in continuity with the distal part, but the duodenal cavity is interrupted by a tough membrane; its site is only recognizable from the outside by the marked discrepancy between the dilated proximal and small distal duodenum. The membrane may have a central hole (*1a*). *II* and *III*: The continuity is maintained by a fibrous cord or not at all. The biliary and pancreatic ducts enter usually the proximal part of the duodenum. A possible modification is the so-called wind-sock web in which a loose membrane is attached to the duodenal wall proximally from its most distal central portion (*1b*). It may also display a central hole (*1a*). The papilla of Vater may be found at the site of insertion or on the proximal or distal surface of the wind sock. Rarely, the proximal and distal part of the duodenum is connected with a narrow segment with communication to the pancreaticobiliary duct system (*2*). Ramification in an *upper* and *lower* pancreaticobiliary duct occurs occasionally in membranaceous duodenal atresia and the complete separated type

In advanced stages, the bilious vomiting may become hemorrhagic due to gastric distension and gastroesophageal reflux and the newborn develops exsiccosis.

Duodenal stenosis may present in *a similar fashion as duodenal atresia, with intermittent vomiting beginning from the neonatal period*, or *with new upper gastrointestinal symptoms* (nausea, vomiting abdominal pain, and weight loss) *any time in childhood or adulthood*. These patients have either a duodenal web, annular pancreas, or both, and peptic ulcer, gastroesophageal reflux, or foreign body ingestion may lead to their recognition.

Today, the quoted median time of diagnosis is 5 days compared to 1–2 days for atresia. Immediate breastfeeding may lead to a delayed recognition.

In addition to prematurity in about 50 % and trisomy 21 in ≤1/3, numerous associated anomalies may be observed in intrinsic duodenal obstruction, and among them, abnormalities of heart and great vessels (up to 37 %) and of intestinal rotation and fixation belong to the most common.

Differential Diagnosis, Work-Ups
Seeming or real bilious vomiting may be observed in premature infants (who bring up few amounts

of yellowish material), meconium gastritis (history of meconium-stained amnion fluid), perinatal cerebral hemorrhage (additional clinical signs), and duodenal duplication. In copious colorless gastric aspirate, neonatal hypertrophic pyloric stenosis, pyloric atresia, or membrane must be considered.

Plain abdominal x-ray in hanging position is diagnostic and shows a large stomach and proximal duodenum with two fluid levels; double-bubble sign or both structures are completely filled with air. If both structures are completely filled with fluid, the double-bubble sign can be provoked by replacement of some of the fluid with the aid of a gastric tube by some air.

In duodenal stenosis, the same findings as in atresia may be encountered together with scattered bubbles throughout the intestinal tract, and upper gastrointestinal contrast study or endoscopy is necessary for diagnosis.

Treatment, Prognosis

After stabilization of the newborn including continuous aspiration and replacement of gastroduodenal secretions, surgery is indicated.

Surgery: After a right transverse supraumbilical incision, the lesser omental sack is opened and the duodenum mobilized by a Kocher maneuver. The gastric tube is advanced to the end of the proximal duodenum to exclude a wind-sock web and later for exclusion of an additional intestinal obstruction by injection of saline. Usually a side-to-side or a diamond-shaped duodenoduodenostomy is performed. In case of a web, occasionally a longitudinal incision over the transition zone is performed with excision of the lateral part of the web and transverse closure. At surgery, the site of the papilla can be seen by pressure on the gallbladder. Laparoscopic repair is quoted in the literature as alternative method.

Postoperative introduction of feeding must be performed slowly and stepwise because normal passage by the duodenum may take a median time of 10 days with an interquartile range of 7–70 days.

Prognosis: Today, survival is 95 %, the overall complication rate 18 %, and median hospital stay 18 days. The prognosis depends mainly on the associated pathologies. Occasionally, functional obstruction occurs many years later due to extreme dilatation of the proximal duodenum combined with atony. It may be possibly prevented by tapering duodenoplasty at initial surgery. Down syndrome does not influence morbidity and mortality of the congenital duodenal obstruction.

15.1.3 Jejunal and Ileal Atresia and Stenosis

Occurrence, Pathoanatomy

Small intestinal atresia and stenosis occur in ≥1:15,000 live births. Ninty-five percent are atresias and 5 % stenoses. Jejunum and ileum are equally involved.

In addition to the **three types of Louw** (arranged in order of increasing frequency) with obstruction by a membrane without interruption of the continuity, with a cordlike structure between the two blind ends, and with a gap in between often including the mesentery (Fig. 15.2), two other and often familial types are encountered in about 10 %:

- **Multiple atresia** with/without mesenteric defects that look like a string of sausages.
- The so-called **apple-peel atresia** in which the proximal jejunum has a blind end and the large mesenteric defect is followed by a distal ileum arranged like a continuous apple peel around and along a mesentery with a feeding artery from the ileocolic, right colic, or inferic mesentery artery (Fig. 15.2).

Especially in the latter two types, increased foreshortened small intestine and prematurity are observed and in apple-peel atresia in addition low birth weights (>50 %) and associated anomalies.

Clinical Significance

- Some atresias (multiple or apple-peel atresia, atresia associated with very low birth weight, with meconium peritonitis, meconium ileus, or

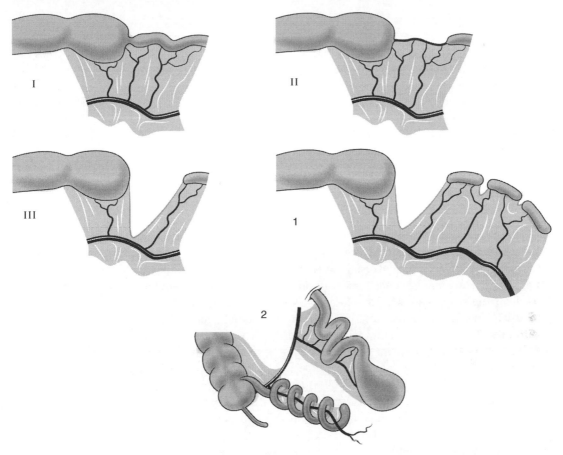

Fig. 15.2 Types of jejunal and ileal atresia: Types *I–III* are similar to those of duodenal atresia. In multiple atresias, several pieces of isolated intestine are observed like a string of sausages that are separated from each other by a gap in the mesentery (*1*). Apple-peel atresia consists of a grossly dilated blind jejunal end, foreshortened small intestine, and residual ileal loops that start from the iliocecum and are arranged around a feeding vessel from the ileocolic artery like a whisk (*2*)

gastroschisis) have a substantial mortality and morbidity including small bowel syndrome.
- Postoperative recovery of intestinal function is often delayed.

Clinical Presentation

Prenatal diagnosis by ultrasound may be difficult in spite of the red flag "polyhydramnios" that may occur in jejunal and ileal atresia as well.

The clinical signs arranged in order of frequency and significance are bilious vomiting, abdominal distension, failure to pass meconium, and jaundice.

Bile-stained vomiting occurs in low obstruction delayed, not forceful, and less copious or is even missing. Site and severity of *abdominal distension* depend as well from the location of the small intestinal obstruction. It may be only moderate, slight, or even absent in high jejunal obstruction whereas low ileal obstruction leads to gross distension with possible RDS due to elevation of the diaphragm and/or visible peristalsis. Often no *meconium* is evacuated or only gray pieces of mucus, and occasionally normal meconium or melena is observed (the latter as a signs of vascular compromise of the intestine). Jaundice due to elevated levels of indirect bilirubin is observed in ≤30 %.

Recognition of **jejunal or ileal stenosis** is often difficult because the already quoted first two signs occur only intermittently.

The clinical examination yields mainly the *site and severity of abdominal distension*. Occasionally, high-pitched intestinal sounds may be auscultated. By gentle introduction of the little finger, *passage of feces may be provoked*.

Although low birth weight is a frequent finding, prematurity and associated anomalies occur much less frequently except for anomalies of rotation and fixation without/with volvulus than in duodenal obstruction.

Differential Diagnosis, Work-Ups
It includes other causes of obstructive ileus or surgical abdomen of the newborn (e.g., adynamic ileus in septicemia) and specifically in low small intestinal obstruction, **colon atresia, intestinal duplication, internal hernia, malrotation, Hirschsprung's disease including total aganglionosis, meconium ileus, and meconium peritonitis**. The last four pathologies may be observed as associated disorders as well.

Colon atresia and stenosis are observed less often than small intestine atresia (≤ 15 % of the latter). Ninty-five percent are atresias, mostly of the Louw type III, and the remaining patients have stenoses. Associated anomalies are observed in $\geq 1/3$ of which musculoskeletal anomalies, abdominal wall midline defects, small intestine atresias, and Hirschsprung's disease are of special interest.

Clinically, a distal obstructive ileus is observed with complete development within 1–2 days that points together with white mucus on rectal examination and the quoted associated anomalies to a possible colon atresia. **Plain abdominal x-ray and contrast enema usually** yield sufficient informations for confirmation of colon atresia (distal cutoff of the air-filled intestine above the pelvis with possible extreme dilatation of the colon proximally to the atresia and absent air in the rectum, distal microcolon up to the site of atresia). In small intestine atresia, additional colon atresia must be excluded by contrast enema and in colon atresia, Hirschsprung's disease must be considered preoperatively by the same examination and careful checking at surgery that may include biopsies. **Surgery** includes primary end-to-oblique anastomosis after resection of the

atresia or stenosis and resection of an extremely dilated proximal colon.

Plain abdominal x-ray in hanging position yields air-fluid levels, a single grossly dilated intestinal loop up to the size of the examiner's thumb, and/or air distal to the supposed obstruction. Number, site, and size of air-fluid levels are useful for approximate determination of the site of obstruction.

Treatment, Prognosis
Preoperative care is similar to other intestinal obstructions. After transverse supraumbilical incision, the whole intestine is inspected for associated malrotation without or with volvulus and/or congenital bands, meconium ileus, or peritonitis. Hidden atresia or stenosis is excluded by saline injection in the intestine distal to the atresia.

The surgical procedure depends on the type of jejunal or ileal atresia (or stenosis) and on the general and surgical implications of the associated disorders and complications.

Surgery: If possible, primary anastomosis(es) is (are) performed using a end-to-oblique anastomosis (if needed, the oblique surface of resection is increased by a short antimesenteric incision) including resection of the dilated proximal part up to the ligament of Treitz in proximal jejunal atresia or up to a segment of jejunum or ileum with 1–1.5 cm in diameter in more distal jejunal and ileal atresia to avoid functional obstruction. The following closure of the mesentery should avoid kinking of the anastomosis.

If the remaining intestine is too short, for example, <50 % of the original length, tapering of the dilated intestine proximal to the atresia is performed in place of resection. In case of associated volvulus, meconium ileus, or peritonitis, gastroschisis or omphalocele, and/or peritonitis with possible impairment of blood supply, some type of exteriorization (e.g., by a Bishop-Koop, Santulli and Blanc, double-barrel [Mikulicz] procedure) with or without intestinal resection is safer than primary anastomosis.

Postoperatively, a nasogastric tube with passive or intermittent slight active suction, TPN, and stepwise enteral nutrition with an appropriate composition is used to overcome the delayed recovery of intestinal motility, secretion, and resorption. The median time to full enteral nutrition in jejunal atresia is 17 days (with an interquartile range of 9–40 days).

Survival in jejunal and ileal atresia is ≥90 %, and the operative morbidity (anastomotic leak and functional obstruction) is low and the mortality <2 %. Very low birth weight, severe associated disorders, and some types of atresias are the main risks for morbidity and mortality. The latter factor may lead to a small intestine of <50 % length (= **short bowel syndrome**) that is combined with diarrhea, malabsorption, and bacterial overgrowth.

15.1.4 Meconium Ileus

Occurrence, Pathoanatomy
It depends on the prevalence of cystic fibrosis that differs somewhat in the western countries and is much less frequent in blacks and Asians. If up to 20 % of newborns with mucoviscidosis have a meconium ileus, its prevalence is 1:8,000 live births in middle Europe.

Secretion of hyperviscous mucus, pathological concentrating process, and exocrine deficiency lead to a tenacious meconium that obstructs the distal ileum. Whereas cecum and several centimeters of the small terminal ileum contain colorless pellets of meconium #, the more proximal part of the distal ileum is grossly dilated and filled with a continuous mass of dark and tenacious meconium #.

Clinical Significance
- Meconium ileus that is mostly caused by mucoviscidosis may be the first clinical manifestation of cystic fibrosis, and only in part of it, familial cases with mucoviscidosis are known.
- Meconium ileus and especially the complicated type may lead to a considerable morbidity and possible mortality already in the neonatal period.
- Meconium ileus of the newborn and the related meconium ileus equivalent (or distal intestinal obstruction syndrome) during childhood belong

to the major abdominal manifestations of cystic fibrosis with great surgical significance.

Clinical Presentation
It depends largely on the type of meconium ileus. In the **simple or uncomplicated type**, obstruction by meconium as quoted above is the sole cause, whereas **complicated meconium ileus** is characterized by additional volvulus without or with perforation followed by meconium peritonitis or with ischemic necrosis of its base, followed by resorption of the involved loop and development of ileal atresia.

Calcifications, dense adhesions, or a pseudocyst with a calcified fibrous wall, or ascites with recognizable pieces of meconium are the sequels of meconium peritonitis depending on whether perforation has occurred during pregnancy or shortly before birth.

Both types of meconium ileus are observed in the same frequency and may be recognized already by **prenatal ultrasound**: polyhydramnios and intestinal echogenicity in the second part of pregnancy, or polyhydramnios, ascites or intra-abdominal calcifications or ascites, dilated intestinal loops, or signs of meconium pseudocyst.

In simple meconium ileus, *bilious vomiting develops slowly within 24 h, several days, or not at all that may lead to a delayed recognition of the meconium ileus. In the first 2 days, mostly no meconium is passed.* Occasionally, gray plugs of mucus or early or delayed small bits of normal meconium may be observed. *The full but not grossly distended belly reveals dilated intestinal loops with visible waves of peristalsis #* and possibly findings corresponding to the described pellets and tenacious meconium on palpation.

Although some cases with **complicated meconium ileus** behave like a distal ileal atresia, early signs of obstructive ileus are mostly observed and possibly combined with a visible and/or palpable mass especially in giant cystic meconium peritonitis.

Differential Diagnosis, Work-Ups
The differential diagnosis includes mainly pathologies of distal obstructive ileus and other causes of meconium peritonitis:

- Ileal or colon atresia
- Hirschsprung's disease including long segment aganglionosis
- Meconium plug syndrome, small left colon syndrome
- Malrotation with volvulus or congenital bands, jejunoileal atresias or stenoses, and intrauterine intussusception
- Immaturity of the myenteric plexus, neuronal intestinal dysplasia (NID), chronic intestinal pseudoobstruction, and other disorders

For work-up, plain abdominal x-ray in hanging position and contrast enema is useful. The former displays in simple meconium ileus distended intestinal loops of varying size without air-fluid levels and possibly the characteristic ground-glass appearance of intestinal loops in the right lower quadrant with coarsely granular radiopaque masses. In complicated meconium ileus, localized impressive bowel distension, air-fluid levels, or signs of a mass may be encountered. Enema with water-soluble contrast shows an unused microcolon and possibly the terminal ileum with pellets and transition zone from the small to the grossly dilated ileum. In addition, it yields informations for the differential diagnosis.

Treatment, Prognosis

In simple meconium ileus, treatment is started with nonoperative measures for resolution of the meconium. It includes i.v. fluids, prophylactic antibiotics, and, under supervision by fluoroscopy, application of N-acetylcysteine by a nasogastric tube and of dilute isotonic gastrografin by a rectal catheter with filling of the dilated ileum. In spite of a success rate of nearly two thirds with one to three attempts over 1–2 days, perforations (<3 %) and other complication are possible.

Surgery is indicated if nonoperative treatment fails or in cases of complicated meconium ileus. It consists in simple meconium ileus either of a tube enterostomy at the transition zone of the terminal ileum with repeated irrigations and removal of the tenacious meconium by enterotomy or of a Roux-en-Y ileostomy without or with resection of the most dilated ileum in case of questionable viability, and postoperative irrigations. Roux-en-Y ileostomy is performed either as modified Bishop-Koop

proximal end-to-distal-side anastomosis with distal enterostomy or as Santulli and Blanc side-to-end anastomosis with proximal enterostomy. In complicated meconium ileus, the surgical procedure must be individualized depending on the findings.

Prognosis concerning survival is up to 100 % for simple and up to 90 % in complicated meconium ileus.

15.1.5 Meconium Peritonitis

Occurrence, Pathoanatomy, Causes

If half of the patients with meconium ileus have meconium peritonitis, the prevalence of meconium peritonitis is probably lower than meconium ileus and depends also on the incidence of the other causes of meconium peritonitis.

Intestinal perforation during the second half of pregnancy or shortly before birth leads to dense intra-abdominal adhesions, yellowish-green nodules, and large masses combined with calcifications as reaction to and composed of outflowing meconium or to ascites.

Meconium peritonitis is caused by intrinsic or extrinsic obstruction of the intestine in 80–90 % and observed without recognizable cause in 10–20 %. Possible obstructions are meconium ileus (leading to volvulus without or with perforation), malrotation with volvulus or congenital bands, atresia or stenosis, and intrauterine intussusception.

Clinical Significance

- Meconium peritonitis itself or the causes of it (may) lead to obstructive ileus of the newborn.
- Some clinical or radiological findings which point to a former meconium peritonitis may be observed by chance without any major clinical relevance, for example, palpable nodules in the scrotum due to an open vaginal process or intra-abdominal calcifications on plain abdominal x-ray.
- Meconium peritonitis may be the first clinical presentation of cystic fibrosis.

Clinical Presentation

In addition to *the clinical signs of obstructive ileus that appear mostly in the following first 3*

*days and are often combined with a grossly dis-
tended abdomen already at birth, the general
condition may be poor with hypothermia and
signs of RDS, the abdominal wall edematous
and discolored, and the scrotum swollen and
reddened.*

Percussion and palpation yields possibly a
tympanic central abdomen with lateral dullness
that changes its site if the examination is repeated
and/or a mass.

Differential Diagnosis, Work-Ups
It includes mainly bacterial peritonitis after intestinal perforation and other causes of surgical
abdomen of the neonate.

Plain abdominal x-ray in hanging position shows
signs of intestinal obstruction and, specifically
in some of the patients, calcifications of various
shape and size from minute to easy recognizable
clods of calcifications and rarely signs of a pseudocyst (air-filled cavity with a calcified membrane,
possible air-fluid level, and with outflow of contrast by diagnostic enema).

Treatment, Prognosis
Treatment is surgical for removal of meconium
masses, not viable parts of intestine, or the wall
of a pseudocyst, and mainly for repair of the
intestinal obstruction. Often a temporary double-barrel enterostomy away from the abdominal incision is necessary instead of primary
anastomosis.

The prognosis depends on the cause of meconium peritonitis and its sequels.

15.1.6 Intestinal Duplications

Occurrence, Types, Pathoanatomy
The precise prevalence is unknown because
duplications are distributed throughout the whole
esophagogastrointestinal tract and handled separately, and some remain symptomless all one's
life.

Duplications are composed of smooth muscles
and an endothelial lining that does not necessarily correspond to that of the adjacent part of
intestine. They form a cyst or a tube of different

length that lies at the mesenteric side, is often
closely interweaved with the wall of the corresponding intestine, and may have a distal or proximal communication with its lumen.

The most common groups are the jejunal and
ileal duplications with >40 % and followed by
cervical and mediastinal or colonic and rectal
types each with approximately 20 %. Gastric or
duodenal duplications amount each to <10 % and
combined thoracoabdominal or multiple duplications each to <5 %.

Clinical Significance
- The possible clinical presentation is variable
  and relates not necessarily to the specific site
  of the duplication.
- Intestinal duplication must be considered in
  the differential diagnosis of almost every disorder of all parts of the intestinal tract independent of clinical presentation.
- Correction of symptomatic and some of the
  asymptomatic duplications may be a challenge
  to the pediatric surgeon.

Clinical Presentation, Differential Diagnosis
Some symptoms and signs are **independent** and
others **dependent on the site** of duplication. To
the former belong a visible, palpable, and/or
space occupying mass or ectopic or orthotopic
gastric mucosa with its inherent inflammation,
ulceration, perforation, or hemorrhage and anemia. Ectopic gastric mucosa is less often encountered in colonic duplication. To the latter belong
a symtomatology that is specific to the site and
clinical and radiological findings of some characteristic associated malformations.

Cervical duplications: RDS, visible or palpable mass of the neck, mainly in infants.

Thoracic duplications: Vertebral anomalies without/with CNS involvement, RDS, chest
pain, other complications of gastric mucosa, or
incidental finding on chest x-ray. Manifestation
is possible at any age. Additional duplication(s)
below the diaphragm and combined thoracoabdominal types must be considered.

Gastric and duodenal duplications: Often
cystic without communication, at the greater
curvature of the stomach or medial to the second

part of duodenum. Gastric outlet or high intestinal obstruction (differential diagnosis of hypertrophic pyloric stenosis or congenital duodenal obstruction), palpable mass, and jaundice or recurrent pancreatitis because of a mass effect or connection to the pancreaticobiliary tree (differential diagnosis of jaundice and recurrent pancreatitis), complications of gastric mucosa.

Jejunal and ileal duplications: Cystic and tubular types. Symptomatic intussusception, obstructive ileus (due to increasing size of communicating duplications) ##, volvulus, and complications of gastric mucosa (differential diagnosis of melena) are observed.

Colonic duplications: Cystic and tubular types (complete duplications up to the peritoneal reflection and communications are possible). Type I: abdominal pain, constipation, palpable abdominal tumor, and obstructive ileus or volvulus. Type II: tubular duplications combined with duplication of the anus, fistulas to the bowel or adjacent organs, or imperforated anus, duplications of the urinary and genital tract, and myelomeningocele and vertebral anomalies. Cosmetic problem arises because of duplication of the external genitals in addition to the same symptoms and signs as in type I.

Rectal duplications: Retrorectal location combined with possible fistulas to the anal channel or perineum, myelomeningocele, and vertebral anomalies. Constipation, rectal bleeding, prolapse, hemorrhoids, perianal fistulas, retrorectal abscess, and urinary tract infection are observed. The differential diagnosis of retrorectal masses and the single signs must be considered: sacrococcygeal teratoma, anterior (myelo-) meningocele, dermoid cyst, chondroma, and other malignancies.

Work-Ups
They include ultrasound with Doppler, upper gastrointestinal study and contrast enema (for evaluation of possible mass effect or communication with the adjacent intestine), contrast CT (demonstrates a typical enhancing rim), MRI (in vertebral anomalies with possible CNS involvement), technetium scan (in suspected heterotopic gastric mucosa), and gastroduodenoscopy or colonoscopy. The single examinations are used dependent on the site of duplication and its clinical presentation.

Treatment, Prognosis
If possible without damage to the adjacent structures (e.g., in duodenal duplications to the pancreaticobiliary tree), complete excision or en bloc segmental excision together with the adjacent intestine should performed. In spite of the possible intimate connection with the wall of the adjacent intestine, resection may be possible either because of a minute dividing plane or by application of the Bianchi technique used for small bowel lengthening.

If resection is impossible or not advisable, stripping of the total (especially gastric) mucosa and leaving a muscular tube which collapses or formation of a proximal and distal communication to the adjacent intestine are possible alternative procedures.

The prognosis depends on the possible radicality of surgery and treatment options of the combined anomalies. The risks of possible carcinomas of the mucosa in adulthood are not yet thoroughly evaluated.

15.1.7 Disorders of Intestinal Rotation and Fixation (Malrotation of Intestine)

Occurrence, Pathoanatomy, Forms, and Types
Malrotation (in a general sense) is either an isolated disorder or an obligatory part of congenital diaphragmatic hernia, omphalocele, and gastroschisis or a possible associated anomaly of cardiovascular or gastrointestinal disorders such congenital duodenal obstruction or anorectal malformation and vice versa, heterotaxia (= abnormal arrangement of body organs with or without congenital heart disease), situs inversus, or other pathologies.

At the beginning of normal development, the primitive gut (= umbilical loop) lies in a median sagittal plane. Between the fourth and twelfth fetal week, an anticlockwise rotation of the intestine occurs along the superior mesenteric artery three times by 90° and temporarily outside of the peritoneal cavity. This process is accompanied or followed by independent rotation of stomach and duodenum, differential growth of the intestine, and mesenteric fixation of ascending and descending colon, and duodenum to the posterior abdominal wall #.

Disorders of these four mechanisms lead to numerous types of malrotation of which three main forms may be described: **nonrotation**, **malrotation** (in a restricted sense, = incomplete or combined normal and inverse rotation), and **incomplete fixation**.

In addition, **separate inverse rotation of the gastroduodenal loop** may occur combined with normal, inverse, or changing torsion of the umbilical loop.

In **nonrotation**, the initial position of the intestine as described above is either maintained (=complete nonrotation) or more commonly followed by an anticlockwise rotation of 90° (=nonrotation Fig. 15.3(1)).

In **nonrotation**, the distal duodenum lies on the right side of the mesenteric vessels with transition to the small intestine that is located on the right, whereas the colon lies on the left side of the peritoneal cavity. The terminal ileum enters mostly the cecum from the right side, and the superior mesenteric vein crosses the artery on its ventral side and follows it along the left side. The relation of the two vessels and their branches to each other is used to define the types of non- and malrotation. Nonrotation is the most common form of disorders of rotation and fixation with 1:1,000 live births.

Due to intensive growth, secondary dislocation, or asymptomatic volvulus of a single part of the umbilical loop after the initial rotation of 90°, numerous modifications of nonrotation are observed; for instance, the proximal colon has a strong tendency of dislocation to the right abdominal side (Fig. 15.3(2)). The same secondary changes may occur in malrotations and may lead to several modifications of the main types. Nonrotation combined with a mesocolic hernia is depicted in Fig. 15.3(3) and also called right paraduodenal hernia in the literature.

In **malrotation**, several types may be encountered. In **malrotation I**, the anticlockwise rotation has stopped at 180°. The distal duodenum lies behind the mesenteric vessels. The proximal colon lies in the midline in front of the mesentery and is separated by it from the distal duodenum. The so-called Ladd's band runs over the third part of duodenum to the right lateral abdominal wall and leads to extrinsic duodenal obstruction. The terminal ileum enters the cecum mostly from the left side. Malrotation I is the second most common disorder of rotation and fixation.

Of the two subtypes of "malrotation I with or without inhibition of growth of the proximal colon," the former is more common; the cecum is located high at the level of the distal duodenum (Fig. 15.3(4)), whereas in the latter subtype, a right colonic flexure has been formed with much lower location of the cecum (Fig. 15.3(5)).

In other types of malrotation, the initial anticlockwise rotation by 90° is followed by an inverse clockwise rotation of 180°. **In malrotation II**, the distal part of duodenum lies in front of the mesenteric vessels and the proximal colon behind the mesentery on the left side of the spine. The terminal ileum enters the cecum mostly from the right side (Fig. 15.3(6)). A translocation of the proximal colon to the right side with or without elevation of the cecum is responsible for several modifications of malrotation II and may lead to a **right mesocolic hernia** (Fig. 15.3(7)) as in the already quoted in nonrotation (though the distal duodenum lies not in front but lateral to the mesentery in the latter).

Retroposition of transverse colon (reverse rotation with colonic obstruction) occurs due to a reverse rotation of 180° (**malrotation III**). The distal duodenum lies in front of the mesenteric root, the proximal colon in the right abdomen, and the transverse colon behind the mesenteric root and the duodenum (Fig. 15.3(8)). If the mesenteric root becomes adherent to the back of the abdominal wall with formation of a tunnel, the transverse colon is compressed. A similar transverse colon obstruction occurs in nonrotation with a secondary volvulus of 180°.

In left mesocolic hernia, the small intestine is partially or completely trapped by the mesentery

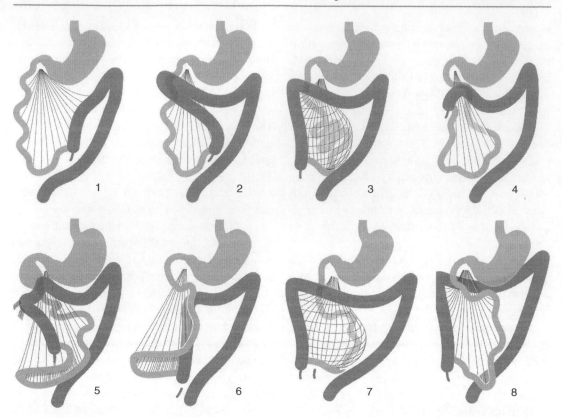

Fig. 15.3 (*1–8*) The drawings from the *left* to the *right* and the *top* to the *bottom* show different disorders of intestinal rotation and fixation. Usually the primitive gut turns from a sagittal position in a counterclockwise direction by tree times 90°. *1*: Nonrotation occurs after one turn by +90°. The small intestine lies on the right and the colon on the left side. *2*: In this example of nonrotation, secondary transfer of the distal end of the proximal colon to the right upper abdomen leads to formation of a hepatic flexure. The terminal ileum enters the cecum from the right side. *3*: Example of nonrotation with secondary transfer of the whole proximal colon to the right side. The terminal ileum enters now the cecum from the left side. The small intestine may be wrapped in the mesentery that corresponds to an example of internal hernia (=hernia mesocolica in nonrotation). *4*: Malrotation I = rotation by +90° + 90°. In this example of incomplete rotation, additional inhibition of growth of the proximal colon has occurred. The duodenojejunal segment lies behind the mesentery, the proximal colon remains short and lies as high cecum in front of the mesentery. *5*: Similar feature is present in this example of malrotation I, but the unrestricted growth of the proximal colon has led to an ascending colon in front of the mesentery. *6*: Malrotation II = rotation by +90°−90°. In this example of malrotation II, the duodenojejunal segment lies in front of the mesentery, the small intestine on the right side of the abdomen, and the terminal ileum enters the cecum from the right side. *7*: In this example of malrotation II, similar findings as in six are encountered, but the secondary transfer of the complete proximal colon has led to an ascending colon and an internal hernia (= hernia mesocolica in malrotation II). *8*: Retroposition of the transverse colon by +90°−90°−90° rotation. The transverse colon lies behind the mesentery and the duodenojejunal segment in front of it

of the descending colon. The inferior mesenteric vein delineates the right margin of the hernia sac and is a part of its neck. It can be interpreted as a type of disorder of fixation in which the ascending or descending colon and duodenum are not fixed to the posterior abdominal wall. If the ascending colon is completely or partially not fixed to the back of the abdominal wall together with a short attachment of the mesentery of the midgut (= **common mesentery**), cecal or ileocolic volvulus may occur.

*The **short attachment of mesentery of the midgut** instead of normal long and oblique insertion leads often to volvulus #. It is together with compression and distorsion of intestine and its vascular supply by **congenital bands, internal*** *hernias, parts of the intestine, and mesenteric vessels, and with torsion due to common mesentery, the main common factor of clinical presentation of disorders of rotation and fixation.*

Clinical Significance
- In all malrotations, the possibility of life-threatening clinical manifestation exists mainly in early life and of chronic recurrent symptoms and signs later in childhood.
- Malrotation is the main cause of abnormal position of the appendix that is encountered in 4 % of appendices and may lead to misinterpretation of heterotopic appendicitis.
- Malposition as incidental finding of x-ray examinations and abdominal surgery may lead to confusion due to the tricky topoanatomical arrangement of the intestine or to the question about the appropriateness of its surgical correction.

Clinical Presentation
Only a part of the patients with malrotation becomes symptomatic during childhood or later in adulthood, and the clinical presentation is not uniform.

Acute obstructive ileus is observed in about 50 % of the patients in the newborn period and only in 15 % beyond infancy. It is caused either by a midgut volvulus or an extrinsic compression or misarrangement (twisting, angulation, kinking) of parts of the intestine such as duodenal obstruction by Ladd's bands, midgut obstruction by a mesocolic hernia, or transverse colon obstruction by a tunnel in the mesentery.

In **midgut volvulus**, *dramatic onset of bilious vomiting is combined with severe abdominal pain (in the middle of the belly) and possibly melena, and the initially scaphoid belly becomes distended and tender and is combined with guarding and signs of septic and hypovolemic shock in advanced stages. #*

The leading sign of **extrinsic obstructive ileus** *is bilious vomiting with the other signs similar to intrinsic duodenal obstruction.*

Chronic and recurrent incomplete or complete obstruction comes to the attention of parents or caregivers of toddlers and schoolchildren.

The symptomatology is explained by chronic or recurrent midgut volvulus, incomplete intestinal obstruction as quoted above, and by torsion of the mesentery. The symptomatology reaches from chronic slight to moderate abdominal pain to severe manifestations as follows: *Recurrent severe abdominal pain, intermittent bilious vomiting, and possible intestinal bleedings are combined with diarrhea, malabsorption, malnutrition, and growth retardation or occur as single cluster of symptoms dependent on whether the intestinal obstruction or the disorder of intestinal blood supply is of predominate importance.* Children with recurrent volvulus complain of *attacks of severe epigastric pain and take a knee-elbow position for relief of pain and possibly recurrent volvulus.*

Many children with chronic and recurrent incomplete have experienced an Odyssey of gastroenterological examinations and psychiatric treatment before the final diagnosis.

Obstruction of transverse colon (reverse rotation with colonic obstruction) becomes rarely symptomatic in children. On the other hand, cecal or ileocolic **volvulus** due to a common mesentery of the midgut may be observed occasionally. *It leads to acute severe abdominal pain of the right lower abdomen combined with nausea and right-sided abdominal distension.*

Work-Ups, Differential Diagnosis
Although **plain abdominal x-ray** in upright position belongs not to the main examinations for work-up of malrotation, some findings may point to it, for example, double-bubble sign combined with sparse and scattered air distal to the obstruction, absence of normal distribution of air in the colon, and displacement of the cecal shadow from the right lower quadrant.

In **acute volvulus**, the already quoted modified double-bubble sign is more frequently observed than proximal small intestine obstruction with distension and thickened wall of the visible loops. In cecal volvulus, an air-filled colonic loop is seen in the left upper quadrant.

In addition to these findings, **ultrasound with color Doppler** shows as specific sign of acute or chronic volvulus a whirlpool pattern of the flow of the mesenteric vessels that have an abnormal position to each other.

The **upper gastrointestinal contrast study** that is mostly used in chronic condition of malrotation displays several characteristics such as distal duodenal obstruction, right-sided location of the site of ligament of Treitz and jejunum, or Z-shaped dilated distal duodenum and proximal jejunum with visible relief of mucosal folds.

The latter sign enables differentiation from **chronic volvulus** in which the same intestinal part has a spiral- or corkscrew-like appearance.

In delayed pictures of the contrast study, entrapment of the small intestine by a mesocolic hernia, abnormal location of proximal colon and cecum, and possible obstruction of the transverse colon may be seen. Contrast enema shows signs of malrotation as displacement of cecum in the epigastrium.

The differential diagnoses of volvulus or extrinsic intestinal obstruction are disorders of surgical abdomen of the newborn (gastric hyperperistalsis points to hypertrophic pyloric stenosis but occurs as well in duodenal obstruction) and older children including peritonitis, and in chronic recurrent or partial obstruction of intestine and mesenteric blood supply, other causes of chronic abdominal pain, malnutrition, and malabsorption.

Treatment, Prognosis

Midgut (and the rare cecal) volvulus and extrinsic obstructive ileus need immediate surgery to prevent short bowel syndrome or death. In chronic symptomatic and in some asymptomatic types (incidental finding at abdominal surgery or due to intended work-ups), elective surgery is indicated.

In both situations, the **Ladd procedure** is performed that includes in case of volvulus reduction, correction of all important abnormalities, and appendectomy. In contrast to Grob's suggestion to restore a normal colonic frame (for relieve of any circulatory disorder), duodenum and small intestine are laid down on the right and the colon on the left side of the abdominal cavity without any or with mesenteric fixation.

Emergency and elective surgery: After a supraumbilical transverse incision, the **volvulus** is reduced outside of the abdomen mostly by a counterclockwise rotation (clockwise torsion is more frequently), the viability of the intestine is checked, and only a truly necrotic segment resected.

After eventration of the whole intestine, the abdomen is checked from the pylorus to the left colonic flexure for form and type of malrotation (the relation of the distal duodenum to the mesenteric root and the topography of proximal colon are useful informations); possible abnormalities and associated duodenal or small intestine obstructions are checked by advancing a gastric tube of sufficient length and air insufflation, and the abnormalities related to malrotation are corrected: **division of Ladd's and other abnormal peritoneal bands**, and of adhesions between duodenum and cecum, and right colon (the proximal duodenum and jejunum should be visible and free except for the site of their vascularization). In **right and left mesocolic hernia**, the lateral peritoneal reflection of the right colon is divided and the sac of the left hernia divided on the right side of the inferior mesenteric vein, respectively. The space behind the colon should be closed to prevent recurrence after mobilization of the small intestine. In **common mesentery**, ascending colon and ileocecal region are sutured to the lateral right abdominal wall. **Reversed torsion with colonic obstruction** need relieve of the constricting tunnel, anterior anastomosis, or completion of inverse rotation by another 90°.

Prognosis

Today, fatal outcome occurs only due to advanced stages of volvulus with septicemia and due to complications of short bowel syndrome after extensive intestinal resection. Obstructive ileus due to postoperative adhesions or intussusception and postoperative infections are infrequent or similar to other laparotomies without peritonitis. Recurrence of volvulus is less than 0.5 % if all needed measures are taken described for Ladd's procedure. In chronic and long-lasting types of malrotation, chronic idiopathic intestinal pseudoobstruction syndrome may be observed in some patients after corrective surgery.

15.1.8 Anorectal Malformations

Occurrence, Types
Anorectal malformations are observed in 1:2,500–3,500 live births. These may occur in well-known syndromes such as Down syndrome, as part of disorders with multiple malformations, associated with one or several anomalies (in up to two thirds), or as familial trait.

Anatomical, embryological, and therapeutic considerations have led to several classifications of which the **Wingspread classification** (1986) uses three main groups: the high, intermediate, and low forms. For therapeutic reasons, **Kiely and Pēna** apply only high (supralevator) and low (infralevator) forms and add the intermediate forms to the former group (Fig. 15.4).

Clinical Significance
- Anorectal malformations may be associated with stool incontinence and/or constipation.

Their incidence depends on the type of anorectal malformation and surgical treatment.
- Cosmesis of the external genitals and perineum may play a role in some of them.
- Anorectal malformations are associated with one or more anomalies in up to two thirds. The major ones are the main cause of mortality of 5–15 %.

Clinical Presentation
The presenting sign is mostly *either a missing normal anus and/or abnormal passage of meconium and gas by a fistula, the urine, or not at all. It leads to a low obstructive ileus in the first days of life if passage of meconium does not occur or only insufficiently.*

Local findings: *The appearance of the perineum does not necessarily permit a diagnosis of high or low type. Flat perineum and adjacent buttocks, shortened sacrum, weak contractions of the external sphincter and pelvic floor muscles, and meconium emerging in the urine or by a fistula of vagina or vestibulum are characteristic of* high **forms** #. And *fistulas of the perineum with absent, sparse, or gross evacuation of meconium and gas* correspond to **low forms** #. In persistent **cloaca** of the girls, *only two instead of three*

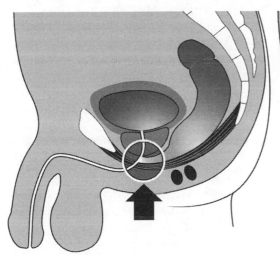
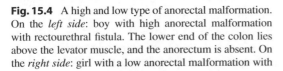
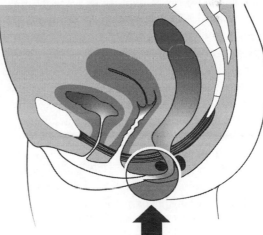

Fig. 15.4 A high and low type of anorectal malformation. On the *left side*: boy with high anorectal malformation with rectourethral fistula. The lower end of the colon lies above the levator muscle, and the anorectum is absent. On the *right side*: girl with a low anorectal malformation with rectovestibular fistula. The rectum passes through the levator muscle and ends above the external sphincter, and its fistula enters the vestibulum by different relations to three portions of the external sphincter

openings are visible at the external genitals and perineum.

General examination must exclude associated malformations and, in case of clinical suspicion, be confirmed by additional examinations. A rare example of an associated malformation is congenital pouch colon (the colon is shorter than normal and the distal end is dilated like a pouch) which is also observed in cloacal malformations.

Differential Diagnosis, Work-Ups

The possibility of another disorder plays only a role if not a careful examination of the local findings is performed, if an associated disorder is present, for example, Hirschsprung's disease or persistent cloaca, or if rectal atresia is present in spite of a normal anus.

Work-ups have two main tools: definition of the form and type of anorectal malformation and exclusion or confirmation of possible associated anomalies.

After introduction of a gastric tube (for exclusion of esophageal atresia and derivation of gastric and intestinal content) and i.v. infusion, the newborn is observed and checked for cardiovascular and for renal malformations by echocardiogram and abdominal ultrasound, respectively.

If thereafter clinical differentiation between high and low form is impossible or the informations are equivocal, lateral plain x-ray is performed of the lower end of the trunk, either in a upside-down position with pelvis and lower extremities held in a right angle or in a prone position with elevated buttocks: The distance between the deepest part of rectum marked by air and the site of anus recognizable by a radiodense tag is used for differentiation; <1 cm=low and >1 cm=high lesion.

In high forms, the specific type is delineated by contrast study through the distal colostoma or by MRI after washing out of meconium. Further work-ups include VCUG (possible vesicoureteral reflux) and ultrasound of lumbosacral region including spinal cord (lumbosacral and CNS anomalies).

Treatment, Prognosis

In **low forms** that include mostly perineal fistulas or anteriorly placed anus, surgery is performed in the neonatal period and in the latter type also in infancy.

Surgery: For **perineal fistulas**, a "cutback" procedure, meticulous excision of the fistulous tract combined with an anastomosis between anorectum and skin at the site of the normal anus, or a minimal posterior sagittal anoplasty (= PSAP) is performed.

In **anteriorly placed anus**, either a minimal PSAP or an anal transposition may be applied. The latter procedure is performed in supine position and includes circumcision of the anus somewhat beyond the mucocutaneous junction, mobilization of the distal anorectum, formation of a tunnel through the external sphincter (the correct site is recognized by equal contraction of the external sphincter on both sides on electrical stimulation), pull-through of the mobilized anorectum, anastomosis between anorectum and skin, and reconstruction of the perineal body. **Analstenosis** is treated either by dilatations or Y-V anoplasty.

In **high and intermediate forms**, colostomy is performed first. A proximal sigmoidal or transverse separate colostoma with maintenance of the arcades has several advantages and leaves the distal sigmoid or colon free for reconstruction. A **posterior sagittal anorectoplasty** (=PSARP) is performed 1–2 months after birth at the earliest.

After introduction of a bladder catheter, a prone position with elevated buttocks is necessary. Following a midline incision from midsacrum to the site of the normal anus or to the perineum depending on the type of anorectal malformation, the parasagittal fibers, the striated muscle complex, and the levator muscle are divided strictly in the midline leaving on each side equal amounts of muscles that are recognizable by the naked eye and electrostimulation and marked with stitches. The posterior rectum is opened at its posterior end, the rectourethral fistula is dissected from the rectum and closed, and the colon mobilized close to its wall from the urethra and the other surroundings until tension-free rectocutaneous anastomosis is possible. After closure of the rectal incision without or with tapering of the rectum, the anterior part of the muscle complex in front of and the levator muscle and the posterior part of the muscle complex are sutured together behind the rectum leaving no dead space and anchoring the rectum to the last muscle layer. A "double diamond" anoplasty is performed after skin closure.

Modifications of PSARP are necessary in the following conditions: In **recto-bladder-neck (bald) fistula**, PSARP is combined with a lower abdominal incision. The site of the rectum is marked by a tube of appropriate size and used for pull-through of rectosigmoid that has been mobilized before. Identification and closure of the fistula are performed from the abdomen. Ligation of the inferior mesenteric vessels is not necessary because sparse division of peripheral branches is sufficient. In **imperforate anus** without fistula, attachment of the rectum to the urethra is all the same as in types with rectourethral fistulas. Nevertheless, PSARP is sufficient. In **rectal atresia or stenosis**, the PSARP access is used for mobilization of the rectum and rectoanal anastomosis. And in **rectovestibular fistula** of the girl and rare rectovaginal fistula, PSARP is modified by continuation of the incision around the fistula into the vestibule. Dissection of the fistula and rectum must consider the difficult separation between rectum and vagina. After sufficient mobilization of the rectum, reconstruction is performed in a similar way without involvement of the levator muscle.

Persistent cloaca needs separation of the rectum from the vagina and of the vagina from the urethra. Rectum and vagina must be mobilized sufficiently to reach the perineum, and the distal urethra is formed by the common channel. If the common channel is longer than 3 cm and in additional genital disorders, PSARP is insufficient and different procedure becomes necessary combined with lower laparotomy.

Prognosis

The specific sequels of the anorectal malformations and postoperative complications are arranged in order of frequency and include mainly disorders of bowel control, constipation, anal stenosis, and bladder voiding disorders and much less frequently rectal mucosal prolapse and bowel retraction. Their reported frequencies depend not only on the number of patients with congenital deficits in anatomy and physiology, the level (high vs low form), the different types, and surgical technique applied but also on the distribution, number, and ages of the reported cases. Outcomes related to psychical and sexual disorders, pregnancy, and delivery are not yet available in a representative number of patients who had the modern surgical methods.

Disorders of bowel control occur in low types in ≤10 %. On the other hand, good bowel control (complete continence with only occasional soiling) has been reported in one fifth to one third and complete incontinence in 25–30 % with the older techniques for high and intermediate types. With posterior sagittal anorectoplasty, totally continent patients were seen in 41 % in a cohort of patients with 92 % high forms and cloaca, and intermediate follow-up. Grade I or more soiling was observed in >50 %. Vestibular fistula and imperforated anus without fistula had the best result with >50 % total continence and only >30 % soiling, and those with bulbar or prostatic fistula, or cloaca less good results with one fourth to one third complete continence and two thirds to three fourths with soiling.

If signs of imminent defecation and straining with no soiling between the defecation are observed in infants and toddlers by the parents, complete continence will probably achieved. On the other hand, amelioration of bowel control and constipation is possible till puberty and adolescence.

Constipation occurs often delayed in the preschool age and in low forms in up to one third. After PSARP, constipation has been observed in >40 %. In high forms, it may be related to a too large rectal volume. **Anal stenosis** is observed in low and high forms and amounts to one third.

The **treatment of disorders of bowel control** depends on the cause and degree of incontinence, child's age, and adherence of the parents: diet with avoiding of diarrhea, training with regular and frequent stool evacuation and methods of biofeedback, regular enemas for complete evacuation of stool, and surgical measures such as anterograde enemas by an intestinal conduit up to a permanent colostoma.

Constipation should be treated by conservative measures (diet, training of stool evacuation habits, laxatives, and enemas) from the beginning and especially the overflow incontinence that aggravates a partial incontinence should be avoided.

Anal stenosis needs regular dilatation from the beginning and sometimes anoplasty. In symptomatic rectal mucosal prolapse, local resection and in bowel retraction, intractable anal stenosis, or former surgery with misplaced bowel, re-pull-through must be considered. For voiding disorder of the bladder, see Chap. 28.

15.1.9 Spontaneous Perforation of the Gastrointestinal Tract

Occurrence, Pathoanatomy
Spontaneous perforation of the stomach or intestine is a rare disorder of the neonatal period, occurs particularly in preterm patients or in neonates with low birth weight, and is caused by localized ischemic necrosis.

Clinical Significance
- Spontaneous perforation must be considered after a pregnancy or birth with amnionitis, placenta previa, or premature detachment of the placenta, in prematurity or low birth weight and in postnatal contributing factors such as additional disorders.
- Spontaneous gastrointestinal perforation is a life-threatening disorder that leads to secondary peritonitis, hypovolemic shock, and possible septicemia.
- Rapid recognition, resuscitation, and surgery are essential for survival.

Clinical Presentation
Spontaneous gastrointestinal perforation is mostly characterized by an acute onset of abdominal distension that is rapidly progressive and has a peak incidence in the second part of the first week of life.

The newborns are apathetic and refuse feeds. The abdomen may be initially tympanitic on percussion, and respiratory distress syndrome and signs of hypovolemic shock develop rapidly.

Work-Ups, Differential Diagnosis
They include plain abdominal x-ray in hanging or lateral decubitus position for confirmation of pneumoperitoneum and laboratory tests (Hb, Lc, platelets count, Quick's test, pH including acid–base balance, and arterial blood gases).

The differential diagnosis must consider gastric perforation from gastric overinsufflation or gastric tube insertion and gastrointestinal perforation proximal to a congenital obstruction, for example, jejunoileal obstruction or Hirschsprung' disease. In addition, secondary pneumoperitoneum during high-pressure ventilation with alveolar rupture and dissection of air from the mediastinum to the abdomen (chest x-ray displays pneumomediastinum) must be taken into account.

Treatment, Prognosis
It consists of resuscitation (i.v. fluid replacement, antibiotics, modest nasogastric suction, and paracentesis for evacuation of air if needed) and emergency laparotomy.

The site of perforation is evaluated after a unilateral supraumbilical transverse incision starting with the stomach with the possible necessity to explore the lesser omental space and ending up with the intraperitoneal part of the rectum. Emanating air bubbles or a site of maximum soiled peritoneum may point to the location of perforation. After debridement of the perforation and resection of the involved wall, the stomach or intestine is reconstructed and closed without or with a primary anastomosis. Temporary enterostomy or exclusive drainage with secondary permanent surgery is considered in extremely premature or very low birth weight neonates although primary surgery is superior to exclusive drainage in necrotizing enterocolitis.

Prognosis depends on the time between perforation and its recognition and treatment, respectively, the degree of prematurity and low birth weight, and the site of perforation.

Prognosis is better in gastric than in intestinal perforation; the site of gastric perforation is either the greater or lesser curvature with involvement of the anterior or posterior wall. Survival in enteric perforation is $> 60\%$ but only $\geq 50\%$ in a group with a median age of 27 weeks and birth weight of 780 g. The latter group displays mostly different postoperative abdominal complications such as recurrence of spontaneous perforation which need laparotomy. Neurodevelopmental impairment may be lower than in surgical necrotizing enterocolitis.

15.2   Surgical Abdomen due to Intestinal Obstruction of Infancy and Thereafter

The disorders that are observed mainly in infancy and later in life are quoted in Table 15.3.

15.2.1 Acute Intussusception (Invagination)

Occurrence, Types
Although intussusception occurs at any age of childhood from the unborn and newborn to the adolescent patient, the preferred age is 3–12 months of age with a prevalence of 4.9 infants with intussusception in 10,000 live births and ≥2/3 of all cases. In addition, the prevalence may differ from country to country or other parts of the world (with very high rates in Africa) and possibly the age distribution as well.

Idiopathic intussusception is observed in ≤90 % (see Fig. 23.1) and in the remainder, the **symptomatic type** with a localized or generalized disorder of the intestine as lead point. **Postoperative invagination** is observed after abdominal or thoracic surgery and the **chronic type of intussusception** mainly in malignant and benign neoplasms. Possible association with rotavirus vaccines or use of antibiotics is actually discussed. Rarely, **appendiceal intussusception** is observed (in which appendectomy may be

Table 15.3 Intestinal obstructions of infancy and thereafter

- Incarcerated inguinal hernia
- Hypertrophic pyloric stenosis
- Intussusception
- Postoperative ileus due to adhesions
- o Rare abdominal wall, pelvic floor, and internal hernias
- o Massive colon dilatation due to fecal impaction
- o Sickle cell disease, vaso-occlusive event (spleen etc.)

insufficient to avoid recurrent intussusception of the cecum at the site of appendiceal stump and resection of a cecal rim including the stump becomes necessary).

Clinical Significance
- Intussusception belongs to the most frequent intestinal obstructions in infants and toddlers.
- Delayed diagnosis leads to an increased morbidity and possibly to a fatal outcome.

In the early and late sixties of the last century, 67 and 33 children died from intussusception in each 6-year period in England and Wales (##).

Clinical Presentation
For early recognition of intussusception, it is important to consider invagination in every acute abdominal disorder because in > 20 % of the patients, the classic symptoms and signs and in > 30 % the corresponding findings may be absent or not discovered.

Sudden onset of intermittent abdominal colics with screaming and drawing up the legs, paleness, and vomiting in an infant or toddler who was fit before or had a simple prodromal disorder (e.g., a cold) belong to the characteristic cluster of initial clinical presentation. In a cohort of consecutive cases, abrupt emesis has been observed in 80 % and pain, and/or red current jelly stool in about 60 %.

Clinical Skills
Careful abdominal examination in a moment in which the child is quiet reveals a resistance or a mass (the so-called invagination tumor) in the right middle or upper quadrant in > 75 %, and the right lower quadrant is void because the cecum cannot be palpated. In addition, *the spontaneous passage of red current jelly stool # may be observed or provoked by rectal examination in > 60 %. It consists of mucus and clear red blood without or with feces. Passage occurs rarely in the early stage, mostly in the intermediate stage and should not be considered as prerequisite for the clinical diagnosis of intussusception. Rectal examination is useful for provocation of stool passage and rarely for palpation of an advanced invagination in the rectum.*

Table 15.4 Time axis of the symptomatology in intussusception

Prodromal stage	Early stage	Late stage
• Respiratory tract Infection	• Abdominal colics	• Obstructive ileus
• Gastroenteritis	• Vomiting	• Peritonitis
• Prodromal disorder not obligatory	• Invagination tumor	• Septicemia
	Red current jelly stool (rarely early sign)	

For didactic reasons, the natural course of intussusception (from the start of invagination in the small intestine and propagation as ileocolic or ileocecal type in the large intestine for a different distance) may be depicted on a time axis:

In the prodromal stage, the patient is either symptomless or suffers from gastroenteritis or upper respiratory tract infection. In the early stage, the already mentioned symptomatology is present. Red current jelly stool is mostly observed in an intermediate stage between the early and late stage. The late stage starts at latest 72 h after the onset of the symptomatology with bilious vomiting, abdominal colics, and constipation combined with abdominal findings of obstructive ileus without or with signs of peritonitis (Table 15.4).

The described clinical presentation does not apply to postoperative and chronic intussusception. In **postoperative intussusception**, the invagination occurs somewhere in the small intestine and *leads to bilious vomiting and abdominal colics about 1 week after surgery. Its recognition may be difficult because the symptomatology falls in a period of starting restoration of postoperative ileus in which the beginning bowel activity may be accompanied by slight colics.* **Chronic invagination** has always a lead point either in the small intestine or colon, the obstruction is incomplete, and it occurs at any age #. *Therefore, the symptomatology is less dramatic with intermittent (not necessarily bilious) vomiting, abdominal pain, and possible deterioration of general health state, for instance, by significant weight loss.*

Chronic intussusception needs special consideration in connection with the abdominal and retroperitoneal non-Hodgkin's lymphoma. It has been called American **Burkitt's lymphoma** in the past and is related to the endemic jaw lymphoma of African children. Clinically, it is observed in two manifestations either as localized intra-abdominal or as extensive and diffuse abdominal and retroperitoneal type. The **localized type** is restricted to one anatomic site, possibly to adjacent lymph nodes, and involves mostly the region of iliocecum and/or Peyer's patches. It presents mostly as surgical abdomen due to chronic intussusception, intestinal obstruction, or acute appendicitis. Complete resection is mostly indicated and possible. The **diffuse and disseminated type** involves the mesenteric root, intestine, and abdominal and retroperitoneal organs and presents as abdominal tumor although surgical abdomen is also possible in some due to intestinal obstruction or perforation. Surgery is not indicated in this type of clinical presentation except for surgical abdomen or diagnostic biopsy if specific diagnosis is not possible otherwise (by paracentesis or thoracocentesis) because surgery delays chemotherapy and debulking is associated with dangerous and unnecessary dissection. Prognosis is better in localized types with complete resection. The new WHO classification of lymphomas is useful for stratification of treatment and prognostication but less for practical clinical needs than the already mentioned clinical typification. The new classification differentiates three pediatric groups: The pediatric follicular lymphoma, pediatric nodal marginal zone lymphoma, and EBV-positive T-cell lymphoproliferative diseases of the child that can be inserted into three classic groups "high-malignant non-Hodgkin's lymphoma group, anaplastic lymphoma group, and lymphoproliferative diseases associated with immunodeficiency." Therefore, Burkitt's tumor belongs to the pediatric follicular lymphoma (high-malignant non-Hodgkin's lymphoma).

In **symptomatic intussusception**, the already described symptoms and signs may be *combined with findings of the underlying disorder*, for

Table 15.5 Important differential diagnoses of acute intussusception

Acute gastroenteritis, enterocolitis	Environmental history
	Enteritic findings, increased transit time
	No invagination tumor
	Bloody stools possible
Decompensated constipation	History of constipation
	Palpable stool masses
Changes of crying habits,	History, behavior of the parents
Wind and evening colic	Observation of feeding and swallowing:
(Three months' colic)	Prolonged feeding, air swallowing,
	Tympanitic belly, excessive wind
Acute appendicitis	In this age group usually perforated,
	Abdominal wall guarding
Postoperative ileus due to adhesions	Previous laparotomy
Urinary tract infection, urolithiasis (urinary tract malformations)	Pyuria, hematuria, and not melena
Inguinal hernia, testicular torsion (first manifestation or incarceration)	Characteristic local findings

example, history of repeated loss of blood by the anus in Meckel's diverticulum or intestinal duplication or general signs in cystic fibrosis. The following pathologies arranged in order of frequency may be encountered as **lead point or cause of intussusception**:

Meckel's diverticulum in ≤ 50 % #, single or generalized polyps in ≤ 40 % #, non-Hodgkin's lymphoma and carcinoid tumor, intestinal duplication #, ectopic pancreas, and systemic diseases such as Henoch-Schönlein-Glanzmann purpura #, cystic fibrosis, and Crohn's disease.

Differential Diagnosis, Work-Ups

The former includes the causes of surgical abdomen in general and more specifically the pathologies quoted in Table 15.5.

Plain x-ray in upright position is not the first line examination in suspected intussusception: Usually only little gas is present in the intestine, and the ascending colon may be visible together with a mass inside. The principal examination is **ultrasound** that has in idiopathic invagination a sensitivity of 98.5–100 %, a specificity of 85–100 %, and a positive or negative predictive value of 100 or 94 %. It demonstrates in the longitudinal direction the so-called pseudokidney # and in the transverse direction, the so-called target sign #. Unfortunately, a pathological lead point is not necessarily recognizable and may be therefore missed.

In equivocal cases, specifically in suspected chronic, postoperative, or symptomatic intussusception (two thirds of the patients with a symptomatic intussusception are older than 2 years; in this age group, >20 % may have a pathologic lead point), **contrast enema #**, **upper GI contrast study**, or **contrast CT** may be diagnostic.

Treatment, Prognosis

1. Nonoperative reposition with air under fluoroscopic guidance or hydrostatic reduction under ultrasound (visible entrance of air or contrast in the distal ileum and sonographic exclusion of a persistent invagination). The latter is recommended by some radiologist in children <3 months and >2 years of age and/or in case of failed pneumatic reduction.

Due to the possibility of vomiting, abdominal pain, fever, and perforation [≤ 3 %], the procedure should be performed after introduction of a nasogastric tube and i.v. line in the presence of an experienced pediatric surgeon.

The success of hydrostatic reposition depends on the time since beginning of the symptoms, the site of the invagination tumor, and the type of intussusception. If reposition is performed within 24 h, the success rate is about 80 % in idiopathic invagination and beyond 24 h about one third [and ≤2/3 in a cohort of successively presenting patients].

2. The indication of surgery is as follows:

- Ileus without/with peritonitis or intestinal perforation
- ≥48 h since beginning of symptomatology (success rate with hydrostatic reposition still one third in some studies)
- Invagination tumor distal to the transverse colon (success rate 40–25 %)
- Intussusception with a recognized or probable pathological lead point (e.g., children beyond 2 years of age)
- Following 1-(2) failure(s) of hydrostatic reposition
- Postoperative and chronic intussusception

Surgery includes i.v. fluid replacement and single shot of triple antibiotics (in case of perforation or intestinal resection antibiotics for several days). After a transverse incision in the right middle abdomen, the intussusception is reduced by milking compression of the intestine immediately behind the invagination tumor #. In case of only partial reduction or perforation, segmental resection of the grossly altered small intestine becomes necessary (in up to 50 %). Surgery is finished by appendectomy and in case of missing fixation of ileocecum and ascending colon, by colopexy to avoid volvulus of the cecum and possibly recurrence of intussusception.

Prognosis

Even today, the mortality may be 0.8 % and postoperative morbidity is about 20 %. The recurrence rate after surgery is 3 % and after nonoperative reduction 5.8–9 %.

A high recurrence rate is observed if all recurrences are considered together: Two thirds have one recurrence, and one third has two or multiple recurrences. The latter occur as isolated episodes or in clusters within up to 8 years. The number of patients with a pathological lead point seems to increase from single to multiple recurrences and the reducibility to decrease. In contrast to the opinion that nonoperative treatment should be continued in two and more recurrences, some recommend after reduction early laparoscopic surgery for exclusion of a pathological lead point and prevention of further intussusception by ileocecopexy.

15.2.2 Postoperative Ileus due to Adhesions

Occurrence

Postoperative obstruction is observed in 2–3 % of laparotomies, but the incidence differs largely depending on the cause of adhesions and the type of initial surgery that has been performed. The role of laparoscopic surgery is not yet fully evaluated in this context (prevention of postoperative adhesions).

Etiopathogenesis, Causes

Postoperative obstruction due to adhesions of childhood is not quoted frequently in the literature, and the incidences related to specific interventions may differ considerably. Several factors lead to a more frequent occurrence of postoperative adhesions. They include rough handling of the intestine, blunt instead of sharp dissection of adhesions, exsiccosis and ischemia of small parts of intestine and mesentery, use of inappropriate suture material and glove powder, etc. (Fig. 15.5).

Nevertheless, open appendectomy is with one fourth the most frequent cause with 0.4–1.2 % postoperative obstruction in simple appendicitis and 0.8–6.2 % in perforated appendicitis. Abdominal surgery of the newborn (gastroschisis, intestinal atresia) and infants (Hirschsprung's disease, anorectal malformations, intussusception), oncological surgery, complicated Meckel's diverticulum, and inflammatory bowel diseases have in order of citation an increasing risk of postoperative ileus due to adhesions with twice to four times higher values than the general 2–3 %.

Two thirds of postoperative obstructions occur within 1 year after surgery (in neonates up to 90 %) and the remainder within 2 to several years afterward.

Clinical Significance

- Postoperative obstruction due to adhesions must be considered in the differential diagnosis of every child with a history of open abdominal or laparoscopic surgery (visible scar(s) of the abdomen) and acute or chronic recurrent abdominal symptoms and signs.

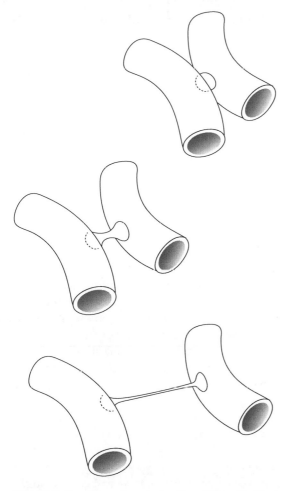

Fig. 15.5 Possible pathogenesis of cord-like adhesions after abdominal surgery. The exudation of fibrin leads to loose broad adhesions between the intestinal loops. Recovery of intestinal motility with to and fro movements of the single loops may lead to formation of fibrinous string-like cords that are replaced by permanent fibrous tissue

- Early recognition and surgical treatment are indispensable to avoid bowel gangrene and peritonitis.

Clinical Presentation

Sudden onset of severe and intermittent crampy abdominal pain of a degree that the child has not experienced hitherto is followed by nausea and vomiting. If a history of abdominal surgery or laparoscopic intervention and a corresponding scar can be recorded at the same time, postoperative obstruction due to adhesions must be

assumed until the proof of the contrary. At the beginning, some stool may be passed and later wind and stool retention occurs.

In a cohort of consecutive patient of different age, cause, stage, and type of postoperative obstruction due to adhesions, nonbilious or bilious vomiting is observed in 85 % and crampy abdominal pain in 75 %, but the medical consultation occurs in >80 % in a period of 1–3 days.

In chronic recurrent postoperative obstruction (<15 % of the cases), the symptomatology is less dramatic or it may end up in a complete obstruction with a clinical presentation as quoted above.

Clinical Skills

Initially (i.e., before development of intestinal gangrene and peritonitis), the abdomen is often not distended. *Percussion and palpation yields localized tenderness and possibly guarding. At the same site or nearby, rushes of hyperactive bowel sounds may be auscultated (in up to 70 % if it is looked for) that are characterized as high pitched and borborygmi (sounds created by a forced passage of some intestinal content through a stenosis). In up to 25 % of children, the clinical, radiological, and operative findings correspond to the same site in the abdomen.*

The interpretation of the clinical presentation may be difficult in **newborns and infants with acute** and **in chronic recurrent obstruction due to adhesions**, and in **early postoperative obstructive ileus** due to twisting and sticking together of single loops.

In **young children**, the clinical presentation seems less dramatic. Nevertheless, sudden onset of vomiting, screaming, frowning, drawing up the legs and/or visible intestinal loops with hyperperistalsis, and stiffening can be observed. In **early postoperative obstruction**, intermittent and crampy abdominal pain, possible bilious vomiting, and the already described local findings are not explained by postoperative paralytic ileus and intestinal atony.

Work-Up, Differential Diagnosis

Work-ups are supine and upright plain abdominal x-ray, upper GI contrast study, contrast enema, and contrast CT.

In contrast to adulthood with the characteristic findings of several or numerous air-fluid levels and no gas in the colorectum in the majority of cases, the same radiological pattern is observed less frequently (50–70 %) in children. Plain x-ray shows often only sparse gas or no gas at all except of one or two intestinal loop(s) distended by gas. This characteristic pattern may be misinterpreted as inconspicuous ##.

In case of equivocal clinical or radiological findings, upper GI study with water-soluble contrast shows immediately or on follow-up contrast stop with prestenotic intestinal dilatation and accentuate circular plicae.

The differential diagnosis includes other causes of acquired surgical abdomen and mainly of obstructive ileus such early postoperative obstructive ileus or intussusception, postoperative paralytic ileus, obstructive ileus due to ascaris infestation, or severe gastroenteritis.

Ascariasis may lead to acute obstructive ileus or intestinal perforation. Poor hygiene, a palpable soft round or oblong mass in the lower belly combined with signs of obstructive ileus, and eosinophilia points to ascariasis as cause of intestinal obstruction and is confirmed by gastrointestinal study with water-soluble contrast (thin, coiled, and tape-like filling defects of the contrast filled intestinal loops). Laparotomy is indicated if an enema and gastric suction does not lead to evacuation of worms with relief of the symptomatology. The mass of worms should be manipulated with fingers similar to intussusception and moved into the cecum. Enterotomy over the obstructing tangle becomes necessary otherwise. Ascaris lumbricoides invades also the biliary tree, pancreatic ducts, and appendix and leads to liver abscess, choledocholithiasis, pancreatitis, and appendicitis. Intestinal perforation leads to fibrinous peritonitis.

Treatment, Prognosis
Urgent surgery is indicated in suspected acute postoperative obstruction due to adhesions because extension and severity of obstruction are not predictable. Exceptions are some chronic recurrent types of postoperative obstruction in which preliminary nasogastric tube and i.v. infusion may be used for clinical follow-up and further work-up.

Surgery: The **expected findings** are as follows: In two thirds of childhood postoperative obstruction due to adhesions, one single cord-like adhesion is encountered either with or without diffuse adhesions. This single adhesion is relevant for intestinal and blood supply obstruction. Exclusive diffuse adhesions, diffuse adhesions with several cord-like adhesions, and the dangerous **volvulus** entrapped by diffuse adhesions occur less frequently.

After rehydration and single-shot antibiotics (that are extended over several days if intestinal resection becomes necessary), **the abdomen is opened** by a transverse incision. The intestinal content is gently squeezed from the small intestine in direction of the stomach where it is removed by suction. The cord-like adhesion is resected and the involved intestine resected if needed (in >15 %, depending on the time since beginning of symptomatology and type of obstruction). The diffuse adhesions should be divided as well to exclude additional cord-like adhesions and volvulus. Afterward, the gastric tube is pushed in the duodenum, lavage is performed, and the intestinal loops are laid back loop by loop according to Grob like a festoon.

Prognosis
The recurrence rate is <10 % and occurs mostly in the first year after surgery. Wound and intraabdominal abscess or delayed postoperative paralytic ileus is observed in ≤5 %. Rarely postoperative malabsorption may occur.

15.2.3   Rare Abdominal Wall, Pelvic Floor, and Internal Hernias

Occurrence, Forms, Pathoanatomy
Internal hernias in malrotation or congenital mesenteric defect are observed occasionally in children, whereas other forms of internal hernias, abdominal wall, or pelvic floor hernias are mainly observed in adults. Rarely, pelvic floor hernias have been observed in newborns. The rare hernias include:

• Spieghel's and lumbar hernias (abdominal wall)
• Obturator, sciatic, and perineal hernias (pelvic floor)

- Treitz's or mesocolic hernias (internal hernias)
- Hernias in congenital mesenteric defect or malrotation (internal hernias)
- Postoperative hernias

In congenital mesenteric defect, a hole in the mesentery of the size 2–3 by 2–3 cm or even larger may lead to internal herniation of intestine and obstructive ileus.

Abdominal wall hernias protrude in the lower abdomen at the lateral edge of abdominal rectus muscle (Spieghel's hernia) or at the lumbocostal (below the 12th rib) or at the ileolumbar triangle (above the iliac crest) in lumbar hernias. In obturator hernia, protrusion occurs through the obturator foramen along the obturator nerve, in sciatic hernias through the sciatic foramens, and in perineal hernias through the pelvic floor. A jejunal loop is entrapped under the mesentery of the transverse mesentery in Treitz's hernia and the ileum under the ileocolic compartment in mesocolic hernia.

Clinical Significance
- Pain and tender swelling at unusual sites of the abdomen, back, gluteal, or perineal region and pain at the inner side of the thigh should alert the surgeon about a rare abdominal hernia.
- The quoted rare hernias should be considered in every case of obstructive ileus in which no common cause is recognizable.

Clinical Presentation
The majority of the described rare hernias are mostly recognized at emergency surgery that is performed because of obstructive ileus.

Such hernias present sometimes with localized pain and tender swelling at unusual sites in the lower abdomen (lateral edge of abdominal rectus muscle in the lower abdomen), back (below the 12th rib and above the iliac crest), at the gluteal fold (sciatic hernias), in the perineal or perivulvar region (perineal hernias). The obturator hernia leads to distinct pain at the inner side of the tight, and no swelling is recognizable except for rectal examination.

Spieghel's hernia is rarely strangulated but all other hernias are often or mostly incarcerated. After large perineal surgery, postoperative perineal hernia may be observed.

Differential Diagnosis, Work-Ups
All causes that lead to obstructive ileus, tender swelling, and obturator or sciatic nerve pain must be considered, for example, postoperative paresis of the flank after lumbotomy or perineal ectopic testis.

Work-ups include ultrasound or MRI in equivocal findings.

Treatment, Prognosis
Obstructive ileus needs emergency surgery and often intestinal resection with possibly primary anastomosis due to the often advanced stage of strangulation. Afterward and in case of the described local findings, the site of hernia must be identified, the content reduced, the neck of the hernia closed, the sack resected, and the causative defect closed by an appropriate method. Laparoscopic repair and surgery from the perineum have been described.

Prognosis depends on the time of herniation and surgery and on the damage to the intestine or other abdominal contents.

15.2.4   Sickle Cell Disease

Occurrence, Pathology
Sickle cell disease is observed in black populations especially in Africa, Middle and North America, and due to the current migration all over the world. It is an autosomally recessively inherited disease that leads to significant quantities of hemoglobin S in the blood. Sickle cell anemia is the most common form of sickle cell disease.

Clinical Significance
- Sickle cell disease is a life-threatening disease with reduced survival.
- Several complications have a differential diagnostic and therapeutic significance in pediatric surgery.

Clinical Presentation
Sickle cell disease is characterized by *chronic hemolytic anemia and intermittent vasoocclusive events* which may involve any organ, lead to acute and chronic pain, and damage of the involved organs, for example, functionally asplenic spleen in early childhood or renal insufficiency later in life.

Dactylitis (swelling of the hands and feet) is the first clinical manifestation in infancy or early childhood. Whereas *stroke, pulmonary artery hypertension, organ insufficiencies, and risk for bacterial infections* have a prognostic significance, other manifestations are of special interest to the pediatric surgeon such as *jaundice, cholelithiasis, priapism, leg ulcers, and vasoocclusive crises* each for differential diagnosis and/or treatment.

Work-Up, Differential Diagnosis

The suspected diagnosis is confirmed by neonatal screening or different tests for demonstration of the presence of significant quantities of Hb S in the blood and/or differentiation of heterozygous carriers of Hb S mutation from patients with sickle cell disease. Depending on history and clinical presentation, complete blood and reticulocyte count, iron status, liver and renal parameters, blood gases, and radiological imaging of lung, brain, and abdominal organs are necessary.

In **splenic sequestration crisis**, the spleen becomes engorged and surgical abdomen must be considered (see Webcode 1703 in Chap. 17). The same is true for other abdominal organ involvement.

Treatment, Prognosis

It consists in case of vasoocclusive events of i.v. hydration, inflammatory agents, and analgetics. Splenectomy is indicated in repeated severe crises and functionally asplenic spleen. It must be followed by appropriate immunizations and prophylactic antibiotics. For treatment of cholelithiasis and priapism, see the index.

Webcodes

The following webcodes can be used on www. psurg.net for further images and data.

1501 Abdominal distension, distal intestinal obstruction	1516 Chronic intussusception, non-Hodgkin's lymphoma
1502 Multiple air-fluid levels	1517 Meckel's diverticulum, lead point
1503 Uncomplicated meconium ileus with	1518 Intestinal polyp, lead point of intussusception

1504 Grossly dilated ileum	1519 Duplication, lead point
1505 Clinical presentation, meconium ileus	1520 Henoch-Schönlein purpura, intussusception
1506 Small intestine duplication with	1521 Ultrasound,' pseudokidney' sign
1507 Obstructive ileus, enlarging duplication cyst	1522 Ultrasound, target sign
1508 Stages of fetal intestinal rotation	1523 Contrast enema, shapes of intussusception
1509 Acute midgut volvulus, early stage	1524 Ileocecal intussusception before reduction
1510 Acute small intestine volvulus, late stage	1525 Plain x-ray, postoperative ileus due to adhesions
1511 Low anorectal anomaly, anovestibular fistula	1526 Plain x-ray, ileus due to adhesions after perforated Meckel's diverticulum
1512 High anorectal anomaly, rectovestibular fistula	1527 Early stage,
1513 Late stage, intussusception with	1528 Intermediate stage,
1514 Small intestine necrosis	1529 Late stage of postoperative ileus due to adhesions
1515 Red current jelly stool	

Bibliography

Section 15.1.2

Bower RJ, Ternberg JL (1972) Preduodenal portal vein. J Pediatr Surg 7:579–584

Ein SH, Kim PC, Miller HA (2000) The late non-functioning duodenal atresia repair – a second look. J Pediatr Surg 35:690–691

Merrot T, Anastasescu R, Pankevych T, Tercier S, Garcia S, Alessandrini P, Guys JM (2006) Duodenal duplications. Clinical characteristics, embryological hypotheses, histological findings, treatment. Eur J Pediatr Surg 16:18–23

Murshed R, Nicholls G, Spitz L (1999) Intrinsic duodenal obstruction: trends in management and outcome over 45 years (1951–1995) with relevance to prenatal counselling. Br J Obstet Gynaecol 106: 1197–1199

Pathak D, Sarin YK (2006) Congenital duodenal obstruction due to a preduodenal portal vein. Indian J Pediatr 73:423–425

Singh SJ, Dickson R, Baskaranathan S, Peat J, Spence K, Kimble R, Cass D (2002) Excisional duodenoplasty: a new technique for congenital duodenal obstruction. Pediatr Surg Int 18:75–78

Spilde TL, St Peter SD, Keckler SJ, Holcomb GW 3rd, Snyder CL, Ostlie DJ (2008) Open vs laparoscopic repair of congenital duodenal obstruction: a concurrent series. J Pediatr Surg 43:1002–1005

Stauffer UG, Schwoebel M (1998) Duodenal atresia and stenosis – annular pancreas. In: O'Neill JA Jr et al (eds) Pediatric surgery, vol II, 5th edn. Mosby, St. Louis

Section 15.3

Casaccia G, Trucchi A, Spirydakis I, Giorlandino C, Aite L, Capolupo I, Catalano OA, Bagolan P (2006) Congenital intestinal anomalies, neonatal short bowel syndrome, and prenatal/neonatal counseling. J Pediatr Surg 41:804–807

Grosfeld JL (1998) Jejunoileal atresia and stenosis. In: O'Neill JA Jr et al (eds) Pediatric surgery, vol II, 5th edn. Mosby, St. Louis

Kumaran N, Shankar KR, Lloyd DA, Losty PD (2002) Trends in the management and outcome of Jejuno-Ileal Atresia. Eur J Pediatr Surg 12:163–167

Piper HG, Alesbury J, Waterford SD, Zurakowski D, Jaksic T (2008) Intestinal atresias: factors affecting clinical outcomes. J Pediatr Surg 43:1244–1248

Prasad TR, Bajpai M (2000) Intestinal atresia. Indian J Pediatr 67:671–678

Sections 15.1.4–15.1.5

Eckoldt F, Heling KS, Woderich R, Kraft S, Bollmann R, Mau H (2003) Meconium peritonitis and pseudo-cyst formation: prenatal diagnosis and post-natal course. Prenat Diagn 23:904–908

Tsai MH, Chu SM, Lien R, Huan IIR, Luo CC (2009) Clinical manifestation in infants with symptomatic meconium peritonitis. Pediatr Neonatol 50:59–64

Section 15.1.6

Bond SJ, Groff DB (1998) Gastrointestinal duplications. In: O'Neill JA Jr et al (eds) Pediatric surgery, vol II, 5th edn. Mosby, St. Louis

Lisi G, Illiceto MT, Rossi C, Broto JM, Jil-Vernet JM, Lelli Chiesa P (2006) Anal canal duplication: a retrospective analysis of 12 cases from two European pediatric surgical departments. Pediatr Surg Int 22:967–973

Teklali Y, Kaddouri N, Barahioui M (2002) Gastrointestinal system duplication in children (19 cases). Arch Pediatr 9:903–906

Section 15.1.7

Antedomenico E, Singh NN, Zagorski SM, Dwyer K, Chung MH (2004) Laparoscopic repair of a right paraduodenal hernia. Surg Endosc 18:165–166

Filston HC (1998) Other causes of intestinal obstruction. In: O'Neill JA Jr et al. (eds) Pediatric surgery, vol II, 5th edn. Mosby, St. Louis

Grob M (1953) Ueber lageanomalien des magendarmtractus infolge störungen der fetalen darmdrehung. Schwabe, Basel

Moran JM, Salas J, Sanjuan S, Amaya JL, Rincon P, Serrano A, Tallo EM (2004) Paramesocolic hernias. Consequences of delayed diagnosis. Report of three new cases. J Pediatr Surg 39:112–116

Schellenberg F, Panagiotis T, Maurer C, Toia D, Steuerwald M (2006) Bauchkoliken: Organische Oder funktionelle Ursache? (Abdominal pain: organic or functional cause?). Schweiz Med Forum 6:253–256

Strouse PJ (2002) Clinics in diagnostic imaging (74). Midgut malrotation with volvulus. Singapore Med J 43:325–328

Touloukian RJ, Smith EI (1998) Disorders of rotation and fixation. In: O'Neill JA Jr et al (eds) Pediatric surgery, vol II, 5th edn. Mosby, St. Louis

Section 15.1.8

Al-Hozaim O, Al-Maary J, Alqahtani A, Zamakhshary M (2010) Laparoscopic-assisted anorectal pull-through for anorectal malformations: a systematic review and the need for standardization of outcome reporting. J Pediatr Surg 45:1500–1504

Banu T, Hannan MJ, Aziz MA, Hoque M, Laila K (2006) Rectovestibular fistula with vaginal malformations. Pediatr Surg Int 22:263–266

Bill AH, Hall DG, Johnson RJ (1975) Position of rectal fistula in relation to the hymen in 46 girls with imperforate anus. J Pediatr Surg 10:361–365

Davies MC, Liao LM, Wilcox DT, Woodhouse CR, Creighton SM (2010) Anorectal malformations: what happens in adulthood? BJU Int 106:398–404

Di Cesare A, Leva E, Macchini F, Canazza L, Carrabba G, Fumagalli M, Mosca M, Torricelli M (2010) Anorectal malformations and neurospinal dysraphism: is this association a major risk for continence? Pediatr Surg Int 26:1077–1081

Hallows MR, Lander AD, Corkery JJ (2002) Anterior resection for megarectosigmoid in congenital anorectal malformations. J Pediatr Surg 37:1464–1466

Hamid CH, Holland AJ, Martin HC (2007) Long-term outcome of anorectal malformations: the patient perspective. Pediatr Surg Int 23:97–102

Kiely EM, Pena A (1998) Anorectal malformations. In: O'Neill JA Jr et al (eds) Pediatric surgery, vol II, 5th edn. Mosby, St. Louis

Lee SC, Chun YS, Jung SE, Park KW, Kim WK (1997) Currinado triad: anorectal malformation, sacral bony abnormality, and presacral mass – a review of 11 cases. J Pediatr Surg 32:58–61

Levitt MA, Pena A (2007) Anorectal malformations. Orphanet J Rare Dis 2:33

Nasr A, McNamara PJ, Mertens L, Levin D, James A, Holtby H, Langer JC (2010) Is routine preoperative 2-dimensional echocardiography necessary for infants with esophageal atresia, omphalocele, or anorectal malformations? J Pediatr Surg 45:876–879

Oldham KT (1998) Atresia, stenosis, and other obstructions of the colon. In: O'Neill JA Jr et al (eds) Pediatric surgery, vol II, 5th edn. Mosby, St. Louis

Patwardhan N, Kiely EM, Drake DP, Spitz L, Pierro A (2001) Colostomy for anorectal anomalies: high incidence of complications. J Pediatr Surg 36:795–798

Pena A, Devries PA (1982) Posterior sagittal anorectoplasty: important technical considerations and new applications. J Pediatr Surg 17:796–809; discussion 809-811

Rangel SJ, de Blaauw I (2010) Advances in pediatric colorectal surgical techniques. Semin Pediatr Surg 19:86–95

Rescorla FJ (1998) Meconium ileus. In: O'Neill JA Jr et al (eds) Pediatric surgery, vol II, 5th edn. Mosby, St. Louis

Rintala RJ, Pakarinen MP (2008) Imperforate anus: long- and short-term outcome. Semin Pediatr Surg 17:79–89

Yilmaz O, Genc A, Ayhan S, Ozcan T, Aygoren R, Taneli C (2011) A female patient with congenital pouch colon (CPC): a case report. Acta Chir Belg 111:335–337

Section 15.1.9

Blakely ML, Gupta H, Lally KP (2008) Surgical management of necrotizing enterocolitis and isolated intestinal perforation in premature neonates. Semin Perinatol 32:122–126

Drewett MS, Burge DM (2007) Recurrent neonatal gastro-intestinal problems after spontaneous intestinal perforation. Pediatr Surg Int 23:1081–1084

Duran R, Inan M, Vatansever U, Aladag N, Acunas B (2007) Etiology of neonatal gastric perforations: review of 10 years experience. Pediatr Int 49:626–630

Hunter CJ, Chokshi N, Ford HR (2008) Evidence vs experience in the surgical management of necrotizing enterocolitis and focal intestinal perforation. J Perinatol 28(Suppl 1):S14–S17

Tarrado X, Castanon M, Thio M, Valderas JM, Garcia Aparicio L, Morales L (2005) Comparative study between isolated intestinal perforation and necrotizing Enterocolitis. Eur J Pediatr Surg 15:88–94

Section 15.2.1

Bai YZ, Chen H, Wang WL (2009) A special type of postoperative intussusception: ileoileal intussusception after surgical reduction of ileocolic intussusception in infants and children. J Pediatr Surg 44:755–758

Bines JE, Ivanoff B, Justice F et al (2004) Clinical case definition for the diagnosis of acute intussusception. J Pediatr Gastroenterol Nutr 39:511–518

Chang YT, Lee JY, Wang JY, Chiou CS, Lin JY (2009) Early laparoscopy for ileocolic intussusception with multiple recurrences in children. Surg Endosc 23:2002–2004

Cortese MM, Staat MA, Weinberg GA, Edwards K, Rice MA, Szilagyi PG, Hall CB, Payne DC, Parashar UD (2009) Underestimates if intussusception rates among US infants based on inpatient discharge data: implications for monitoring the safety of rotavirus vaccines. J Infect Dis 200(Suppl 1):S264–S270

Daneman A, Alton DJ, Lobo E, Gravett J, Kim P, Ein SH (1998) Patterns of recurrence of intussusception in children: a 17-year review. Pediatr Radiol 28:913–919

Filston HC (1998) Other causes of intestinal obstruction. In: O'Neill JA Jr et al. (eds) Pediatric surgery, vol II, 5th edn. Mosby, St. Louis

Henry MCW, Breuer CK, Tashjian DB et al (2006) The appendix sign: a radiologic marker for irreducible intussusception. J Pediatr Surg 41:487–489

Holcomb GW 3rd, Ross AJ 3rd, O'Neill JA Jr (1991) Postoperative intussusception: increasing frequency or increasing awareness? South Med J 84:1334–1339

Hviid A, Svanstrom H (2009) Antibiotic use and intussusception in early childhood. J Antimicrob Chemother 64:642–648

Kaiser G (1976) Früherfassung und Therapie der Darminvagination im Kindesalter. Chir Praxis 21: 239–250

Kaiser AD, Applegate KE, Ladd AP (2007) Current success in the treatment of intussusception in children. Surgery 142:469–475; discussion 475-477

Kong FT, Liu WY, Tang YM, Zhong L, Wang XJ, Yang G, Chen HP (2010) Intussusception in infants younger than 3 months: a single center's experience. World J Pediatr 6:55–59

Ong NT, Beasley DW (1990) The leadpoint in intussusception. J Pediatr Surg 25:640–643

Page MP, Ricca RL, Resnick AS, Puder M, Fishman SJ (2008) Newborn and toddler intestinal obstruction owing to congenital mesenteric defects. J Pediatr Surg 43:755–758

Reijneveld SA, Brugman E, Hirasing RA (2001) Excessive infant crying: the impact of varying definitions. Pediatrics 108:893–897

Stringer MD, Pledger G, Drake DP (1992) Childhood deaths from intussusception in England and Wales, 1984–1989. BMJ 304(6829):737–739

Swerlow EC, Harris NL, Jaffe ES et al (2008) WHO classification of tumours of haematopoietic and lymphoid tissues, 4th edn. International Agency for Research on Cancer, Lyon

Vogetseder A, Gengler C, Reineke T, Tinguely M (2011) Pädiatrische Lymphom-diagnostik Aktuelles aus der Sicht der Pathologen. Schweiz Med Forum 11:73–78

Whitehouse JS, Gourlay DM, Winthrop AL, Cassidy LD, Arca MJ (2010) Is it safe to discharge intussusception patients after successful hydrostatic reduction? J Pediatr Surg 45:1182–1186

Young DG (1998) Intussusception. In: O'Neill JA Jr et al (eds) Pediatric surgery, vol II, 5th edn. Mosby, St. Louis

Zmora O, Shin CE (2008) Multiple surgical interventions due to recurrent intussusception in a patient with Henoch-Schönlein purpura: a case report. Eur J Pediatr Surg 18:340–341

Section 15.2.2

Filston HC (1998) Other causes of intestinal obstruction. In: O'Neill JA Jr et al. (eds) Pediatric surgery, vol II, 5th edn. Mosby, St. Louis

Osifo OD, Ovueni ME (2010) Is nonoperative management of adhesive intestinal obstruction applicable in a resource-poor country? Afr J Paediatr Surg 7:66–70

Soravia C, Kaiser G (1990–1991) Postoperativer Bridenileus beim Kind. Anlass zur ver-zögerter Erkennung? Chir Praxis 43:661–667

Differential Diagnosis: Obstructive Ileus due to Ascariasis Infestation

Maletin M, Veselinovic I, Stoijlijkovic GB, Vapa D, Budakov B (2009) Death due to unrecognized ascariasis infestation: two medicolegal autopsy cases. Am J Forensic Med Pathol 30:292–294

Section 15.2.3

Dulucq JL, Wintringer P, Mahajna A (2011) Occult hernias detected by laparoscopic totally extra-peritoneal inguinal hernia repair: a prospective study. Hernia 15:399–402

Losanoff JE, Richman BW, Jones JW (2002) Spigelian hernia in a child: case report and review of the literature. Hernia 6:191–193

Petrie A, Shane Tubbs R, Matusz P, Shaffer K, Loukas M (2011) Obturator hernia. Anatomy, embryology, diagnosis, and treatment. Clin Anat 24:562–569

Prada Arias M, Dargallo Carbonell T, Estévez_Martinez E, Bautista Casasnovas A, Varela Cives R (2004) Handlebar hernia in children: two cases and review of the literature. Eur J Pediatr Surg 14:133–136

Soto-Pérez-de-Celis E, Gonzales-Pezzat I (2011) Letter to the editor. Obturator hernia, an uncommon cause of intestinal obstruction. Rev Esp Enferm Dig 103: 48–51

Stamatiou D, Skandalakis JE, Skandalakis LJ, Mirilas P (2010) Perineal hernia: surgical anatomy, embryology, and technique of repair. Am Surg 76:474–479

Steffensen TS, Opitz JM, Gilbert-Barness E (2009) Congenital perineal hernia in a fetus with trisomy 18. Fetal Pediatr Pathol 28:95–99

Section 15.2.4

Al-Salem AH (2006) Indications and complications of splenectomy for children with sickle cell disease. J Pediatr Surg 41:1909–1915

Bender MA, Hobbs W (2009) Sickle cell disease. In: Pagon RA, Bird TC, Dolan CR, Stephens K (eds) GeneReviews [internet]. University of Washington, Seattle [updated 2009 Sep 17]

Pack-Mabien A, Haynes J Jr (2009) A primary care provider's guide to preventive and acute care management of adults and children with sickle cell disease. J Am Acad Nurse Pract 21:250–257

Surgical Abdomen due to Abdominal Trauma and Foreign Bodies

16

16.1 Abdominal Trauma

16.1.1 General Features of Abdominal Trauma

Occurrence, Clinical Significance

Abdominal trauma may play an important role in the differential diagnosis of surgical abdomen although it is only the third most common site of trauma similar to thoracic injury and a corresponding history is often available.

- Isolated injury to the abdomen is often underestimated because it is mentioned in the history only incompletely or not at all and the primary care provider does not consider the possibility of an abdominal injury.
- In multisystemic organ injury that is observed in up 50 % of major trauma, a single severe injury such as trauma to the head may be in the forefront.
- Mortality may be observed in up to 15 % of abdominal trauma.

Causes

It is important to know possible causes of abdominal trauma and their specific conditions because it permits to consider the corresponding patterns of injury, for example, frontal motor vehicle accident versus lateral impact as occupant or passenger who is not restraint by a belt versus a small child placed in a seat belt.

In motor vehicle accident, and depending on age and circumstances as occupant, pedestrian, cyclist, or motorcyclist, in adventure and agricultural activities, and falls from the height (in stairwells and from storeys), often multisystemic organ injuries are observed.

On the other hand, falls from a standing position or play and sports activities lead more frequently to isolated abdominal trauma. The large number of such injuries and involved small children is caused by increasing development and diversification of locomotor and occupational tools.

Extremely dangerous or not considered at first are assaults and clashes, blows to a pregnant woman, birth trauma, and child abuse, hoof kicks, gunshots, and stab (impalement) injuries.

Clinical Presentation, Resuscitation

Ascertainment of time, cause, and precise mechanism of injury is very important and should be completed by informations about possible symptoms and signs originating after the time of trauma and of the measures that have already been taken.

The **clinical examination** by a pediatric or trauma surgeon should be **simultaneously** performed with **resuscitation** by an anesthesiologist or emergency care pediatrician and some **routine work-ups** (including blood and urine examinations and plain chest and abdominal x-rays). The clinical examination can be divided chronologically in a general survey, evaluation of specific organ injuries, and follow-up of general and local findings. In spite of continuous teamwork with regular arrangements among the participating staff, the **final lead and responsibility should be in one hand.**

G.L. Kaiser, *Symptoms and Signs in Pediatric Surgery*,
DOI 10.1007/978-3-642-31161-1_16, © Springer-Verlag Berlin Heidelberg 2012

The **general survey** includes evaluation and documentation of respiration, consciousness, and blood circulation, and possible multisystemic organ injury and immediate life-threatening conditions.

Evaluation of specific organ injuries: Correlation exists not always between the reported history about the severity of trauma mechanism and the severity of the findings, for example, unspectacular fall to the edge of a bed is followed by a splenic rupture.

In multisystemic organ injury, first major injuries should be excluded. Symptoms and signs of the respiratory system may be caused by abdominal injury, dilated stomach, or distended belly due to pneumo- or hemoperitoneum. A GCS ≤8 corresponds to a severe head injury. In children, imminent shock remains longer compensated than in adults. Recapillarization time, pulse frequency, and age-dependent shock index=pulse frequency/blood pressure (1.4–1.2 at age 1–2, 1.0 at age 4–6, and 0.9–0.7 at age 8–14 years) are useful.

The possible **abdominal findings** include vague, diffuse, localized, radiating, or not traceable spontaneous pain and/or tenderness on percussion and palpation and/or general distension or suppleness. Findings of the abdominal wall, back, lower thoracic wall, pelvic region, or beyond it that point to a specific local or generalized impact such as ecchymosis, abrasion, laceration (including gunshot or stab wound), contusion or specific marks from a handlebar or tire track, and petechial head and neck bleedings and scleral hemorrhages after thoracoabdominal compression are important. The abdominal findings may be caused by a dilated stomach or paralytic ileus, abdominal wall contusion or hematoma, or intra-abdominal visceral or vascular lesion.

In addition, clinical signs of fractures of the lower ribs, of the spine, and the pelvis should be excluded because they may lead to findings of a surgical abdomen. On the other hand, multisystemic organ injury and head injury may hide the clinical presentation of abdominal trauma.

After clinical evaluation of specific organ injuries, corresponding radiological imaging is performed for confirmation and precise evaluation.

Clinical follow-ups should be performed in short-term intervals especially in case of equivocal or absent abdominal findings to exclude changes to the worse.

Resuscitation includes i.v. lines (and depending on the severity also central and arterial access) for fluid and blood replacement, blood examinations (chemistry including myocardial enzymes and hematological examinations including coagulation studies and blood testing), and monitoring; intubation and artificial respiration; introduction of nasogastric tube (in case of suspected frontobasal fractures, orogastric tube) for relief of gastric dilatation; bladder catheter for urine examination and measurement of output; and possibly tube thoracostomy (pneumo- and/or hemothorax), needle aspiration of gross pneumoperitoneum or mini-laparotomy for peritoneal drainage of hemoperitoneum or diagnostic lavage etc.

Work-ups are performed at different stages of resuscitation and clinical examination, and dependent on the severity of injury. In severe multisystem injury or isolated organ injuries, a battery of blood tests and plain chest and abdominal x-rays including cervical spine are performed as measure of routine at the beginning and whole body CT with i.v. contrast shortly after stabilization and clinical evaluation of specific organ injuries.

Abdominal ultrasound, peritoneal lavage, and diagnostic laparoscopy are alternative methods to define the need and urgency of laparotomy if both types of injury are less dramatic and/or the abdominal findings are normal or equivocal and/or if the whole body CT is not available and/or urgent extra-abdominal surgery is indicated. Ultrasound shows immediately intra-abdominal fluid corresponding to hemorrhage; injury to the parenchymatous organs is often recognized after 24 h that renders sonography useful for follow-ups.

Treatment

Laparotomy in abdominal trauma is indicated in the following conditions:
- Unstable vital signs despite adequate fluid resuscitation
- Transfusion requirements of half and more of the child's blood volume
- Pneumoperitoneum (after exclusion of a trauma to the tracheobronchial tree)

- Peritoneal signs on physical examination
- Abnormal peritoneal lavage effluent
- Gross abdominal distension with arterial hypotension
- Specific intra-abdominal injuries
- Stab and gunshot wounds with peritoneal penetration

Penetrating Abdominal Trauma
It occurs less frequently than blunt trauma although the quoted incidence of 5 % may be much higher depending on the catchment area and part of the world. The penetrating injury leads often to severe hemorrhage and complex organ injury, and the local findings at the site of penetration depend on the used instrument. Whereas in stab wounds the possible injuries depend on the track of the applied corpus delicti and are therefore more or less predictable, in gunshot wounds, the site and extent of intra-abdominal trauma are not predictable #.

After resuscitation, short clinical examination, and torso CT, emergency laparotomy is indicated in gunshot (except for grazing shots) and in stab wounds with signs of major blood loss or peritonitis. All other stab wounds including those of flank and back need only laparotomy or retroperitoneal revision if the wound track extends into the abdominal cavity or the retroperitoneal space. In case of equivocal findings, either peritoneal lavage or diagnostic laparoscopy can be performed to avoid an unnecessary laparotomy.

Surgery includes debridement and excision of the wound tract and repair of the encountered organ and vascular injuries.

16.1.2   Injury of the Kidney

Occurrence, Grading
In blunt abdominal trauma of childhood, renal trauma is observed most frequently because the kidneys are more exposed and mobile in this age group. A blow to the left or right flank or upper and middle belly and rapid deceleration are the mechanisms of direct and indirect impact. Combined involvement of the spleen in up to one quarter in direct trauma and injury to the renovascular bundle or ureteropelvic junction in indirect

trauma are possible consequences. In malformed or tumor kidneys, minor injuries may lead to gross hematuria or retro- or intraperitoneal rupture.

Renal injuries are classified either in minor, major, and complicated types or in five **grades** to which belong a precise description of the pathoanatomical findings. In grades I, II, and III (=minor injuries accounting for about 85 % of all injuries), there is no urinary extravasation and rupture of the collecting system. In grade I, contusion (with only microscopic lesions) or subcapsular hematoma; in grade II, perirenal hematoma or laceration of <1 cm depth; and in grade III, >1 cm depth of renal cortex are observed #. Major injuries are observed in about 10 %; they correspond to grade IV with either laceration of the renal parenchyma from cortex and medulla to the collecting system # and/or renovascular injury to the main artery or vein. Complex or grade V injuries (about 5 %) are a shattered kidney or avulsion of the hilum with devascularization of the kidney (or other severe renovascular injuries, rupture of a single kidney, trauma to a malformed or tumor kidney, and rupture of pelvis or ureter).

Clinical Significance
- Major and complex kidney injuries may lead to the loss of one kidney (or rarely of both kidneys) and to early and late morbidity.
- These impacts are even more life threatening in children with an anatomically or functionally single kidney.
- Symptoms and signs of renal trauma may be the first manifestation of renal malformation or tumor.

Clinical Presentation
Severe pain, tenderness, and guarding concern the involved flank and/or upper and middle belly with possible contusional marks, and in case of a large perirenal hematoma or extravasation of urine, a mass of the flank is visible and palpable. Gross or microscopic hematuria is not necessarily present, and the former correlates only partly with the severity of the injury (the risk of severe renal injury amounts to >70 % in gross hematuria # and only to 10 % [except for renovascular

injury] in microscopic hematuria). On the other hand, already minor trauma is sufficient for gross hematuria in malformed kidneys.

Work-Ups, Differential Diagnosis

Depending on the suspected severity, either contrast CT or color Doppler ultrasound is performed. Renovascular injury must be suspected in case of central hematoma and/or lack of renal enhancement or excretion. Ultrasound can be used in suspected isolated renal trauma with stable general conditions and moderate to mild local findings ##. Doppler ultrasound should be always performed because intima laceration with arterial thrombosis occurs often in children with seemingly minor injury. Urinalysis is useful for confirmation of a possible trauma to the kidney and recognition of an accidental urinary tract infection.

The differential diagnosis has a major significance in minor (or major) trauma to a malformed or tumor kidney that should not be missed.

Treatment, Prognosis

Renal injuries of grades I–III are treated nonoperatively, and grade V and some grade IV need surgery.

In **nonoperative treatment**, close follow-up with ultrasound and urinalysis is necessary. Beginning of enteral nutrition, length of bed rest and hospitalization, and further reevaluation with contrast CT and hematological examinations depend on the clinical symptomatology and development of the original renal injury.

In grade IV injury, early operative treatment (for prevention of related morbidity) or nonoperative treatment (for prevention of nephrectomy) with secondary surgery if needed is controversially discussed. All patients need an i.v. line to deal with paralytic ileus, shock and anemia, and infection (prophylactic antibiotics).

Indications for immediate or early surgery are hemodynamic instability, suspected renovascular injury, fracture of the upper or lower pole with dislocation and diminished vascularization #, and large urine evacuation, and all grade V renal injuries. Intervention for renal fracture and large urine evacuation can be performed a few days after trauma; for urine evacuation, ultrasound-guided catheter drainage is possible.

Surgery: After transabdominal access with colon mobilization, first the vascular peduncle is checked. The main artery and/or vein are repaired (segmental arteries and veins including the left main vein may be ligated if needed). Afterward, Gerota's fascia is opened followed by evacuation of hematomas, debridement of lacerations, ligation of major vessels, and sutures of the collecting system with monofilamentous and absorbable sutures. Finally, closure of renal capsule, if needed with the aid of an absorbable mesh and drainage is performed.

Renovascular injuries belong to two main groups: Children with severe trauma (multisystemic organ injury, renal grade IV or V injuries, penetrating and blunt abdominal trauma) and children with seemingly moderate trauma (isolated renal injury, blunt abdominal trauma). In the second group, intima laceration of the left >right main renal artery has led to a complete or incomplete obliteration of the artery # (this mechanism may be observed in the first group as well in addition to others). In general, a complete occlusion time up to 8 h has a good chance of renal recovery after revascularization. For different reasons, the second group comes mostly too late to surgery.

Prognosis

Early complications are prolonged paralytic ileus, persistent bleeding with ureteric colics and anemia, and urine extravasation, septicemia, and perinephritic abscess.

Diminished renal function, **pseudocyst** of the kidney #, dilatation of the collecting system (e.g., upper calyx syndrome), and arterial hypertension are possible late complications. In contrast to the mostly complete recovery of the kidney in grades I–III lesions, preservation of the kidney or major parts of it is possible in about 80 % of operative cases with good function. **Hypertension** is observed in <5 %.

Because of the possibility of late complications, clinical and sonographic follow-ups should be performed in increasing intervals in grades III–IV injuries without or with surgery up to the puberty #.

Hypertension may be observed already 1 month after trauma and at latest after 15 years. The growth pattern and the morphology of the injured kidney makes possible to estimate the final renal damage and to perform the necessary renal function test.

16.1.3 Injury of the Spleen

Occurrence, Grading, and Types
Among all intra-abdominal organs, the spleen is the most frequently injured (30–40 %).

Involvement of spleen and kidney is observed in up 25 %.

Grading includes five types: In types I–III, the hilus is not involved; the rupture of the capsule is combined with a <1 cm deep, <3 cm, and >3 cm deep laceration of the parenchyma. In grade IV, the hilus is involved too and in grade V, multiple fragmentations and devascularizations correspond to a shattered spleen.

Two-time splenic rupture means a clinically relevant posthemorrhage that is observed a few days up to 1½ month after the trauma and is caused by resolution of the staunching hematoma at the fracture site. Splenic rupture may occur after minor trauma in splenomegaly due to Hodgkin's disease or mononucleosis.

Clinical Significance
- Splenectomy should be avoided whenever possible due to the risk of overwhelming postsplenectomy infection or septicemia (=OPSI) that occurs in 1.5 % and has a mortality of 50 % if prophylactic measures are not taken.

Clinical Presentation
The history yields often a blow to the left lower thoracic cage, left upper abdomen, or flank, and *the children may complain of left upper quadrant or shoulder pain. In addition to possible contusional marks, the left upper belly displays tenderness and guarding on percussion and palpation.*

Work-Ups, Differential Diagnosis
In severe multisystemic organ injury and isolated abdominal trauma, contrast CT of the abdomen should be performed. In not urgent or moderate or slight trauma, ultrasound with subsequent follow-ups on the second day and thereafter may be sufficient ##.

If plain abdominal x-ray has been performed, displacement of stomach and left colonic flexure, absent splenic shadow, and left lower rib fractures are possible indications of splenic rupture.

In suspected injury of the spleen, the possibility of diaphragmatic rupture and/or left lower lobe lung contusion must be considered, especially in indistinct delineation of the diaphragmatic contour and abnormal position of the tip of a gastic tube on routine plain x-rays and/or in rib fractures, tachypnea and dyspnea.

Unexpected splenic rupture in splenomegaly leads to left upper abdominal pain. It is observed in several other disorders, for instance, in intestinal incarceration of a left-sided or bilateral Morgagni hernia that has not been recognized hitherto.

Treatment, Prognosis
With blood replacement and close clinical and radiological follow-up, nonoperative treatment may be possible in >90 %.

Indications for surgery are transfusion requirement of half or more of the child's blood volume and/or severe involvement of the hilus or shattered spleen (grades VI and V), multisystemic organ injury with the need of urgent extra-abdominal surgery, or coagulopathy.

Surgery: If technically possible and not too time-consuming, splenorrhaphy (by sutures or wrapping) or segmental resection is performed #. For reconstructive surgery and splenectomy, mobilization is necessary by incision of all splenic attachments, and continuous blood loss can be avoided by temporary compression of the hilus with the fingers. In segmental resection at least one third of the spleen should be preserved to avoid OPSI. Prevention of OPSI needs appropriate vaccination (polyvalent pneumococcal vaccination with booster doses after 3 years) and chemoprophylaxis (aminopenicillin) or presumptive medication in adolescence in case of infection.

Hospitalization depends on the severity of spleen injury, its treatment, and associated injuries. Left-sided hemorrhagic pleural effusion and two-time splenic rupture belong to the early complications. The former needs evacuation by pleural punction or tube thoracostomy if symptomatic and the latter surgery with preservation of the spleen.

Because of the possibility of development of a **pseudocyst** of the spleen, long-term clinical and sonographic follow-up is necessary after nonoperative treatment of severe spleen rupture with gross hematoma.

16.1.4 Injury of the Liver

Occurrence, Grading

If slight types of liver injury with increase of liver enzymes and without sonographic findings are included, liver trauma has the same frequency as spleen injury. In >50 % of liver trauma, multisystemic organ injury is observed of which right lung contusion and hemopneumothorax are particularly tricky because they may mask liver trauma.

Clinical Significance

- Liver injury leads more frequently to a life-threatening hemorrhage than the other visceral organs.
- Severe liver injury is the main cause of lethality in abdominal trauma.
- After nonoperative and operative treatment, significant complications may occur.

Clinical Presentation

A blow to the right side or front of the lower thoracic cage, to the right upper quadrant or flank may be recorded in the history combined with *a visible corresponding contusional mark. Right upper abdominal pain with possible radiation to the right shoulder, tenderness, and guarding on percussion and palpation with possible extension to the left side are the main clinical findings. Abdominal distension with dullness on percussion that persists in spite of introduction of a nasogastric tube points to a possible trauma to the liver.*

Work-Ups

Contrast CT is the first-line examination, whereas ultrasound is useful for initial screening (confirmation and estimation of amount of hemoperito-neum) and follow-up in nonoperative treatment. Of the laboratory tests, hemoglobin, coagulation factors, liver enzymes, bilirubin, alkaline phosphatase, amylase, lipase, and cross-reaction of blood preserve are important.

Treatment

The majority of liver injuries can be treated nonoperatively in children if the already quoted conditions for intra-abdominal bleedings are met, anemia and coagulation disorders have been treated effectively from the beginning, and the precise type of injury is known.

Surgery is indicated in blood requirement of half or more of the child's blood volume and/or in injury to the retrohepatic vessels (inferior vena cava, hepatic veins = grade V) and avulsion of the liver (grade VI). For grading, see Fig. 16.1.

Surgery: Appropriate sites of i.v. lines should be available above the diaphragm. After a midline abdominal incision (with possible extension to a midline sternotomy), the free blood is sucked away and temporary control of the bleeding is performed before evaluation of the rupture site (manual compression or packing of the bleeding site, compression of aorta at the hiatus, or Pringle maneuver [occlusion of the porta hepatis by a vascular clamp]). Afterward, debridement, ligation of large vessels, staunching of diffuse bleeding (by cauterization or hemostatic fleeces), and drainage is performed.

In permanent and severe bleeding (e.g., in large lobar fractures or extensive disruptions of parenchyma including major vessels) and/or grade V and VI types of injury, complete mobilization and medial reflection of the liver and total vascular occlusion are necessary, or alternatively a caval shunt (sternotomy for introduction of a supradiaphragmatic and mobilization of right colonic flexure and Kocher maneuver of an infradiaphragmatic caval vascular loop and caval shunt).

Except for limited segmental resection of devascularized liver tissue, major liver resection is usually not performed in the acute stage.

Prognosis for survival depends on the time between trauma and appropriate treatment, the severity of the initial liver trauma, and the postoperative complications.

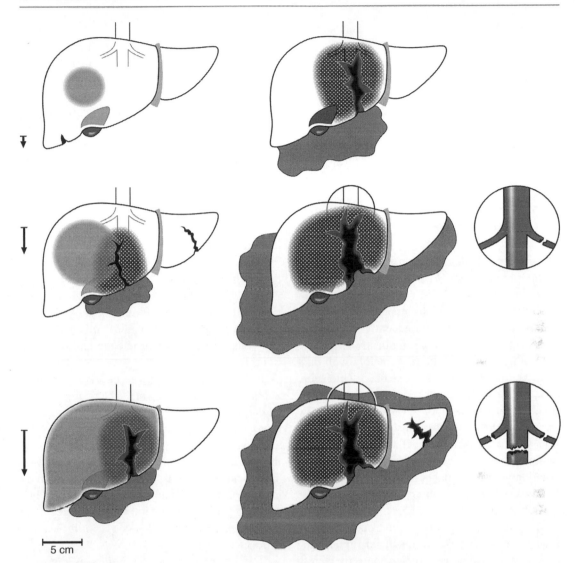

Fig. 16.1 Grading of liver injury from the *top* on the *left side* to the *bottom* on the *right side*. Classification uses degree of hematoma and laceration in the lower grades and laceration and vascular injury in the higher grades to describe the severity. In the *left row*, the drawing at the *top* corresponds to **grade I** and includes a subcapsular hematoma of <10 % of the surface area and/or a capsular tear of <1 cm depth, in the *middle* corresponds to **grade II**, and includes a subcapsular hematoma of 10–50 % of the surface area, an intraparenchymal hematoma <10 cm in diameter, and/or capsular tear of 1–3 cm depth and <10 cm length with active bleeding, at the *bottom* corresponds to **grade III** and the subcapsular hematoma includes >50 % of the surface area or is expanding, a ruptured subcapsular or intraparenchymatous hematoma with active bleeding, and/or a laceration of >3 cm depth. In the *right row* at the *top*, grade **IV injury** is depicted: It includes an intraparenchymatous ruptured hematoma and/or parenchymal disruption that involves 25–75 % of hepatic lobe or 1–3 segments within a lobe; in the *middle*, **grade V** injury is depicted: The parenchymal disruption involves >75 % of hepatic lobe or >3 segments and juxtahepatic venous injury (central major hepatic veins or retrohepatic vena cava), and at the **bottom grade VI** in which avulsion of the liver has occurred

The latter are mainly responsible for the postoperative morbidity.

Coagulopathy and metabolic disorder of albumin and glucose, infection, and accumulation of bile at the site of injury and in the peritoneum belong to the early complications. **Hemobilia** is an intermediate or late complication: Recurrent bleeding in the depth of the liver is responsible for it that leads to evacuation of blood into the gastrointestinal tract by the bilious tract. Hematemesis or drainage of blood by the nasogastric tube, recurrent abdominal pain and icterus, and/or passage of blood by the anus are the clinical presentations. Selective arteriography is used to determine the site of the bleeding artery; selective embolization or resection of the involved segment is necessary to cure the complication.

16.1.5 Injuries of Pancreas and Duodenum

Occurrence, Types
Although injuries of pancreas and duodenum occur in general much less frequently than trauma to kidney, spleen, and liver, pancreatic trauma occurs somewhat more frequently in children than in adults and is more frequently associated with other abdominal injuries, mainly with duodenal trauma due to its close spatial relationship.

Grading in four types permits a quick description and comparison of severity of pancreatic injuries. Grade I means contusion without laceration of the main duct, grade II and III transsection with possible duct laceration, and grade IV combination with duodenal trauma. Complete laceration is less frequently observed in children.

Duodenal contusion leads to an intramural hematoma that may obstruct the duodenal passage for a few weeks. In duodenal rupture, the intraperitoneal type is observed more frequently than the retroperitoneal.

Clinical Significance
• Recognition of injuries of pancreas and duodenum may be difficult. Therefore, it must be looked for in case of minimal suspicion up to the proof of the contrary.
• Injuries of pancreas and duodenum may lead to several complications of which some are time-consuming or even life threatening.

Clinical Presentation
A history of a perpendicular or oblique impact to the epigastrium that squeezes the pancreas or parts of it against the spine or posterior abdominal wall arouses the suspicion of possible pancreatic trauma. Typical examples are impacted by a handlebar of a bicycle or punch to the epigastrium.

On clinical examination, a contusional mark of the region of the navel #, tenderness, and guarding may be observed in the upper median abdomen that corresponds to site of abdominal pain. Later, the findings may migrate to the back or whole belly in case of pancreatitis or bilious peritonitis.

Complications include posttraumatic pancreatitis, pseudocyst of the pancreas, duodenal hematoma, bilious peritonitis, rarely laceration of the main pancreatic or obstruction of the common bile duct, and left-sided pleural effusion. Not all children have a specific clinical presentation, and in all of them, it must be looked for by laboratory tests and radiological imaging in the follow-up of suspected pancreatic and duodenal injuries.

In **posttraumatic pancreatitis**, persistent abdominal pain radiating in the back or migrating in the lower abdomen and mainly continuously increased or increasing values of serum amylase and lipase and fluid accumulation in and around the pancreas on ultrasound are diagnostic. Treatment consists of continuous drainage by a nasogastroduodenal tube, fluid and electrolyte replacement, and parenteral nutrition except for necrotizing pancreatitis that needs antibiotics and if infected surgery.

The **pseudocyst of the pancreas** develops within the first 3–4 weeks after trauma. It is best recognized by follow-ups with ultrasound before clinical manifestation occurs.

By similar treatment options as in posttraumatic pancreatitis, the natural course may be affected positively, or the cyst is drained by ultrasound- or CT-guided percutaneous intervention if a critical size is reached or no signs of spontaneous involution are evident. Drainage has a reliable chance of permanent cyst collapse.

Space-occupying effect on the gastric outlet with vomiting or on renal artery with hypertension, perforation into the peritoneum with chemical peritonitis, life-threatening spontaneous hemorrhage (selective arteriography and embolization of bleeding arteries are diagnostic and therapeutic options if the superior mesenteric or splenic artery is not involved), and abscess are possible complications that may be possibly avoided by early drainage as well as by internalization of the mature cyst that does not respond to catheter drainage.

In contrast to advanced pseudocysts of the pancreas, most **pancreaticoduodenal fistulas** heal by the same nonsurgical treatment as in pancreatitis. **Left-sided pleural effusion** needs tube thoracostomy if large.

In **duodenal hematoma,** that is recognizable by ultrasound, upper gastroduodenal contrast study (coiled-spring signs), or contrast CT, vomiting occurs or the gastrointestinal content drained by a nasogastric tube does not decrease with time, and/or the start of enteral nutrition is impossible. The obstruction disappears under TPN within few weeks.

Work-Ups

The sensitivity of ultrasound to recognize **pancreatic injury** is with 70 % less than contrast CT with at least 90 %. **Ultrasound** is more suitable for follow-ups with resolution of contusion and temporarily dilated main duct as indirect sign of obstruction, or development of the already quoted complications including duodenal hematoma.

Determination of **serum amylase and lipase**, calcium, glucose, liver enzymes, bilirubin, alkaline phosphatase, and hematological examinations is used either as adjunct of diagnosis with elevated or short-term increasing values or as starting point of developing complications such as posttraumatic pancreatitis. Unfortunately, normal findings of amylase are found in spite of pancreatic injury, and elevated values may be caused by other disorders, for example, trauma to the salivary glands in craniofacial injury in the first posttraumatic hours.

If **plain abdominal x-ray** has been performed, effacement of the psoas shadow and air around the right kidney or at an unusual site may point to **duodenal perforation**. In the latter type of trauma, CT with contrast applied by a nasogastric tube and egress of contrast from the duodenum is more suitable.

If obstruction of the **common bile duct or laceration of the main duct** is suspected, **ERCP or MRI** with cholangiopancreaticography should performed before surgery.

Treatment, Prognosis

Injuries of pancreas and duodenum are treated in children mostly expectantly with nasogastric tube, fluid and electrolyte replacement, and TPN **except for** type IV pancreatic injuries, duodenal perforation, common bile duct obstruction, or main duct laceration.

If **surgery** is indicated or performed within the context of multisystemic organ injury, it is or may be necessary to evaluate pancreas and duodenum step by step: Localized emphysema or bilious imbibition may point to a trauma. Palpation of the head of pancreas and duodenum through the foramen of Winslow and inspection of the pancreas after division of the gastrocolic ligament, of the head of pancreas and proximal duodenum by a Kocher maneuvre, and of the distal duodenum after release of the cecal and small intestinal mesentery are performed.

Type IV injury needs depending on the severity of pancreas and duodenal trauma either diverticularization of the duodenum with proximal disconnection, vagotomy, distal gastrectomy and Billroth II reconstruction, and drainage of duodenum, gallbladder and the site of surgery or a pyloric exclusion procedure, and only rarely total pancreatoduodenectomy. Distal pancreatectomy is performed in case of **disruption of the main duct** beyond the superior mesenteric artery including ligation of the duct, inversion of the edges of the pancreas with nonabsorbable sutures, drainage, and preservation of the spleen. **Duodenal perforation** needs immediate debridement and suture.

Lethality is usually related to multisystemic organ injury or complications. Early complications are posttraumatic pancreatitis, especially the necrotizing and infected variation and the development of a pancreas pseudocyst (autodigestion of pancreas and fatty tissue leads to confluent tissue necrosis and liquefaction that is encapsulated by granulations tissue) with the inherent complications or a pancreaticoduodenal fistula.

If a posttraumatic or any other pancreatitis is not recognized, the possible development of a **pseudocyst** is not considered until its manifestation as a visible and/or palpable abdominal tumor with nausea, vomiting, epigastric pain and compression of the adjacent organs, peritonitis, intra-abdominal abscess, or hemorrhage.

Except for severe types, pancreas and duodenal trauma have a favorable outcome.

16.1.6 Perforations of the Gastrointestinal Tract

Occurrence, Etiopathogenesis, Pathoanatomy
This type of organ injury occurs less frequently than those of parenchymatous abdominal organs. Perforation of the stomach is observed more frequently in children than in adults.

Stomach: Rupture is mainly observed if the impact occurs in a full stomach or by forceful introduction of a nasogastric tube, overinflation in reanimation, or introduction of anesthesia, etc. Endoscopy must also be considered as cause of injury. Traumatic ruptures occur particularly at the greater curvature close to the fundus.

Small intestine: Intestinal rupture is one possible injury of the lap belt complex (intestinal and lumbar spine injury) and must be considered in child abuse with blows to the belly #. Intestinal impact may be followed by rupture or contusion with delayed rupture or intestinal stenosis at the site of decreased vascularization. Rupture occurs mainly at the antimesenteric site and proximal to the ligament of Treitz, in the middle of small intestine or in its distal part. In contusion, the secondary rupture occurs few days and intestinal stenosis approximately 1 month after trauma leading to obstructive or posttraumatic ileus due to adhesions.

Colon and rectum: Traumatic perforation occurs less often than in small intestine and mostly by penetrating abdominal trauma or by endoscopy, reduction of intussusception (small bowel and colon), forceful enemas, etc. Rectal injuries occur by impalement injuries or sexual abuse and are often combined with trauma to the

perineum and vagina. Perforation of the extraperitoneal part must be considered specifically.

Clinical Significance
- Perforations of the gastrointestinal tract should be treated as soon as possible because they lead unavoidably to peritonitis or pararectal abscess and possibly to septicemia.
- The possibility of delayed perforation or obstructive ileus should be considered in the management of patients with a history of possible injury to the gastrointestinal tract.

Clinical Findings
Specific informations from the history and a contusional mark of the belly are often the only indications of a possible gastrointestinal perforation. The sites of such ecchymoses, abrasions, or wounds correspond to the site of perforation in colonic and gastric lesions and less in small bowel perforation. A bloody tip of a gastric tube may be an indication of perforation.

Pneumoperitoneum is not observed in all perforations. In general, the more proximal the perforation is, the more probable is a pneumoperitoneum. *The epigastrium or belly becomes grossly enlarged and tympanitic on percussion.*

Signs of peritonitis are not present at the beginning and develop within 24 h or are only minimal due to encapsulation of the perforation site. *The abdominal pain, tenderness, and guarding on percussion and palpation are diffusely or localized.* These signs are delayed in secondary perforation by several days.

Perineal and perianal contusions and lacerations, or hemorrhage from anus or vagina, point to a colonic perforation which can be felt or suspected by gentle rectal examination (blood at the finger tip, palpable rectal wall hematoma, or interruption of its continuity).

Work-Ups, Differential Diagnosis
Plain abdominal x-ray in lateral recumbent or upright position # may show intra-abdominal air. In suspected gastric perforation, visualization is possible by insufflation of air through the nasogastric tube.

As in the former examination, CT shows often no air. Peritoneal fluid and enhancement of the intestinal wall at the site of perforation indicate in absence of parenchymatous abdominal organ injury intestinal perforation.

In suspected rectal injury, rectosigmoidoscopy is the first-line examination; it should be combined with colposcopy in girls.

The differential diagnosis plays only a role in delayed perforation or posttraumatic obstructive ileus. A history of antecedent abdominal trauma and an abdominal scar are the most important informations for differentiation from other causes of surgical abdomen.

Treatment, Prognosis

It includes immediate triple antibiotic medication and laparotomy with debridement of the site of perforation, closure (or segmental resection if needed), and drainage of the site of perforation. A gastric or gastroduodenal tube eliminates the accumulating gastrointestinal fluid till resolution of paralytic ileus.

In rectal injury, debridement and primary closure are performed either by the transanal route or by laparotomy (in case of perforation above the peritoneal reflection) combined with presacral drainage and in severe cases with a diverting colostomy, revision of the rectal injury, and suture of a possible vaginal tear.

Prognosis depends on the promptness of treatment and the cause of injury. The risk of postoperative ileus due to adhesion is increased similar to other causes of peritonitis. Severe rectal injuries lead possibly to early infectious complications such as pararectal abscess and late sequels, for instance, fecal incontinence and stenosis of anus, introitus, and vagina.

16.1.7 Injuries to the Diaphragm or Pelvis

Occurrence, Clinical Significance

Injuries of the diaphragm and/or pelvis must be considered always in severe abdominal trauma.

Pelvic fractures may be observed in up to one fifth of severe blunt abdominal trauma and diaphragmatic injury somewhat less frequently. The clinical significance is as follows:

- Both injuries must be excluded deliberately in every severe trauma of the torso although some findings may indicate them as quoted below.
- Diaphragmatic rupture may lead to tachypnea and dyspnea and pelvic fracture to severe occult hemorrhage with shock, and both clinical presentations can lead to an erroneously interpretation in the context of abdominal and thoracic trauma.

Clinical Presentation

A history of direct and forceful blow to the lower chest or upper abdomen on one side, a corresponding contusional mark, and decreased breath and unexpected intestinal sounds in the lower chest and some findings on routine chest x-ray point to a possible **diaphragmatic rupture.** Such findings are effacement or elevation of the diaphragmatic contour, intrathoracic site of a nasogastric tube, atypical pneumothorax or gas pattern, and plate-like atelectasis in the lower lung field. Diaphragmatic rupture may escape clinical recognition. Herniation of stomach or intestine through the rupture site is confirmed by contrast application and of the spleen only by CT.

In **pelvic fracture**, a fall from the height or an overrunning motor vehicle accident, contusional marks and hematomas of the suprapubic region, below the iliac crest, and at the external genitals are possible findings. Anterior and lateral compression and palpation of the pelvis on rectal examination may be painful, and a pelvic mass corresponding to a hematoma may be felt. Blood at the external urethral meatus, difficult or impossible bladder catheterization, and elevation of the prostate in boys at rectal examination are indications of a pelvic fracture complicated by urethral rupture.

The main clinical significance for blunt abdominal trauma is the possibility of major hemorrhage associated with pelvic fracture and its persistence in case of instability. A routine abdominal x-ray that includes the pelvis permits a preliminary diagnosis.

Treatment

In diaphragmatic rupture, early transabdominal reduction of possibly herniated stomach, intestine, or spleen and debridement and overlapping closure of the diaphragmatic injury with two rows of nonabsorbable sutures are necessary to correct the associated morbidity and avoid delayed surgery with the inherent difficulties because of posttraumatic adhesions.

In pelvic fracture, external fixation is necessary in case of instability in addition to blood replacement and possible arteriography with selective embolization of bleeding arterial vessels.

16.2 Foreign Bodies of the Gastrointestinal Tract

Occurrence

Infants, toddlers, retarded children, or those with psychiatric disorders, and even every child may swallow every object that they stick in the mouth and that is not too large (foreign body ingestion).

If the foreign bodies have reached the stomach, about the majority of them pass the gastrointestinal tract and are evacuated by the anus without any sequels.

Clinical Significance

- Nevertheless, all children with a history of a swallowed foreign body need clinical and possibly radiological follow-up.
- All disabled or children with psychiatric disorders (e.g., with self-mutilation) and with a large foreign body (e.g., pocketknife) must be referred to a tertiary care center for treatment and evaluation of the underlying cause.

Clinical Presentation

Large objects including trichobezoar (in trichotillomania) # lead to a voiding disorder of the stomach with vomiting and impossibility of food intake.

Some foreign bodies may get stuck in the duodenum (e.g., coins), at the level of Treitz ligament, somewhere in the small intestine (e.g., not chewed fresh fruits [pieces of mandarin] or swelling up of dried fruits), in the ileocecal region including appendix (e.g., pins or toothpicks) #, or at the site of congenital or acquired stenoses or evaginations of the intestine. The foreign bodies may lead to complete obstruction of the intestine, to a pressure score of the intestinal wall, and/or to a direct perforation with signs of obstructive ileus or localized peritonitis.

All in all, up to 99 % of all foreign bodies pass the gastrointestinal tract within <1 month without any symptoms and signs.

Work-Ups, Differential Diagnosis

In addition to a careful history and clinical examination of the oral cavity, neck (observation of swallowing), and belly (signs of obstructive ileus or peritonitis) by the pediatrician or general practitioner, the parents should check every stool for the swallowed foreign body.

If no spontaneous evacuation of the foreign body is observed, plain abdominal x-ray should be performed to recognize the foreign body and its possible site or to exclude it, although its evacuation has not been observed by the parents (compliance).

The differential diagnosis of obstructive ileus or peritonitis must always consider a complicated swallowed foreign body because the history of a swallowed foreign body may not be remembered or foreign body ingestion has not been observed by the caregivers.

Treatment

Foreign bodies of stomach and duodenum should be removed by endoscopy immediately if they are dangerous (e.g., button battery) or delayed if they remained there longer than 1 week. Large gastroduodenal objects # and complicated foreign bodies of the small intestine need urgent enterotomy by laparotomy or laparoscopy and after 1 week if symptomless.

Outcome is mostly uneventful except for complicated foreign bodies.

Webcodes

The following webcodes can be used on www. psurg.net for further images and data.

1601 Gunshot injury, evisceration	1611 Grade III splenic injury, ultrasound
1602 Grade III renal injury, arteriography	1612 Grade III splenic injury, CT
1603 Grade IV renal injury, CT	1613 Grade III splenic injury, operative finding
1604 Hematuria in renal injury	1614 Contusional mark
1605 Grade II renal injury, ultrasound	1615 Jejunal perforation, child abuse
1606 Grade II renal injury, follow-up	1616 Pneumoperitoneum, lateral recumbent position
1607 Grade III renal injury, devitalized part	1617 Trichobezoar, stomach
1608 Thrombotic obstruction renal artery(arteriography)	1618 Pin, perforation appendix
1609 Renal pseudocyst after grade IV injury	1619 Metallic foreign bodies, stomach
1610 Upper calix syndrome after grade III injury	

Bibliography

Section 16.1 Textbook Articles, Occurrence, Injury Grading, Radiological Imaging, Treatment

Baka AG, Delgado CA, Simon HK (2002) Current use and perceived utility of ultrasound for evaluation of pediatric compared with adult trauma patients. Pediatr Emerg Care 18:163–167

Eichelberger MR, Moront M (1998) Abdominal trauma. In: O'Neill JA Jr et al (eds) Pediatric surgery, vol I, 5th edn. Mosby, St. Louis

Gaines BA (2009) Intra-abdominal solid organ injury in children: diagnosis and treatment. J Trauma 67(2 Suppl):135–139

Holmes JF, Gladman A, Chang CH (2007) Performance of abdominal ultrasonography in pediatric blunt trauma patients: a meta-analysis. J Pediatr Surg 42:1588–1594

Kiankhooy A, Sartorelli KH, Vane DW, Bhave AD (2010) Angiographic embolization is safe and effective therapy for blunt abdominal solid injury in children. J Trauma 68:526–531

Knudson MM, Maull KI (1999) Nonoperative management of solid organ injuries. Past, present, and future. Surg Clin North Am 79:1357–1371

Moore EE, Shackford SR, Pachter HL et al (1989) Organ injury scaling: spleen, liver, and kidney. J Trauma 29:1664–1666

Ozturk H, Dokucu AI, Onen A, Otcu S, Gedik S, Azal OF (2004) Non-operative management if isolated solid organ injuries due to blunt abdominal trauma in children: a fifteen-year experience. Eur J Pediatr Surg 14:29–34

Schroeppel TJ, Croce MA (2007) Diagnosis and management of blunt abdominal solid organ injury. Curr Opin Crit Care 13:399–404

Wang MY, Kim KA, Griffith PM, Summers S, McComb JG, Levy ML, Mahour GH (2001) Injuries from falls in the pediatric population: an analysis of 729 cases. J Pediatr Surg 36:1528–1534

Yen K, Gorelick MH (2002) Ultrasound application for pediatric emergency department: a review of the current literature. Pediatr Emerg Care 18:226–234

Section 16.1.2

Carvajal MI, Müller C, Kaiser G (1993) Operative versus konservative Behandlung der kindlichen Milzverletzung – Aufwand und Ausgang. Chir Gastroenterol 9(suppl 2):139–141

Perez-Brayfield MR, Gatti JM, Smith EA et al (2002) Blunt traumatic hematuria in children: is a simplified algorithm justified? J Urol 167:2543–2547

Section 16.1.3

Hansen K, Singer DB (2001) Asplenic-hyposplenic overwhelming sepsis: postsplenectomy sepsis revisited. Pediatr Dev Pathol 4:105–121

Mühlemann K, Francioli P (2000) Die Prävention von Pneumokokkeninfektionen durch die Impfung. Schweiz Aerztezeitung 81:554–560

Styllianos S (2002) Compliance with evidence-based guidelines in children with isolated spleen or liver injury: a prospective study. J Pediatr Surg 37:453–456

Section 16.1.4

Badger SA, Barclay R, Campbell P, Mole DJ, Diamond T (2009) Management of liver trauma. World J Surg 33:2522–2537

Ciraulo DL, Luk S, Palter M, Cowell V, Welch J, Cortes V, Orlando R, Banever T (1998) Selective hepatic arterial embolization of grade IV and V blunt hepatic injuries: an extension of resuscitation in the nonoperative management of traumatic hepatic injuries. J Trauma 45:353–358; discussion 358-359

Feichter S, Esslinger P, Schwöbel M-G (2011) Ausgedehnte Leberruptur mit Ver-letzung der Gallenwege Auch im Kindesalter nicht immer eine Operationsindikation. Schweiz Med Forum 11:142–143

Landau A, van As AB, Numanoglu A, Millar AJ, Rode H (2006) Liver injuries in children: the role of selective non-operative management. Injury 37:66–71

Moore EE, Cogbill TH, Jurkovitch GJ, Shackford SR, Malangoni MA, Champion HR (1995) Organ injury scaling – spleen, liver (1994 rev). J Trauma 38: 323–324

Stracieri LD, Scarpelini S (2006) Hepatic injury. Acta Cir Bras 21(Suppl 1):85–88

Nellensteijn D, Porte RJ, van Zuuren W, ten Duis HJ, Hulscher JBF (2009) Paediatric blunt liver trauma in a Dutch level 1 trauma center. Eur J Pediatr Surg 19:358–361

Section 16.1.5

Jobst MA, Canty TG, Lynch FP (1999) Management of pancreatic injury in pediatric blunt abdominal trauma. J Pediatr Surg 34:818–824

Karagüzel G, Senocak ME, Büyükpamukcu N, Hicsönmez A (1995) Surgical management of pancreatic pseudocyst in children: a long term evaluation. J Pediatr Surg 30:777–780

Keller MS, Stafford PW, Vane DW (1997) Conservative management of pancreatic trauma in children. J Trauma 42:1079–1100

Linsenmaier U, Wirth S, Reiser M, Körner M (2008) Diagnosis and classification of pancreatic and duodenal injuries in emergency radiology. Radiographics 28:1591–1602

Patty I, Kalaoui M, Al-Shamali M, Al-Hassan F, Al-Naqeeb B (2001) Endoscopic drainage for pancreatic pseudocyst in children. J Pediatr Surg 36:503–505

Rosenthal R, Vogelbach P (2001) Posttraumatische Pankreaspseudozyste beim Kind (Posttraumatic Pancreatic Pseudocyst in children – case report and discussion). Swiss Surg 7:225–228

Sections 16.1.6–16.1.7

Galifer RB, Forgues D, Mourregot A, Guibal MP, Allal H, Mekki M, Rized D (2001) Blunt traumatic injuries of the gastrointestinal and biliary tract in childhood. Analysis of 16 cases. Eur J Pediatr Surg 11:230–234

Kim SH, Shin SS, Jeong YY, Heo SH, Kim JW, Kang HK (2009) Gastrointestinal tract perforation: MDCT finding according to the perforation sites. Korean J Radiol 10:63–70

Williams H (2006) Perforation–how to spot free intraperitoneal air on abdominal radiograph. Arch Dis Child Educ Pract Ed 91:ep54–ep57

Section 16.1.7

Scharff JR, Naunheim KS (2007) Traumatic diaphragmatic injuries. Thorac Surg Clin 17:81–85

Shehata SM, Shabaan BS (2006) Diaphragmatic injuries in children after blunt abdominal trauma. J Pediatr Surg 41:1727–1731

Section 16.2

Arana A et al (2001) Management of ingested foreign bodies in childhood and review of the literature. Eur J Pediatr 160:468–472

Chronic Abdominal Pain

Occurrence

Chronic abdominal pain is a frequent cause of medical consultation. One possible definition is recurrent abdominal pain that lasts during more than 3 months. Nevertheless, conditions which last less than this period must be considered in the differential diagnosis as well. An organic cause can be discovered only in less than 20 %.

Clinical Significance

- It is a challenge to recognize those patients with chronic abdominal pain in whom an organic cause is responsible.
- Therefore, it happens relatively frequently that even pathologies with a significant morbidity are not recognized for a long time because evaluation is focused on the chronic abdominal pain and its probable functional origin.

Clinical Presentation

Waking up at night, precise description and anatomically compatible sites, radiation, and possible triggering mechanisms of pain, and associated symptoms, signs, and local findings are characteristics for organic abdominal pain. Anamnestic important criteria are familiality of some disorders and informations about the occurrence of abdominal pain (e.g., before or during menstruation in developed girls) or previous surgery.

Examples of associated signs and local findings are vomiting and its content, passage of blood by the anus, change of defecation habits and stool consistency, dysuria, hematuria, and primary amenorrhea, weight loss, growth arrest, or anemia and inflammatory blood signs, localized tenderness and guarding, abdominal wall scar, observation of the patient at the moment of abdominal pain (e.g., presentation of specific body position such as knee-elbow position in intestinal volvulus), and abnormal findings at general examination (e.g., anal fissure).

Imperforate hymen is a relatively frequent and characteristic example of congenital or acquired gynatresia which leads to chronic abdominal pain and is associated with other characteristic findings: The pain is acute, recurrent, and abdominopelvic and occurs in schoolchildren and specifically in adolescents at the time of menarche which does not occur, and the pain may be associated with disorders of micturition (e.g., acute urinary retention).

Differential Diagnosis, Work-Ups

The surgically relevant pathologies leading to chronic abdominal pain are described among the presenting symptoms and signs of the thoracic, abdominal, and urogenital compartments, and some are listed in Table 17.1. The differential diagnosis must consider functional pain according to the Rom II criteria. It concerns mostly children older than 4 years; the pain is vague and poorly localized and misses the criteria of organic abdominal pain quoted above. According to pediatric gastroenterologists, 80 % of all children with chronic abdominal pain have functional or dysfunctional disorders; they occur mainly in

Table 17.1 Surgically relevant pathologies leading to chronic abdominal pain

o Morgagni and Bochdalek's	● Recurrent testicular torsion
Diaphragmatic hernia #	● Intermittent PUJ obstruction #
● Gastroesophageal reflux	o Nephrolithiasis
	● Cystitis
o Epigastric hernia	o Other Urological malformations
● Recurrent inguinal hernia	
o Rare abdominal wall, pelvic floor, and internal hernias	● Imperforate hymen #
o Primary peptic ulcer	● Torsion of ovarian cyst/tumor
o Chronic pancreatitis	● Premenstrual syndrome
o Cholelithiasis	o Endometriosis
o Adult type of choledochal cyst	o Other gynatresias (muco-/hematometrocolpos)
o Liver echinococcosis	
o Obstructive ileus due to postoperative adhesions	● Primary dysmenorrhea
● Disorders of intestinal rotation and fixation	
o Chronic intestinal pseudoobstruction	
o Crohn's disease	
o Chronic recurrent Appendicitis	
o Constipation	
o Sickle cell disease #	

schoolchildren (5–15 years of age) and disappear in 30–50 % within several weeks after the first consultation. But in some children, they continue up to adolescence and adulthood.

The work-ups depend on the suspected organic cause.

Webcodes

The following webcodes can be used on www. psurg.net for further images and data.

1701 Chronic abdominal pain ending up with surgical abdomen	1704 Chronic recurrent abdominal pain, normal IVU and IVU
1702 Incarcerated left colonic flexure, Bochdalek's hernia	1705 After fluid load, intermittent pyeloureteral junction obstruction
1703 Splenic infarctions, sickle cell disease	1706 Chronic lower abdominal pain, imperforate hymen

Bibliography

Cleckner-Smith CS, Doughty AS, Grossman JA (1998) Premenstrual symptoms: prevalence and severity in an adolescent sample. J Adolesc Health 22:403–408

Corazziari E (2004) The Rome criteria for functional gastrointestinal disorders: a critical reappraisal. J Pediatr Gastroenterol Nutr 39:S754–S755

Davis AR, Westhoff CL (2001) Primary dysmenorrhea in adolescent girls and treatment with oral contraceptives. J Pediatr Adolesc Gynecol 14:1–2

Miele E, Simeone D, Marino A et al (2004) Functional gastrointestinal disorders in children: an Italian prospective study. Pediatrics 114:73–78

Thakkar K, Chen L, Tatevian N, Shulman RJ, McDuffie A, Tsou M, Gilger MA, El-Serag HB (2009) Diagnostic yield of oesophagogastroduodenoscopy in children with abdominal pain. Aliment Pharmacol Ther 30:662–669

Disorders of the Abdominal Wall Recognizable from the Outside (Excluding Abdominal Wall Hernias)

Depending on the region of the world, malformations of the abdominal wall are present already at prenatal ultrasound examination and the remainder shortly after birth.

Abdominal wall defects of the midline combined with abdominal eviscerations and abnormal findings during the physiological healing process of the navel are the presenting signs.

The prevalence of these malformations is different and extends from frequent ≥1: 1,000 live births to relatively frequent ≥1:5,000, to rare ≥1:10,000, and to very rare ≥1:50,000. This phenomenon of variable prevalence applies to all anomalies. Reliable figures can demonstrate changes in occurrence of single malformation and permit epidemiological conclusions. In the last decades, an increased prevalence has been observed in gastroschisis all over the world that is an important pathology in the differential diagnosis of abdominal wall malformations (Table 18.1).

Table 18.1 Differential diagnosis of disorders of the abdominal wall (excluding abdominal wall hernias)

- Pathologies of the umbilicus
  - Variations of normal healing process
  - Umbilical granuloma and omphalitis
  - Omphalomesenteric and urachal duct remnants
  - Miscellaneous congenital and acquired disorders of navel
- Gastroschisis and omphalocele
- Bladder exstrophy
- Vesicointestinal fissure (cloacal exstrophy)

18.1 Pathologies of the Navel (Excluding Umbilical Hernia)

Disorders of the umbilicus are frequent. They concern mostly the natural healing process of the navel and less frequently congenital abnormalities.

Separation of the umbilical stump occurs at a mean age of 2 weeks (3 days to 2 months) with 10 % after the third week. It leaves a granulomatous surface of 1–10-mm diameter behind that epithelizes usually in a few days.

Depending on the location of the limit between abdominal wall skin and umbilical cord surface, different types of navel may be observed in the newborn. In contrast to the usually encountered type with a limit at the level of the abdominal wall, the normal skin covers a small part of the cord (cutis navel #), or a small circular rim around the navel is not covered by skin (amniotic navel). Spontaneous correction of the two last-mentioned types occurs in infancy.

18.1.1 Umbilical Granuloma, Omphalitis

Occurrence
Large and persistent umbilical granulomas are observed frequently, whereas omphalitis has become rare (<1 % of live births) in developed but not in third world countries.

G.L. Kaiser, *Symptoms and Signs in Pediatric Surgery*, DOI 10.1007/978-3-642-31161-1_18, © Springer-Verlag Berlin Heidelberg 2012

Clinical Significance

- Umbilical granuloma is a bothersome disorder and may be mixed up with omphalomesenteric or urachal remnants or other disorders.
- Omphalitis may lead to a life-threatening necrotizing fasciitis, septicemia, portal vein thrombosis, and extrahepatic portal hypertension.

Clinical Presentation

In **umbilical granuloma**, *the normal granulomatous surface of the navel center persists after 1 week and leads to a wetting and bleeding wound* (see Fig. 19.2) (see Webcode 1922 of Chap. 19).

Purulent discharge and signs of periumbilical cellulitis with swelling and redness are typical for **omphalitis**.

In necrotizing fasciitis and umbilical gangrene, *the local findings* "progression of periumbilical cellulitis, violaceous discoloration, blistering of the skin, and bloody discharge" *are combined with general signs* such as tachycardia, pyrexia, or hypothermia, and abdominal distension.

Work-Ups, Differential Diagnosis

In omphalitis, inflammatory blood signs should be determined, and blood cultures and Gram stain and cultures of the secretion should be performed.

The differential diagnosis of umbilical granuloma must consider the already quoted malformations and their local findings, and possibly initiate the corresponding work-ups.

Treatment, Prognosis

Umbilical granuloma needs repeated cauterization with silver nitrate and prophylaxis of infection. In omphalitis, i.v. antibiotic treatment is indicated that considers the possible germs (polymicrobial infection, Gram-negative germs, *Staphylococcus aureus*, or *Streptococcus pyogenes*).

In necrotizing fasciitis, urgent surgery is indicated with debridement and wide excision of all involved tissue including the preperitoneal umbilical vessels and amniotic remnants.

After healing, abdominal wall and navel reconstruction is necessary.

Prognosis

In umbilical granuloma and early omphalitis, complete healing is achieved. The morbidity and mortality of advanced omphalitis and necrotizing fasciitis are still high.

18.1.2 Remnants of the Omphalomesenteric (Vitellointestinal) Duct

Types, Occurrence

The embryonal vitellointestinal tract is a communication between the entoderm and the secondary yolk sac. Partial or complete remnants of this duct lead to different pathoanatomical structures as follows:

Meckel's diverticulum is a proximal remnant that originates from the ileum and ends blindly # and is the most frequent type (observed in about 2 % of the population). All other forms occur rarely. In **congenital bands** without or with intervening cyst, a connection exists between the undersurface of the navel and the antimesenteric side of the ileum # (or rarely the tip of the appendix). The torsion, angulation, or internal herniation of an intestinal loop is a possible complication of congenital bands. **Persistence of omphalomesenteric duct** # or of **its distal part** is followed by the fistula in the center of the navel and bilious discharge or watery secretion. In the former type, eventration of the duct without or with parts of the intestinum to the outside is a possible sequel. **Umbilical polyp** or **preperitoneal cyst** (Roser's cyst) is another type of omphalomesenteric remnants.

Clinical Significance

- Dependent on the type of omphalomesenteric remnants and their inherent complications, a large variation of the clinical manifestation is possible.

Clinical Presentation

Lower gastrointestinal bleeding and other complications of peptic ulceration, *obstructive ileus, and diverticulitis* are the three main clinical manifestations of **Meckel's diverticulum. In the other types**, *a visible and/or palpable pathology of the navel, obstructive ileus, or peritonitis* corresponds to the presenting symptoms and signs.

In umbilical pathologies, *an enlarged navel with seemingly granulation tissue; discharge of bile, air, and stool (if feeded), or a watery secretion; an opening in the center of the navel that can be probed, and protrusion of a fleshy mass or eventration of intestine may be visible, or a cystic mass underneath the navel may be palpable.*

Work-Ups, Differential Diagnosis

The knowledge of the possible clinical manifestation is indispensable for recognition of omphalomesenteric remnants. In patent omphalomesenteric duct or distal fistula, contrast fistulography with lateral X-ray of the abdomen may be useful although not absolutely necessary in completely patent omphalomesenteric duct. Ultrasound of navel and abdominal wall permits confirmation of a suspected Roser's cyst. Sometimes, surgical revision with inspection of the undersurface of the navel by an infraumbilical incision confirms the diagnosis.

Except for patent omphalomesenteric duct with bilious discharge, other congenital or acquired disorders of the navel must be considered in the differential diagnosis of such malformations (e.g., dermoid cyst or umbilical granuloma) and those of obstructive ileus or localized or diffuse peritonitis.

Treatment, Prognosis

Intra-abdominal complications need emergency surgery with complete resection of the omphalomesenteric remnants and possibly intestinal resection in advanced obstructive ileus.

For a patent omphalomesenteric duct and pathologies restricted to the navel, a semicircular incision of the umbilicus that may be extended by an infraumbilical midline incision permits extraperitoneal preparation and resection of the navel structures from behind in Roser's cyst, distal fistula, and umbilical polyp and is followed by intra-abdominal resection of a patent duct including a small border of normal ileum wall and an adequate two layer suture to avoid ileum stenosis and adhesions at the suture site.

Permanent healing is possible if adequate and complete resection of the omphalomesenteric remnant is performed except for possible intra-abdominal complications with possible subsequent postoperative ileus due to adhesions.

18.1.3 Urachal Remnants

Types, Occurrence

Urachal remnants are derived from the embryological communication between urinary bladder and allantois.

Persistence of the proximal part that starts from the bladder vertex and ends blindly like a diverticulum is probably the most frequently observed type, for instance, at surgery #. A distal sinus tract with an opening at the navel center or a completely patent urachal duct without or with an intervening cyst or an isolated cyst at the site or lateral of the former urachal duct # is the less frequently observed form.

Clinical Significance

- Except for purulent inflammation of an urachal cyst and recurrent cystitis of urachal diverticulum, urachal remnants lead to less severe complications than the cranial counterpart.

Clinical Presentation

A wetting umbilicus is the presenting sign of a completely **patent urachal duct** or a **distal sinus tract**. *The discharge leads to dermatitis and is recognized by its urinous smell.*

An **urachal cyst** manifests either as *midline* or lateral *hypogastric abdominal tumor*, or as *phlegmonous or purulent infection of the abdominal wall.*

On close observation, a specific sign with *retraction and effacement of the navel* after micturition may be observed in urachal remnants with normalization after filling of the bladder.

Work-Ups, Differential Diagnosis

The main diagnostic tools and aims are ultrasound for confirmation of an urachal cyst, fistulography for delineation of a distal sinus tract, and voiding cystourethrography (VCU) and cystoscopy for recognition of a bladder diverticulum. Indentation of the bladder vertex by an urachal cyst or exclusion of an infravesical obstruction is an additional finding of endoscopy and VCU.

The differential diagnosis must consider in case of urachal cyst the much more frequent acute or chronic recurrent bladder retention or an abdominal tumor, and in case of abdominal wall infection, an infection due to a suprapubic dermoid sinus tract, other causes of recurrent urinary tract infection in case of suspected urachal diverticulum, or an omphalomesenteric sinus tract in case of a wetting navel.

Suprapubic dermoid sinuses start from the pubic skin, follow the superior bladder surface, and end in the region of the umbilicus. Resection is indicated to avoid infectious complications.

Treatment, Prognosis
Surgery: A fistulous tract including the umbilical opening, patent urachal tract, or urachal cyst is completely excised by a periumbilical or lower abdominal midline incision that remains extraperitoneally. The urachal diverticulum is best completely resected at surgery that is performed for other reasons.

In case of an infected urachal cyst, resection is best performed after healing of infection.

Outcome is permanent healing if all urachal remnants are removed completely. Adenocarcinoma originating from urachal remnant has been observed in adults.

18.1.4 Miscellaneous Congenital and Acquired Disorders of the Navel

Dysmorphology and unusual location of the navel may point to specific syndromes. In congenital thoracic and abdominal midline defects, the umbilicus is either high or low set, partially integrated, and often combined with umbilical hernia or omphalocele, especially in the more severe type of such malformations.

Protrusions of the navel are based on ectopic tissue (pancreatic or hepatic tissue, or endometriosis), hamartoma, or on a benign or malignant primary or metastatic tumor (epidermoid cyst #, malignant melanoma).

There are numerous mostly acquired **causes of inflammation and infection of the umbilicus.** Inserted or endogenous foreign bodies such as piercing, omphalolith, talc or pilonidal disease,

enteric fistulas to the navel (perforated appendicitis, Crohn's disease), infection from the outside of the navel, and systemic dermatoses are encountered in chronically inflamed navels.

18.2 Omphalocele and Gastroschisis (Common Topics I)

Occurrence, Types
In both malformations, an abdominal wall defect in the area of the umbilicus is combined with eventration of abdominal viscera (Fig. 18.1).

Although omphalocele is observed more frequently with about 1 in 5,000 live births than gastroschisis, the latter malformation has been observed increasingly in the past decades.

Whereas eventration occurs in omphalocele into a persistent sac outside of the peritoneal cavity through the umbilical ring, in gastroschisis, an open eventration through an abdominal midline cleft to the outside of the abdomen is observed.

Omphalocele may be divided into three types: In **congenital hernia of the umbilical cord**, the omphalocele sac contains only few intestinal loops, and the diameter of the mass exceeds not more than 4 cm #. In **giant omphalocele**, the very large sac contains almost every abdominal viscera including urinary bladder and possibly genitals #. The most frequent **common type** has a 4–12-cm-wide umbilical ring with different sizes of the omphalocele sac that contains in up to 50 % liver in addition to the intestine. In ≥10 % of the cases, the omphalocele is either pre- or perinatally ruptured.

In **gastroschisis**, the abdominal cleft is mostly smaller than 4 cm (range of length 2–5 cm), and the eventration consists mostly of small and large intestine that is usually covered by thick membrane # (prenatal gastroschisis). In the so-called perinatal gastroschisis, the intestine has a nearly normal appearance.

Clinical Significance
- In both malformations, the major surgical challenge is to reduce the abdominal viscera in a small abdominal cavity.

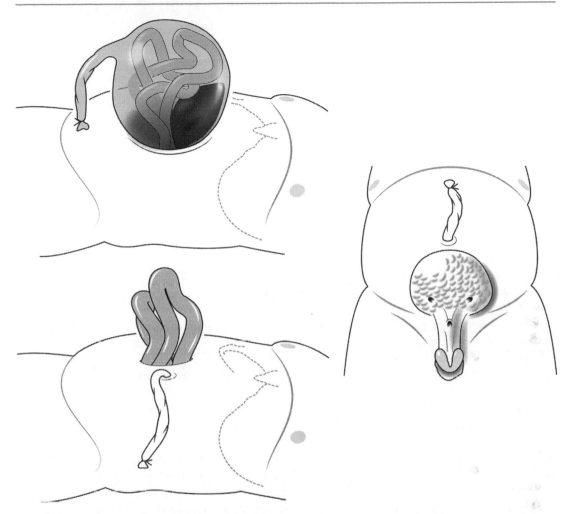

Fig. 18.1 The diagrammatic drawings on the *left side* show an omphalocele and laparoschisis (gastroschisis) that are seen from the left side of the patients, and the drawing on the *right side* demonstrates a bladder exstrophy seen from the legs of a newborn. *Top left*: The omphalocele is a sack that protrudes through the site of the navel and contains intestine of normal caliber and appearance and parenchymatous organs like the liver. The umbilical cord inserts eccentrically on the sack. *Bottom left*: In laparoschisis (gastroschisis), a short midline cleft with insertion of the umbilical cord mostly on the right side allows protrusion of intestine in the amniotic cavity before birth. The intestine is often large and short with adhesions of the loops to each other. *Right side*: The observer pulls the residual prepuce on the ventral side in a caudal direction (not shown in the drawing). Bladder and penis are open on its dorsal side and lie below the low-set navel. The mucous membrane of the bladder displays secondary changes like small polyps. Trigonum with the ureteral orifices, bladder neck, verumontanum, urethral plate, and split glans and prepuce are recognizable, and the latter correspond to grade 3 epispadias

- In omphalocele, those with associated malformations that are encountered in 40–80% have an increased morbidity, mortality, and less favourable final outcome.
- In gastroschisis, a prolonged postoperative ileus combined with decreased absorptive capacity and prematurity or low birth weight have a substantial influence on early and late outcome.

Prenatal diagnosis of omphalocele and gastroschisis is possible by ultrasound already in the first trimester (as early as in the tenth week of gestation). It is used together with Doppler for recognition of associated major anomalies in omphalocele (supplemented by amniocentesis for chromosomal analysis), growth retardation, and intestinal distortion especially in gastroschisis (intrauterine torsion of the extraperitoneal intestine or its impingement at the level of the abdominal wall cleft), and for timely referral of the unborn child with the mother to a tertiary center. Increased levels of maternal alpha-fetoprotein in the second trimester may indicate gastroschisis and somewhat less probably omphalocele. But it must be differentiated from myelomeningocele and other disorders.

18.2.1 Omphalocele

Clinical Presentation

The *large individual variation of omphalocele* concerns size and content of the sac, diameter of umbilical ring (=defect of abdominal wall), volume of the abdominal cavity, intact or ruptured sac, and number and types of associated malformations. An inverse proportional relation exists between size of the sac and volume of the abdominal cavity.

The omphalocele sac lies in front of and is in continuity with the umbilical ring, and the umbilical cord starts eccentrically from it #. Prior and immediately after birth, the sac is transparent and permits recognition of its content. Later, it gets opaque and whitish. The eventrated liver has a roundish shape with elongation of the hepatic veins.

The following associated anomalies may be encountered either solitary or in combination and are arranged in order of frequency:
- Cardiovascular malformations and autosomal trisomies 13–15, 18, and 21, each in about 20 %
- Beckwith-Wiedemann syndrome (macroglossia, visceromegaly, specific craniofacial feature, and episodes of hypoglycemia), in ≥10 %
- Gastrointestinal malformations, among them malrotation in 100 % and other anomalies that are however much less frequently than in gastroschisis
- As part of a lower midline syndrome or pentalogy of Cantrell with hypo- or epigastric location of the omphalocele

18.2.2 Gastroschisis

Clinical Presentation

The *individual variation of clinical presentation is less striking* than that of omphalocele and concerns length of the abdominal cleft, presentation of the eventrated intestine, possible intestinal malformations, and prematurity or low birth weight.

A short abdominal midline cleft is visible with protrusion of the unprotected intestine. The cleft is mostly on the right side of insertion of a normal umbilical cord including a small strip of skin #.

The intestinal loops are dilated, their wall is thickened, and the malrotated intestine has a reduced length. If the eventration has occurred early in gestation, the intestinal loops stick together and are covered by an adherent membrane because of alteration by the amniotic fluid, ischemia, and constriction. Therefore, recognition of intestinal malformations may be difficult.

Prematurity or low birth weight and length is observed in up to 70 % of the cases. The mean maternal age, birth order, birth weight, and gestational age of the newborn are significantly lower than in omphalocele. Associated malformations concern mainly the intestine and occur in about 20 %. In addition to the obligatory malrotation, atresia, or stenosis #, Meckel's diverticulum and duplications are encountered in 10–15 %.

18.3   Omphalocele and Gastroschisis (Common Topics II)

Work-Ups, Differential Diagnosis

Omphalocele and gastroschisis are usually clinical diagnoses if the characteristics of each disorder are known. Work-ups are necessary in omphalocele for suspected cardiovascular malformations (echocardiography), autosomal trisomies (genetic consultation, chromosomal examination), **Beckwith-Wiedemann syndrome** (microcephalia with protruding occipital region, vascular nevus of the face, and slit-like transverse retraction of the auricle, episodic hypoglycemia), and anomalies in which omphalocele is a possible part of a chest or abdominal wall defect. Prematurity or low birth weight in gastroschisis needs the expertise of neonatologists.

The differential diagnosis between omphalocele, gastroschisis, bladder exstrophy, and vesicointestinal fissure is usually possible by precise clinical examination although evaluation of incomplete types of bladder exstrophy and the specific pathoanatomy of vesicointestinal fissure are only possible by further work-up (VCU, cystoscopy, contrast studies, CT/MRI).

If remnants of the sac, an asymmetric insertion of the cord, and a midline umbilical ring are detectable, the differentiation between a ruptured omphalocele and gastroschisis is possible. After a spontaneous epithelization of a hernia of the umbilical cord, it may be mixed up with a cutis navel. Clamping immediately after birth or later resection is dangerous because of interruption of the few intestinal loops within the hernia.

In midline chest or abdominal wall defects, the diagnostically relevant findings are usually in the forefront, and omphalocele is a possible additional trait.

Treatment, Prognosis

The following topics must be considered:

- Time and mode of delivery
- Resuscitation and urgent work-ups
- Decision to treat or not to treat
- Mode of treatment
- Treatment of early and late complications

Whenever possible, **delivery** should be performed at term after referral of the pregnant mother to a tertiary care center. Although in giant omphalocele or in severe intestinovascular compromise of gastroschisis delivery is best performed by cesarean section, there are no prospective and well-controlled studies that confirm that c-section provides substantial benefit for neonates with abdominal wall defects. In case of overt intestinovascular compromise during gestation, preterm delivery is indicated in gastroschisis if possible after lung maturation.

Resuscitation includes introduction of a nasogastric tube, an i.v. line at the upper extremities for maintenance and replacement of fluid and electrolytes, intubation and artificial ventilation, insertion of a bladder catheter, placement of the eventration in a transparent and sterile bowel bag, of the neonate in a lateral position, and under a radiation heater or in an infant care island. It is very important that the initial steps include inspection of the intestine in gastroschisis for possible distorted vascularization and compression at the level of the abdominal wall cleft. Correct positioning and support of the eventrated intestine and possible untwisting or emergency enlargement of the abdominal cleft belongs to the first steps.

Urgent **work-ups** include plain chest X-ray, consultation of cardiologist and other pediatric specialists, and further work-ups only if major malformations of the cardiovascular system, the airways, or the diaphragm are suspected.

The indication for surgery should be discussed in a first step with the involved team and in a second step together with the parents with the possibility of a final **decision to treat or not to treat** in case of the quoted trisomies with poor prognosis or severe associated anomalies and extreme prematurity. If surgery is indicated, either **primary closure** # of the abdominal wall defect or **staged silo closure** # is the main procedure. Although each of them has advantages and disadvantages, the current opinion prefers primary closure whenever possible.

For **primary closure** of omphalocele, the skin division around the sac leaves only a small rim and may be started with a small transverse incision on the right or left lateral side that facilitates mobilization from the omphalocele. After ligation of the umbilical vein, arteries, and former urachus, the sac is carefully dissected from the liver surface if it is a part of eventration. In gastroschisis, a small rim of the short abdominal wall cleft must be resected and enlarged in a cranial and caudal direction with preservation of the umbilical stump.

Revision of the viscera and abdominal cavity permits recognition and treatment of intestinal obstructions and other abnormalities in the setting of malrotation (e.g., Ladd's bands), of omphalomesenteric remnants, of intestinal duplications, and specifically of intestinal atresia and stenosis in gastroschisis. Their diagnosis is facilitated with careful milking out the intestine in a caudal direction. Appendectomy avoids diagnostic difficulties later in life. Finally, the diaphragms should be proved for possible congenital diaphragmatic hernia.

Before reduction of the viscera, additional space in the abdomen may be achieved by stretching the abdominal wall muscles in lateral and other directions, careful evacuation of the small intestine (air and secretions by the nasogastric tube) and of the large intestine (meconium by a rectal tube), and muscle relaxation. Reduction must avoid twisting of the intestine and the in- and outflow of the hepatic veins if the liver is eventrated.

The abdominal wall is closed in two layers with nonabsorbable sutures with preservation of the umbilical stump or reconstruction of a navel.

In **staged silo closure**, preparation of the abdominal wall defect, resection of the omphalocele, and revision of the intestine are the same as in primary closure. Correction of an intestinal atresia may be delayed till secondary closure of gastroschisis. The borders of the prosthetic silo are sutured to the rectus muscle and fascia with nonabsorbable sutures avoiding any gap between the stitches after careful reposition of the viscera into the silo. Sutures and permanent traction at the top of the silastic sac should permit a vertical upright position of the sac and its content in relation to the abdominal wall. Gravitation and repeated diminution of the silo volume by sutures or stapling devices in 12–24-h intervals lead to reduction of the viscera into the abdominal cavity within ½–1 week. After surgery, the silo is wrapped with sterile gauze soaked in povidone-iodine solution.

Primary and staged silo closure need peri- and postoperative systemic antibiotics and pre- and especially postoperative intensive care with relaxation and artificial ventilation with positive end-expiratory pressure, replacement of high fluid losses, total parenteral nutrition, and monitoring after primary closure (abdominal compartment syndrome) or staged silo closure (wound care and reduction procedures).

Early complications: A **too tight closure** is avoided by measurement of the intra-abdominal pressure and by the expertise of the pediatric surgeon who should remain in close contact with the pediatric anesthesiologist during surgery and specifically during abdominal wall closure. Intra-abdominal pressure may be estimated by values of the intravesical or intragastric pressure and should not exceed 20 mmHg for primary closure. The same applies to an airway pressure exceeding 25 mmHg.

Respiratory and hemodynamic compromises are the sequels of a too tight closure and lead to severe morbidity and possible mortality. Specifically, necessity of high pressure ventilation and respiratory distress syndrome, renal failure including renal vein thrombosis, and intestinal necrosis are the possible disorders and need **immediate release of the primary closure.**

In **premature complete separation of the silastic silo**, resuturing should be avoided and after removal of the silo, an alternative procedure can be performed, for example, closure of the skin with or without interposition of an appropriate synthetic sheet and secondary closure of muscles and skin. In omphalocele, occasionally nonoperative topical treatment of the omphalocele sac # may be an alternative procedure followed by secondary resection and abdominal wall closure.

Whereas prognosis of omphalocele is restricted in a giant type or major associated anomalies, prognosis of the gastroschisis is restricted by a persistent postoperative ileus with prolonged transit time, decreased absorption, and disorder of defecation. Although normalization occurs within 6 months, the infant needs a central venous catheter for total parenteral nutrition with the inherent danger of catheter-related septicemia and liver disease. The differential diagnoses of postoperative ileus are missed atresia, Ladd's band, and other mechanical obstructions that are best excluded by gastrointestinal contrast studies.

Causes of fatal outcome are associated anomalies in omphalocele, prematurity and complications of the intestine, or TPN in gastroschisis. Long-term survival is >90 % in omphalocele and >95 % in gastroschisis.

18.4 Bladder Exstrophy

Pathoanatomy, Occurrence

Bladder exstrophy belongs to the epispadias-exstrophy complex that includes pubic diastasis, continent and incontinent epispadias, pubovesical cleft, classic bladder exstrophy, superior vesical fistula, duplex exstrophy, bladder exstrophy with imperforate anus, and vesicointestinal fissure and has as common feature different degrees of abdominal wall and/or dorsal wall deficiency of the urethra. In classic bladder exstrophy, the abdominal wall defect concerns the hypogastrium directly below the umbilical cord and is combined with a defect of the anterior bladder wall, a dorsally split urethra and external genitals, and diastatic symphysis.

Bladder exstrophy occurs in 1:10,000–50,000 live births. Girls are much less frequently involved.

Clinical Significance

- At best, a normal bladder function is achieved by reconstructive surgery only in two thirds of the patients.

Clinical Presentation

The midline of the hypogastrium is filled up with a longitudinal oval area of a red, velvet-like, and increasingly polypous mucous membrane of the posterior bladder wall that differs in size, is leaking urine, and becomes prominent on straining and crying (= bladder plate). *The bladder neck continues to a dorsally split penis that is deviated in a dorsal direction, short, and disproportionate #* (Fig. 18.1).

By seizing the apron-like prepuce and traction to the penis, the trigonum and the dorsal wall of the penis become visible with the ureteral orifices, verumontanum with the entrance of the ejaculatory ducts, foreshortened urethra with a possible dorsal chordee, and relatively large glans with its everted halves. In girls, the separated halves of the vulva and clitoris and its glans are the most prominent features #.

The diastatic and outward rotated ends of the pubic rami are palpable in the medial part of the groin in both sexes. In addition, an anteriorly displaced anus is recognizable.

The variation of the **incomplete form of bladder exstrophy** is even greater than that of classic bladder exstrophy, and differentiation of specific subtypes is more difficult.

In **duplicate exstrophy** (exstrophic double bladder) #, the exstrophic bladder plate looks like a classic bladder exstrophy although neither urine is leaking nor ureteral orifices are recognizable. Underneath, a normal or somewhat smaller bladder exists, and the penis is either foreshortened and epispadic or normal combined with some diastasis of symphysis and abdominal wall muscles.

In **pseudoexstrophy**, the bladder is normal, but it bulges between the separated abdominal wall muscles and is covered only by a cicatricial skin retraction. The epispadic penis is short. **The superior vesical fissure** (suprapubic cleft bladder) # shows a circumscript opening of the bladder with possible prolapse of bladder mucosa. The penis is usually intact with a superficial epispadic sulcus and dermal sinuses. In other incomplete forms to which the **covered exstrophy** belongs, the bladder (and penis) is to a great extent normal but may have a small fistula and/or is covered by a small area of wrinkled skin or a large zone of thin fascia and skin leading to some prolapse.

Associated malformations and disorders are uncommon in classic bladder exstrophy except for **unilateral and bilateral inguinal hernia**, **cryptorchidism**, and **umbilical hernia**. Inguinal hernias need an additional technique of repair because they are indirect and direct in combination. Because of abnormal spatial arrangement of the pelvis, the **gait** is initially waddling and later normal. The **anteriorly displaced anus** together with abnormal arrangement of the pelvic floor may be initially combined with some fecal incontinence and rectal prolapse with spontaneous resolution. In addition, **recurrent prolapse of the uterus** may be observed initially in girls.

In severe forms of epispadias-exstrophy complex, for example, vesicointestinal fissure, prematurity and associated malformations including omphalocele are observed more frequently.

Work-Ups, Differential Diagnosis

In classic bladder exstrophy, careful clinical examination is sufficient for diagnosis and planning of reconstructive surgery if the properties and size of the bladder, the distance between the pubic rami, and the quality of the penile structures are considered. Ultrasound of the kidneys and upper urinary tract should be performed initially and on follow-up for exclusion of primary or secondary obstructive uropathies or reflux and renal abnormalities.

Plain abdominal X-ray including pelvis and CT with 3D reconstruction may be used for measurement of the interpubic distance and planning of osteotomy combined with bladder reconstruction.

Differential diagnosis must be considered in some rare forms of bladder exstrophy, for example, incomplete form of bladder exstrophy.

Treatment, Prognosis

Surgery is indicated in almost all cases and includes **staged functional reconstruction of bladder and epispadias** that should be performed whenever possible, or some type of urinary diversion if staged reconstruction is impossible due to not available resources or a defective bladder plate, or if efforts of reconstruction have failed. Alternatively, complete primary repair using penile disassembly technique has been proposed.

The **first step of functional reconstruction** is performed in the first few days after birth and converts the exstrophic bladder to an incontinent epispadias. The incision follows the periphery of the bladder plate and includes above the bladder a triangle with the umbilical cord (with resection of the stump and repair of a possible umbilical hernia or omphalocele) and below a sufficient large plate of the bladder neck and prostatic urethra with the verumontanum. It is completed by a paraexstrophic skin flap of either side. After complete mobilization of the bladder plate and dissection of the corpora cavernosa off the inferior pubic rami with preservation of their neurovascular supply, the corpora cavernosa are approximated in the midline and the paraexstrophic flaps closed in the midline. Afterward, the plate of bladder and prostatic urethra are tubularized leaving a catheter in the bladder, urethra, and ureters. Finally, the pubic halves are approximated by a nonabsorbable suture depending on the age without or with pelvic osteotomy (e.g., anterior iliac

osteotomy with external fixator pins) followed by fascia and skin closure.

In girls, the same first step of functional reconstruction is performed but supplemented by mobilization and downward fixation of the vagina.

The **second step** concerns epispadias repair in boys at the age of 6–12 months for which several techniques are available, for example, Cantwell-Ransley and Mitchell-Bagli procedure.

The **third step** at the age of 4 years includes usually ureteral reimplantation in a cephalad position, bladder neck reconstruction, for example, according to Young-Dees-Leadbetter, and correction of the bifid clitoris and vaginoplasty in girls (in whom it has not been performed in first stage).

Follow-ups are necessary after each step. They include clinical assessment of lower abdomen, penis and continence (being dry for at least 3 h), uroflowmetry, and ultrasound (upper urinary tract, bladder capacity). Adequacy of the urinary control is known within 1 year after repair.

If the children remain **incontinent and/or have a small bladder capacity**, the following procedures must be discussed combined with possible augmentation cystoplasty: increase of the outlet resistance by bladder neck injections analogous to reflux, repeated bladder neck reconstruction, wrap around sling, or artificial urinary sphincter. If continence cannot be achieved, augmentation cystoplasty with ileum is performed. It is usually supplemented by a continent catheterizable stoma (e.g., Mitrofanoff procedure) that permits clean intermittent catheterization (CIC) and closure of the bladder neck. Urinary diversion that has been commonly used in former times with very high rates of long-term continence (e.g., ureterosigmoidostomy) must be discussed as well.

The possible complications of staged reconstruction include rarely complete or partial wound dehiscence, bladder prolapse or bladder outlet obstruction, and glans or corporal loss. Hydroureteronephrosis and renal scarring (15–25 %), nephrolithiasis and bladder calculi, and increased risk of bladder carcinoma in the fifth decade of life belong to the main long-term complications. Complete primary repair is associated with increased need for secondary surgery and possible hypospadias and glans or corporal loss.

Urinary continence and volitional voiding is achieved with staged reconstruction in 70–85 % (40 % in adults combined with loss of volitional voiding with time). The penis and lower abdomen are cosmetically and functionally acceptable in up to 85 % (with more than one intervention for reconstruction in ≥25 %).

At least 15–30 % needs secondary surgery due to incontinence and/or insufficient bladder capacity.

18.5 Cloacal Exstrophy (Vesicointestinal Fissure)

Pathoanatomy, Occurrence

Although cloacal exstrophy has various forms, mostly two exstrophic hemibladders on either side of the hypogastrium are encountered combined with an exstrophic part of the large intestinum in between usually corresponding to the ileocecum.

The exstrophic intestinum communicates in its superior part with the ileum, in its intermediate part possibly with a duplicated appendix, and its distal part possibly with colon of different length that ends blindly up to an imperforate anus, continues to an anteriorly displaced anus, or is sometimes combined with colonic duplication.

Vesicointestinal fissure is a very rare malformation accounting for about 10 % of all forms of bladder exstrophy.

Clinical Significance

- Although 90 % of all children with cloacal exstrophy survive today with proper treatment, physiological fecal and urinary continence and reconstruction of the male external genitals are only possible in a small proportion of the patients.
- Treatment needs a coordinated multidisciplinary early and staged treatment in a tertiary center of pediatric surgery and possibly gender assignment already in the neonatal period.

Clinical Presentation

The hypogastrium is completely filled up with the ballooning mucous membranes of the two posterior bladder walls on either side and of the exstrophic midline ileocecum.

The ureteral orifices and the already quoted intestinal apertures become visible either as openings or as evaginations by close inspection if the evisceration is pushed in a superior direction. In its superior border, a low-set umbilical cord and mostly an associated omphalocele are recognized. The external genitals are often rudimentary in males and possibly split in both sexes (e.g., bifid scrotum or clitoris).

Split symphysis anomaly and possible abdominal wall deficiency are specific parts of cloacal exstrophy.

Associated malformations occur more frequently than in bladder exstrophy. The most frequent are quoted below:

- Prematurity and small weight for date, cryptorchidism, and inguinal hernia.
- In addition to the specific intestinal malformations quoted above and to the common types, malabsorption may be observed with or without a foreshortened small intestine.
- Vertebral and spinal cord anomalies, for example, myelomeningoceles occur in up to 50 %.
- The less frequent urogenital anomalies include renal agenesis or aplasia, fusion disorder, ectopy, obstructive uropathy, and duplication or atresia of the female internal genitals.
- Orthopedic disorders such as clubfoot, dislocation of the hip, and scoliosis.

Prenatal diagnosis and evaluation of possible major anomalies is possible.

Differential Diagnosis, Work-Ups

Differentiation between cloacal and bladder exstrophy may be difficult if one half or both halves of the bladder are covered with skin in the former and in incomplete forms of the latter disorder.

Work-ups are necessary for precise description of the individual case and exclusion of associated malformations. The precise description concerns presence and length of colon distal to the exstrophic intestine, and description of the external and internal genitals, and gender assignment by endoscopy, contrast CT, ultrasound, and karyotyping. For exclusion of associated malformations (e.g., bilateral renal agenesis, obstructive uropathy, atresia of vagina, or minimal spinal dysraphism), ultrasound and MRI are used.

Treatment, Prognosis

In general, treatment is indicated except in cases with extreme prematurity and/or severe associated anomalies. It must consider the individual form and the associated malformations and takes place in stages.

Reconstruction should be performed shortly after birth. It includes (1) separation of the exstrophic intestine from the two hemibladders, tubularization, and creation of a terminal colostomy away from the site of abdominal wall closure with preservation of all available intestine including appendices; (2) reconstruction of the bladder with approximation of the symphysis (or staged procedures); (3) omphalocele and abdominal wall repair; (4) orchiectomy if conversion to a female sex is necessary due to rudimentary male external genitals.

Staged silo closure or primary skin closure in giant omphalocele or primary or delayed repair of myelomeningocele is possibly an additional procedure early in infancy.

Complete bladder reconstruction including epispadias or continent urinary diversion, complete intestinal reconstruction, continent fecal diversion, or anorectal reconstruction, and reconstruction of female internal genitals are performed in later stages.

Prognosis

Except for physiological fecal continence, sexual intercourse, and fertility in boys, physiological or social urinary continence can be achieved for the majority of patients and sexual intercourse, pregnancy, and birth for the majority of girls.

Webcodes

The following webcodes can be used on www. psurg.net for further images and data.

1801 Cutis navel	1812 Characteristics of gastroschisis
1802 Meckel's diverticulum	1813 Associated intestinal anomalies
1803 Congenital band	1814 Primary closure
1804 Patent vitellointestinal duct	1815 Staged silo closure
1805 Bladder diverticulum	1816 Nonoperative topical treatment
1806 Urachal cyst	1817 Characteristics of bladder exstrophy
1807 (Epi) dermoid cyst navel	1818 Female bladder exstrophy
1808 Hernia of the umbilical cord	1819 Duplicate bladder exstrophy
1809 Giant omphalocele	1820 Superior vesical fissure
1810 Intestine, prenatal gastroschisis	1821 Cloacal exstrophy (vesicointestinal fissure)
1811 Characteristics of omphalocele	

Bibliography

Section 18.1

Allen JW, Song J, Velcek FT (2004) Acute presentation of infected urachal cysts: case report and review of diagnosis and therapeutic interventions. Pediatr Emerg Care 20:108–111

Amoury RA, Snyder CL (1998) Meckel's diverticulum. In: O'Neill JA Jr et al (eds) Pediatric surgery, vol 2, 5th edn. Mosby, St. Louis

Chawla Y, Duseja A, Dhiman RK (2009) Review article: the modern management of portal vein thrombosis. Aliment Pharmacol Ther 30:881–894

Cilley RE, Krummel TM (1998) Disorders of the umbilicus. In: O'Neill JA Jr et al (eds) Pediatric surgery, vol 2, 5th edn. Mosby, St. Louis

Rowe PC, Gearhart JP (1993) Retraction of the umbilicus during voiding as an initial sign of an urachal anomaly. Pediatrics 91:153–154

Upadhyay V, Kukkady A (2003) Urachal remnants: an enigma. Eur J Pediatr Surg 13:372–376

Section 18.2

Cooney DR (1998) Defects of the abdominal wall. In: O'Neill JA Jr et al (eds) Pediatric surgery, vol 2, 5th edn. Mosby, St. Louis

Novotny DA, Klein RL, Boeckman CR (1993) Gastroschisis: an 18-year review. J Pediatr Surg 28: 650–652

Sapin E, Lewin F, Baron JM, Bargy F, Wakim A, Helardot PG (1993) Prenatal diagnosis and management of gastroschisis. Pediatr Surg Int 8:31–33

Section 18.3

Baird AD (2011) Exstrophy in the adolescent and young adult population. Semin Pediatr Surg 20:109–112

Brock JW III, O'Neill JA Jr (1998) Bladder exstrophy. In: O'Neill JA Jr et al (eds) Pediatric surgery, vol 2, 5th edn. Mosby, St. Louis

Chalmers D, Ferrer F (2011) Continent urinary diversion in the epispadias-exstrophy complex. Semin Pediatr Surg 20:102–108

Corroppolo M, Zampieri N, Pietrobelli A, Giacomello L, Camoglio FS (2007) Bladder exstrophy variants. Minerva Urol Nefrol 59:109–113

Dave S, Salle JL (2008) Current status of bladder neck reconstruction. Curr Opin Urol 18:419 424

Hernandez DJ, Purves T, Gearhart JP (2008) Complications of surgical reconstruction of the exstrophy-epispadias complex. J Pediatr Urol 4:460–466

Husmann DA (2006) Surgery insight: advantages and pitfalls of surgical techniques for correction of bladder exstrophy. Nat Clin Pract Urol 3:95–100

Johnston JH (1982) The exstrophic anomalies. In: Williams DI, Johnston JH (eds) Paediatric urology, 2nd edn. Butterworths, London

Oesterling JE, Jeffs RD (1987) The importance of a successful initial bladder closure in the surgical management of classical bladder exstrophy: analysis of 144 patients treated at the Johns Hopkins Hospital between 1975 and 1985. J Urol 137:258

Ransley PG, Duffy PG, Wollin M (1988) Bladder exstrophy closure and epispadias repair. In: Spitz L, Nixon HH (eds) Paediatric surgery, 4th edn. Butterworths, London

Woodhouse CR, North AC, Gearhart JP (2006) Standing the test of time: long-term outcome of reconstruction of the exstrophy bladder. World J Urol 24: 244–249

Section 18.4

Levitt MA, Mak GZ, Falcone RA Jr, Pena A (2008) Cloacal exstrophy – pull-through or permanent stoma? A review of 53 patients. J Pediatr Surg 43:164–168; discussion 168–170

Mathews R (2011) Achieving urinary continence in cloacal exstrophy. Semin Pediatr Surg 20:126 129

O'Neill JA Jr (1998) Cloacal exstrophy. In: O'Neill JA Jr et al (eds) Pediatric surgery, vol 2, 5th edn. Mosby, St. Louis

Swelling of the Groin and Navel

Tumefaction of the groin # or navel # is a very frequent presenting sign. Its differential diagnosis is listed in Table 19.1.

Such findings are being confirmed by the family doctor at the first consultation if they exist already for a long time or have occurred recently. If the clinical course is intermittent, he has to rely on precise informations of the caregivers because the described finding cannot be proved; at best, the reliability of the parenteral findings may be concluded from additional findings and provocation tests.

The differential diagnosis is even more difficult if mostly older children complain of pain in the groin with possible radiation.

Table 19.1 Differential diagnosis of swelling of the groin or navel

- Congenital and acquired inguinal hernia
- o Hydrocele of the cord
- Testicular hydrocele (Fig. 19.2)
- Cryptorchidism and related disorders
- Inguinal lymphadenopathies
- Pain in the groin
- Umbilical hernia
- o Paraumbilical and epigastric hernia
- o Cutis navel
- o Early and late stage of hernia of the umbilical cord
- o Umbilical hernia associated with congenital abdominal wall defect
- o Tumors of the umbilicus

19.1 Swelling and Pain of the Groin Including Scrotum

19.1.1 Inguinal Hernia

Pathoanatomy, Occurrence

The majority of inguinal hernia is congenital in childhood although direct and acquired inguinal hernias are observed as well, for example, in bladder exstrophy. For their manifestation, a combination of a patent processus vaginalis and additional factors is necessary. Examples of such factors are undescended testis, several congenital and acquired disorders, ventriculoperitoneal shunt, and peritoneal dialysis. Prior birth, the processus vaginalis is open in all individuals, remains so after birth in many for several months, and is about one fifth in adults.

Up to 25 % of premature infants develop inguinal hernia #. The highest incidence is in the first year of life (about 80 % of all childhood inguinal hernias) with a peak in the first month of life. In infancy, boys are six times more involved than girls, >50 % concern the right and >25 % the left side, and >10 % are bilateral at first manifestation. If the left side is affected initially, the chance of a right-sided inguinal hernia is about 60 % on follow-up.

Clinical Significance

- Congenital inguinal hernia belongs with 1–4 % to the most frequent pathologies in

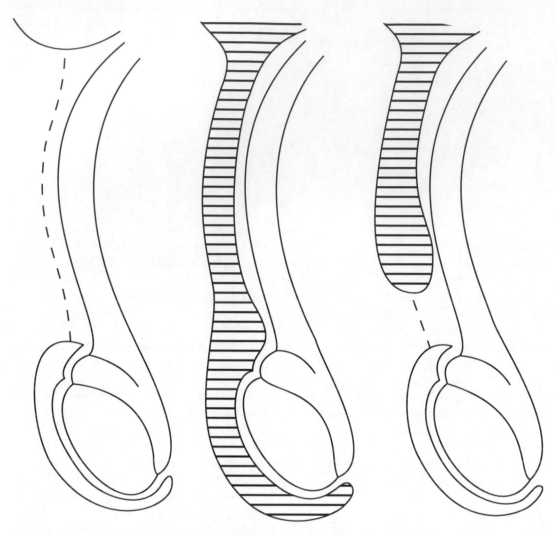

Fig. 19.1 Types of congenital inguinal hernias. Drawing on the *left side* shows obliteration of the patent processus vaginalis that occurs in the majority of children. Complete or inguinoscrotal inguinal hernia manifests in some of the children as shown in the *middle* drawing if the processus remains completely open. Common inguinal hernia may occur in some of the children if the processus remains partly open combined with obliteration of its distal end up to the tunica vaginalis of testis as shown in the *right* drawing

pediatric surgery, especially in prematurity, in the first month and in the first year of life, and in boys # and Fig. 19.1.
- Inguinal hernia is prone to incarceration, especially in the first year of life, and is a continuous source of inguinal pain.
- Incarcerated or strangulated inguinal hernia belongs together with intraperitoneal adhesions to the most common causes of mechanical bowel obstruction in developing countries.

- Umbilical hernia belongs also to the most frequent disorders of pediatric surgery. The clinical significance of umbilical hernia is less well delineated due to the quoted frequent spontaneous resolution.

Clinical Presentation, Clinical Skills
Recurrent manifestation of inguinal hernia may lead to inguinal pain. Inguinal pain may also be quoted in teenagers in sports, prolonged walking, and standing without an overt inguinal hernia.

The leading sign of inguinal hernia is a smooth and firm swelling of the medial groin (inguinal hernia #) with possible continuation into the scrotum (complete inguinal hernia, inguinoscrotal hernia #) that becomes narrower in the lateral direction of the groin, and larger or first manifests on crying or straining. The overlying skin is nonirritable, the tumefaction is painless on palpation, and a gorgling intestinal loop may be felt and heard on examination.

Reduction of an inguinal hernia can be used as diagnostic sign. It is important to know that a special technique is necessary for reduction, and reduction may become more difficult the younger the child.

If consultation takes place in an intermittent stage of inguinal hernia, provocation tests and additional findings may be used: *Stretching of the infant with extended legs and the arms held straight above the head increases the intra-abdominal pressure as well as coughing and blowing up a balloon or examination in standing position in older children. Palpation of the spermatic cord and rolling it over the pubic tubercle can be used to estimate its diameter and to compare it with the contralateral side (silk glove sign, if the size is much larger than a Spaghetti number 3 on one or both sides, an open processus vaginalis is likely). In girls beyond infancy, examination in upright position permits recognition of effacement of the groin structures, especially in unilateral inguinal hernia #.*

Complications
They include irreducibility of inguinal hernia, manifestation of an inguinal hernia after herniotomy, and postoperative complications.

In irreducibility, differentiation between **incarceration** and **strangulation** is used. An incarcerated inguinal hernia means that the content cannot be easily reduced where as strangulation tells an imminent or ongoing gangrene of its content. Progress from incarcerated to strangulation is often rapid, especially in infants and small children. In clinical practice, an **early stage or irresponsibility** is often observed in which reduction seems impossible due to application of an inadequate technique or inconvenient conditions such as a constantly crying infant.

Clinical differentiation between these stages is important for the decision if a trial of manual reduction is still permitted.

Strangulation is observed in ≥ 10 % of childhood inguinal hernia. It concerns boys as well as girls, and two thirds occur in the first year of life with a maximum strangulation rate of about 30 % in the first and second month of life. The somewhat lower incidence in premature infants may be explained by the closer observation in this age group. In contrast to adults, strangulation concerns the intestine # as well as the testis #, or ovary and fallopian tube. About 10 % of such male patients have their necrotic testicle removed at the time of emergency herniorrhaphy or diminished growth or atrophy of the testicle on follow-up. A cyanotic testis at surgery does not predict long-term damage. In girls, either strangulation or torsion leads to interruption of blood supply of the ovary.

There is a continuous transition from **incarceration to strangulation**. On clinical examination, *the groin or inguinoscrotal swelling is painful and tender on palpation; the overlying skin exhibits signs of cellulitis with possible continuation to the scrotum #. Irritability, groin and abdominal pain, and vomiting are the symptoms followed by signs of obstructive ileus and secondary peritonitis.*

Work-Ups, Differential Diagnosis
Ultrasound is only necessary if a clinical differentiation from other disorders is not possible and relevant for the indication of surgery. Plain abdominal x-ray in upright (hanging) position confirms the suspicion of obstructive ileus and permits modifications of the surgical access.

Mainly in difficult reduction maneuvers, incarceration, or complete inguinal hernia, the following differential diagnoses must be considered:
• Hydrocele of the cord or canal of Nuck in girls
• Testicular torsion in undescended testis
• Inguinal lymphadenopathy
• Direct inguinal hernia
• Femoral hernia
• Testicular hydrocele
• Causes of testicular and scrotal swelling

Direct inguinal hernia is encountered in some congenital malformations, for example, in bladder exstrophy in combination with congenital hernia or in disorders with connective tissue deficiency. After hernia repair, an additional direct inguinal hernia may be misinterpreted as recurrence. *The shape of the groin mass is semi-roundish; it lies medially to the epigastric vessels and does not taper off in direction of the inguinal channel, and reduction is easy.* At surgery, there is a weakness of the transverse fascia and high insertion of the internal oblique muscle, resection of the hernia sac is usually not necessary in infants, and suture of the oblique internal muscle to the inguinal ligament is sufficient.

Femoral hernia occurs rarely in children and is observed in girls, boys, and female teenagers. *It may be painful and tender due to strangulation of preperitoneal fat or parts of intestine or bladder. The swelling is below the inguinal ligament and somewhat more lateral than inguinal hernia. Its reduction from below is diagnostic.*

Surgery consists of inguinalization of the hernia sac, resection of its content if strangulated, ligature, and resection. The McVay technique sutures the internal oblique and transverse muscle and its fascia to the ligament of Cooper (pecten of pubic bone).

Treatment, Prognosis

Rapid reduction is necessary in case of acute manifestation of an inguinal hernia except for older children with intermittent manifestations and spontaneous reductions.

For **manual reduction**, the fingers of the left hand form a funnel at the site where the groin swelling tapers off in a lateral direction and those of the right hand compress the swelling in a concentric manner. Sedation or quitenting of the patient and elevation of the buttocks are the most important prerequisites of success of such a maneuver.

In case of difficult reduction or a residual finding of the hernia after reduction, immediate hernia repair is necessary. On the other hand, manual reduction is contraindicated in overt obstructive ileus and/or peritonitis.

Diagnosis of an inguinal hernia in childhood is tantamount to an indication of surgery because spontaneous resolution does not occur and incarceration remains a lifelong risk. In general, the younger the child, the more urgent is surgery.

Especially in infants with unilateral inguinal hernia, **simultaneous revision** of the contralateral side for patent processus vaginalis should be discussed with the parents. Although revision of an unconspicuous groin is an unnecessary operation in at least 85 % of the cases, it is annoying from a psychological viewpoint if an infant needs later a second intervention for inguinal hernia of the other side because most contralateral hernias occur within a few years of the first surgery at the latest.

Therefore, simultaneous contralateral revision may be indicated for the following reasons:

- A second anesthesia is a high risk, for example, in prematurity with lung disorder.
- A distant place of residence that can be reached only by roundabout route.
- Anomalies with increased risk of bilaterality, such as omphalocele, gastroschisis, bladder exstrophy, or disorders with ventriculoperitoneal shunt or peritoneal dialysis.
- Patient with advanced stage of incarceration.

Because of the increased risk of general anesthesia, hernia repair should not be performed as outpatient before 4 months of age. The **principles of repair of congenital inguinal hernia** are the following: Transverse incision in a skin creases above and lateral to the pubic tubercle and incision of the external oblique aponeurosis without/with the external ring; preparation of the inguinal ligament and separation of fascia and muscle fibers of the cremasteric muscle; lifting of the hernia sac that is dissected free to the inner ring; after inspection of the inner side of the sac, it is twisted, ligated at the level of the inner ring, and completely resected; before closure of the external oblique aponeurosis, Scarpa's fascia, and skin, additional sutures may be placed: Sutures for narrowing of a wide or incised internal ring inferiomedially and/or sutures of the high insertion of the internal oblique muscle to the inguinal ligament for prophylaxis or cure of a **direct inguinal hernia** (Girard's technique #). At surgery, damage to the ilioinguinal nerve, vas deference, or spermatic vessels should be avoided. Occasionally, a small yellow piece of ectopic adrenal gland tissue is encountered at surgery that should be removed. At the end of the surgery, a check for correct position of the testis in the scrotum is necessary.

At **surgery of girls**, the possibility of testicular feminization should always be considered (1 in 200 girls with inguinal hernia). Traction to the round ligament shows usually a fallopian tube and regular ovary. In equivocal cases, biopsy of the gonad and postoperative work-ups are necessary #. The fallopian tube and ovary may lie in the wall of the hernia sac (sliding type of inguinal hernia). Nevertheless, the sac is always ligated distal to fallopian tube by a tobacco suture, resected, and the stump (corresponding to the base of the sac) is sutured to undersurface of the transverse abdominal muscle. In addition, the internal ring may be closed with sutures through transverse fascia.

In **incarceration**, the inguinal approach may be extended and the internal ring enlarged. In case of intestinal resection or if the strangulated intestinal part is slipped back prior to inspection, an additional abdominal incision in the corresponding lower abdomen may become necessary. Resection is only necessary if the incarcerated intestine is freed and observed showing neither recovery of its blue and dark color, nor mesenteric arterial pulse, nor peristalsis.

Prognosis

After surgery, some scrotal swelling may be observed either because of a seroma or hematoma. It is usually followed by spontaneous resolution.

More severe complications include undescended testis, recurrence, and injury to the vas deferens and testicular vessels. Mortality is unusual even in incarceration and results of associated disorders and/or lack of experience of the surgeon or anesthesiologist.

Undescended testis observed in <1 % results from not replacement of the testis in the scrotum, not recognition of undescended testis, especially in premature infants, and late ascending testis. Orchidopexy is indicated after the diagnosis.

Recurrence observed in <1 % (and more frequently after incarceration) is mostly a recurrence of the original inguinal hernia # (due to technical problems at surgery concerning the hernia sac and predisposing factors) and less frequently because of a direct inguinal hernia that has not

been recognized at primary surgery or developed thereafter, or a femoral hernia. Repair is necessary after the diagnosis.

The figures of **injury to the vas deferens and/or testicular vessels** are unknown (<1 %) and result more likely from forceful dissection or inappropriate use of instruments than from frank division. After compression and occlusion of the vas deferens, entrance of spermatozoa into the lymphatics and development of sperm-auto-agglutinating antibodies are possible. After division of these structures, immediate reconstruction is possible by microsurgical techniques.

19.1.2 Hydrocele of the Cord or Canal of Nuck (Girls)

Pathoanatomy, Clinical Significance

A part of the processus vaginalis remains open and is filled with fluid that enters from the peritoneal cavity through a narrow part of the processus # and Fig. 19.2. Occasionally, the narrow part is widely open in its most proximal part and leads to an additional inguinal hernia.

- Hydrocele of the cord is an important differential diagnosis of inguinal hernia.
- If a hydrocele of the cord is not recognized as such, any trial of reduction leads to unnecessary pain.

Clinical Findings

The swelling is a well-defined roundish mass with a sharply delineated lateral end. It is nontender, cystic, supple, and somewhat movable on palpation and translucent #. The clinical diagnosis may be difficult if it is combined with an inguinal hernia.

In girls, *the swelling concerns mainly the upper part of the vulva and adjacent groin #.*

Work-Ups

In equivocal cases, ultrasound of the groin demonstrates the diagnosis.

Treatment, Prognosis

Excision is indicated already in infancy because no spontaneous resolution can be expected. Surgery should include the whole processus vaginalis. Permanent cure is the rule.

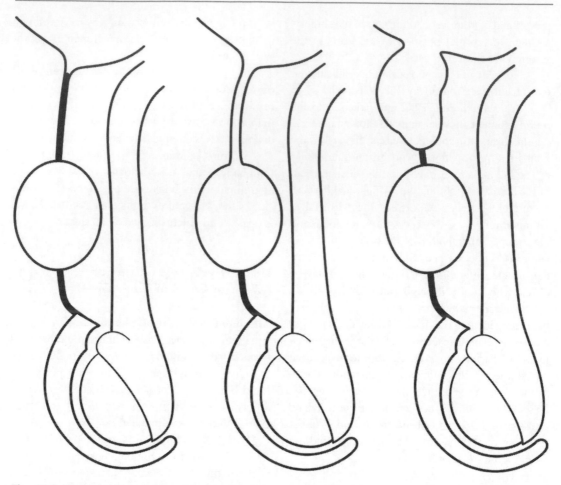

Fig. 19.2 Drawings of variations of hydrocele of the cord. *Left side*: The processus peritonei vaginalis is atretic except for a residual cavity of the size of a walnut. Spontaneous resolution does not occur. In the *middle*: The hydrocele of the cord is connected with the peritoneal cavity by a minute tract. *Right side*: The hydrocele of the cord is associated with a small sack of a possible inguinal hernia. This variation and that quoted in the drawing in the *middle* must be looked for at surgery and treated accordingly to avoid manifestation of inguinal hernia or recurrence of hydrocele of the cord

19.1.3 Cryptorchidism Including Torsion of Undescended Testis

Clinical Significance

- Canalicular, prefascial, or high scrotal testis, sliding testis, and iatrogenic undescended testis may all mimic inguinal hernia, especially in neonates and premature infants. The same is true for torsion of an undescended testis.

Clinical Findings

In the **already quoted presentations of an undescended testis**, *the groin mass is solid and well delineated. If* **torsion** *has occurred, sudden onset of pain, nausea, and vomiting are reported. The mass in the groin is tender, solid, and tough on palpation #.*

Recognition of torsion may be difficult in retarded children because the acute onset has often not been noticed.

19.1.4 Inguinal Lymphadenopathy

Pathoanatomy, Clinical Significance

The superficial inguinal lymph nodes lie below the inguinal ligament and drain the leg, vulva, perineum, and the skin of scrotum and penis. Its clinical significance is as follows:

- Enlargement of the size of a lent up to a peanut is a frequent accidental finding beyond infancy.
- Clinical significance arises if enlargement is acute, exceeds the quoted size, or is combined with inflammatory findings in the draining area.

Clinical Findings

The inguinal lymph nodes are located lateral to the external ring or below the inguinal ligament and are depending on the cause and its stage either tender, firm, fixed, or fluctuant with inflammatory sign of the overlying skin #, or painless on palpation. The draining area may demonstrate an infectious focus.

Differential Diagnosis, Work-Ups

Differentiation from other pathologies may be difficult in obese children, especially if the overlying skin is swollen and the lesion is painful. History and clinical examination for possible site of entrance of the infection, other involved node groups, possible enlargement of liver and spleen are important. In addition to search for inflammatory blood signs, ultrasound permits diagnosis of lymphadenopathy and description of its morphologic characteristics (see cervical lymphadenopathies as well). A typical example of usefulness of ultrasound is suspected inguinal hernia in the girls (prolapse of ovary versus inguinal lymphadenopathy).

Treatment, Prognosis

Prognosis depends on the cause and stage of lymphadenopathy. In purulent lymphadenitis, incision and drainage are needed.

19.1.5 Pain in the Groin

Occurrence, Clinical Significance

Pain in the groin is a frequent complaint in the daily practice of family physicians. It presents in different ways:

- Combined with an overt local finding in the groin
- Explained by a distant disorder with radiation of the pain
- Without a concrete cause at the first glance

- The last presentation becomes significant with increasing age and bothers parents and family physician.

Clinical Presentation

In case of **pain in the groin combined with local findings**, an incarcerated (congenital) inguinal hernia, torsion or another disorder of undescended testis, inguinal lymphadenopathy, and disorders with testicular and/or scrotal swelling must be looked for.

Less frequently is the direct inguinal or femoral hernia, and if a scar after hernia repair is present, a recurrent inguinal hernia, a localized pain due to a neuroma after injury to the ilioinguinal nerve, or diffuse pain because of the scar must be considered.

In case of a **distant disorder**, additional findings point to specific locations such as scrotum, retroperitoneum, hip joint, or adjacent musculoskeletal system.

If **no concrete cause** seems to be present at first glance, recurrent manifestation of inguinal hernia, uni- or bilateral testicular torsion, meralgia paresthetica, or stress to musculoskeletal system by sports and dance must be evaluated by history and specific clinical skills.

Work-Ups, Differential Diagnosis

They depend on the disorders that should be excluded and the suspected disorders according to history and local findings, for example, recurrent sudden onset of testicular pain with spontaneous recovery is characteristic for recurrent testicular torsion.

Treatment

It depends on the causal disorder.

19.2 Swelling and Pain of the Navel and Linea Alba

19.2.1 Umbilical Hernia

Occurrence, Pathogenesis

Umbilical hernia is a frequent finding in infancy, especially in black children. In most cases, spontaneous resolution occurs by cicatricial retraction of the connective tissue in the umbilical plate after separation of the umbilical cord that closes the facial ring.

Because this healing process is delayed in some infants and small children due to adverse factors such as malnutrition and respiratory and intestinal disorders and since the natural history cannot be predicted in the individual case, umbilical hernia may become a case of illness during this period.

Clinical Significance

- The frequency of umbilical hernia, the disfiguring appearance especially on crying, the imagination of suffering of the child, and the uncertainty in the individual case that relates to the time of spontaneous healing worry and bother parents and family physician although spontaneous resolution occurs mostly in infancy and even up to the age of 5 years.
- Complications of umbilical hernia in older children such as strangulations are increasingly observed.

Clinical Findings

Umbilical hernia manifests in the first few weeks usually after cord separation up to 6 months of life. *The swelling concerns the center of the navel, increases on straining and crying, and reaches a size of fingertip # to nut and more. The larger the umbilical hernia, the more the ballooning mass includes the adjacent skin; the structure of the navel is effaced or lost #. The shape may vary between semispherical and tail-like protrusion #.*

The content of the sac can be easily reduced by gentle finger pressure if the child is calmed down. It consists of parts of intestine and/or omentum *that can be felt and recognized by its smooth or granular consistency and its gurgling sounds in the former. After reduction, the fascial ring and its size are palpable.*

If the diameter is <1 cm, the probability and time of spontaneous resolution are greater and shorter than if it is >1.5 cm.

Differential Diagnosis

The differential diagnosis includes cutis navel and omphalocele of cord after spontaneous epithelization and less probable other congenital and acquired disorders of the navel #.

Treatment, Prognosis

Absolute indications of hernia repair are incarceration and persistence of an umbilical hernia until preschool age. In incarceration, spontaneous pain, obstructive ileus, and tenderness of the hernia are present. Incarceration is increasingly observed in children. Spontaneous resolution is unlikely in umbilical hernia that persists till preschool age.

Relative indications are large types, umbilical hernias with an umbilical ring >1.5 cm diameter, and umbilical hernias in which the parents are considerably stressed at any age or beyond 6 months of age, respectively.

Surgery includes semicircular incision close to the navel, preparation and division of the hernia sac, and closure at its neck. It is followed by transverse closure of the fascia including the umbilical ring with interrupted sutures. After possible resection of superfluous skin in large umbilical hernia, the undersurface of the center of the umbilicus skin is sutured to the fascia and the skin incision closed.

Permanent cure if appropriate surgery is performed and no local infection arises.

19.2.2   Epigastric Hernia

Pathoanatomy, Occurrence, Clinical Significance

Epigastric hernia is rarely reported in children although precise examination of the epigastriums yields often one or several small congenital gaps of the midline fascia from the xiphoid process to the umbilicus. Initially, pieces of preperitoneal fat prolapse through the small holes and are followed latter by evaginations of peritoneum.

- Epigastric hernia leads to vague upper abdominal pain, its recognition needs specific attention and clinical skills and is therefore often missed.
- Types with close vicinity to the umbilicus may be misinterpreted as umbilical hernia and left to spontaneous resolution by mistake (paraumbilical hernia)

Clinical Findings

Occasionally, *an epigastric tender, granular, and flat mass of the size of lentil is felt on palpation in a supine position. Provocation of spontaneous midline pain and the characteristic finding that can be palpated or even seen in a sitting up maneuver without the aids of the arms.*

Differential Diagnosis, Work-Ups

In diastasis of the abdominal rectus muscles, the midline is wide, gets wider, and develops to a longitudinal gap in a sitting up maneuver with both muscles prominent on either side of the gap. Other differential diagnoses are small abdominal wall tumors and intra-abdominal causes of epigastric abdominal pain (chronic abdominal pain). Ultrasound of the midline soft tissue may be useful for imaging of small masses, their characteristics, and relation to the different layers.

Treatment, Prognosis

Surgery is indicated in case of specific clinical and/or ultrasound findings and related to the epigastric pain because spontaneous resolution does not occur. It consists of resection of the prolapsed fatty tissue and peritoneum and closure of the fascial defects and leads to permanent cure.

Webcodes

The following webcodes can be used on www. psurg.net for further images and data.

1901 Tumefaction right groin	1912 Testicular feminization, gonad
1902 Tumefaction navel	1913 Recurrent l inguinal hernia, left side
1903 Bilateral inguinal hernia, prematurity	1914 Operative finding, hydrocele of the cord
1904 Age and sex distribution inguinal hernia	1915 Right hydrocele of the cord
1905 Right inguinal hernia	1916 Left hydrocele of the canal of Nuck
1906 Right complete inguinal hernia	1917 Operative finding, torsion undescended testis
1907 Right inguinal hernia, girl	1918 Purulent inguinal lymphadenitis
1908 Intestinal strangulation	1919 Small umbilical hernia
1909 Testicular necrosis, incarceration	1920 Large umbilical hernia
1910 Incarcerated inguinal hernia	1921 Umbilical hernia, tail-like shape
1911 Girard's technique	1922 Umbilical hernia, umbilical granuloma

Bibliography

Section 19.1

Chan KL, Tam PK (2004) Technical refinements in laparoscopic repair of childhood inguinal hernias. Surg Endosc 18:957–960

Cooke A, Deshpande AV, La Hei ER, Kellie S, Arbuckle S, Cummins G (2009) Ectopic nephrogenic rests in children: the clinicosurgical implications. J Pediatr Surg 44:e13–16

Garvey JF, Read JW, Turner A (2010) Sportsman hernia: what can we do? Hernia 14:17–25

Högger C (1978) Schädigung des Hodens und des Ovars bei eingeklemmten Leistenbrüchen im Säuglings- und Kleinkindesalter. Z Kinderchir 23:293–301

Hutson JM (1998) Undescended testis, torsion, and varicocele. In: O'Neill JA Jr et al (eds) Pediatric surgery, vol II, 5th edn. Mosby, St. Louis

Lloyd DA, Rintala J (1998) Inguinal hernia and hydrocele. In: O'Neill JA Jr et al (eds) Pediatric surgery, vol II, 5th edn. Mosby, St. Louis

Madziga AG, Nuhu AI (2008) Causes and treatment outcome of mechanical obstruction in north eastern Nigeria. West Afr J Med 27:101–105

Momoh JT (1985) External hernia in Nigerian children. Ann Trop Paediatr 5:197–200

Moore CP, Marr JK, Huang CJ (2011) Cryptorchid testicular torsion. Pediatr Emerg Care 27:121–123

Pisacane A, de Luca U, Vaccaro F et al (1995) Breastfeeding and inguinal hernia. J Pediatr 127:109–111

Ris H-B et al (1987) 10 Jahre Erfahrung mit einer modifizierten Operationstechnik nach Shouldice für Inguinalhernien bei Erwachsenen. I. Methode und Resultate bei 716 nachkontrollierten Operation. Chirurg 58:93–99

Senayli A, Senayli Y, Sezer E, Sezer T (2007) Torsion of an encysted fluid collection. Sci World J 7:822–824

Section 19.2

Albanese CT, Rengal S, Bermudez D (2006) A novel laparoscopic technique for repair of pediatric umbilical and epigastric hernias. J Pediatr Surg 41:859–862

Ameh EA (2004) Incarceration of umbilical hernia in children: is the trend increasing? letter to the editors. Eur J Pediatr Surg 14:218

Cilley RE, Krummel TM (1998) Disorders of the umbilicus. In: O'Neill JA Jr et al (eds) Pediatric surgery, vol II, 5th edn. Mosby, St. Louis

Coats RD, Helikson MA, Burd RS (2000) Presentation and management of epigastric hernias in children. J Pediatr Surg 35:1754–1756

Vomiting, regurgitation, and dysphagia belong to the typical presenting symptoms and signs of the disorders listed in Table 20.1.

For vomiting, time after food intake or during the 24-h cycle, content, and associated symptoms are important additional informations. Regurgitation is often interpreted as vomiting; a precise history and observation yields however that indigestible pieces of food or foreign bodies are brought up in case of regurgitation which get stuck in the esophagus. Dysphagia is defined as getting stuck of a piece of food or as difficult swallowing and is often accompanied by hypersalivation (slobbering, drooling). Some drooling is normal during infancy.

Table 20.1 Differential diagnosis of vomiting, regurgitation, and dysphagia

Vomiting, regurgitation

- Esophageal atresia, isolated tracheoesophageal fistula
- Gastroesophageal reflux, hiatus hernia
- Hypertrophic pyloric stenosis
- Gastric voiding disorders
- Surgical abdomen
- Urinary tract infection (pediatric urological disorders)
- Hydrocephalus, shunt dysfunction → macrocephalia
- Brain injury → unconsciousness

Dysphagia

- Esophageal stenosis (congenital, acquired)
- Achalasia, neurological disorders of swallowing
- Volvulus of the stomach, upside-down stomach, paraesophageal hernia (primary, secondary), and Morgagni diaphragmatic hernia (with gastrointestinal symptomatology)
- Foreign body ingestion
- Chemical injury of the upper gastrointestinal tract

The quoted presenting signs occur often combined in the same disorder. They may also be caused by pathologies outside of the upper gastrointestinal tract.

20.1 Esophageal Atresia, Isolated Tracheoesophageal Fistula

Occurrence, Pathoanatomy

Esophageal atresia is a classic, relatively frequent pediatric surgical disorder with 1 in 2,500 to 5,000 live births.

The common classifications (Gross, Vogt-Ladd, Waterston, and Spitz) describe either the anatomical types or prognostic factors such as associated birth weight of < or >1,500 g and major cardiovascular anomalies.

The following anatomical types are arranged in order of frequency (I–IV and A–E correspond to the Vogt-Ladd and Gross classification):

Esophageal atresia with distal fistula	IIIb/C	>80 %
Esophageal atresia without fistula	Ib/A	<10 %
Tracheoesophageal fistula without esophageal atresia	IIIa/E	<5 %
Esophageal atresia with fistula to both pouches	IV/D	<2 %
Esophageal atresia with proximal fistula	II/B	<1 %

In Vogt-Ladd's classification, type Ia corresponds to a complete aplasia of the esophagus and IIIa to a long-gap esophageal atresia that

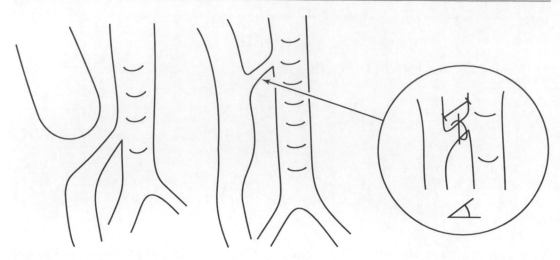

Fig. 20.1 Two types of esophageal atresia are recognizable. The drawing on the *left side* shows the most common type 3b according to Vogt. The dilated proximal esophagus has a blind end, and a fistula from the trachea runs to the small distal esophagus. The drawing on the *right side* displays an isolated tracheoesophageal fistula (type 4 according to Vogt). The esophagus is intact, but a fistula runs from a more proximal site of the trachea to a more distal site of the esophagus (N-fistula)

occurs usually in esophageal atresia without fistula and infrequently in the other types.

In the most common type "esophageal atresia with distal fistula," the proximal esophagus ends in a pouch somewhat below the thoracic inlet. The distal fistula originates from the trachea and continues to the distal esophagus (Fig. 20.1).

Four variations and types are of practical significance:

- In the long-gap esophageal atresia, the distance between the two parts of the esophagus is too large; a primary anastomosis is impossible in spite of minor additional measures at surgery. This variation can be observed in almost all newborns with esophageal atresia without fistula and occasionally in the other types of esophageal atresia. In addition, radiological imaging confirms a long-gap atresia; a distance more than 2–3 cm is only a numerical approximation of it.
- The esophageal atresia without fistula exhibits, in addition to the long-gap variety, more frequently the known associated anomalies including tracheomalacia than the other types.
- In types with proximal and fistula to both pouches and in tracheoesophageal fistula without esophageal atresia (Fig. 20.1), difficulties arise in the pre- and intraoperative recognition and need variation of surgical technique

Clinical Significance

- It is very important that esophageal atresia is recognized early after birth before a respiratory distress syndrome becomes manifest.
- Long-term follow-up and care demands a great deal of expertise on part of the pediatrician and pediatric surgeon.

Clinical Findings

Esophageal atresia may be suspected by prenatal ultrasound if polyhydramnion is combined with a small or absent stomach.

Hypersalivation combined with episodes of regurgitation, chocking, coughing, and possible cyanosis are observed already in the first hours after birth. They occur spontaneously or immediately after the first trial of feeding with tea. Froth in front of the nostrils and mouth corresponds to regurgitated saliva or tea mixed with air. Dependent on the severity of reflux of gastric acid, elevation of the diaphragm because of overinflation of the stomach, and aspiration of saliva and possibly food, signs of respiratory distress develop. A first confirmation of the diagnosis can be attained if a tube cannot be introduced through the mouth in the stomach.

In **esophageal atresia without tracheoesophageal fistula**, *there is no air in the abdomen and the belly remains therefore under the level of the thorax.*

The **clinical presentation in isolated tracheoesophageal fistula** is somewhat different, and it *may remain unrecognized initially. At feeding, chocking and cyanotic spells may be observed initially without regurgitation and later recurrent right upper pneumonia and intermittent abdominal distension after coughing and crying.*

Associated anomalies are observed in 50–70 % of the cases and include the following anomalies:

Cardiovascular in	35 %
Gastrointestinal and urogenital each in	25 %
Skeletal, neurological and other each in	≥10 %

VACTERL is the most common association of several malformations in esophageal atresia and includes vertebral, anorectal, cardiovascular, tracheoesophageal, renal, and radial limb abnormalities. Trisomy 13 and 18 are representatives of chromosomal aberrations. Potter's syndrome including bilateral renal agenesis is an extreme example of anomalies that decide against treatment.

Work-Ups, Differential Diagnosis

Work-Ups concern confirmation and typification of esophageal atresia and of suspected associated malformations.

Plain chest and abdominal x-ray shows an air-filled upper pouch and air in stomach and intestine in the classic type of esophageal atresia and possible causes of respiratory impairment. No air in the abdomen assumes the possibility of esophageal atresia without distal fistula, with a proximal fistula, or a hidden distal fistula in the classic type #. The upper pouch and its level is visible on a plain x-rax with a radiopaque catheter tip and more precisely by introduction of some water-soluble **contrast** combined with lateral x-ray including the neck (a small and short upper pouch or connection to the trachea are indications

of an upper fistula). The upper fistula may be also recognized by preoperative broncho- and esophagoscopy. For diagnosis of isolated tracheoesophageal fistula, contrast application in prone position and lateral view may demonstrate the N-fistula ascending from the esophagus into the trachea # or its direct visualization is possible by esophagoscopy and/or bronchoscopy. After performance of a gastrostomy, the distance between the two parts of the esophagus can be measured after contrast application in possible long-gap esophageal atresia.

The indication of additional work-ups for associated anomalies depends largely on a careful and expert clinical examination and on the possibility of interference in the planned surgery. Echocardiogram, abdominal ultrasound, and genetic consultation belong to the most urgent examinations (severe cardiovascular anomaly, bilateral renal agenesis in Potter's syndrome, and trisomies or associations such as VACTERL).

The differential diagnoses are those of vomiting, regurgitation, and dysphagia in the early stage and those of respiratory distress in later stages.

Treatment, Prognosis

The **common type of esophageal atresia** is usually operated within 24–48 h to avoid further impairment of the respiratory system after stabilization of the newborn and exclusion of major associated anomalies.

General anesthesia for **surgery** should avoid major gas flow through the distal fistula. The posterior mediastinum is approached by a subscapular posterolateral incision through the 4th intercostal space with expleural dissection whenever possible.

After preparation of the proximal pouch, distal tracheoesophageal fistula, adjacent trachea, and vagus nerves, a vessel loop is passed around the fistula that is divided close to the trachea. The trachea is closed including a small rim of the former fistula with interrupted sutures, and its tightness is checked with by a water bath.

The proximal pouch is gently mobilized to the thoracic inlet and the distal esophagus to a lesser degree using traction sutures at their ends. As soon as both ends can be approached without major traction, both ends are sparsely incised and resected, and an end-to-end anastomosis is performed starting with to stay sutures to both edges and interrupted sutures of the back wall including both layers of the esophagus. After introduction of a feeding tube in the stomach, the anterior wall is closed in the same way. A chest tube with the tip away from the anastomosis is left, and the incision is closed stepwise.

In **esophageal atresia without esophageal fistula**, a gastrostomy is performed within 24 h that permits enteral nutrition and further confirmation of the type of esophageal atresia by distal and proximal contrast application.

Repair is delayed first for 2–3 months because growth may diminish the distance between the proximal and distal part of the esophagus in some patients and permit secondary anastomosis, especially if extensive mobilization and additional procedures are performed (circular myotomy, opening of the hiatus, proximal pouch-flap esophagoplasty or advancement of a part or the whole stomach into the thorax after laparotomy).

If the distance between the two parts is still too large for these measures, either a primary gastric transposition to the esophagus is performed without thoracotomy or a left cervical esophagostomy followed by esophageal replacement in a later stage (colonic inter-position).

In **isolated tracheoesophageal fistula** #, repair is mostly possible by a low-cervical access on the right side with the head extended and turned to the left side. After retraction of the sternomastoid muscle in a posterior direction, the dissection follows medially to the carotid sheet to the trachea and esophagus with retraction of the inferior thyroid artery and the middle thyroid vein and preservation of the right and left recurrent laryngeal nerve. After careful passing of two vessel loops around the esophagus proximally and distally to the fistula, traction sutures are placed at the upper and lower base of the fistula close to esophagus and trachea. The fistula is resected and the trachea closed in a longitudinal and the esophagus in a transverse direction with interrupted sutures with the same technique as in the common esophageal atresia. Before stepwise

closure, a gastric tube is advanced through the esophagus and a soft drain left in the site of surgery.

In **esophageal atresia with proximal pouch** (either as double form in classic esophageal atresia or as esophageal atresia with proximal pouch), the proximal end of the esophagus is carefully dissected to recognize the preoperative suspected or confirmed fistula. The fistula may be tiny or in a very high position. Repair follows the already quoted principles. In case of missed double fistula at first operation, a cervical approach can be used.

Patient with operated tracheoesophageal fistula need lifelong follow-ups (gastroesophageal reflux with the inherent complications, recurrent respiratory tract infections, and sequels of the associated anomalies and performed interventions). The overall long-term survival is 85–90 % because of some subgroups with greater risk of death (birth weight <1,500 g), major associated malformations, and long-gap length variety.

20.2 Gastroesophageal Reflux, Hiatus Hernia

Occurrence, Pathoanatomy, and Grouping
Gastroesophageal reflux belongs to the most frequent causes of vomiting in the 1st year of life.

Two groups of children may be differentiated:
- Children in whom the gastroesophageal transition is normal (acute angle of His) or shows an obtuse angle in the upper gastrointestinal contrast study #, and reflux is not recognizable during the radiological examination or exhibits different degrees of reflux (reflux to the distal, middle, or proximal esophagus with possible entrance into the respiratory tract).
- Children in whom different parts of the stomach herniate intermittently or permanently into the thorax combined with a visible reflux # – hiatus hernia, present in <10 % of children with gastroesophageal reflux.

Clinical Significance
- The frequent occurrence of reflux in the daily life bothers parents and those close to them

and leads to failure to thrive if the reflux is severe and long-standing.

- If not treated and/or no spontaneous resolution occurs, reflux may lead to a lifelong physically disabling disease (recurrent respiratory impairment and/or dysphagia due to esophageal stenosis including brachyesophagus) or life-threatening complication (ALTE, sudden infant death)

Clinical Presentation

Repeated bringing up of a part of the swallowed milk or tea either during or some time after feeding combined with an acid smell is the characteristic sign of **uncomplicated reflux**. *Vomiting may occur in a bow although the bringing up is less projectile than in hypertrophic pyloric stenosis (Fig. 20.2), may start already in the first days after birth, and increases in severity during early infancy. In time, vomiting may decrease or disappear either because of spontaneous recovery or due to changes of nutrition (semiliquid or solid meals) and motor development (upright position).*

In toddlers and schoolchildren, *vomiting is less frequently observed or only in intermittent episodes, and abdominal and thoracic pain, pyrosis, and dysphagia may be observed* that have no regular correlation with possible esophagitis.

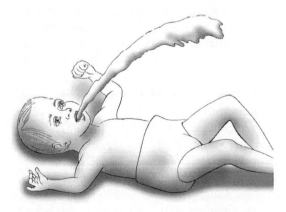

Fig. 20.2 The drawing shows a young infant with projectile vomiting. It occurs during or shortly after feedings and is a very forceful ejection which travels in a flat arc shape for several feet as shown in the drawing, and there is a large amount of milk, formula, or tea

In addition to the described symptomatology, the following complications occur with decreasing frequency – **complicated reflux**:

- *Failure to thrive* with insufficient or stop of weight gain, malnutrition, and insufficiently increasing body length #.
- *Reactive airway disease* consists of chronic and possibly asthmoid bronchitis and aspiration pneumonias of different location including lung abscess, laryngitis, and pharyngitis, sinusitis, and otitis. *Laryngospasm, hoarseness and stridor, fever and dyspnea, chronic cough and chocking at night, apnea, and deterioration of asthma and ALTE are the possible signs.*
- *Hematemesis* (upper gastrointestinal bleeding), *evacuation of blood by the anus* (lower gastrointestinal bleeding), and *chronic anemia* are important sequels of complicated reflux. Hematemesis is observed *either as a trace of fresh blood or brownish hematin or as corresponding discoloration of the gastric content that is brought up #.*
- *Dysphagia* is, as the already quoted complications and the following unspecific symptoms, a sequel of reflux of gastric acid that occurs intermittently between the meals, on lying down for sleeping, and on straining. *Circular stenosis or stenosis of long distance, or brachyesophagus develops depending on the main direction of shrinkage (observed in 60 % of children with significant esophagitis and in 6 % of children with surgery for reflux). Irritability and food rejection may be a sign of esophagitis in infants.*
- *Unexplained crying, abdominal, epigastric, or retrosternal pain, bad breath, and torticollis.*

In contrast to the described symptoms and signs, reflux cases without overt signs also occur in children who sometimes end up with severe complications in child- or adulthood.

Differential Diagnosis, Work-Ups

The differential diagnoses of uncomplicated reflux are those of vomiting in infants and small children. In complicated reflux, the most impressive sign may be the reason for different groups of differential diagnosis, for example, in hematemesis or torticollis.

The observation that multiple symptoms and signs occur in the same patient in two thirds of reflux cases is a useful tool in the differential diagnosis.

Confirmation of a suspected reflux is obtained best by **continuous (24-h) pH monitoring** that has a sensitivity of 100 % and a specificity of 94 %. Diagnostic is a pH≤4 in more than 5 % of the recorded time #. Because the **upper gastrointestinal contrast study** is less sensitive and specific, reflux may be overlooked. On the other hand, hiatus hernia, antral dysmotility or obstruction, stricture of the esophagus and its characteristics, and disorders of esophageal motility is only or best depicted by it. **Esophagoscopy** is not very useful for reflux diagnosis, but for esophagitis together with biopsy (only 50 % of esophagitis # are recognized by endoscopy alone) and for treatment of strictures.

In selected cases, **scintiscan** can be applied for proof of aspiration and antral dysmotility and **manometry** of the esophagus for confirmation of achalasia.

Treatment, Prognosis

The uncomplicated gastroesophageal reflux is treated today with **nonoperative measures**, especially with drugs for a limited time, this on the assumption that spontaneous recovery occurs. Resolution has been observed in 60 % in the 1st year of life and afterward in a smaller percentage. Useful adjuncts are semi-upright position combined with frequent, small, and thickened feedings. Often, a stepwise procedure is used depending on the severity of reflux and success of treatment: Starting with postural therapy and dietary measures, prokinetic drugs are added (cisapride) if the former fails. In case of failure of prokinetics, esophagitis, and respiratory symptoms, antacids or histamine H2 receptor blocker are introduced. The beneficial role of upright position especial of the sitting position is controversially discussed.

The **indications of surgery** are controversial because of the effectiveness of modern drugs and the possibility of recurrence after surgery. On the other hand, lifelong medication is necessary in some patients, and only the gastric acid production is interrupted and not the reflux as such.

Indications of surgery are the following conditions:

- Complicated reflux in which nonoperative treatment fails.
- Hiatus hernia and severe sequels of aspiration (chronic lung disease) and esophagitis (severe esophageal stenoses).
- Reflux in esophageal atresia, congenital diaphragmatic hernia, omphalocele, and laparoschisis.
- Reflux in neurological disorders such as cerebral palsy and psychomotor retardation
- Chronic diseases in which failure to thrive and recurrent respiratory tract infection play an important role become worse by reflux and are therefore a possible indication for surgery.

If surgery is planned, feeding problems, motility disorders of the esophagus, and voiding disorders of the stomach should be excluded. Otherwise, a gastrostomy, a not too tight fundus wrap, or a pyloroplasty should be added to fundoplication.

Surgery can be performed either minimally invasive or open and consists of Nissen fundoplication, Thal semi-fundoplication, Thal-Ashcraft or Boix-Ochoa procedure, or their modifications.

Nissen fundoplication # is a substitute of the insufficient antireflux mechanism. After a high transverse incision in the left upper abdomen, the peritoneal reflection between diaphragm and cardia is divided, and the esophageal hiatus and abdominal esophagus dissected with preservation of the vagus nerves. The upper part of the triangular ligament and lesser omentum is incised, and the abdominal esophagus pulled in a caudal and left direction with the aid of a catheter inserted around the cardia. The diameter of the esophageal hiatus is diminished with sutures of the crura that include muscle and peritoneum, and a wrap of appropriate length (2–3 cm in infants) is formed around the abdominal esophagus by pulling a part of fundus behind the esophagus. Both parts of the fundus are brought together anteriorly with two layers of interrupted and nonabsorbable sutures of which the deep layer includes the anterior esophageal wall. A gastric tube of 1–2 cm diameter avoids a too tight cuff. After sutures of the upper fundus border to the diaphragm and insertion of normal gastric tube, the incision is closed.

Boix-Ochoa and Thal-Ashcraft procedures correct the abnormal anatomy with the aim to restore the biological antireflux mechanism. The **Thal-Ashcraft technique** consists of an anterior 180-degree semi-fundoplication (the anterior portion of the gastric fundus is attached to the anterior abdominal esophagus). After closure of the enlarged hiatus, the greater curvature of anterior portion of fundus is fixed along the left side of the abdominal esophagus from the greater curvature-gastroesophageal junction for a distance of 2 (4–5) cm. Following fixation of the upper end of the wrap to the anterior esophagus and rim of the hiatus, the lesser curvature is sutured to the right lateral abdominal eso-esophagus down to the lesser curvature-gastroesohageal junction.

Prognosis

No studies until adulthood are available about possible drawbacks of long-term medication of the histamine H2 receptor antagonists. It is not excluded that some adults with symptomatic reflux have in fact a persistence of infantile reflux that was treated or not treated during infancy and later not appreciated because of the natural history with amelioration at the time of walking and eating from the table. Episodic vomiting in case of travelling and stress and abdominal pain has been referred to other causes till the fifth decade when the complaints become again prominent.

No symptoms and normal x-ray findings have been reported in >90 % after Nissen fundoplication and 1 % recurrence and 7 % mostly clinically silent radiological abnormalities of which herniation of the fundoplication was the most common and the less frequent paraesophageal hernia and peptic stenosis often needed further operative treatment. In general, recurrences that need reoperation are observed in >2–8.5 %, and belching is possible in more than 60 % after a few weeks and <5 % displays severe inflation of the stomach. Similar results are reported after laparoscopic fundoplication. The results of fundoplication in neurologically disabled children with about 70 % success are less favorable.

20.3 Hypertrophic Pyloric Stenosis

Occurrence

Hypertrophic pyloric stenosis is a frequent cause of vomiting in early infancy (1–4 in 1,000 live births) and is observed more frequently in boys. It occurs rarely immediately after birth and the 4th month of life.

Clinical Significance

- If not recognized as cause of vomiting in early infancy, dangerous exsiccosis and, in case of less severe clinical presentation, failure to thrive may develop.

Clinical Presentation

Some vomiting at or after feeding starts in the 2nd to 4th week of life (initially not after every feed and not forceful) and develops gradually or rapidly to the complete clinical presentation. Although the infant drinks greedily, its milk is brought up with considerable force (projectile vomiting for distance of up to one meter or more, Fig. 20.2) at and/or after every meal. The vomitus consists of gastric juice, fresh, or ingested milk and may sometimes contain traces of fresh or altered blood. The infants develop signs of exsiccosis, the body weight remains the same (in a period of rapid increase) or decreases, and dark-green splashes of a so-called hunger stool # are evacuated.

Depending on the severity and duration of vomiting, *a sunken fontanel, dry skin and mucous membranes, picked up fold of the belly, upper arm, or thigh that does not snap back if released are recognizable* as sign of exsiccosis.

In case of clinical presentation in the first two weeks or between the 2nd and 3rd month of life, combined with hematemesis, jaundice (indirect hyperbilirubinemia), and/or prematurity, the diagnosis may be masked. Associated gastroesophageal reflux is either a sequel of hypertrophic pyloric stenosis (that disappears after pyloromyotomy) or second disease.

Clinical Skills

After feeding of some sweetened tea with a bottle, a **distinct gastric peristalsis** can be seen running from the left upper belly to the umbilicus #.

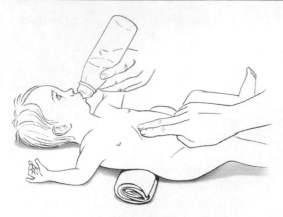

Fig. 20.3 The technique of palpation of the pyloric tumor is demonstrated in the drawing. The most important conditions are (1) sedation of the infant with artificially sweetened tea and (2) examination of the infant with warm index and middle fingers without any haste. A firm olive-like mass (pyloric tumor) can be palpated in the right upper abdomen that is elevated by a roll, by smoothly moving both fingertips to and fro. Students should perform such an examination preoperatively in the anesthetized and relaxed patient for the first time

It is accompanied by frowning and followed by projectile vomiting.

Palpation of an **olive-shaped mass** is possible in the quietened child with a roll under his back on the right side of the abdominal rectus muscle at the level of the navel that corresponds to the hypertrophic pyloric muscle. The mass can be rolled under the finger. This diagnostic sign can be palpated in >90 % if an appropriate technique, experience, and patience is applied (Fig. 20.3).

Differential Diagnosis, Work-Ups

It includes all causes of vomiting in early infancy. Of special interest are gastroesophageal reflux, rarely pyloric atresia, complete/incomplete antral web, duplication cyst, ectopic pancreatic tissue, duodenal obstruction above ampulla of Vater, antral dysmotility disorders, congenital adrenal hyperplasia (CAH) with salt loss, gastroenteritis, and feeding mismanagement.

Work-ups include electrolytes including bicarbonate. Hypochloremic and hypokalemic alkalosis is typical for hypertrophic pyloric stenosis (whereas adrenogenital syndrome with salt loss leads to hyperpotassemia and hyponatremia and hypochloremia).

The next step is **ultrasound** # that needs an expert radiologist, but has a sensitivity and specificity close to 100 % if no olive-shaped pyloric tumor is palpable or for confirmation of the clinical diagnosis. A thickness of the pyloric muscle of ≥4 mm is diagnostic (≥3 mm in the 1st month of life) and of ≤1 mm excludes hypertrophic pyloric stenosis. In case of values between >1 and <4 mm, ultrasound should be repeated some days later or completed by an upper gastrointestinal contrast study because hypertrophic pyloric stenosis may be become symptomatic several days before the pathological ultrasound findings. The **contrast study** shows an indirect sign elongation of the pyloric channel and indentation on the antral contour (so-called shoulder sign) #.

Treatment, Prognosis

Surgery should not be performed before fluid and electrolyte loss is corrected, among other things, because metabolic alkalosis leads to hypoventilation after surgery. The correction of the deficits takes one or more days depending on the severity of exsiccosis and base excess (<25 to >35 mEq/L) and needs substitution and replacement by 5–10 % glucose containing saline without correction of serum potassium and surveillance of urine output and serum electrolytes including bicarbonate.

Ramstedt pyloromyotomy # is performed after lavage and aspiration of gastric content. After a transverse incision over the right abdominal rectus muscle above the navel with retraction of the muscle to the midline, the stomach is grasped with the right hand, and the pylorus is delivered by traction on the stomach and pressure on the adjacent belly. Following an incision of the serosa along an avascular zone of the pylorus from the pyloric vein or a white line at this site to the antrum as far as the hypertrophied antrum muscle extends, the muscle layer is divided by careful spreading movements till all fibers are divided. Special care is necessary in this maneuver close to the duodenum. Integrity of the gastric mucous membrane is proved by injection of air in the stomach by the anesthetist and observation of the surgeon if air bubbles escape from the pylorus with the bulging mucosa in a saline bath. In case of perforation, the mucosa is closed with absorbable fine interrupted sutures and covered with a piece of omentum.

Access by the umbilicus or laparoscopic myotomy have been described.

Postoperative care needs a feeding schedule by which frequent and increasing amounts of tea and milk are given 6–12 h after surgery. Depending on the regime and the possible care at home, hospitalization after surgery is 1–2, 3–4, or more days.

Advanced cases with gross gastric dilatation or associated gastroesophageal reflux need special care because early postoperative vomiting may occur because of disorders of gastric peristalsis and reflux.

Prognosis is excellent in the majority of cases, and former patients have no gastrointestinal symptoms, gastric emptying disorders, or abnormal ultrasound findings in adulthood. The early perioperative complications include perforation of the gastric mucosa recognized or missed at surgery, incomplete separation of the muscle layer (it occurs usually in the area close to the antrum), wound infection, and prolonged postoperative vomiting (for different causes). The single surgical complications do and should occur in less than 1 %, and lethality is unusual. Prolonged vomitus after surgery combined with (e.g., peritonitis in missed perforation) or without local findings needs work-ups. The necessity of additional surgery depends on the results of work-up and especially on the cause.

20.4   Gastric Emptying Disorders

Occurrence
Delayed gastric emptying is observed either as **structural disorder** in congenital anomalies or acquired disorder (gastroduodenal ulcer, neoplasms, or as complication of abdominal trauma or ingestion of acid substances), or as **functional disorder.** The latter form of gastric emptying disorder has no mechanical cause, is infrequent, and occurs as isolated entity or as part of a neurodevelopmental disability (with oral motor dysfunction, dysphagia, and constipation) that is observed in neuromuscular diseases, cerebral palsy, spina

bifida, gastroesophageal reflux, and inborn errors of metabolism (e.g., pyruvate dehydrogenase deficiency).

Clinical Significance
- In infants and children of any age with neurological disorders and vomiting or other signs of the upper gastrointestinal tract, functional gastric emptying disorders must be considered in the differential diagnosis, work-ups, and treatment.
- The same applies to suspected classic pediatric surgical and other structural pathologies leading to vomiting.
- Gastroesophageal reflux may be associated with functional gastric emptying disorder, especially in children with cerebral palsy.

Clinical Presentation
Jodhpur disease is an example of isolated functional gastric emptying disorder and is characterized by *nonbilious vomiting, abdominal pain, and visible gastric peristalsis that lead to weight loss, dehydration, and dyselectrolytemia in infants and toddlers* between 1 month and 6 years of age. The clinical presentation of other forms of functional gastric emptying disorders is similar.

Differential Diagnosis, Work-Ups
The differential diagnosis includes causes of structural disorders leading to gastric emptying and functional dyspepsia similar to ulcer disease.

Possible work-ups include upper gastrointestinal contrast study (large stomach and delayed gastric emptying), application of milk or standardized meal radiolabeled with (13)C-octanoid acid and determination of the half-life of the isotope in the stomach, or the (13)C-octanoid breath test.

Treatment, Prognosis
Gastric endoscopy and surgical exploration including histology have been normal in Jodhpur disease, and pyloroplasty (Heineke-Mikulicz) was initially successful, whereas the same treatment or forceful dilatation had only uneventful long-term results in ≥50 % of other cohorts with functional gastric emptying disorder. Functional gastric emptying is not a uniform disorder with different

causes, severity of presentation, results of work-ups, and variable results of surgery or dilatation.

20.5   Esophageal Stenosis

Esophageal stenosis is either congenital or acquired. Differentiation is not always easy because the former comes sometimes to the attention later in childhood and the responsible cause is occasionally not remembered in the latter.

20.5.1 Congenital Esophageal Stenosis

Occurrence, Types, and Forms
Congenital esophageal stenosis is a rare malformation. The intrinsic form is observed in 1 of 25,000–50,000 live births and consists of three types which are somewhat different in diagnosis and treatment:
- Esophageal stenosis due to tracheobronchial remnants (distal esophagus)
- Esophageal stenosis due to fibromuscular hypertrophy (at any site, of any length)
- Membranaceous esophageal stenosis (middle and distal esophagus) #
The extrinsic form includes vascular ring anomalies, intestinal duplication, and congenital tumors.

Clinical Significance
- Congenital esophageal stenosis is often a difficult diagnosis and should therefore be considered in every infant and small child with vomiting, dysphagia, and failure to thrive.

Clinical Presentation
Infants become often symptomatic after introduction of semisolid and solid feed with vomiting, dysphagia, signs of reactive airway disease, and failure to thrive.

Vomiting and reactive airway disease may occur already in the neonatal period or failure to thrive may be the sole sign depending on the type of congenital esophageal stenosis.

*It is useful to know that **intrinsic** esophageal stenosis may be associated with esophageal atresia of any type and with other anomalies.*

The symptomatology is variable in the **extrinsic form** and depends on the site and the cause of obstruction. If the proximal esophagus is obstructed by intestinal duplication, *respiratory distress syndrome or signs of the respiratory tract occur*, whereas obstruction of the middle or distal esophagus leads to *dysphagia and other upper gastrointestinal signs or to the incidental finding of a posterior mediastinal tumor*. Whereas dysphagia and respiratory signs with deterioration by stress is observed in duplication of the aortic arch, aberration of the right subclavian artery leads only to dysphagia.

Differential Diagnosis, Work-Ups
It includes all disorders with dysphagia and other sign of the upper gastrointestinal tract, RDS and signs of reactive airway disease, and incidental findings of a posterior neck and mediastinal tumor, and especially **esophageal achalasia** and **leiomyoma of the esophageal wall** that have similar clinical and radiological findings.

Work-ups include upper gastrointestinal contrast study including cineradiography, esophago-scopy, and CT including contrast. The **contrast study** shows an abrupt narrowing or a tapered narrowing (membranaceous or esophageal steno-sis due to fibromuscular hypertrophy) and a possible dilatation of the esophagus proximally to the stenosis, or in vascular ring anomalies, an offset of the longitudinal axis of the esophagus. **Esophagoscopy** demonstrates the stenosis, its site, and morphology (and is diagnostic for membranaceous stenosis). **CT** is useful for imaging of the intrinsic and extrinsic causes of stenosis and its lengths.

Treatment, Prognosis
Intrinsic esophageal stenoses are treated initially with dilations, either with tapered dilators under endoscopic guidance or with fluoroscopically guided forceful pneumatic distension. The possibility of esophageal perforation followed by mediastinitis must be taken into account.

In intrinsic esophageal stenoses resistant to bouginage or as initial procedure in esophageal stenosis with suspected tracheobronchial remnant, segmental esophageal resection or rarely replacement of the esophagus is indicated. The access is either a right or left thoracotomy or laparotomy depending on the site and length of the stenosis. Segmental resection is possible if the length is less than 3 cm; the distal end of the stenosis can be marked with a catheter by traction after inflation of its distally situated balloon; resection and end-to-end anastomosis must preserve the phrenic and vagal nerves, and surgery close to the cardia must consider the possibility of secondary reflux and fundoplication is necessary in the same session.

Extrinsic causes need resection (intestinal duplication, congenital tumors) or vascular surgery (vascular ring anomalies).

Permanent cure is possible if the site and cause of stenosis is completely resectable, and there is no traction on the anastomosis from the adjacent segments.

20.5.2 Acquired Esophageal Stenosis

Occurrence, Causes
Acquired esophageal stenoses are more frequent than congenital forms. Their prevalence depends on the frequency of the responsible causes. **Gastroesophageal reflux (peptic stenosis) #, caustic stricture**, and **stenosis due to ingested foreign body** are the most common causes, especially in developing countries.

Postoperative and **postinterventional stenoses** (repair of esophageal atresia, segmental resection, and replacement procedures of the esophagus and endoscopy, bouginage, endoscopic sclerotherapy, and other procedures) and less frequent disorders e.g., bullous epidermolysis or paraesophageal tumors are additional important causes.

Clinical Significance
- Acquired esophageal stenosis is a lengthy and difficult to treat disorder and represents a life-long defective healing process.
- After healing of the responsible cause, the clinical manifestation of esophageal stenosis occurs after a symptom-free interval unexpectedly, insidiously, and gradually.

Clinical Presentation
The first manifestation of a developing stenosis may be a piece of food or foreign body that gets stuck in the esophagus, drooling, and slackened drinking and eating. It is followed by dysphagia and regurgitation (masked as vomiting).

For early recognition of a developing stenosis, the surgeon must pay attention to its possibility and its early signs.

Differential Diagnosis, Work-ups
It encompasses all disorders that lead to the quoted symptomatology. The possibility of secondary esophageal stenosis must be considered always if an ingested foreign body has been removed especially if ulceration has been present and/or the foreign has been left there for a long time.

Upper gastrointestinal contrast study # and endoscopy belong to the main diagnostic tools and permit to describe the site, severity, and extension of stenosis and the follow-up after treatment.

Treatment, Prognosis
Repeated bouginage, localized resections, and esophageal replacement procedures belong to the therapeutic tools possibly completed by a gastrostomy.

The prognosis depends on cause and severity of the esophageal stenosis.

20.6 Achalasia

Occurrence, Pathophysiology
Achalasia is a rare disorder in childhood. A not very well-known cause leads to a motility disorder of the whole esophagus combined with insufficient reflex opening (relaxation) of the cardia at swallowing.

Achalasia is already observed in infancy # with gradual development of the disorder in contrast to the somewhat more frequent involvement of schoolchildren and adults with the possibility of sudden onset of incapacity to proper swallowing.

Clinical Significance

- Early recognition of achalasia is difficult because of its possibly gradual development and rarity in childhood.
- On the other hand, treatment in an early stage is more effective and seems to be related with a better long-term outcome.

Clinical Presentation

Regurgitation of undigested food, possible aspiration with reactive airway disease, and failure to thrive are the main clinical signs of achalasia.

Regurgitation in small children may be interpreted as reaction of defiance, and dysphagia can be articulated only in a certain age. *In infancy, regurgitation looks like vomiting, and the clinical presentation is misjudged as gastroesophageal reflux.*

In spite of the intermittent, wavelike course of achalasia, deterioration is observed from stage I (without) to stage III (with grotesque dilatation and tortuosity of the middle and proximal esophagus).

Work-Ups, Differential Diagnosis

The **upper gastrointestinal contrast study and fluoroscopy** shows a smooth and conical narrowing of the distal esophagus that ends in thread-like, hardly visible segment #. In advanced stages, the middle and proximal esophagus is dilated and may display tortuosity, an air-fluid level, or retained food. The peristalsis is poor, and the esophagus does not empty on fluoroscopy.

Esophageal manometry is diagnostic and characterized by absent propulsive peristalsis, insufficient relaxation of the lower esophageal sphincter, and increased pressure of the sphincter

Continuous pH monitoring may be used as adjunct if manometry is not available and demonstrates absent acid reflux episodes and emptying of an acid fluid bolus.

In contrast to the typical esophageal stenosis, the instruments for **esophagoscopy** can be passed into stomach without difficulties and show possible retention esophagitis of the middle and proximal esophagus.

Treatment, Prognosis

Forceful pneumatic distension is an example of a nonoperative measures and leads to some success especially in older schoolchildren and if applied repeatedly. The danger of esophageal rupture or reflux is ≤5 or ≥10 %.

Permanent cure is achieved in 90 % with a **modified Heller esophagocardiomyotomy**. The procedure is best performed by an open abdominal or laparoscopic access and includes resection of a longitudinal, 1-cm wide strip of the whole anterior muscle layer including 2 cm of the cardia and a variable length (4–8 cm) of the distal esophagus and leaving an intact mucosa. Surgery is completed by a semicircular fundoplication that does not compromise the site of myectomy. The length of myectomy depends on the stage of achalasia and the distance of narrowing of the esophagus.

In case of recurrence, incomplete myectomy must be considered, and dependent on the clinical and morphological severity of achalasia and duration of symptomatology, a repeated myectomy or esophageal replacement is performed. The necessity of the latter is unusual in childhood.

If surgery is performed in an early stage, permanent cure is possible. The motility disorder of the esophagus remains, but normalization of esophageal dilatation and amelioration of the narrow segment and esophageal emptying is achieved. In adulthood, a risk of squamous cell carcinoma of the esophagus exists.

20.7 Functional Disorders of Swallowing

They are mainly observed in children with neurodevelopmental disability who are poor feeders and display other symptoms and signs of the gastrointestinal tract.

20.8 Gastric Volvulus, Paraesophageal Hernia, and Upside-Down Stomach

Occurrence, Types, and Pathoanatomy

Gastric volvulus, congenital and acquired paraesophageal hernia, and upside-down stomach are rare disorders.

Gastric volvulus takes place in three different directions along the longitudinal gastric axis (cardiopyloric line, organoaxial volvulus), the short axis (middle line between lesser and greater curvature, mesentericoaxial volvulus), or combined along both axes (mixed biplanar volvulus). The gastric antrum rotates upward and from left to right in organoaxial volvulus, and the antrum rotates upward and from right to left in mesentericoaxial volvulus producing an upside-down stomach. Gastric volvulus is possible due to a deficit of gastric fixation and malformation of the diaphragm (congenital diaphragmatic hernia, diaphragmatic eventration) and other adjacent organs. **Paraesophageal hiatus hernia** and **intrathoracic upside-down stomach** are related disorders of hiatus hernia in which a part of the stomach herniates through the hiatus not exclusively as axial hiatus hernia but as paraesophageal or mixed type or herniates completely as final stage of hiatus hernia into the same space and gets thereby an additional volvulus (upside-down stomach). The two conditions are possible because the esophageal hiatus is extremely wide, and/or secondary brachyesophagus has occurred.

Clinical Significance

- Acute gastric volvulus and to a lesser degree upside-down stomach may lead to gangrene of the stomach.
- In gastric volvulus, paraesophageal hiatus hernia, and upside-down stomach, vomiting is not in the foreground of acute presentation but dysphagia and regurgitation because of kinking of the gastroesophageal junction and of a posterior mediastinal mass effect in the latter two conditions which may also lead to cardiorespiratory signs.

Clinical Presentation

Acute gastric volvulus presents with *epigastric pain. Dysphagia and regurgitation may be combined with impossibility to pass a gastric tube in the stomach. Regurgitation after a meal that is followed by persistent retching has been quoted as suggestive of gastric volvulus. The epigastrium is tender and tympanitic on clinical examination. Depending on the time since beginning and the degree of volvulus, shock, peritonitis, and septicemia develop. The clinical presentation is unspecific in chronic recurrent volvulus except for epigastric pain.*

In paraesophageal hiatus hernia, *preexisting vomiting due to the gastroesophageal reflux may be combined with dysphagia and especially with cardiorespiratory signs.*

Differential Diagnosis, Work-Ups

Disorders of epigastric pain and tenderness and/or mediastinal tumor must be considered and specifically congenital diaphragmatic hernias (Morgagni or Bochdalek's hernia) with delayed and abdominal clinical presentation.

Chest and/or abdominal x-ray displays air accumulation in the upper abdomen with a possible double air-fluid level in gastric volvulus and air-filled supradiaphragmatic structure in paraesophageal hiatus hernia or upside-down stomach. Esophagogastric contrast study is diagnostic in all three disorders except for complete obstruction of gastroesophageal junction.

Treatment, Prognosis

Emergency surgery is indicated in acute gastric volvulus and as soon as possible elective surgery in chronic volvulus and the other two disorders. The transabdominal access includes retorsion of gastric volvulus, fundophrenicopexy and corpoventropexy (along the esophageal axis), and repair of possible associated anomalies. In the other two disorders, the herniated stomach is reduced, the hiatus repaired (a possible common hiatus for esophagus and aorta must be considered), and the stomach fixated in the same way as in gastric volvulus (possibly combined with semifundoplication).

The outcome is uneventful if the general condition of the child is good and the quoted principles of surgery are applied.

20.9 Foreign Body Ingestion

Occurrence, Types of Foreign Bodies

Foreign body ingestion is a frequent event in the daily medical practice. In contrast to caustic injuries with a peak of occurrence in small children (mean age 3 years), foreign body ingestion

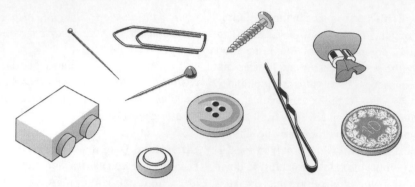

Fig. 20.4 The drawing shows common ingested foreign bodies. All objects are visible on plain x-ray except for the LEGO particle and the piece of sausage. The dangerous knob battery is recognizable at the *bottom* on the *left side*

is more evenly distributed from late infancy to adolescence and includes a large variety of objects that are taken into the mouth and swallowed unintentionally.

Frequent objects are coins, parts of toys, nails, needles and pins, hairslides, buttons, and disc batteries, and insufficiently chewed or unchewable parts of food as seen in Fig. 20.4.

Extraordinary and/or large amounts of foreign bodies point to a psychiatric disorder combined with self-mutilating or suicidal intentions, or with mental retardation #.

Some foreign bodies that got stuck in the upper or lower gastrointestinal tract point to a latent obstruction of the alimentary tract in congenital or acquired disorders with or without former surgery, for instance, stenosis and motility disorder after repair of esophageal atresia, peptic esophageal stenosis in gastroesophageal reflux, etc.

Clinical Significance
- Swallowed foreign body is a frequent disorder at any age and without or with mental disorder.
- Every foreign body that got stuck at any segment of the gastrointestinal tract may point to a latent obstruction.

Clinical Presentation
The following reasons of possible foreign body ingestion may lead to consultation:
- A caregiver of the child is missing an object.
- The caregiver observes that the child takes an object into the mouth that is not available afterward with or without symptoms.

- The same observation applies to schoolchildren, adolescents, and their mates.
- The child is observed while eating or playing and starts immediately coughing, retching, and having to force down something in the esophagus, and this episode is followed by drooling and refusal of swallowing.
- The already quoted presentation has been observed neither by a caregiver nor by the patient.

If the foreign body got stuck in the esophagus, a relatively unspecific symptomatology develops with pain in the throat, neck, retrosternal, or interscapular region; drooling; and dysphagia, much later with hematemesis or signs of the respiratory tract. If the foreign body got stuck in the stomach, duodenum, or lower gastrointestinal tract, often, no symptoms and signs are present and only in case of complications. Spontaneous passage occurs more frequently after swallowing of the foreign body with entrance in the stomach than getting stuck; the quoted figure of 90 % is possibly to optimistic.

Differential Diagnosis, Work-Ups
The diagnosis may be difficult in the last of the quoted reasons for consultation because a link to possible foreign body ingestion has initially not been noticed or has been forgotten. The differential diagnosis includes therefore all disorders with similar clinical presentation.

The work-ups start with a lateral plain x-ray of the neck (that may be completed with a contrast swallow if a radioparent object is suspected, e.g., a plastic toy #) and are followed by plain chest and/or abdominal x-ray ## for confirmation of a foreign body, its site, and exclusion of its possible aspiration. Rarely, CT is necessary. Sometimes, esophagoscopy is diagnostic as well as therapeutic.

Treatment, Prognosis

In the recent literature, procedures are increasingly proposed which try to avoid general anesthesia and endoscopic extraction and to save time and expenses, for instance, by extraction of the foreign body by a Foley catheter with an inflatable balloon or advancement into the stomach by bougies. Such procedures do not consider the anxiety of children and variety of clinical presentation of foreign bodies.

Foreign bodies that got stuck in the esophagus should be removed as soon as possible under guidance of a rigid or flexible endoscope. The same applies to disc batteries and to persistent foreign bodies of the upper gastrointestinal tract. Because three fourths of the esophageal foreign bodies get stuck in the cricopharyngeal region, careful inspection is necessary after intubation and before introduction of the esophagoscope; it is often possible to remove them by an appropriate instrument. The introduced esophagoscope should be advanced only slowly to avoid that the foreign body is pushed into the stomach before he can be grasped and extracted.

20.10 Corrosive Ingestion (Caustic Stricture of the Upper Gastrointestinal Tract)

Occurrence, Pathophysiology, and Anatomy

Although severe caustic injuries are observed less frequently in the developed countries due to prevention measures, less severe accidents are still a matter of concern. In developing countries, however, corrosive ingestion of all grades is still a burden of the public health system.

Small children are mostly involved in corrosive ingestions, whereas this type of injury occurs less frequently in schoolchildren or adolescents and if so by mistake or as an act of suicide or self-mutilation.

Location, severity, and extension of corrosive injuries depend largely on the concentration, physical form (liquid or granular [crystalline]), and pH of the caustic substances. **Acid substances** are often expectorated or pass rapidly the esophagus and remain in the gastric antrum, whereas **alkaline liquid or granular substances** may damage the oral cavity and oropharynx and involve mostly the esophagus, especially the cricopharyngeal area, the middle part, and the distal segment of esophagus close to the cardia or sites where the granular substances adhere. Simultaneous involvement of larynx or respiratory tract is possible by spillage, aspiration, or development of fumes.

Acids lead to a **coagulation necrosis** that limits further penetration, whereas alkaline substances may penetrate through all layers of the esophageal wall due to the accompanying **liquefactive necrosis** that constitutes no barrier.

The **sequels of caustic injury** are edema, hyperemia, fibrinous membranes, erosions, ulcers, and scattered or extended necroses and become visible 24–48 h after injury. The edema is resolved and the necrotic tissue sloughed after 1–2 weeks and between the third and sixth week re-epithelization, and scarring takes place leading to possible adhesions of the wall, stricture, and shortening of the esophagus.

Clinical Significance

- The early evaluation of severity and extension of caustic injuries and prognostication of possible late sequels is a challenge for the pediatric surgeon.
- Caustic strictures of the upper gastrointestinal tract, especially of the esophagus. lead to a lifelong morbidity.

Clinical Presentation

In developed countries, the physician is often rapidly consulted, and only few symptoms and signs may be present in this early stage. Although the ingested material or the corresponding container is known, precise informations about the circumstances of ingestion (for instance, amount of swallowed caustic substance) are often not available.

Contact with a poison center and a careful examination are the next steps if immediate resuscitation are not necessary for stridor, dyspnea, and/or shock.

The large number of possible caustic agents includes cleaning substances for the household and liquids or granular materials for industry, trade, agriculture, and gardening.

The clinical presentation on follow-up varies from hardly recognizable signs to drooling and refusal to swallow and to overt dysphagia, regurgitation of bloody saliva, or pain at the inside of mouth, throat, chest, belly, and back. Inspection of the mouth including tongue and oropharynx for localized or diffuse swelling, redness, or formation of eschar is very important because severe involvement of mouth and oropharynx is accompanied in 90 % by similar findings of the esophagus.

Stridor and other respiratory signs point to spillage of alkaline fluid to larynx and respiratory tract and shock and abdominal signs to mediastinitis, peritonitis, and septicemia.

Work-Ups, Differential Diagnosis
Appropriate informations about the ingested caustic substance and distinct involvement of oral cavity and oropharynx are the indication of esophagoscopy that confirms the diagnosis of corrosive ingestion and allows description of its severity and extension (grades 0–IIIb) if the examination is performed 12–24 h after the trauma.

Plain x-rays of neck (lateral view), chest, or abdomen (upright position) are only necessary in case of suspected mediastinitis, respiratory disorder, or esophagogastric perforation.

Differential diagnosis is only important in cases in which the history of caustic injury is not known or got lost and concerns mainly children with a developing stricture leading to drooling, dysphagia, and regurgitation e.g., a foreign body that got stuck in the esophagus.

Treatment, Prognosis
Initial treatment depends on the severity and extension of caustic injury. The role of prophylactic antibiotics, antifungal drugs, and steroids remains controversial. Antibiotics may be restricted to severe grades with extensive necrosis, perforation, and/or concomitant respiratory tract infection or septicemia.

In all grades, oral intake of fluid and appropriate food is withheld as long as swallowing does not function and is replaced by a nasogastric tube, gastrostomy, or jejunostomy tube for feeding.

Whereas grade I lesions (edema and hyperemia) are discharged as soon as normal food intake is possible and need only clinical follow-up and only radiological follow-up if they get symptomatic, all other grades (grade IIa with hemorrhages, blisters, whitish membranes, and superficial ulcers and grades IIb and IIIa and b with deep ulcers and necroses) receive a permanent nasogastric tube, a gradual peroral nutrition, and a 1st upper contrast study 10–14 days after trauma.

Beginning strictures are treated with repeated dilatations as soon as they are recognized radiologically. The concomitant medication of antacids or antisecretory drugs should be considered. Dilatations are performed in general anesthesia under endoscopic surveillance, guided for instance by a transesophageal string that connects the oral cavity with the gastrostomy and continued until normal swallowing and caliber of the esophagus is achieved (visualized by endoscopy and upper GI contrast study). If dilatations fail, segmental esophageal resection or esophageal replacement without or with esophageal resection is performed.

The **prognosis** depends on the severity and extension of caustic injury and concerns the disorder and its progress and the chosen procedures.

About one fourth of the children with caustic injury need prolonged hospitalization and <10 % develops strictures. At least 40 % of the children respond to dilatations, and the remainder need surgery. In cases with successfully dilated esophagus or that is otherwise left behind, long-term clinical, endoscopic including biopsy, and contrast studies are necessary because gastroesophageal reflux and dysmotility dysfunction persist often, and Barrett's esophagus or esophageal carcinoma may develop after one to several decades.

Repeated dilatations are necessary for 9–12 months. They hold the danger of perforation that occurs in up to 10 % of the cases. Perforation is treated with antibiotics and possible drainage if recognized immediately after the bouginage.

Webcodes

The following webcodes can be used on www. psurg.net for further images and data.

2001 Esophageal atresia type II or III a	2013 Ultrasound, pyloric stenosis
2002 Isolated tracheoesophageal fistula	2014 Upper GI contrast study, pyloric stenosis
2003 Isolated tracheoesophageal fistula at surgery	2015 Pyloromyotomy
2004 Obtuse angle of His	2016 Membranaceous esophageal stenosis
2005 Hiatus hernia	2017 Circular peptic stenosis
2006 Failure to thrive, gastroesophageal reflux	2018 Long-distance peptic stenosis
2007 Hematemesis, gastroesophageal reflux	2019 Achalasia esophagus, infancy
2008 Ph-recording, gastroesophageal reflux	2020 Achalasia, before and after surgery
2009 Reflux esophagitis	2021 Upside-down stomach, hiatus hernia
2010 Nissen fundoplication	2022 Gastric foreign body, psychiatric disorder
2011 Hunger stool, pyloric stenosis	2023 Esophageal foreign body
2012 Gastric peristalsis, pyloric stenosis	2024 Disc battery, abdominal x-ray
	2025 Swallowed and native disc battery

Bibliography

General, Chest Pain, and Differential Diagnosis

Chial HJ, Camilleri M, Williams DE et al (2003a) Rumination syndrome in children and adolescents: diagnosis, treatment, and prognosis. Pediatrics 111:158–162

Garza JM, Kaul A (2010) Gastroesophageal reflux, eosinophilic esophagitis, and foreign body. Pediatr Clin North Am 57:1331–1345

Section 20.1

Bruch SW, Hirschl RB, Coran AG (2010) The diagnosis and management of recurrent tracheoesophageal fistulas. J Pediatr Surg 45:337–340

Burgos L, Barrena S, Andrés AM, Martinez L, Hernandez F, Olivares P, Lassaletta L, Tovar JA (2010) Colonic interposition for esophageal replacement in children remains a good choice: 33-year median follow-up of 65 patients. J Pediatr Surg 45:341–345

Burjonrappa SC, Youssef S, St-Vil D (2010) What is the incidence of Barret's and gastric metaplasia in esophageal atresia/tracheoesophageal fistula (EA/TEF) patients? Eur J Pediatr Surg 21:25–29

Harmon CM, Coran AG (1998a) Congenital anomalies of the esophagus. In: O'Neill JA Jr et al (eds) Pediatric surgery, vol II, 5th edn. Mosby, St Louis

Harrison J, Martin J, Crameri J, Robertson CF, Ranganathan SC (2010) Lung function in children with repaired tracheo-esophageal fistula using the oscillation technique. Pediatr Pulmonol 45:1057–1063

Holland AJ, Fitzgerald DA (2010) Oesophageal atresia and tracheo-oesophageal fistula: current management strategies and complications. Paediatr Respir Rev 11:100–106, quiz 106–107

Holland AJ, Ron O, Pierro A, Drake D, Curry JI, Kiely EM, Spitz L (2009) Surgical outcomes of esophageal atresia without fistula for 24 years at a single institution. J Pediatr Surg 44:1928–1932

Hunter CJ, Petrosyan M, Connelly M, Ford HR, Nguyen NX (2009) Repair of long-gap esophageal atresia: gastric conduits may improve outcome – a 20-year single center experience. Pediatr Surg Int 25:1087–1091

Petrosyan M, Estrada J, Hunter C, Woo R, Stein J, Ford HR, Anselmo DM (2009) Esophageal atresia/tracheoesophageal fistula in very low-birth-weight neonates: improved outcomes with staged repair. J Pediatr Surg 44:2278–2281

Nasr A, McNamara PJ, Mertens L, Levin D, James A, Holtby H, Langer JC (2010) Is routine preoperative 2-dimensional echocardiography necessary for infants with esophageal atresia, omphalocele, or anorectal malformations? J Pediatr Surg 45:876–879

Scott DA (1993–2009) Esophageal atresia/tracheoesophageal fistula overview. In: Pagon RA, Bird TC, Dolan CR, Stephens K (eds) Gene reviews [internet]. University of Washington, Seattle

Serhal L, Gottrand F, Sfeir R, Guimber D, Devos P, Bonnevalle M, Storme L, Turck D, Michaud L (2010) Anastomotic stricture after surgical repair of esophageal atresia: frequency, risk factors, and efficacy of esophageal bougie dilatations. J Pediatr Surg 45:1459–1462

Shah AR, Lazar EL, Atlas AB (2009) Tracheal diverticula after tracheoeosphageal fistula repair: case series and review of the literature. J Pediatr Surg 44:2107–2111

Sistonen SJ, Koivusalo A, Nieminen U, Lindahl H, Lohi J, Kero M, Kärkkäinen PA, Sarna S, Rintala RJ (2010)

Esophageal morbidity and function in adults with repaired esophageal atresia with tracheoesophageal fistula: a population-based long-term follow-up. Ann Surg 251:1167–1173

Tannuri U, Tannuri AC, Goncalves ME, Cardoso SR (2008) Total gastric transposition is better than partial tube esophagoplasty for esophageal replacement in children. Dis Esophagus 21:73–77

Section 20.2

Allal H, Captier G, Lopez M, Forgues D, Galifer RB (2001) Evaluation of 142 consecutive laparoscopic fundoplications in children: effects of the learning curve and technical choice. J Pediatr Surg 36: 921–926

Al-Salem AH (2007) Congenital pyloric atresia and associated anomalies. Pediatr Surg Int 23:559–563

Berkowitz D, Naveh Y, Berant M et al (1997) "Infantile Colic" as the sole manifestation of gastroesophageal reflux. J Pediatr Gastroenterol Nutr 24:231–233

Boix-Ochoa J, Rowe MI (1998) Gastroesophageal reflux. In: O'Neill JA Jr et al (eds) Pediatric surgery, vol II, 5th edn. Mosby, St Louis

Campanozzi A, Boccia G, Pensabene L, Panetta F, Marseglia A, Strisciuglio P, Barbera C, Magazzu G, Pettoello-Mantovani M, Staiano A (2009) Prevalence and natural history of gastroesophageal reflux: pediatric prospective survey. Pediatrics 123:779–783

Cohen MC, Ashok D, Gell M, Bishop J, Walker J, Thomson M, Al-Adnani M (2009) Pediatric columnar lined esophagus vs Barrett's esophagus: is it the time for a consensus definition. Pediatr Dev Pathol 12:116–126

Da Dalt L, Mazzoleni S, Montini G, Donzelli F, Zacchello F (1989) Diagnostic accuracy of pH monitoring in gastro-oesophageal reflux. Arch Dis Child 64: 1421–1426

El-Serag HB, Gilger M, Carter J, Genta RM, Rabeneck L (2004) Childhood GERD is a risk factor for GERD in adolescents and young adults. Am J Gastroenterol 99:806–812

El-Serag HB, Gilger MA, Shub MD, Richardson P, Bancroft J (2006) The prevalence of suspected Barrett's esophagus in children and adolescents: a multicenter endoscopic study. Gastrointest Endosc 64:671–675

Engelmann C, Gritsa S, Gratz KF, Ure BM (2010) Laparoscopic anterior hemifundoplication improves key symptoms without impact on GE in children with and children without neurodevelopmental delays. J Pediatr Gastroenterol Nutr 51:437–442

Estevao-Costa J, Fragoso AC, Prata MJ, Campos M, Trindade E, Dias JA, Brazao AM (2011) Gastric emptying and antireflux surgery. Pediatr Surg Int 27: 367–371

Fonkalsrud EW, Ashcraft KW, Coran AG et al (1998) Surgical treatment of gastro-esophageal reflux in children: a combined hospital study of 7467 patients. Pediatrics 101:419–422

Gilger MA, El Serag HB, Gold BD, Dietrich CL, Tsou V, McDuffie A, Shub MD (2008) Prevalence of endoscopic findings of erosive esophagitis in children: a population-based study. J Pediatr Gastroenterol Nutr 47:141–146

Gold BD (2006) Is gastroesophageal reflux disease really a life-long disease: do babies who regurgitate grow up to be adults with GERD complications? Am J Gastroenterol 101:641–644

Hassall E (2008) Step-up and step down approaches to treatment of gastroesophageal reflux disease in children. Curr Gastroenetrol Rep 10:324–331

Hoffman I, Tertychnyy A, Ectors N, De Greef T, Haesendonck N, Tack J (2007) Duodenogastroesopgageal reflux in children with refractory gastroesophageal reflux disease. J Pediatr 151:307–311

Numanoglu A, Millar AJ, Brown RA, Rode H (2005) Gastroesophageal reflux strictures in children, management and outcome. Pediatr Surg Int 21:631–634

Ramenofsky ML (1986) Gastroesophageal reflux: clinical manifestations and diagnosis. In: Ashcraft KW, Holder TM (eds) Pediatric esophageal surgery. Grune & Stratton, Orlando

Ravelli AM, Panarotto MB, Verdoni L, Consolati V, Bolognini S (2006) Pulmonary aspiration shown by scintigraphy in gastroesophageal reflux-related respiratory disease. Chest 130:1520–1526

Saedon M, Gourgiotis S, Germanos S (2007) Is there a changing trend in surgical management of gastroesophageal reflux disease in children? World J Gastroenterol 13:4417–4422

Soyer T, Karnak I, Tanyel FC, Senocak ME, Ciftci AO, Büyüpanmukcu N (2007) The use of pH monitoring and esophageal manometry in the evaluation of results of surgical therapy for gastroesophageal reflux disease. Eur J Pediatr Surg 17:158–162

Tasker A, Dettmar PW, Panetti M et al (2002) Reflux of gastric juice glue ear in children. Lancet 9: 359(9305)–439

Van der Pol RJ, Smits MJ, van Wijk MP et al (2011) Efficacy of proton-pump inhibitors in children with gastroesophageal reflux: a systematic review. Pediatrics 127:925–935

Tovar JA, Luis AL, Encinas JL, Burgos L, Pederiva F, Martinez L, Olivares P (2007) Pediatric surgeons and gastroesophageal reflux. J Pediatr Surg 42: 277–283

Vanderhoof JA, Moran JR, Harris CL et al (2003) Efficacy of a pre-thickened infant formula: a multicenter, double-blind, randomized, placebo-controlled parallel group trial in 104 infants with symptomatic gastroesophageal reflux. Clin Pediatr (Phila) 42:483–495

Vicente Y, Hernandez-Peredo G, Molina M, Prieto G, Tovar JA (2001) Acute food bolus impaction without stricture in children with gastroesopgahegal reflux. J Pediatr Surg 36:1397–1400

Section 20.3

Cooper WO, Griffin MR, Arbogast P et al (2002) Very early exposure to erythromycin and infantile hypertrophic pyloric stenosis. Acta Pediatr Adolesc Med 156:647–650

Friedman JN, Goldman RD, Srivastava R et al (2004) Development of a clinical dehydration scale for use in children between 1 and 36 months of age. J Pediatr 1445:201–207

Hernanz-Schulman M, Sells LL, Ambrosino MM, Heller RM, Stein SM, Neblett WW III (1994) Hypertrophic pyloric stenosis in the infant without a palpable olive: accuracy of sonographic diagnosis. Radiology 193:771–776

Lüdtke FE, Bertus M, Michalski S, Dapper FD, Lepsien G (1994) Long-term analysis of ultrasonic features of the antropyloric region 17–27 years after treatment of infantile hypertrophic pyloric stenosis. J Clin Ultrasound 22:299–305

Mandell GA, Wolfson PJ, Adkins ES et al (1999) Cost-effective imaging approach to the nonbilious vomiting infant. Pediatrics 103:1198–1202

Miozzari HH, Tönz M, von Vigier RO, Bianchetti MG (2001) Fluid resuscitiation in infantile hypertrophic pyloric stenosis. Acta Paediatr 90:511–515

Okoye BE, Parikh DH, Buck RG, Lander AD (2000) Pyloric atresia: five new cases, a new association, and a review of the literature with guidelines. J Pediatr Surg 35:1242–1245

Pfendner EG, Lucky AW (1993–2008 [updated 2009]) Epidermolysis bullosa with pyloric atresia. In: Pagon RA, Bird TD, Dolan CR, Stephens K (eds) Gene reviews [internet]. University of Washington, Seattle

Scherer LR III (1998a) Peptic ulcer and other conditions of the stomach. In: O'Neill JA Jr et al (eds) Pediatric surgery, vol II, 5th edn. Mosby, St Louis

Schwartz MZ (1998) Hypertrophic pyloric stenosis. In: O'Neill JA Jr et al (eds) Pediatric surgery, vol II, 5th edn. Mosby, St Louis

Wathen JE, MacKenzie T, Bothner JP (2004) Usefulness of the serum electrolyte panel in the management of pediatric dehydration treated with intravenously administered fluids. Pediatrics 114:1227–1234

Section 20.4

Barohn RJ, Levine EJ, Olson JO, Mendell JR (1988) Gastric hypomotility in Duchenne's muscular dystrophy. N Engl J Med 319:15–18

Jawaid W, Abdalwahab A, Blair G, Skarsgard E, Webber E (2006) Outcomes of pyloroplasty and pyloric dilatation in children diagnosed with nonobstructive delayed gastric emptying. J Pediatr Surg 41:2059–2061

Machado RS, Yamamoto E, da Silva Patricio FR, Reber M, Kawakami E (2010) Gastric emptying evaluation in children with erosive gastroesophageal reflux disease. Pediatr Surg Int 26:473–478

Medhus AW, Bjornland K, Emblem R, Husebye E (2007) Liquid and solid gastric emptying in adults treated for Hirschsprung's disease during early childhood. Scand J Gastroenterol 42:34–40

Sharma KK, Ranka P, Goyal P, Dabi DR (2008) Gastric outlet obstruction in children: an overview with report of Jodhpur disease and Sharma's classification. J Pediatr Surg 43:1891–1897

Singh SJ, Gibbons NJ, Blackshaw PE, Vincent M, J Wakefield, Perkins AC (2006) Gastric emptying of solids in normal children – a preliminary report. J Pediatr Surg 41:413–417

Struijs MC, Lasko D, Somme S, Chiu P (2010) Gastric emptying scans: unnecessary preoperative testing for fundoplications? J Pediatr Surg 45:350–354, discussion 354

Sullivan PB (2008) Gastrointestinal disorders in children with neurodevelopmental disabilities. Dev Disabil Res Rev 14:128–136

Section 20.5

Ashcraft KW (1986) Vascular ring. In: Ashcraft KW, Holder TM (eds) Pediatric esophageal surgery. Grune & Stratton, Orlando

Harmon CM, Coran AG (1998b) Congenital anomalies of the esophagus. In: O'Neill JA Jr et al (eds) Pediatric surgery, vol II, 5th edn. Mosby, St Louis

Jones DW, Kunisaki SM, Teitelbaum DH, Spigland NA, Coran AG (2010) Congenital esophageal stenosis: the differential diagnosis and management. Pediatr Surg 26:547–551

Section 20.6

Burke CA, Achkar E, Falk GW (1997) Effect of pneumatic dilation on gastroesophageal reflux in achalasia. Dig Dis Sci 42:998–1002

Eckhardt VF, Hoischen T, Bernhard G (2008) Life expectancy, complications, and causes of death in patients with achalasia: results of a 33-year follow-up investigation. Eur J Gastroenterol Hepatol 20:956–960

Jolley SG, Baron HI (1998) Disorders of esophageal function. In: O'Neill JA Jr et al (eds) Pediatric surgery, vol I, 5th edn. Mosby, St Louis

Karnak I, Senocak ME, Tanyel FC, Büyükpamukcu N (2001) Achalasia in childhood: surgical treatment and outcome. Eur J Pediatr Surg 11:223–229

Levine ML, Moskowitz GW, Dorf BS, Bank S (1991) Pneumatic dilation in patients with achalsia with modified Gruntzig dilator (Levine) under direct endoscopic control: results after 5 years. Am J Gastroenterol 86:1581–1584

Orlandi M, Inauen W (2007) "…und plötzlich konnte ich nicht mehr schlucken!" ("…and suddenly I couldn't swallow any more!"). Schweiz Med Forum 7:333–335

Ortiz A, de Haro LF, Parrilla P, Lage A, Perez D, Munitiz V, Ruiz D, Molina J (2008) Very long-term objective evaluation of Heller myotomy plus posterior partial fundoplication in patients with achalasia of the cardia. Ann Surg 247:258–264

Pasricha PJ, Rai R, Ravich WJ et al (1996) Botulinum toxin for achalasia: long-term outcome and predictors of response. Gastroenterology 110:1410–1415

Tsuboi K, Omura N, Yano F, Kashiwagi H, Kawasaki N, Suzuki Y, Yanaga K (2009) Preoperative dilatation does not affect the surgical outcome of laparoscopic Heller myotomy and Dor fundoplication for esophageal achalasia. Surg Laparosc Endosc Percutan Tech 19:98–100

Section 20.7

Chial HJ, Camilleri M, Williams DE et al (2003b) Rumination syndrome in children and adolescents: diagnosis, treatment, and prognosis. Pediatrics 111:158–162

Mbonda E, Claus D, Bonnier C et al (1995) Prolonged dysphagia caused by congenital pharyngeal dysfunction. J Pediatr 126:923–927

Section 20.8

Campbell JB, Rappaport LN, Skerker LB (1972) Radiology 103:153–156

Jetley NK, Al-Assiri AH, Al Awadi D (2009) Congenital paraesophageal hernia: a 10 year experience from Saudi Arabia. Indian J Pediatr 76:489–493

Mc Intyre RC Jr, Bensard DD, Karrer FM, Hall RJ, Lilly JR (1994) The pediatric diaphragm in acute gastric volvulus. J Am Coll Surg 178:234–238

Scherer LR III (1998b) Peptic ulcer and other conditions of the stomach. In: O'Neill JA Jr et al (eds) Pediatric surgery, vol II, 5th edn. Mosby, St Louis

Stiefel D, Willi UV, Sacher P, Schwöbel MG, Stauffer UG (2000) Pitfalls in therapy of upside-down stomach. Eur J Pediatr Surg 10:162–166

Section 20.9

Aslan A, Unal I, Karaguzel M, Melikoglu M (2003) A case of intestinal obstruction due to phytobezoar – an alternative surgical approach. Swiss Surg 9:35–37

Chen X, Milkovich S, Stool D, van As AB, Reilly J, Rider G (2006) Pediatric coin ingestion and aspiration. Int J Pediatr Otorhinolaryngol 70:325–329

Johnson DG (1998) Esophagoscopy and other diagnostic techniques. In: O'Neill JA Jr et al (eds) Pediatric surgery, vol I, 5th edn. Mosby, St Louis

Kelley JE, Leech MH, Carr MG (1993) A safe and cost-effective protocol for the magement of esophageal coins in children. J Pediatr Surg 28:898–900

Little DC, Shah SR, St Peter SD, Calkins CM, Morrow SE, Murphy JP, Sharp RJ, Andrews WS, Holcomb GW 3rd, Ostlie DJ, Snyder CL (2006) Esophageal foreign bodies in the pediatric population: our first 500 cases. J Pediatr Surg 41:914–918

Marom T, Goldfarb A, Russo E, Roth Y (2010) Battery ingestion in children. Int J Pediatr Otorhinolaryngol 74:849–854

Paul RI, Jaffe DM (1988) Sharp object ingestions in children: illustrative cases and literature review. Pediatr Emerg Care 4:245–248

Sénéchaud C, Robert JH, Bertin D, Spiliopoulos A (1996) Perforation oesophagienne: quel traitement dans quelle situation? Swiss Surg 2:187–190

Sharp RJ (1986) Esophageal foreign bodies. In: Ashcraft KW, Holder TM (eds) Pediatric esophageal surgery. Grune & Stratton, Orlando

Section 20.10

Elicevic M, Alim A, Tekant GT, Sarimurat N, Adaletli I, Kurugoglu S, Bakan M, Kaya G, Erdogan E (2008) Management of esophageal perforation secondary to caustic esophageal injury in children. Surg Today 38:311–315

Gupta SK, Croffie JM, Fitzgerald JF (2001) Is esophagogastroduodenoscopy necessary in All caustic ingestions ? J Pediatr Gastroenterol Nutr 32:50–53

Kulick RM, Selbst SM, Baker MD, Woodward GA (1988) Thermal epiglottitis after swallowing hot beverages. Pediatrics 81:441–444

Millar AJW, Cywes S (1998) Caustic strictures of the esophagus. In: O'Neill JA Jr et al (eds) Pediatric surgery, vol I, 5th edn. Mosby, St Louis

Nuutinen M, Uhari M, Karvali T, Kouvalainen K (1994) Consequences of caustic ingestion in children. Acta Paediatr 83:1200–1205

Sanchez-Ramirez CA, Larrosa-Haro A, Vasquez Garibay EM, Larios-Arceo F (2011) Caustic ingestion and oesophageal damage in children: clinical spectrum and fee-ding practices. J Paediatr Child Health 47:378–380

Schärli A, Kummer M (1972) Ueber Säureverätzungen des Magens im Kindesalter: Z Kinderchir 11(suppl):493–503

Tokar B, Cevik AA, Ilhan H (2007) Ingested gastrointestinal foreign bodies: predisposing factors for complications in children having surgical or endoscopic removal. Pediatr Surg Int 23:135–39

Smith MT, Wong RK (2006) Esophageal foreign bodies: types and technique for removal. Curr Treat Options Gastroenterol 9:75–84

Constipation

21

Constipation is a very frequently observed presenting sign. In addition to the common idiopathic form of constipation, several pathologies exist that lead to constipation and can be cured by surgery or in which surgery is an adjuvant measure of their treatment.

Constipation can be determined by a combination of the following observations:

- The disorder lasts longer than 1 month.
- The interval between stool evacuations lasts longer than 3 days.
- Evacuation of hard stool like goat excrement or of loamy and malodorous stool.
- Stool masses that are palpated by abdominal or rectal examination.
- Change of the defecation pattern that was typical for the involved child up to now.

The rectal examination that is a taboo nowadays belongs still to the gold standard in suspected constipation, especially in Hirschsprung's disease like in Douglas abscess. Breastfeed infants who evacuate fresh stools relatively rarely and small children with daily hard stools like goat excrements do not have constipation.

The common idiopathic constipation starts in approximately two thirds of the children in the 2nd half of infancy and may exacerbate after inadequate fluid supply, during bowel training, or after an extraordinary event. Severe constipation leads to long-term dilatation of the rectum ampulla # and grotesque stool accumulation that is followed by encopresis because of overflow incontinence starting at 3 years of age and occasionally by volvulus of the sigmoid flexure.

In addition to consultation for the important differential diagnostic delineation of constipation (Table 21.1), the pediatric surgeon may be consulted for manual stool evacuation, in suspected surgical abdomen because of acute decompensation of constipation or of volvulus of the sigmoid flexure, in abdominal tumor, and in rectal prolapse or anal fissure.

Table 21.1 Differential diagnosis of constipation from a surgical point of view

• Disorders of intestinal innervation
– **Hirschsprung's disease**
– Intestinal neuronal dysplasia
– Immaturity of intramural plexuses
– **Anal sphincter achalasia**
• Anal and rectal stenosis (intrinsic and extrinsic)
• Anterior displaced anus
o Postoperative anorectal malformation and Hirschsprung's disease
o Spina bifida and other neurological disorders
o Small left colon syndrome
o Meconium plug syndrome
o Chronic idiopathic intestinal pseudoobstruction[a]
o Megacystis-microcolon-intestinal hypoperistalsis syndrome
• Pediatric disorders

[a]The term "chronic idiopathic intestinal pseudoobstruction" is used in the literature in a restricted or a more general sense

G.L. Kaiser, *Symptoms and Signs in Pediatric Surgery*,
DOI 10.1007/978-3-642-31161-1_21, © Springer-Verlag Berlin Heidelberg 2012

21.1 Disorders of Intestinal Innervation

21.1.1 Hirschsprung's Disease (Congenital Megacolon)

Occurrence, Cause

Hirschsprung's disease is quite frequently observed (1:5,500 live births). It occurs sporadically or in children with a family history. Whereas the common classic form has a distinctly male preponderance, more females are observed in the long-segment types.

The intestinal motility disorder and relative obstruction is caused by absence of ganglion cells of the intramural plexuses #, hypertrophy of the submucous parasympathetical nerve fibers, and increased number of neuroendocrinous cells. Hirschsprung's disease is an inherited disease that is modified by sex and results from several mutations of the RET proto-oncogen in chromosome 10 and other chromosomes.

Clinical Significance

- Constipation as leading sign of Hirschsprung's disease can be cured permanently by a pull-through procedure with elimination of the aganglionic part in the majority of cases.
- Untreated Hirschsprung's disease is a source of lifelong morbidity and possible death due to enterocolitis.
- Operated Hirschsprung's disease needs lifelong follow-ups in a minority of cases because of persistent gastrointestinal symptoms.

Types, Pathoanatomy

The aganglionic part extends from the anal channel in a cranial direction for a differently long distance. Depending on the length of the aganglionic segment, several types of Hirschsprung's disease can be differentiated and arranged according to their frequency of occurrence (Fig. 21.1):

• Classic type: Extension to the rectum and sigmoid #	73–81 %
• Long-segment type: Extension beyond the rectosigmoid	10–26 %
• Long-segment type: Total colonic involvement	3–12 %

• Long-segment type: Total colonic and variable small intestinal involvement = Zuelzer-Wilson syndrome #	≤3 %
• Ultrashort type: Extension up to 3 cm from the anocutaneous line	≤3 %

The aganglionic segment remains relatively narrow and is followed by a funnel-shaped transitional zone of variable length in cm. Both parts have an abnormal pattern of ineffective motility. They continue in a seemingly normal proximal part that exhibits hypertrophy, dilatation, and occasionally an intervening segment of intestinal neuronal dysplasia. The visible dilated part develops with increasing age grotesque dimensions (megacolon) with diminished propulsive motility despite of normal innervation.

Clinical Presentation

The majority of newborns with Hirschsprung's disease are symptomatic, but only a few develop early complications such as **ileus of the newborn** # or peritonitis due to **spontaneous intestinal perforation**, or **symptomatic enterocolitis**.

Recognition of Hirschsprung's disease needs special attention and observation: Delayed passage of meconium that is evacuated in portions and in a stuttering way beyond 24–48 h (passage occurs in 95 % of full-term infants within 24 h). In addition, some poor feeding, posseting, abdominal distension, and diarrhea may be observed in the following days in spite of breastfeeding #.

Constipation takes a prominent place beyond the neonatal period *possibly accompanied by some abdominal distension # and malodorous stools. Commencement of formula instead of mother milk leads to deterioration of constipation, diminished passage of winds, and in older infants and toddlers, failure to thrive.* Toddlers with aganglionosis develop abnormal abdominal distension that contrasts with signs of failure to thrive #. This clinical presentation is today unusual in the developed countries with a clinical diagnosis in the neonatal period or infancy but is still observed in developing countries and resembles sprue.

Clinical Skill

The stool is loamy and malodorous. The abdomen is distended with visible intestinal loops,

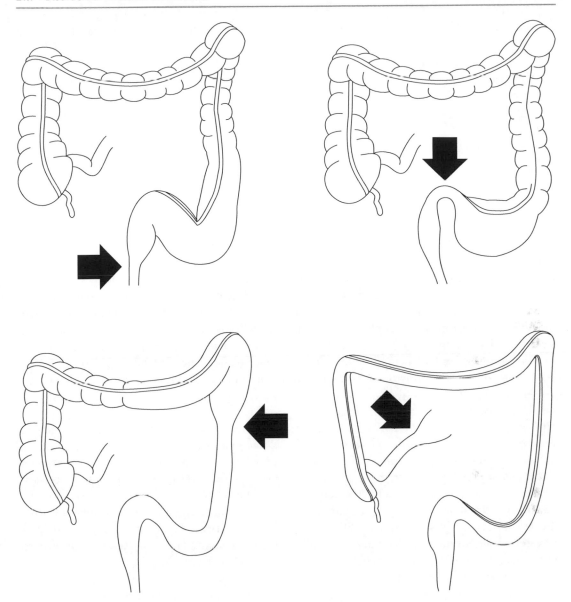

Fig. 21.1 Types of Hirschsprung's disease. The four single drawings demonstrate from the *top left* to the *bottom right* an increasing length of involved large and possible small intestine. *Top left*: Ultrashort type of Hirschsprung's disease with maximum involvement of the rectum of 3 cm from the anocutaneous line (≤3 %). Megacolon as shown in the drawing develops in advanced stages. *Top right*: Involvement of rectum or rectum and sigmoid colon – classic type of Hirschsprung's disease (in more than three fourths). *Bottom left*: Involvement of the colon beyond the sigmoid colon for a variable distance – long-segment type of Hirschsprung's diseases with partial colonic involvement (in up one fourth). *Bottom right*: Long-segment types of Hirschsprung's disease with either involvement of the total colon or with involvement of the total colon and a variable distance of the small intestine (Zuelzer-Wilson syndrome [≤3 %]). The radiological and operative appearance is similar in both types. The arrows mark the site of transition from aganglionic to ganglionic intestine. Notice the loss of haustration and the smaller caliber of the involved intestine and the deconfiguration of the megacolon

hypersonoric on percussion, and with burbling sounds on auscultation. The percentile of body weight may be below the normal body length.

A careful rectal examination with an appropriate finger size yields an empty rectal ampulla, and after withdrawal of the finger, explosive expulsion of wind or meconium and wind, breast-feeding or formula milk stool is observed with some relief of abdominal distension.

The clinical presentation is different in the long-segment and ultrashort type of Hirschsprung's disease, surgical abdomen of neonatal megacolon, and enterocolitis.

Associated anomalies are unusual and concern mainly Down syndrome (<10 → 15 %), anorectal malformation (3 %), and atresia of small intestine or colon (<1 %). Trisomy 18 and MEN type 2A are examples of rare associated disorders.

The prognosis of megacolon is less favorable if associated with Down syndrome: higher incidence of enterocolitis or less continence (night-time incontinence) and failure of compensatory mechanisms at puberty to overcome stool incontinence. In atresias, the diagnosis of megacolon may be missed before and after correction of the structural obstruction.

The **long-segment type** is difficult to diagnose. *Although some obstructive signs are mostly present in the neonate, meconium and stools are passed spontaneously, and the diagnosis of Hirschsprung's disease is often delayed. A history of familial aganglionosis and female sex of the index patient and his relatives should draw the attention to a long-segment type.*

Contrast enema: Instead of a microcolon as in distal small intestinal atresia or meconium ileus, the colon is possibly somewhat dilated, the flexures are not tortuous, and a transition zone is not recognizable. The postevacuation x-rays show significant contrast retention and retrograde passage in the more proximal part of ileum. Most cases are recognized at exploratory laparotomy or laparoscopy.

The **ultrashort type** is often not recognized in infancy and small children and may be even treated as psychiatric disorder in school age for the following reasons: *Constipation starts insidiously, is combined with encopresis, and defecation can be provoked by simple measures. In children with grotesque stool retention, missing urge of defecation, and evacuation periods of 10 and more days, ultrashort type of Hirschsprung's disease must be excluded.*

Diagnostic is an absent relaxation reflex of the internal sphincter. Contrast enema (missing transitional zone) and biopsy (possible presence of ganglion cells) are not reliable. Treatment consists of subcutaneous posterior myectomy. A 1–2-cm-wide piece of the internal muscle is resected for the length of 5 cm from the anocutaneous line. In long-standing, gross megacolon, a pull-through procedure is necessary with resection of the dilated rectum.

Enterocolitis occurs either pre- or postoperatively and concerns the aganglionic or ganglionic part of large or small intestine. Invasion of intestinal germs in the intestinal wall is made possible by stasis and local humoral and cellular immunodeficiency, and long-segment types are a risk factor. Mortality has been quoted in the 1970s to 1990s of the last century in up to 30 %.

The clinical presentation includes arranged in order of frequency: *explosive diarrhea (stool is possibly intermingled with traces of blood), vomiting, fever, and lethargy. The belly is distended and possibly tender.*

Diagnostic may be an upright plain abdominal x-ray with multiple air-fluid levels of which the lowest and largest show a horizontal interruption (so-called cut-off sign at the upper pelvic border). Treatment consists of repeated washouts with saline solution and a large rectal tube, i.v. triple antibiotics (including metronidazole), and possible enterostomy and sphincterotomy in unoperated and operated patients.

Work-Ups, Differential Diagnosis
Diagnosis of Hirschsprung's disease and its typification (extension of aganglionosis) is best achieved by a combination of contrast enema, anorectal manometry, and surgical (full-thickness) or suction biopsy because mainly false-negative data may result from a single examination depending on the age (prematurity or full-term neonates), type of aganglionosis (long-segment or ultrashort types), and experience of the radiologist and pediatric surgeon.

Radiological imaging: Plain x-ray in supine or upright position shows numerous intestinal loops that are somewhat distended by air with possible absence of gas at the site of the rectum.

Multiple air-fluid levels that are of different size consist mainly of gas and fill up nearly the whole abdomen point to a low intestinal obstruction, especially to an ileus of the newborn in Hirschsprung's disease #, and free or localized intramural air indicates spontaneous perforation # or enterocolitis in this context.

Contrast enema including postevacuation x-rays shows a small distal part, a cone-shaped transitional zone, and a proximal dilated part of the large intestine #. The pathognomonic transitional zone is or may be absent in ultrashort or long-segment types, young infants, or after rigorous washouts or overlooked (e.g., due to an overlapping contrast-filled loop). A constantly recognizable colonic loop # (megacolon #) or significant contrast retention in postevacuation x-rays are highly suggestive of aganglionosis and irregularities of the intestinal wall of enterocolitis.

Anorectal manometry needs special equipment and experience. The normal relaxation reflex of the internal sphincter may not yet be developed in premature and young full-term newborns or in functional obstruction. Its absence is pathognomonic for aganglionosis and isolated anal achalasia #.

Surgical **biopsy** needs general anesthesia, is performed by laparotomy, laparoscopy, or transanal approach, and yields full-thickness specimens, possibly informations about the extension of aganglionosis, and is combined with the danger of perforation or hemorrhage. Suction biopsy is performed without anesthesia, and complications occur less frequently (<2‰). Additional acetylcholinesterase staining permits excellent results in diagnosis of classic Hirschsprung's disease #.

The **differential diagnosis** must consider other causes of constipation and delay of meconium evacuation, and especially in newborns and infants, causes of low intestinal obstruction (meconium ileus, distal ileal and colonic atresia, small intestinal stenosis, anorectal malformations, and rarely congenital segmental dilatation) and functional obstruction such as prematurity, hypothyroidism, and septicemia. Depending on

the place of pediatric surgical activity or the familial origin and the age of the child, **Chagas disease** must be considered in the differential diagnosis.

Chagas disease is an infection by the protozoon Trypanosoma cruzi that occurs mainly in Bolivia, Argentina, and Brazil (South and Central America) but is observed today worldwide. Vector is the bug Triatoma infestans in endemic zones and accidentally in the USA. In the rest of the world, transmission occurs from the infected mother to the unborn child, by food in involved family members, and by transfusion of blood products or transplantation of biological tissue.

The acute stage is followed by a chronic stage after a latent period of several years without any symptoms and protozoons in the blood. The chronic stage is characterized by possible reactivation of the infection and by disorders of heart (20–40 %) and/or gastrointestinal tract (10–20 %).

The disorders of the heart concern the conduction system (arrhythmia) or myocardium (tachycardia) with multifocal fibrosis, secondary dilatation of the heart or the left ventricle, and possible sudden lethal heart failure. The disorders of gastrointestinal tract concern the esophagus (dysphagia) and/or the colon (constipation). Activity of Trypanosoma cruzi leads to destruction of the autonomic nerve cells of the intestinal plexuses with secondary achalasia of the esophagus and/or acquired megacolon similar to Hirschsprung's disease.

Diagnosis is possible in the acute stage or in reactivation by microscopical detection of protozoons in the blood or in the biological tissue and fluid, respectively, and in the latent and chronic stage, best by two methods of specific polymerase chain reaction (in the chronic stage, serological screening may become negative).

Chagas disease is treated with benzimidazole (decreasing effectiveness with increasing duration of the disease) and its complications accordingly. Depending on the time of infection and due to increased survival in general, children may also suffer from heart disorders, acquired achalasia of esophagus, and aganglionosis of rectum and colon. They need similar surgical interventions as in the congenital types of achalasia and megacolon.

Treatment

For permanent cure, surgery is necessary. After diagnosis of Hirschsprung's disease, either a diverting colostomy or a nonoperative approach is chosen.

Although **the latter procedure** is less commonly applied, it permits postponement of final surgery to the age of 4–6 months without the need of a colostomy. Nurses carry out washouts twice a day. They teach the technique to the parents (use of saline and rectal tubes of appropriate size). The procedure is facilitated by breastfeeding or tested mother's milk. Regular follow-ups by the family doctor and pediatric surgeon avoid an ineffective technique and a possible enterocolitis.

The diverting colostomy is performed in the left lower quadrant for classic aganglionosis whereas long-segment types need colostomy or enterostomy at the site of the transitional zone. It is used to confirm the diagnosis and its extension by frozen and full-thickness biopsies that are taken from the upper end of aganglionosis, transitional zone, and lower end of ganglionic intestine. Diverting enterostomies are often closed at the time of final surgery.

The time of final surgery (neonatal period vs. 1st or 2nd part of infancy), access (transanal vs. abdominoperineal approach [open or laparoscopically]), and technique are a matter of discussion. The commonly used abdominoperineal procedures are modifications of Soave, Duhamel, or Swenson technique. The perineal one-stage pull-through and transanal endorectal pull-through have gained acceptance by many since the last 10–15 years.

In **Soave endorectal pull-through**, the rectal mucosa and submucosa is removed, and the ganglionic colon pulled through the remaining aganglionic muscular cuff and after dilation of the anus anastomosed to the lower end of the muscular cuff and lower edge of the divided anal mucous membrane 1 cm above the dentate line. Possible functional stenosis (constipation, enterocolitis) is avoided by shortening of the muscular cuff with an upper end 1–2 cm above the levator muscle.

In **Duhamel pull-through**, the anterolateral wall of about 6-cm aganglionic rectum is used for an anastomosis with the ganglionic colon that contributes its posterolateral wall to the conduit. The mobilized ganglionic colon is brought behind the original rectum, and after incision of the posterior rectal wall, its lower edge is anastomosed with the posterior lower end of the ganglionic colon 1 cm above the dentate line. Mechanical stapling devices facilitate resection of the common walls and performance of anastomosis.

In **Swenson procedure**, surgery is simultaneously started after left lower laparotomy with performance of surgical biopsies for frozen sections (at the same locations as in enterostomy) and mobilization of the intraperitoneal rectosigmoid with maintenance of blood supply of the ganglionic colon foreseen for pull-through. After incision of the peritoneal reflection, the ureters and vasa deferentia are marked, and dissection of the rectum is performed very close to its wall and with stanching of the small blood vessels. The distal preparation ends posteriorly close to the dentate line of the anus and anteriorly 3–4 cm above it (Grob's 1st modification) after forceful anal dilatation, a pull-through is performed with an instrument that ends in a conical knob and is introduced by the anus to the transitional zone where the colon is ligated over the knob #. After pull-through, an oblique anastomosis is performed outside of the anus between the lower end of the ganglionic colon and everted anal channel (Grob's 2nd modification #). After reduction of the anastomosis and peritonealization of lower peritoneal cavity, the abdominal incision is closed.

Prognosis

All patients with Hirschsprung's disease need regular follow-ups by a pediatric surgeon up to puberty, and in some, lifelong observations are necessary. If an appropriate technique is carefully applied, neither incontinence nor functional voiding disorders of clinical relevance or disorders of erection are observed at the time of puberty.

Figures of a large multicenter study that have been published in the 1980s of the last century displayed following percentages of symptoms and signs after a mean follow-up time of 5.9 years (mean time at surgery 11 months, mean age at last follow-up 8.0 years):

Constipation	9.4 %	(7.9–10.4)[a]
Diarrhea	7.6 %	(3.8–13.2)
Diarrhea and constipation	1.5 %	(1.6–1.9)
Enterocolitis	7.3 %	(3.7–13.6)
Encopresis	13.6 %	(10.0–17.6)
Enuresis	10.9 %	(5.4–15.3)

[a]The percentages in the brackets correspond to variation of the different surgical techniques

The quoted results are probably better today because surgery is performed earlier with an increased refinement of technique and follow-ups are more extensive. In addition, the beneficial effects of puberty have not been considered in these figures.

If only the open abdominoperineal procedures are considered, postoperative ileus due to adhesions occurs in 11–12 % (caused by surgery and/or enterocolitis). The overall mortality of ≤5 % is caused by long-segment aganglionosis, enterocolitis, functional and structural ileus, and rarely by associated anomalies.

21.1.2 Intestinal Neuronal Dysplasia (IND)

Occurrence, Definition

IND has been recognized as an independent disorder after histopathological evaluation of rectal suction biopsies of children with constipation. In contrast to the much less frequent type A, type B is observed in 2.3 % of such biopsies. Type B IND occurs as isolated disorder or in combination with Hirschsprung's disease (involvement of the ganglionated colon of variable length proximally to the transitional zone) in at least 6 %. The quantitative definition is ≥5 giant ganglia in 30 serial sections including the submucosa (or ≥15–20 % giant ganglia [>8 nerve cells] of all submucous ganglia counted). In addition, incomplete or morphologically deviating forms must be discussed. In type A IND, the intramural sympathetic system is absent or hypoplastic.

Clinical Significance
- Recognition of IND permits to relate the gastrointestinal symptoms to a specific disorder

with implications for clinical course, treatment, and prognosis.
- IND associated with Hirschsprung's disease may be a cause of postoperative constipation or enterocolitis.

Clinical Presentation

The symptomatology of type A IND *starts early, is usually severe, and needs mostly surgical intervention. Intestinal obstruction, diarrhea combined with blood and mucus, or perforation of intestine is observed.*

In contrast to type A IND, the clinical presentation of type B is *variable in relation to its severity and time of onset. In the majority of cases, a benign course is observed: delayed passage of meconium, occasionally hidden by a meconium plug syndrome, retention of stool in spite of feeding with human milk, and intermittent abdominal distension. It may be followed by a more severe constipation in which overflow incontinence leads to fecal soiling that precedes each bowel movement. Less frequently, obstructive symptoms, symptoms similar to chronic intestinal pseudoobstruction, overt obstructive ileus, enterocolitis #, peritonitis, and perforation are observed.*

Due to maturation, spontaneous recovery of the disease is possible up to the age of 1 year. On the other hand, severe irreversible changes may be observed in single schoolchildren, adolescents, and adults such as segmental dilatations without any propulsive activity, enterocolitis, or large or small bowel ischemia.

Work-Ups, Differential Diagnosis

They are dictated by the clinical presentation. For the initial diagnosis, rectal suction biopsy at 9cm above the dentate line is diagnostic and demonstrates the already quoted criteria for a quantitative diagnosis. Anorectal manometry yields abnormal, absent, or normal internal sphincter relaxation reflex; it may be applied if sphincter myectomy is considered. Radiological imaging techniques (plain abdominal x-ray in upright position, contrast enema, anterograde GI contrast study, or peroral scintiscan) and intestinal manometry are used in emergency (e.g., obstructive ileus, enterocolitis, perforation) or chronic cases (segmental dilatations, slow transit, absent propulsive activity).

The differential diagnosis includes all **pathologies with constipation** and occasionally disorders with constipation resistant to nonoperative measures, **surgical abdomen**, and **chronic intestinal obstruction**. At surgery of the latter cases, full-thickness biopsies should be taken depending on the age for exclusion of total aganglionosis of the colon, immaturity of the enteric nervous system, and aplastic desmosis in neonates and young infants and of atrophic desmosis and hypoganglionosis in older children.

Treatment, Prognosis

Most children with type B IND can be treated conservatively up to the age of 4 years with prokinetic drugs, diet, laxatives, and washouts. On the other hand, aggressive treatment is dictated by the clinical presentation in few cases. Myectomy of the internal sphincter is indicated in severe constipation, especially if repeated anal dilatations had only a temporary effect in the past or in manometric abnormal findings.

Children of any age with acute or chronic intestinal obstruction, severe enterocolitis, perforation, and peritonitis and older children with persistent constipation need surgery. The interventions include temporary colostomy or enterostomy up to rectodescendectomy and segmental resections of involved intestinal parts.

It seems that the majority of cases with type B IND have a good outcome with regular stool evacuation on long-term follow-up. On the other hand, the question arises if the severe cases observed in school age and adolescence could have been avoided by early selection and treatment.

21.1.3 Immaturity of the Enteric Nervous System (Plexus Immaturity)

Occurrence

Immaturity of the intramural plexuses that is observed in preterm and term neonates occurs with or without associated malformations. Some of the patients with small left colon syndrome and microcolon of prematurity belong probably to the same entity that is observed less frequently than the well-known dysganglionoses.

Clinical Significance

- Clinical, radiological, and intraoperative confusions is possible with a long-segment Hirschsprung's disease especially with Zuelzer-Wilson syndrome.

Clinical Presentation

If the entire colon with or without parts of the small intestine is involved, signs of a low small intestinal obstruction develops that lead to laparotomy. At surgery, the small intestine is dilated proximally to the ileocecal valve or apart from it in a more oral direction depending on the length of the involved small intestine #. The whole intestine is filled with air, and the colon does not look like a microcolon.

Work-Ups, Differential Diagnosis

Those of low small intestine obstruction: Contrast enema and anterograde GI study show slow and insufficient transit and emptying of the involved part. At surgery, full-thickness biopsies must be taken at, above, and below the transitional zone that demonstrates in nitroxide synthase and picric acid/sirius red-staining immature nerve cells and connective tissue.

The **differential diagnosis** includes mainly ileal atresia or stenosis, long-segment aganglionosis, and theoretically all histological diagnoses leading to constipation.

Treatment, Prognosis

Long-segment involvement needs usually temporary colostomy or enterostomy that should be performed proximally and adjacent to the transitional zone with a separate proximal and distal stoma. Maturation is observed by instillation of increasing amounts of stool into the distal stoma and observation of the transit of contrast by the same route. Feeding is maintained by parenteral nutrition and/or application of peroral adapted milk. Enterostomies are closed if passage is normalized, clinically by evacuation of regular stools and radiologically by normal contrast transit. At the same time, biopsies are repeated.

Permanent cure is possible. Occasionally, **classic Hirschsprung's disease** or a **chronic intestinal pseudoobstruction** may be hidden behind and associated with it.

21.1.4 Anal Sphincter Achalasia

Occurrence, Types
Reflectory relaxation of the internal anal sphincter muscle may be absent or abnormal for several reasons. It leads to blockage of stool evacuation and is a frequent cause of constipation. The following types are observed:

- Myogenic achalasia: It is mostly caused by inflammatory processes which spread to the internal sphincter muscle such as anal fissure, fistula-in-ano, and cryptitis.
- Neurogenic achalasia: It is either an obligatory part of Hirschsprung's disease or an isolated type of aganglionosis (internal anal sphincter neurogenic achalasia).
- Neurovegetative-psychogenic achalasia: It is a discoordination in which the voluntary sphincter muscles contract instead of relaxing during defecation.

Clinical Significance
- Anal sphincter achalasia plays an important role in constipation, either as isolated or as combined factor that must considered in the its treatment.

Clinical Presentation
A specific history and careful local examination yields already the suspicion of achalasia and its type without the necessity of proving it by defecography, anorectal manometry, electromyography in every case, for example, in myogenic achalasia.

Work-Ups, Differential Diagnosis
Anorectal manometry and biopsy are necessary for isolated neurogenic achalasia.

In every case of constipation especially in those cases with disorders of stool evacuation, achalasia must be considered in the differential diagnosis.

Treatment, Prognosis
Neurogenic achalasia is, and myogenic achalasia may be, surgical if the underlying cause needs optimum treatment. Internal sphincter myectomy leads to a permanent cure in the majority cases of neurogenic and in selected cases of myogenic achalasia. In neurovegetative-psychogenic achalasia, behavioral therapy and other nonoperative treatments may lead to success.

21.2 Anal and Rectal Stenosis

Occurrence, Causes, and Pathoanatomy
Anorectal stenosis is a quite frequent cause of constipation.

Anal or rectal stenosis is either functional or organic, intrinsic or extrinsic, and congenital or acquired.

Different types of spina bifida, sacrum aplasia, and other neurological disorders belong to the functional stenoses and are examples of congenital origin. Perianorectal pathologies with sphincteric hypertonicity because of pain are acquired stenoses of which anal fissure, perianal and rectal abscess, fistula-in-ano, symptomatic hemorrhoids and thrombosis of the external hemorrhoids, and perianal condyloma acuminatum are the most common.

The causes of organic anorectal stenosis are quoted in Table 21.2. In intrinsic stenoses, site

Table 21.2 Differential diagnosis of organic anorectal stenosis

Congenital pathologies
o Anal and rectal stenosis (*anorectal malformations*)
• Sacrococcygeal teratoma
o Rectal duplication
o Anterior (myelo)meningocele (*spina bifida*)
o Enteric and neuroenteric cyst (*enteric cyst*)
Acquired pathologies
• Postoperative anorectal malformations and Hirschsprung's disease
o Rectal and pararectal tumor
• Pelvic, abdominal, and retroperitoneal tumor (*abdominal tumor*)
o Stenosis after impalement injury or child abuse
o Fecaloma
o Perianal and perirectal abscess

and extension is somewhat different depending on the specific cause: Congenital stenoses are either short (membranaceous stenosis) or long and lie in the upper anal canal, above it, or at the level of dentate line. On the other hand, postsurgical stenoses are short and are at the site of the former anastomosis (usually above the dentate line) or concern the anocutaneous transition zone. In case of rectal or pararectal neoplasm, the mass cannot be delineated completely by rectal palpation except for a polypus of the rectum or colon or the leading point of intussusception. Pelvic tumors or abdominal tumors with pelvic extension display other symptoms as well.

Clinical Significance
- Anorectal stenosis is an easy recognizable cause of constipation if it is considered at all.
- Functional stenosis should be taken into account as well, especially in the frequently observed perianal pathologies for which treatment of constipation may be an integral part.

Clinical Presentation
In addition to constipation and difficult defecation, reduction of the caliber of the stool column up to the diameter of a pencil or a dentistry paste may be observed. The stenosis and its characteristics may be felt *with the small finger in newborns or the index finger in schoolchildren. Hegar's dilators are used for precise quantification, and the results compared with a table of normal values for age and sex.* In addition, careful inspection and palpation of the lower abdomen, pelvis, perineum, external genitals, and anorectum are indispensable.

Work-Ups, Differential Diagnosis
A specific history and clinical examination including calibration permits recognition of several causes of functional and organic stenosis. Plain x-ray of the lower abdomen including the whole pelvis and sacrum in two planes, contrast enema and cinedefecography, CT or MRI, and anorectoscopy confirms the suspected clinical diagnosis and delineates, in case of specific malformations and tumors, their extension and dignity.

The differential diagnosis includes all disorders with constipation and specifically the causes that lead to anorectal stenosis.

Treatment, Prognosis
In extrinsic causes, their surgical removal is necessary. Intrinsic causes need local resection with anastomosis or widening plasty (short stenoses) after a posterior midline access, or a pull-through procedure (long-segment stenoses), if repeated dilatations in general anesthesia fail.

The outcome depends on the cause.

21.3   Anterior Ectopic (Perineal) Anus

Occurrence
Anterior ectopic anus is quite frequently observed. It may be associated with severe constipation.

Clinical Significance
- Anterior ectopic anus that is associated with stenosis or mid-anal sphincter malformation is associated with severe constipation that can be permanently relieved by surgery.

Clinical Presentation
Constipation exists since birth or early infancy. But recognition of this specific cause of constipation may be delayed till adulthood. Mainly, female patients are involved.

The demonstration of an anteriorly displaced anus # and its quantification by the so-called anal position index is probably not sufficient for recognition of the clinically important subgroup anterior ectopic anus with stenosis or mid-sphincter malformation because an abnormal index with <0.34 in girls and <0.46 in boys may be observed in >two fifths of girls and >one fifth of boys, and the incidence of constipation is not significantly different from those with a normal index. The anal position index x/y is calculated by division of x, distance between the scrotal end in boys or the posterior labial commissure in girls, and the tip of the coccyx by y, distance between the same starting point and mid-anus.

Therefore, specific additional information and clinical findings are necessary to pick up the quoted subgroup such as *excessive strain and pain at defecation, defecation intervals up to 1 week and more, and soiling. At clinical examination, the anus is surrounded by the circular fibers of the external sphincter that are visible anteriorly. The posterior aspect is depressed and bordered on either side by diverging skin folds coming from the anal verge. The depressed area lies eccentrically in the pigmented zone and bulges out during straining. In severe cases, an inverted crescently shaped skin fold is recognizable anteriorly.*

On rectal examination, *a shelf is felt just above the anal verge with a gap like a cul-de-sac above it and below the sling of the puborectalis muscle.*

Work-Ups, Differential Diagnosis

Calibration of the anal canal, endosonography, CT, or MRI belong to the work-ups to recognize anal stenosis or mid-anal sphincter malformation (identification of absence or hypoplasia of the middle portion the external sphincter muscle).

If contrast enema is performed in long-standing disease, the findings are similar to those of idiopathic constipation.

The clinical delineation includes the common not symptomatic anterior ectopic anus, all causes with persistent constipation and not overt local findings at first glance such as ultrashort type of Hirschsprung's disease.

Treatment, Prognosis

In addition to a posterior anoplasty after a butterfly incision combined with posterior external sphincterotomy of the subcutaneous circular fibers, several other procedures have been published.

Immediate relief of pain and soiling and gradual normalization of defecation without laxatives in long-standing disease are usually observed after surgery. Best results are achieved in infants below the age of 6 months.

21.4 Postoperative Anorectal Anomalies, Hirschsprung's Disease, and Spina Bifida

Occurrence, Causes

Although the diseases quoted in the headline occur much less frequently than constipation in general, chronic stool retention belongs to the postoperative and non-postoperative morbidity of these disorders.

The possible causes of constipation are many and diverse in these disorders. In postoperative anorectal malformations, anorectal stenosis, delay of maturation of the defecation mechanism, and congenital or acquired neurological deficit are possible causes, whereas in postoperative Hirschsprung's disease, sphincter achalasia, residual primary or secondary aganglionic segment, associated IND, and idiopathic constipation play a significant role.

Clinical Significance

- Constipation may be a troublesome complication of all three disorders because it leads to possible obstructive symptoms such as attacks of abdominal pain, to paradoxical diarrhea, encopresis, and soiling and necessitates time-consuming and demanding measures.

Clinical Presentation

It is or may be similar to idiopathic constipation.

Work-Ups, Differential Diagnosis, Treatment, and Prognosis

The necessary tools must consider the most probable cause(s) of constipation and include history and clinical examination including anorectal findings, contrast enema and defecography, rectal suction and laparoscopic full-thickness biopsy, and anorectal manometry.

The differential diagnosis must include the already quoted causes of constipation and to a lesser degree all other disorders with constipation.

Treatment must consider the individual cause of constipation and the possibility of deterioration of a fecal incontinence and includes operative, for example, anal sphincter myectomy in anal sphincter achalasia or nonoperative measures.

Prognosis depends on the cause of constipation.

21.5 Meconium Plug Syndrome, Small Left Colon Syndrome

Occurrence

Each of the two disorders occur less frequently than jejunoileal atresia, both are functional obstructions of the colon with spontaneous resolution within several days or in case of small left colon syndrome more frequently within 1 month or more, and a clinical and radiological overlap of both disorders can be observed.

Clinical Significance

- Both disorders have a differential diagnostic significance because they resemble clinically and, in case of small left colon syndrome, also radiologically Hirschsprung's disease.
- Both disorders have occasionally an underlying diagnosis of Hirschsprung' disease and cystic fibrosis.

Underlying Diseases

In **meconium plug syndrome**, the following disorders may be encountered in order of decreasing frequency: isolated meconium plug syndrome (up to 80 %), aganglionosis of all types (13 %), small left colon syndrome, maternal diabetes (8 %), and cystic fibrosis that is observed most frequently in meconium ileus and meconium plug syndrome.

Small left colon syndrome: At least 5 % of the mothers have diabetes mellitus. Known risk factors are toxemia of pregnancy, C-section, hypothyroidism, psychotropic drugs, and prematurity. Immaturity of the intramural plexuses of left colon and rectum plays a major role. Hirschsprung's disease and cystic fibrosis belong to the most important underlying diseases.

Clinical Presentation

In **meconium plug syndrome**, *meconium evacuation is delayed for >48 h and abdominal distension develops. Meconium evacuation takes place only after spontaneous or provoked passage of a so-called meconium plug that consists of a glutinous meconium plug combined with a mucous, whitish extension like the tail of Halley's comet #.*

In **left small colon syndrome**, *the symptomatology is variable and extends from delayed meconium passage and abdominal distension like in the meconium plug syndrome to obstructive symptoms and signs for up to 1 month and more that need parenteral nutrition and daily washouts or lead to spontaneous colon perforation and necessitate temporary colostomy.*

In **premature infants**, meconium evacuation may be delayed for days to weeks. In case of obvious prolongation and association with obstructive signs such as distention and vomiting, the following three disorders must be considered: **necrotizing enterocolitis, microcolon of prematurity, and the related meconium plug syndrome of the premature infant**. *The latter differs from the common meconium plug syndrome by its extension into the ascending colon, its late diagnosis after birth, and some mothers with eclampsia.*

Work-Ups, Differential Diagnosis

Although both disorders may be suspected by plain abdominal x-ray in hanging position, contrast enema is diagnostic and shows meconium plug as intraluminal defect of the contrast column. Small left colon syndrome is a description of a narrow descending colon with transition in a dilated transverse colon as characteristic finding of the contrast enema #. Distinct haustration of the descending colon permits differentiation from long-segment Hirschsprung's disease.

The differential diagnosis includes all disorders with delayed passage of meconium, low obstructive ileus, or spontaneous intestinal perforation and peritonitis.

Treatment, Prognosis

Contrast enema is often therapeutic with relief of functional obstruction in meconium plug syndrome and slight small left colon syndrome. The latter needs often parenteral nutrition and washouts, or even colostomy for 1 month and more.

Prognosis is excellent, if no underlying disease is present.

21.6　Chronic Idiopathic Intestinal Pseudoobstruction

Occurrence, Classification

Chronic idiopathic intestinal obstruction includes rare disorders in which the obstructive symptomatology is not caused by an internal or external pathoanatomical obstacle of the intestine.

The classification includes mainly visceral neuropathies (abnormalities of the intestinal nervous system) and visceral myopathies (involvement of the intestinal smooth muscle). These disorders may be congenital or acquired, primary or part of a systemic disease, and familial or spontaneous. The already quoted Hirschsprung's disease, IND, hypoganglionosis, or immaturity of the intramural plexuses are well-known disease entities for which the term idiopathic intestinal pseudoobstruction does not apply.

Clinical Significance

- Disorders of chronic idiopathic intestinal pseudoobstruction are troublesome and expensive because of their long-term symptomatology, difficulties of diagnostic work-up, and only restricted therapeutic options.
- They must be considered in the differential diagnosis of constipation and obstructive intestinal symptomatology.
- Intestinal pseudoobstruction may be a part of a paraneoplastic syndrome.

Clinical Presentation

The history should consider possible familiality, excessive drug use, or exposure to infectious diseases, for example, Chagas disease caused by Trypanosoma cruzi that occurs in Middle and South America and leads among other things to a Hirschsprung's-like disease due to destruction of the myenteric plexus, or urological abnormalities.

A chronic disease is often observed with unpredictable deteriorations and ameliorations that is characterized by abdominal distension, constipation and gas retention, intermittent attacks of abdominal pain, and signs of intestinal obstruction including vomiting and dysphagia. Up to one third of the children have disorders of urine transport and voiding leading to urinary tract infection, megavesica, and other signs.

Several familial types of visceral neuropathies or myopathies are described without or with other organ involvement. In the latter category, the degenerated smooth muscle may be replaced by connective tissue. **Megacystis-microcolon-intestinal hypoperistalsis syndrome** is a related disorder in which the colon remains unused because the content of the small intestine cannot be transported; the outcome of its neonatal ileus is bad with a high mortality rate.

Work-Ups, Differential Diagnosis

It includes contrast enema and study of the upper gastrointestinal tract and small intestine for visualization of pathological intestinal contractility and emptying and their site, and for exclusion of any pathoanatomical obstruction. For quantitative analysis, scintiscan after peroral isotope intake can be used. After exclusion of possible dysganglionosis by rectal suction biopsies, laparotomy or laparoscopy becomes necessary for full-thickness biopsies (for histology and electron microscopy with different staining techniques) of the probably involved parts of intestine according to the radiological imaging studies and intraoperative findings. Visceral neuropathies display intestinal loops that are small and have a strong but uncoordinated motility, whereas visceral myopathies have grossly dilated loops with weak contractility.

In addition, ultrasound is necessary for recognition of possible megavesica, hydroureteronephrosis, etc.

The **differential diagnosis** must consider theoretically all disorders with vomiting, regurgitation, and dysphagia, constipation, surgical abdomen (especially abdominal distension), and chronic abdominal pain.

Treatment, Prognosis

In general, intestinal resections or bypass and reconstructive interventions are not useful in the majority of visceral neuropathies or myopathies except for small intestine transplantation in selected cases. Treatment options are prokinetics, parenteral or selective enteral nutrition, laxatives and washouts, and measures against bacterial overgrowth. Nutrition needs vascular access, gastrostomy, or jejunostomy that is also useful for venting of intestinal gas.

Depending on the type of chronic idiopathic intestinal pseudoobstruction and its course, prognosis may be fatal in the long term.

Webcodes

The following webcodes can be used on www.psurg.net for further images and data.

2101 Functional constipation, postevacuation contrast enema	2112 Constantly recognizable colonic loop
2102 Aganglionic colon, histology	2113 Corresponding megacolon
2103 Aganglionic, transitional zone, normal part	2114 Anorectal manometry, missing relaxation
2104 Zuelzer-Wilson syndrome including ileum	2115 Suction rectal biopsy, hypertrophic nerve fibers
2105 Newborn with surgical abdomen	2116 Swenson-Grob pull-through
2106 Abnormal breast fed stool	2117 Swenson-Grob, preanal anastomosis
2107 Abdominal distension	2118 Enterocolitis, intestinal neuronal dysplasia
2108 Failure to thrive	2119 Immaturity of intramural plexuses
2109 Ileus of the newborn, plain x-ray	2120 Anterior ectopic anus
2110 Spontaneous perforation, plain x-ray	2121 Meconium plug syndrome
2111 Hirschsprung's disease, contrast enema	2122 Small left colon syndrome

Bibliography

General and Differential Diagnosis

Biggs WS, Dery WH (2006) Evaluation and treatment of constipation in infants and children. Am Fam Physician 73:469–477

Borowitz SM, Cox DJ, Kovatchev B et al (2005) Treatment of childhood constipation by primary care physicians: efficacy and predictors of outcomes. Pediatrics 115:873–877

Feichter S, Meier-Ruge WA, Bruder E (2009) The histopathology of gastrointestinal motility disorders in children. Semin Pediatr Surg 18:206–211

Felt B, Wise CG, Olson A et al (1999) Guideline for the management of pediatric idiopathic constipation and soiling. Arch Pediatr Adolesc Med 153:380–385

Holschneider A (1977) Elektromanometrie des enddarmes: diagnostik der inkonti-nenz und chronischen obstipation, 1. Auflage. Urban und Schwarzenberg, München

Loening-Baucke V (2005) Prevalence, symptoms and outcome of constipation in infants and toddlers. J Pediatr 146:359–363

Tafazzoli K, Soost K, Wessel L, Wedel T (2005) Topographic peculiarities of the submucous plexus in the human anorectum – consequences for histopatho-

logical evaluation of rectal biopsies. Eur J Pediatr Surg 15:159–163

Vargas-Gonzalez R, Paniagua-Morgan F, Victoria G, de la Torre-Mondragon L, Manuel-Aparicio J (2008) Currarino syndrome. A rare cause of severe constipation. Case report and literature review. Rev Gastroenterol Mex 73:80–84

Youssef NN, Peters JM, Henderson W et al (2002) Dose response of PEG 3350 for the treatment of childhood fecal impaction. J Pediatr 141:410–414

Section 21.1.1

Albanese CT, Jennings RW, Smith B et al (1999) Perineal one-stage pull-through for Hirschsprung's disease. J Pediatr Surg 34:377–380

Bagwell CE, Langham MR Jr, Mahaffey SM, Talbert JL, Shandling B (1992) Pseudomembraneous colitis following resection for Hirschsprung's disease. J Pediatr Surg 27:1261–1264

Borchard F, Meier-Ruge W, Wiebecke B, Briner J, Müntefering H, Födisch HF, Holschneider AM, Schmidt A, Enck P, Stolte M (1991) Innervationsstörungen des dickdarms – klassifikation and diagnostik. Ergebnisse einer Kon-sensus-tagung der arbeitsgemeinschaft für gastroenteropathologie vom 01.12.1990 In frakfurt/main. Pathologe 12:171–174

De La Torre-Mondragon L, Ortega A (2000) Transanal versus open endorectal pull-through for Hirschsprung's disease. J Pediatr Surg 35:1630–1632

De Lorijn F, Kremer LC, Reitsma JB, Benninga MA (2006) Diagnostic tests in Hirschsprung disease: a systematic review. J Pediatr Gastroenterol Nutr 42:496–505

Holschneider AM (1982) Clinical and electromanometric studies of postoperative continence in Hirschsprung's disease: relationship to the surgical procedures. In: Holschneider MA (ed) Hirschsprung's disease. Hippokrates/Thieme-Stratton, Stuttgart/New York

Kaiser G, Bettex M (1982) Clinical generalities. In: Holschneider MA (ed) Hirschsprung's disease. Hippokrates/Thieme-Stratton, Stuttgart/New York

Lynn HB, van Heerden JA (1975) Rectal myectomy in Hirschsprung's disease: a decade of experience. Arch Surg 110:991–994

Meier-Ruge WA, Bruder E, Holschneider AM, Lochbühler H, Piket G, Posselt HG, Tewes G (2004a) Diagnosis and therapy of ultrashort Hirschsprung's disease. Eur J Pediatr Surg 14:392–397

Qualman SJ, Murray R (1994) Aganglionosis and related disorders. Hum Pathol 25:1141

Rintala RJ (2003) Transanal coloanal pull-through with a short muscular cuff for classic Hirschsprung's disease. Eur J Pediatr Surg 13:181–186

Schulten D, Holschneider AM, Meier-Ruge W (2000) Proximal segment histology of resected bowel in Hirschsprung's disease predicts postoperative bowel function. Eur J Pediatr Surg 10:378–381

Teitelbaum DH, Coran AG, Weitzman JJ, Ziegler MM, Kane T (1998) Hirschsprung's disease and related neuromuscular disorder of the intestine. In: O'Neill JA Jr et al (eds) Pediatric surgery, vol II, 5th edn. Mosby, St. Louis

Differential Diagnosis

Irving IM, Lister J (1977) Segmental dilatation of the ileum. J Pediatr Surg 12:103–112

Mathur P, Mogra N, Surana SS, Bordia S (2004) Congenital segmental dilatation of the colon with ano-rectal malformation. J Pediatr Surgery 39:e18–20

Montedonico S, Piotrowska AP, Rolle U, Puri P (2008) Histochemical staining of rectal suction biopsies at the first investigation in patients with chronic constipation. Pediatr Surg Int 24:785–792

Schmunis GA, Yadon ZE (2009) Chagas disease: a Latin American health problem becoming a world health problem. Acta Trop 115(1–2):14–21

Section 21.1.2

Bruder E, Meier-Ruge WA (2007) Intestinal neuronal dysplasia type B: how do we understand it today? Pathologe 28:137–142

Koletzko S, Ballauff A, Hadziselimovic F, Enck P (1993) Is histological diagnosis of neuronal intestinal dysplasia related to clinical and manometric findings in constipated children? Result of a Pilot Study. J Pediatr gastroenterol Nutr 17:59–65

Meier-Ruge WA, Ammann K, Bruder E, Holschneider AM, Schärli AF, Schmittenbe-cher PP, Stoss F (2004b) Updated results on intestinal neuronal dysplasia (IND B). Eur J Pediatr Surg 14:384–391

Schärli AF (1992) Neuronal intestinal dysplasia. Pediatr Surg Int 7:2–7

Schimpl G, Uray E, Ratschek M, Höllwarth ME (2004) Constipation and intestinal neuronal dysplasia type B: a clinical follow-up study. J Pediatr Gastroenterol Nutr 38:308 311

Section 21.1.3

Ament ME, Vargas J (1988) Diagnosis and management of chronic intestinal pseudo-obstruction syndromes in infancy and childhood. Arq Gastroenterol Sao Paulo 25:157–165

Burge D, Drewett M (2004) Meconium plug obstruction. Pediatr Surg Int 20:108–110

Cassaccia G, Trucchi A, Nahom A, Lucidi V, Giorlandino C, Bagolan P (2003) The impact of cystic fibrosis on neonatal intestinal obstruction: the need for prenatal/neo-natal screening. Pediatr Surg Int 19:75–78

El Haddad M, Corcery JJ (1985) The anus of the newborn. Pediatrics 76:927–928

Fuchs JR, Langer JC (1998) Long-term outcome after neonatal meconium obstruction. Pediatrics 101:E7

Glassman M, Spivak W, Mininberg D, Madara J (1989) Chronic idiopathic intestinal pseudoobstruction: a commonly misdiagnosed disease in infants and children. Pediatrics 83:603–608

Heaton ND, Howard ER, Garrett JR (1991) Small left colon syndrome: an immature enteric plexus. J R Soc Med 84:113–114

Herek O, Polat A (2004) Incidence of anterior displacement of the anus and its relationship to constipation in children. Surg Today 34:190–192

Hirsig J, Hanimann B, Willi U, Xiao X (1988) Bedeutung des anterioren ektopen anus und anderer anorektaler fehlbildungen für die kindliche obstipation (significance of the anteriorly displaced anus and other anorectal malformations in constipated children). Schweiz Rundsch Med 77:527–532

Hugot JP, Ferkdajdi L, Faure C, Lachassine E, Bellaiche M, Bocquet L, Gaudelus J, Navarro J, Cézard JP (1992) Chronic intestinal pseudo-obstruction and delayed myenteric ganglion cell maturation. Arch Fr Pediatr 49:721–723

Hyman PE (1995) Chronic intestinal pseudo-obstruction in childhood: progress in diagnosis and treatment. Scand J Gastroenterol Suppl 213:39–46

Hyman PE, McDiarmid SV, Napolitano J, Abrams CE, Tomomasa T (1988) Antroduodenal motility in children with chronic intestinal pseudoobstruction. J Pediatr 112:899–905

Keckler SJ, Peter SD, Spilde TL, Tsao K, Ostlie DJ, Holcomb GW 3rd, Snyder CL (2008) Current significance of meconium plug syndrome. J Pediatr Surg 43:896–898

Krasna IH, Rosenfeld D, Salerno P (1996) Is it necrotizing enterocolitis, microcolon of prematurity, or delayed meconium plug? J Pediatr Surg 31:855–858

Langer JC (2004) Persistent obstructive symptoms after surgery for Hirschsprung's disease: development of a diagnostic and therapeutic algorithm. J Pediatr Surg 39:1458–1462

Lassmann G, Kees A, Körner K, Wurnig P (1989) Transient functional obstruction of the colon in neonates: examination of its development by manometry and biopsies. Prog Pediatr Surg 24:202–216

Meier R, Beglinger C, Dederding JP, Meyer-Wyss B, Fumagalli M, Rowedder A, Turberg J, Brignoli R (1992) Alters- und geschlechtsspezifische normwerte der dick-darmtransitzeit bei gesunden. Schweiz med Wschr 122:940–943

Navarro J, Sonsino E, Boige N, Nabarra B, Ferkadji L, Mashako LMN, Cezard JP (1990) Visceral neuropathies responsible for chronic intestinal pseudo-obstruction syndrome in pediatric practice: analysis of 26 cases. J Pediatr Gastroenterol Nutr 11:179–195

Nonaka M, Goulet O, Arahan P, Fekete C, Ricour C, Nezelof C (1989) Primary intestinal myopathy, a cause of chronic idiopathic intestinal pseudoobstruction syndrome (CIPS): clinicopathological studies of seven cases in children. Pediatr Pathol 9:409–424

Rolle U, Piaseczna-Piotrowska A, Puri P (2007) Interstitial cells of cajal in the normal gut and in intestinal motility disorders of childhood. Pediatr Surg Int 23:1139–1152

Shah AJ, Bhattacharjee N, Patel DN, Ganatra JR (2003) Anal shift: preliminary results. J Pediatr Surg 38:196–198

Stafford PW (1998) Other disorders of the anus and rectum. Anorectal function. In: O'Neill JA Jr et al (eds) Pediatric surgery, vol II, 5th edn. Mosby, St Louis

Upadhyaya P (1984) Mid-anal sphincteric malformation, cause of costipation in anterior perineal anus. J Pediatr Surg 19:183–186

Wildhaber B, Niggli F, Stallmach T, Willi U, Stauffer UG, Sacher P (2002) Intestinal pseudoobstruction as a paraneoplastic syndrome in ganglioneuroblastoma. J Pediatr Surg 12:429–431

Hematemesis

If blood is brought up (hematemesis) or evacuated by the anus (melena) that is recognizable clearly us such, the parents and the child are very frightened and the physician is consulted immediately. Other forms of gastrointestinal blood evacuation must be ascertained by asking or even tested for it.

A precise history and inspection of vomited material or the evacuated intestinal content are particularly important. They permit to differentiate the common disorders that must be considered.

Fresh or older blood may be vomited, regurgitated, or emptied from the oral cavity combined with blood clots in a large or small amount. In the latter condition, the amount of blood seems larger than really because of the mixture of saliva. **Vomiting of hematin** is often not payed attention to, mainly if only splashes of hematin mixed up with mucus or milk are distributed over the sheets. The same applies to **gastric aspirate** with fresh blood or coffee-ground.

Evacuation of **occult blood** must be excluded occasionally, for instance, in case of cryptogenetic anemia. Tests for occult blood may show false-positive or false-negative results. A factor calculated by the blood urea nitrogen and creatinine makes possible at best to differentiate between upper and lower gastrointestinal hemorrhage.

For differential diagnostic reasons and estimation of the inherent emergency, the **general condition** of the child (shock signs), the hemoglobin, and other **blood values** must be checked as well.

Table 22.1 Differential diagnosis of hematemesis from a pediatric surgical viewpoint

- Swallowed blood
- Gastric tube, prolonged vomiting
- Complicated gastroesophageal reflux
- Erosive gastritis, gastroduodenal ulcer
- o Esophageal varices
- o Foreign body ingestion, caustic injury
- o Volvulus of the stomach, Morgagni or hiatus hernia, and paraesophageal hernia

In Table 22.1, the pediatric surgically relevant disorders leading to hematemesis are listed and weighted. Hematemesis of the newborn needs special attention because some causes of hematemesis are specific for this age group as hemorrhagic disease, swallowed maternal blood, erosive gastritis, and coagulopathy. In infancy, reflux esophagitis and erosive gastritis; between 1 and 2 years peptic ulcer disease; and beyond 2 years, esophageal varices appear as new and depending on the catchment area prominent cause of hematemesis. If the frequency of the causes of hematemesis is not considered, nearly every disorder may be encountered during childhood, for instance, peptic ulcer disease in the newborn because of maternal gastrin.

22.1 Swallowed Blood

Occurrence, Causes
Swallowed blood is one of the most common causes of hematemesis in childhood. The swallowed blood

in newborns comes from the mother either caught at birth or during breastfeeding from the nipple.

Later in life, the following sources of swallowed blood may be found:

- Epistaxis
- Trauma to the structures of vestibulum, oral cavity, oropharynx, and nasopharynx, for instance, dentoalveolar lesions, tongue bite, stab injury after a fall with a rodlike object in the mouth, or severe craniofacial trauma.
- Oronasopharyngeal surgery or instrumentation, for example, tonsillectomy with afterbleeding or intubation and endoscopies.
- Rarely, spontaneous hemorrhage stems from congenital anomalies or neoplasms, for example, from malignant pharyngeal fibroma.

Clinical Significance

- The amount of bleeding is difficult to assess and may be under- or overestimated.
- The possibility of blood aspiration or inherent shock must be considered.

Clinical Findings

History and clinical examination permit often recognition of swallowed blood and its origin that is vomited (hematemesis), visible in the gastric aspirate, or nasogastric tube. If some time has elapsed since bleeding, it is difficult to attribute hematemesis or hemorrhagic aspirate to swallowed blood at first glance.

In newborns with swallowing of blood at birth, mostly large amounts of gastric content stained with blood may be aspirated. After epistaxis, trauma, or surgery, splashes of dried blood around the nostrils and in the face are recognizable, blood in the nasogastric tube #, or aspirate. The brought up masses consist either of fresh blood mixed up with saliva and clots or denatured blood.

Differential Diagnosis, Work-Ups

In newborns, hematemesis of fresh or coffee-ground blood and melena is a relatively frequent finding and may be unrelated to swallowing of blood, for instance, in acute **erosive gastritis** due to stress or rarely to maternal gastrin. Often no obvious cause is encountered. In addition, **hemorrhagic disease of the newborn** (skin bleedings, cephalhematoma, hematoma of the orbit, intrac-

ranial hemorrhage, hematemesis, and melena; third to seventh day after birth because of vitamin K deficiency) and less frequently a **coagulopathy** (hematoma of the orbit, intracranial hemorrhage, umbilical bleeding) must be considered.

The differential diagnosis of hematemesis of older children is different. In postoperative hemorrhage, consultation of the responsible surgeon or pediatric specialist is necessary for definition of type, site, and significance of hemorrhage. Some after-bleedings have characteristic patterns, for example, after-bleeding in tonsillectomy occurs in 1–2 % and mostly in the first 24 h or 7–10 days after surgery.

Epistaxis is a frequent cause of hematemesis. Epistaxis occurs either anteriorly or posteriorly. The source of the former and more common type is the plexus of Kiesselbach and of the latter, a branch of the phenopalatal artery.

Work-ups include Abt test in newborns with suspected swallowed maternal blood and blood tests in suspected hemorrhagic disease or coagulopathy. For hematemesis after trauma or in congenital malformations or neoplasms, endoscopy and radiological imaging are necessary, and generally in severe bleedings, hemoglobin, coagulation tests, and blood preserves are indispensable.

Treatment, Prognosis

Treatment and prognosis depend on the cause of swallowed blood and hematemesis, and blood substitution and/or surgical stanching may become necessary. In **epistaxis**, emergency measures include forward inclination of the head, compression of the involved side of the nose against the midline structure for 5 min, and introduction of an appropriate gauze soaked with vasoconstrictive agent. In case of failure of these measures and/or posterior epistaxis, emergency consultation by an ENT specialist is necessary for specific tamponade or another form of blood stanching.

22.2 Gastroesophageal Reflux

Occurrence

Although bringing up of gastric content with traces of fresh blood or coffee-ground is mostly caused by reflux esophagitis in infancy,

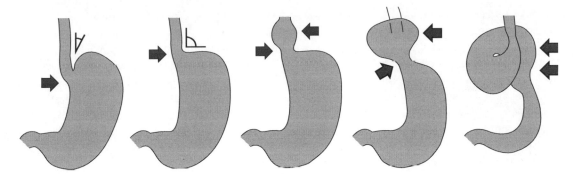

Fig. 22.1 Gastroesophageal reflux and hiatus hernia in relation to radiological and intraoperative findings. The drawings show from *left* to *right* the following findings: (1) normal anatomical findings with an acute angle of His. Gastroesophageal reflux (=reflux) is not excluded, even if no reflux of contrast is observed; (2) angle of His is obtuse; reflux is most probable (chalasia, gaping cardia); (3) a small pouch of stomach is intermittently or permanently above the diaphragm (epiphrenic pouch); (4) a large pouch is permanently above the diaphragm; and (5) large amounts of stomach lie twisted above the stomach (upside-down stomach). The forms with permanent gastric pouch above the diaphragm (4) and (5) are called hiatus hernia and combined with reflux and in (5), in addition with possible dysphagia and inability to vomit right sixth row: The uppder arrow corresponds to the site of the epiphrenic pouch and the lower to the site of the esophageal hiatus

vomiting and recurrent aspirations are in the foreground of clinical presentation and attract more attention.

In the neonate and young infant, there is a continuous transition between "physiological" and pathological reflux with delayed maturation or abnormality of the lower esophageal "sphincter." The pathological reflux reveals persistent vomiting and especially symptoms and signs of complicated reflux.

Clinical Significance

- Hematemesis is an indication that the suspected reflux is more than physiological, needs work-up, appropriate treatment, and follow-up.
- It may be the cause of chronic anemia, occult or gross blood evacuation by the anus.

Clinical Presentation

It may be a discrepancy between inconspicuous hematemesis # and the spectacular findings at endoscopy #.

Work-Ups, Differential Diagnosis

The reader is referred to Sect. 20.2. If esophagogram and fluoroscopy are performed, astonishing findings may be recognized in 10 % and more of the patients with reflux (Fig. 22.1) that can be cured permanently only with surgery.

Treatment, Prognosis

Infants and older children with hematemesis because of reflux need in addition to an appropriate diet H2 receptor antagonists. Surgery is indicated in unresponsive esophagitis, severe and continuous stricture formation, and/or distinct failure to thrive.

22.3   Peptic Ulcer Disease (Gastric and Duodenal Ulcer)

Occurrence, Types

Gastric or duodenal ulcers occur at any age of childhood and are quite frequent under specific conditions or in a specific age group.

In **primary ulcer**, a prepyloric or duodenal ulcer is the main disease that is observed preferentially in the second decade. Primary ulcer will drastically decrease with increasing eradication of Helicobacter pylori in developed countries if Helicobacter gastritis is considered as main cause of primary ulcer.

Secondary ulcers occur because of stress and are observed at any age from the neonatal period to adolescence. Difficult labor, resuscitation, and low Apgar scores are examples of neonatal stress leading to erosive gastritis or secondary ulcer with hematemesis. Later in life, trauma (especially head injury, multisystemic organ injury, and burns), septicemia, oncological diseases, and long-term medications (e.g., NSAID, steroids, etc.) are common stressors. The majority of secondary ulcers are observed in children below school age; they tend to be multiple and confined to the fundus with relation to erosive gastritis in very young patients and to be solitary in older children with a location similar to the primary ulcer. Rare secondary ulcers are those combined with chronic hypertrophic pyloric stenosis or duodenal obstruction, and other rare gastric outlet obstructions (incomplete antral or prepyloric web).

Clinical Significance
- Secondary ulcers manifest out of the blue either with severe hemorrhage leading to hematemesis, possible shock, and/or perforation and surgical abdomen. Prophylactic treatment with antacids avoids their occurrence to a large extent.
- Primary peptic ulcer disease is an important differential diagnosis of diffuse abdominal or epigastric pain that is related to daytime and food intake.

Clinical Presentation
The history yields possibly familiality, extraordinary drug administration, or psychic problems.

The younger the child, the less specific is the symptomatology. *In infancy, vomiting, refusal to drink, and crying are possible indications of peptic ulcer disease. Schoolchildren and teenagers* with primary ulcer *complain of unspecific abdominal or epigastric, nocturnal, and postprandial pain; poor digestion; vomiting; and occasionally hematemesis.*

On clinical examination, diffuse or epigastric tenderness and weight loss are possible findings.

In case of familiality, a mean age of 11 years (4–15 years), characteristic abdominal pain and weight loss, duodenal or prepyloric ulcus is very probable.

The majority of secondary ulcers manifest because of complications to which belong bleeding (hemorrhagic gastric aspirate, hematemesis, and shock) or perforation (signs of peritonitis and surgical abdomen).

Work-Ups, Differential Diagnosis
Gastroduodenoscopy is the first-line diagnostic tool because radiological imaging is less reliable for ulcer diagnosis and should be reserved for suspected gastric outlet obstruction and ulcer with closed perforation or penetration in the surrounding organs (upper GI study, CT, or MRI with contrast).

In newborns and infants, endoscopy is used for location of hemorrhage and possibly for stanching. It is used in older children for confirmation of a clinically suspected ulcer and for biopsy (exclusion of Helicobacter pylori [=H. pylori] gastritis).

The differential diagnosis includes other disorders with hematemesis depending on the age and presentation of hemorrhage and/or abdominal pain.

Zollinger-Ellison syndrome is a rare differential diagnosis. Multiple ulcers and other endoscopic findings point to this disorder that is confirmed by spontaneous and induced hypergastrinemia. In children, total gastrectomy should be avoided whenever possible. H2 receptor antagonists and complete resection of the responsible tumor of the pancreas if possible are the primary options. **Functional abdominal pain** is usually not combined with complaints specific for peptic ulcer. It is also true for **other causes of chronic abdominal pain** that have other clinical characteristics.

Treatment, Prognosis
The primary ulcer is treated with antacids and H2 receptor antagonists and if necessary with eradication of H. pylori. Proton pump inhibitors and cytoprotective agents are other options of medical treatment.

Secondary ulcer is best avoided by antacids and if present, by alleviation of its cause and H2 receptor antagonists.

Hemorrhage and hematemesis is initially treated by a nasogastric tube of appropriate size, repeated warm saline lavage (or iced saline) for evacuation of the clots, and volume replacement. Endoscopic stanching depends on the individual experience.

The **indications of surgery** are:

- Massive hemorrhage (blood loss in 24 h equal to the estimated blood volume or equal to half of it (in children <2 or >2 years of age)) or persistent hemorrhage
- Perforation including closed perforation and penetration
- Persistent gastric outlet obstruction
- Secondary ulcer in which cure of the underlying cause is not possible at present
- Progressive secondary ulcers (e.g., Cushing's and Curling's ulcer)

Emergency treatment consists of oversewing (or plication) of the base of the bleeding ulcer or point, or closure of the perforation possibly combined with pyloroplasty. Although resections should be avoided in children occasionally, partial resection may be necessary in large perforated ulcers. If ulcer surgery is indicated, selective vagotomy and pyloroplasty has the least disadvantages in children.

The prognosis concerning permanent cure is best for secondary ulcers if the underlying cause can be treated within a foreseeable future. In primary ulcers, the early prognosis is favorable due to the available modern drugs. Intermediate and long-term prognosis is uncertain because of the high risk of recurrences that continues up to adulthood. In adults, only one third has no recurrences for a longer time and eradication of H. pylrori has improved the prognosis of primary ulcer.

22.4   Esophageal and Gastric Varices

Occurrence, Types

Esophageal varices develop in portal hypertension as a sequel of portocaval bypass.

In portal hypertension, the portal pressure increases to >12–15 cm H_2O that is normally 8–12 cm H_2O, and the gradient between vena porta and cava becomes > 7 cm H_2O (>5 mmHg). The risk of bleeding from esophageal varices starts with 10–12 mmHg (13.6–16 cm H_2O).

In the past, up to 70 % of childhood portal hypertension was based on a **prehepatic block** of the portal vein because of thrombosis after omphalitis, umbilical catheterization, or abdominal infection, for example, liver abscess and septicemia in developed countries; the liver function is not impaired in the early stages of such cases. Preoperative work-up must consider isolated portal vein occlusion in two thirds and combined with splenic or superior mesenteric vein involvement in one fourth or <5 %. Extrinsic tumor compression is a rare cause in children.

Today, the majority of portal hypertension is due to an **intrahepatic** or post-sinusoidal **block** due to liver disease with increase in hepatic resistance, whereas in developing countries, the prehepatic block is still an important type of portal hypertension like the **suprahepatic block** (hepatic vein or suprahepatic vena cava). Budd-Chiari syndrome plays a role in Middle and South America or Asia; it is related in its primary form to thrombosis of hepatic veins or the terminal portion of inferior vena cava.

Surviving children with biliary atresia and portoenterostomy, sporadic or familial congenital hepatic fibrosis (autosomal recessive disease with cholangitis and portal hypertension), cystic fibrosis (10–15 % with biliary cirrhosis), α1-antitrypsin deficiency, posthepatic cirrhosis, cirrhosis in thesaurismoses, and cystic liver disease are the most important causes of portal hypertension with intrahepatic block; they have different degrees of liver involvement.

Clinical Significance

- One of the main causes of severe and repeated hematemesis in childhood is portal hypertension with esophageal varices.
- The type with intrahepatic block of esophageal varices is increasingly prominent in developed countries. It needs individualization of therapeutic options and is a great challenge of treatment.

Clinical Presentation

Unexpected, life-threatening, and severe hematemesis is the leading sign of esophageal varices: fresh and denatured blood mixed up with clots and gastric juice is brought up or regurgitated in large amounts, possibly combined with imminent shock. In prehepatic block, hematemesis may start in the first year and is encountered mostly at the age of 2–3 years, and about four fifth will have at least one episode in their life. Hematemesis may be precipitated by upper airway infections or acetylsalicylic acid. Later, hematemesis may be due to gastric varices.

Isolated splenomegaly is the first presenting sign in one third of such cases. Abdominal pain and/or complications of hypersplenism are encountered less often.

In addition, the following signs may be encountered *spider angiomas* (cirsomphalos), *ascites* (transient or permanent*), hemorrhoids #, and occult blood loss from the anus (chronic anemia)*. Melena is observed with commencement of hematemesis. Hemorrhoids are usually of grade III. Although they bleed rarely, hemorrhage is often severe.

The clinical presentation of portal hypertension with intrahepatic obstruction differs from that of classic extrahepatic block by possibly *earlier onset of hematemesis that is more difficult to control, variable hepatic signs depending on the underlying liver disease (e.g., hepatomegaly), its grade* (according to Child's classification)*, and the usual knowledge of the cause*. In suprahepatic block, the liver is involved as well.

Sequels of advanced prehepatic and intrahepatic portal hypertension are growth retardation, portal biliopathy (strictures, dilatations, and stones in the biliary tree leading to cholangitis and biliary cirrhosis), protein-C deficiency, and abnormal cell-mediated immunity, hepatopulmonary syndrome, and encephalopathy.

Differential Diagnosis, Work-Ups

It includes all disorders with hematemesis, splenomegaly, and/or pancytopenia. Major hemorrhages leading to hematemesis are mainly encountered in peptic ulcer disease and with large amounts of swallowed blood after trauma or less frequently after surgery. In the differential diagnosis, infectious, parasitic, and oncohematological diseases should be considered as well, for example, **Kalazar** (visceral leishmaniasis) that leads to cholestasis and acute or chronic liver disease, or **Schistosomiasis japonica** in which hepatosplenomegaly and portal hypertension

may occur. In addition, hepatic complications of **autosomal recessive polycystic kidney disease** (biliary disease and portal hypertension) must be considered.

Work-ups are indicated after initial or repeated **hematemesis**, in **isolated splenomegaly**, **other signs of portal hypertension**, and **diseases associated with possible portal hypertension**.

They include esophagogastroscopy for visualization of esophageal and gastric varices; abdominal Doppler ultrasound with demonstration of cavernomatous transformation of the occluded portal vein, reversal of flow in the portal system, and liver morphology (sensitivity up to 100 % and specificity up 96 %); percutaneous splenoportography, angiography of the mesenteric artery, retrograde transjugular portography; MD-CT for illustration of the whole portal system, its site of obstruction, and its bypass circulation; and MRI for parenchymal characterization and biliary tract evaluation.

In addition, hepatic fibrosis scan for liver stiffness score measurement (for fibrosis and possible varices also ultrasound, albumin values, platelet count, spleen length can be used), quantitative tests, and liver biopsy may be used as preendoscopic screening tests of esophageal varices or for estimation of the functional reserve of the involved liver. The Child-Turcotte-Pugh system (CTP) or model for end-stage liver disease (MELD) permits grading of the involved liver.

Blood examinations include determination of albumin, bilirubin, liver enzymes, hemoglobin, leukocytes, platelets, and coagulation profile (prothrombin time). Whereas prehepatic portal hypertension shows usually normal values except for anemia, leukopenia, and thrombocytopenia, intrahepatic portal hypertension leads to decreased albumin levels and increased values of the other parameters. The same may be true for advanced stages of prehepatic portal hypertension due to prolonged decrease in portal circulation or for albumin shortly after hematemesis and following ascites formation.

Treatment, Prognosis

It concerns **the first or recurrent bleeding(s) from the varices**, possible shock, and primary or secondary coagulation disorder. After central venous access, introduction of a nasograstic tube, and gastric lavage with iced saline, treatment is started with i.v. glypressin combined with nitroglycerin (instead of vasopressin) or alternatively with octreotide (instead of somatostatin) as continuous infusion and with blood transfusion. Balloon tamponade has only a temporary effect and should be only used after endotracheal intubation.

For **primary prophylaxis** in case of high risk for hematemesis, **further treatment in case of persistent bleeding**, and **secondary prophylaxis** in children with a history of hematemesis, **endoscopic sclerotherapy** of the varices or banding is performed with possible medication of propranolol or β-blockers:

With the aid of a rigid or flexible endoscopy, clusters of varices are treated by direct or indirect injection of a sclerosant. Several sessions are usually necessary during more than 2–4 months. Hemorrhage, ulceration, dysmotility, stricture, and perforation of the esophagus are possible complications of topical treatment. Symptoms of hypersplenism, portal biliopathy, or liver dysfunction occur in few patients before adolescence, and treatment does not influence the progression time of esophageal varices in case of cirrhosis. Although elastic banding is a more difficult technique, eradication of esophageal varices is possible in a shorter time frame with less sessions, rebleedings, and complications. After eradication, regular endoscopic follow-up is necessary.

Bleeding from gastric varices needs special attention especially on follow-up of eradicated esophageal varices. Balloon-occluded retrograde transvenous obliteration possibly combined with partial splenic embolization or injection of tissue adhesive agents is a possible treatment option.

Depending on the type of portal hypertension, the grade of hepatic involvement, and the outlook of the underlying disorder, **shunt treatment** should be performed, especially if endoscopic therapy fails to control recurrent variceal hemorrhage.

Shunt treatment is indicated in symptomatic esophageal varices due to **classic prehepatic type** with cavernomatous transformation because spontaneous resolution of portal hypertension does not occur, the decreased portal blood flow and natural shunts may lead to clinical manifestation, and anxiety toward repeated hematemesis is not resolved. In small children with small diameters of the vessels, the time before surgery may be bridged by repeated sclerotherapy.

Of the available portosystemic shunts, the side-to-side splenorenal shunt without splenectomy, the mesocaval shunt with jugular vein interposition, or the mesentericoportal shunt (meso-Rex shunt: vein graft between the umbilical segment of left portal vein in the rex recess and the superior mesenteric vein) are options (Fig. 22.2)

In **intrahepatic obstruction** with Child-Pugh's criteria A or B, portocaval shunt with interposition of a jugular vein graft and meso-Rex shunt are options. These shunts preserve some portal hepatic perfusion, avoid hepatic encephalopathy, and do not grossly interfere with a possible liver transplantation. Placement of a transjugular intrahepatic portosystemic shunt in children needs specific skills, and its role for long-term shunting is not yet clarified. This life-preserving technique is useful for stabilization of critically ill patients while awaiting liver transplantation.

In **ascites** resistant to medical treatment, a peritoneal venous shunt (LeVeen valve, placement in the superior vena cava through the internal jugular vein) can be performed.

Acute thrombosis of the portal vein needs special consideration. In case of conspicuous umbilical catheterization, omphalitis, intra-abdominal septicemia of the newborn, after splenectomy (<10 %), and antineoplastic chemotherapy, evaluation of the possibly involved vessels and intestine is necessary. After exclusion of intestinal ischemia, the umbilical catheter is removed and thrombolytic therapy started with urokinase or heparin for 6 months to prevent intestinal ischemia and prehepatic portal hypertension. Intestinal ischemia needs immediate laparotomy for thrombectomy or intestinal resection.

Because of the large variability of hepatic involvement, some patients with the intrahepatic

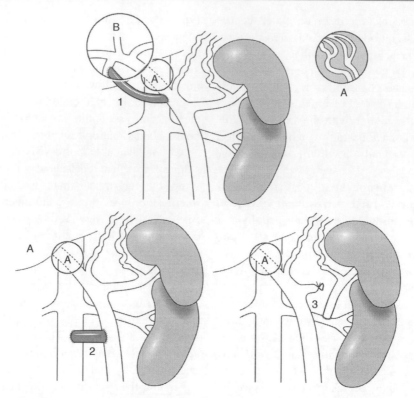

Fig. 22.2 Types of shunt surgery for childhood esophageal varices with prehepatic block. The drawing on the *top* shows a mesentericoportal shunt using a jugular vein graft between the superior mesenteric vein and the umbilical segment of the right portal vein (=meso-Rex shunt). The

drawings at the *bottom* show on the left side a mesentericocaval shunt with jugular vein interposition and on the right side an end-to-side splenorenal shunt. *A* shows vascular transformation of the prehepatic portal block. *B* the umbilical segment of the right portal vein

type may have a good long-term outcome, although mortality is two thirds within the first 5 years after shunt surgery in such cases. In contrast, survival rate after 10-year postoperative follow-up in prehepatic portal hypertension is 96 % with only 2 % complications (shunt thrombosis or stenosis with recurrent hematemesis), no hepatic encephalopathy, and remarkably improved quality of life including growth. The results of single institutes with smaller numbers of patients are 80–96 % long-term shunt function with median follow-ups of 50 months (0.5–13.2 years) and 8 years (0.4–14.2 years). In surgical shunting for bleeding varices of children with portal hypertension and cirrhosis (Child classes A and B), the 2-year survival is significantly better with less frequent shunt failure than the transjugular intrahepatic portosystemic shunting with less survival and more shunt failure.

Webcodes

The following webcodes can be used on www. psurg.net for further images and data.

2201 Swallowed blood, head injury	2203 Reflux esophagitis
2202 Splashes of hematin	2204 Hemorrhoids, portal hypertension

Bibliography

General and Differential Diagnosis

Arensman RM (1998) Gastrointestinal bleeding. In: O'Neill JA Jr et al (eds) Pediatric surgery, vol II, 5th edn. Mosby, St Louis

Boyle JT (1983) Gastrointestinal bleeding. In: Fleisher G, Ludwig S et al (eds) Text-book of pediatric emergency medicine. Williams & Wilkins, Baltimore/London

Section 22.1

der Meulen J, for the National Prospective Tonsillectomy Audit (Royal College of Surgeons of England, London; et al) (2004) Tonsillectomy technique as a risk factor for postoperative Van Haemorrhage. Lancet 364:697–702

McGarry G (2006) Nosebleeds in children. Clin Evid 15:496–499

Section 22.2

Ramenofsky ML (1986) Gastroesophageal reflux: clinical manifestations and diagnosis. In: Ashcraft KW, Holder TM (eds) Pediatric esophageal surgery. Grune & Stratton, Orlando

Section 22.3

Murphy MS, Eastham EJ (1987) Peptic ulcer disease in childhood: long-term prognosis. J Pediatr Gastroenterol Nutr 6:271–724

Murphy MS, Eastham EJ, Jimenez M, Nelson R, Jackson RH (1987) Duodenal ulceration: review of 110 cases. Arch Dis Child 62:554–558

Scherer LR (1998) Peptic ulcer and other conditions of the stomach. In: O'Neill JA Jr et al (eds) Pediatric surgery, vol II, 5th edn. Mosby, St Louis, p Mosby

Differential Diagnosis

Kibiki GS, Thielman NM, Maro VP, Sam NE, Dolmans WM, Crump JA (2006) Hookworm infection of the duodenum associated with dyspepsia and diagnosed by oesophagoduodenoscopy: case report. East Afr Med J 83:689–692

Sauseng W, Benesch M, Lackner H, Urban C, Kronberger M, Gadner H, Höllwarth M, Spuller E, Aschauer M, Horcher E (2007) Clinical, radiological, and pathological findings in four children with gastrointestinal stromal tumor of the stomach. Pediatr Hematol Oncol 24:209–219

Section 22.4

Altman RP (1998) Portal hypertension. In: O'Neill JA Jr et al (eds) Pediatric surgery, vol II, 5th edn. Mosby, St Louis

Brisse H, Orbach D, Lassau N, Servois V, Doz F, Debray D, Helfre S, Hatmann O, Neuenschwander S (2004) Portal vein thrombosis during antineoplastic chemotherapy in children: report of five cases and review of the literature. Eur J Cancer 40:2659–2666, Comment in: Eur J Cancer (2004) 40:2643–2644

Chardot C, Darani A, Dubois R, Mure PY, Pracros JP, Lachaux A (2009) Modified technique of meso-Rex shunt in case of insufficient length of the jugular vein graft. J Pediatr Surg 44:E9–12

Chawla Y, Duseja A, Dhiman RK (2009) Review article: the modern management of portal vein thrombosis. Aliment Pharmacol Ther 1(30):881–894

Clarc W, Hernandez J, McKeon B, Villadolid D, Al-Saadi S, Mullinax J, Ross SB, Rosemurgy AS II (2010) Surgical shunting versus transjugular intrahepatic portasystemic shunting for bleeding varices resulting from portal hypertension and cirrhosis: a meta-analysis. Am Surg 76:857–864

Clatworthy HW Jr (1990) Big shunts for small patients with portal hypertension: a bit of history. J Pediatr Surg 25:1082–1084

Fonkalsrud EW (1982) Long-term results following surgical management of portal hypertension in childfren. Z Kinderchir 35:57–61

Khuroo MS, Khuroo NS, Farahat KL, Khuroo YS, Sofi AA, Dahab ST (2005) Meta-analysis: endoscopic variceal ligation for primary prophylaxis of oesophageal variceal bleeding. Aliment Pharmacol Ther 15(21):347–361

Lillegard JB, Hanna AM, McKenzie TJ, Moir CR, Ishitani MB, Nagorney DM (2010) A single-institution review of portosystemic shunts in children. HPB Surg 2010, 2010: 964597

Lorenz JM (2008) Placement of transjugular intrahepatic portosystemic shunts in children. Tech Vasc Interv Radiol 11:235–240

Meisheri IV, Kothari PR, Kumar A, Deshmukh A (2010) Splenic artery embolisation for portal hypertension in children. Afr J Paediatr Surg 7:86–91

Mileti E, Rosenthal P (2010) Management of portal hypertension in children. Curr Gastroenterol Rep 13.10–16

Mrad SM, Boukhthir S, Oubich F, Gharsallah L, Basaoui S (2007) Treatment of upper gastrointestinal bleeding in portal hypertension in children. Tunis Med 85:184–188

Plessier A, Valla DC (2008) Budd-Chiari syndrome. Semin Liver Dis 28:259–269

Prasad R, Singh UK, Mishra OP, Jaiswal BP, Muthusami S (2010) Portal hypertension with visceral leishmaniasis. Indian Pediatr 7(47):965–967

Schettino GCM, Fagundes EDT, Roquete MLV, Ferreira AR, Penna FJ (2006) Portal vein thrombosis in children and adolescents. J Paediatr (Rio J) 82:171–178

Sharif K, McKierman P, de Ville de Goyet J (2010) Mesoportal bypass for extrahepatic portal vein obstruction in children: close to a cure for most! J Pediatr Surg 45:272–276

Wolff M, Hirner A (2003) Current state of portosystemic shunt surgery. Langenbecks Arch Surg 388:141–149

Yachha SK, Chetri K, Lal R (2002) Management of portal hypertension. Indian J Pediatr 69:809–813

Lower Gastrointestinal Bleeding (Melena)

23

The blood that is lost by the anus may be fresh or denaturated # and associated with # or without mucus. The blood may lie on the stool, or the stool may be intermingled with blood – in the former case, often added during defecation. Several components of ingested food such as beetroots may feign melena or the blood originates from a urethral, vaginal, or perianal lesion. Therefore, a specific history and precise local inspection including the stool are very important. The causes of melena relevant to pediatric surgery are listed in Table 23.1.

23.1 Disorders with Upper Gastrointestinal Bleeding

The majority of the disorders with hematemesis may lead to pitch stools or at least to occult blood loss and severe esophagogastric hemorrhage is usually followed by recognizable blood loss from the anus though with some time delay. Although upside-down stomach and gastric volvulus may lead to upper gastrointestinal bleeding, hematemesis is not necessarily present in the stool for mechanical reasons.

23.2 Disorders with Lower Gastrointestinal Bleeding

23.2.1 Intestinal Volvulus

Occurrence, Causes

Torsion of the small intestine or colon and of a part of them occurs pre- and postnatally and in different congenital or acquired disorders:

Table 23.1 Differential diagnosis of lower gastrointestinal bleeding in pediatric surgery

- Disorders with upper gastrointestinal bleeding
- Intestinal volvulus
- Acute and chronic intussusception
- Henoch-Schönlein purpura
- Meckel's diverticulum
- o Intestinal duplication
- Necrotizing enterocolitis
- Intestinal polyps
- o Incarcerated inguinal hernia
- o Hemorrhoids
- Anal fissure
- Injuries of perineum and anorectum
- Ulcerative colitis and Crohn's disease
- o Rare causes of lower gastrointestinal bleeding
- o Intestinal Bilharziasis

- Anomalies of intestinal rotation and fixation
- Meconium ileus
- Congenital atresia of small intestine or colon
- Meckel's diverticulum
- Intestinal duplication
- Internal Hernias
- Mesenteric cyst and other masses
- Obstructive ileus due to postoperative adhesions

23.2.1.1 Volvulus of the Small Intestine

Clinical Significance

- In every intestinal volvulus, the danger of irreversible intestinal damage exists # and if the involved intestine is long enough or combined

G.L. Kaiser, *Symptoms and Signs in Pediatric Surgery*,
DOI 10.1007/978-3-642-31161-1_23, © Springer-Verlag Berlin Heidelberg 2012

with a specific function, of short bowel syndrome and/or absorptive deficits.

• The early recognition and treatment is therefore mandatory.

Clinical Presentation
Although melena may be an important presenting sign, it may be missing. Acute abdominal colics, nausea, and vomiting or the equivalents of colics (restlessness, bouts of unexplained crying, and drawing up of the legs) are in the foreground of clinical presentation combined with other signs of obstructive ileus.

A *history* of former abdominal surgery or temporary bouts of abdominal pain and *localized abdominal pain and tenderness* may point to the cause, site, and type of obstruction, for example, obstructive ileus due to postoperative adhesions or volvulus in anomalies of intestinal rotation #. The volvulus of these causes is often not recognized before surgery.

In chronic or recurrent volvulus due to anomalies of rotation, the less frequently observed melena is mostly caused by congestion of the veins that have an abnormal course. The chronic and recurrent melena of intestinal duplication or Meckel's diverticulum is mostly because of peptic ulceration.

Differential Diagnosis, Work-Ups
It includes disorders of surgical abdomen, obstructive ileus, and acute or recurrent lower gastrointestinal bleeding of any age.

For work-ups, the reader is referred to Sect. 15.1.7.

Treatment, Prognosis
Emergency surgery is indicated in confirmed or suspected intestinal volvulus. Surgery includes, whenever possible, retortion of the volvulus or intestinal resection if the damage is irreversible.

In case of early surgery, the outcome is favorable. If intestinal resection is necessary, small bowel syndrome may occur. Volvulus belongs together with NEC and gastroschisis to the main causes of small bowel syndrome.

23.2.1.2 Volvulus of the Colon

Occurrence, Types, Causes
In contrast to the elderly man, colonic volvulus is a rare disorder in childhood. It is observed at most five times less frequently than small intestine volvulus.

The following types are encountered arranged in order of decreasing frequency: **sigmoid colonic volvulus**, **iliosigmoid knotting** (the distal ileum is twisted firmly around the sigmoid colon and its mesentery), **cecal, and transverse colon volvulus**.

Whereas a narrow attachment of the mesosigmoid is combined with a redundant colon in sigmoid volvulus, abnormal or missing fixation, or common ileocecal fixation is causally related to volvulus in the other types.

Clinical Significance
• Volvulus of the colon is potentially a life-threatening disorder, especially iliosigmoid knotting because it is less well known than appendicitis in the population and not always considered in the differential diagnosis of surgical abdomen.

Clinical Presentation
Volvulus of the sigmoid is observed either as acute or recurrent disorder with spontaneous or nonoperative reduction (≥10 %).

The median age at presentation is 7 years with possible involvement of newborns or adolescent patients, and male predominance. *A history of abdominal colics (possibly in the left lower abdomen), distension, vomiting, and constipation may be recorded lasting since 1–4 days, and the following signs are encountered in order of decreasing frequency: abdominal tenderness, distension, absent stool in the anorectum, guarding, decreased or increased bowel sounds, and bloody mucoid discharge by the anus with location of tenderness and guarding in the left lower abdomen.*

Advanced cases show *symptoms and signs of peritonitis and septic shock because of gangrene or perforation* of the large intestine.

The clinical presentation of the other types of volvulus is similar. In **iliosigmoid knotting**, *signs of low small intestinal obstruction are combined with those of colonic obstruction*, and transverse colon volvulus may be combined with sigmoid volvulus.

The reported high rate of emergency surgery (up to three fourths) and mortality (<10 to ≥ 20 %) are caused by delayed referrals. Because associated congenital megacolon has been reported in >15 %, screening for Hirschsprung's disease is indicated.

Work-Ups, Differential Diagnosis

Work-ups include plain abdominal x-ray in upright position (coffee bean sign or distended colonic loop extending upward from the pelvis), contrast enema (confirmation of volvulus or complete contrast stop), and colonoscopy (used at the same time for reduction with or without placement of a rectal tube).

Because the diagnosis may be missed by radiological imaging, a high degree of clinical attention is necessary to perform colonoscopy or diagnostic laparoscopy or –laparotomy.

The following two disorders are of special interest in the differential diagnosis: **acute manifestation of stool impaction** as a common complication of constipation and **fecal impaction following ingestion of prickly pears (Opuntia ficus India)**: The cactus is cultivated in the Middle East (Mediterranean basin), Middle America, Australia, and South Africa. *1–2 days after ingestion of large amounts of the cactus fruit, the children start with low abdominal pain, acute constipation, difficulties in walking, and possible lower GI hemorrhage. The left lower quadrant is tender with the outline of a tender left colonic loop. Rectal examination is extremely painful and exhibits dense granular masses.* The masses must be evacuated manually and with NaCl enemas in general anesthesia with the possibility of a second procedure afterward.

Treatment, Prognosis

Nonoperative reduction with enema, contrast enema, or colonoscopy is indicated in sigmoid volvulus if neither gangrene nor perforation is present. This approach is problematic in iliosigmoid knotting.

Surgery is absolutely indicated if nonoperative reduction fails and in case of intestinal necrosis, perforation, recurrent sigmoid, or another type of volvulus. It is also recommended as semi-elective procedure after successful nonoperative reduction due to the risk of recurrence and the high morbidity in case of delayed admittance.

Although Ladd's procedure (widening of the mesosigmoid base), sigmoidopexy, and extraperitonealization of the sigmoid have been proposed, only sigmoid resection and colorectal anastomosis eliminate permanently recurrences. At surgery, the sigmoid is twisted in a clockwise or counterclockwise direction and by 360° in two fifths. In cecal or transverse volvulus, nonresectional methods should be applied for fixation.

Intestinal gangrene or perforation needs colonic (and possibly ileal) resection combined with primary anastomosis or temporary enterostomy(ies).

In sigmoid, cecal, or transverse colon volvulus, prognosis depends on the stage of volvulus. In early cases of sigmoid volvulus with prompt reduction and resection (by the time of emergency surgery or after nonoperative reduction as semi-selective intervention), permanent cure is achieved whereas some risk of recurrence exists in nonoperative reduction.

23.2.2 Acute and Chronic Intussusception

Although the characteristic red current jelly stools may be observed occasionally as early sign and more frequently after the classic early signs, the diagnosis of acute intussusception should not exclusively rely on it because melena is not observed in >40 % and is mostly not an early sign. The classic symptomatology consists of a well-nourished infant in his second to fourth trimenon in whom a sudden onset of intermittent abdominal colics, paleness, and vomiting is observed and a mass is palpated in the right

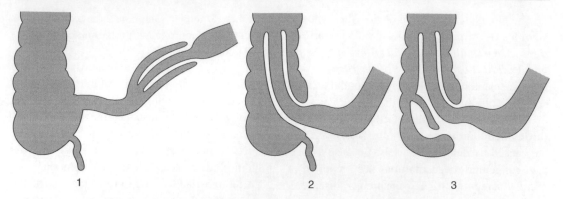

Fig. 23.1 Pathoanatomical forms of intussusception encountered at surgery. (*1*) On the *left side* of the row: Ileoileal intussusception is the initial stage in most of childhood invaginations including the idiopathic. Ileoileal intussusceptions are mainly encountered at surgery in symptomatic, postoperative, and chronic invaginations with the primary cause in symptomatic forms in the small intestine, for example, Meckel's diverticulum as one of the most common causes. (*2*) Ileocolic intussusception is observed most frequently in idiopathic invagination. Appendix and cecum are omitted from the intussusception. (*3*) In the ileocecal intussusception that is also observed in idiopathic intussusception, the appendix and cecum is included in the intussusception

middle or upper belly. In chronic intussusception, melena is more likely a sign of the underlying disorder. The pathoanatomical forms of intussusception seen at surgery are depicted in Fig. 23.1.

23.2.3 Henoch-Schönlein Purpura (Palpable Purpura with Normal Thrombocytes)

Occurrence, Cause
Henoch-Schönlein syndrome occurs at a median age of 5 years. It is caused by allergic vasculitis leading to bleeding and edema.

Clinical Significance
- Henoch-Schönlein purpura is important in pediatric surgery due to the possible acute or recurrent abdominal symptoms and signs, joint swellings, and scrotal involvement with testicular and scrotal swelling and hematoma.

Clinical Presentation
The following signs and symptoms belong to Henoch-Schönlein purpura: *petechial skin bleedings and ecchymoses #, skin edemas, periarticular joint swellings, abdominal colics (in two thirds), lower gastrointestinal bleeding (in one third) #, and in >40 % involvement of the kidneys with microscopic hematuria. The intermittently occurring symptoms and signs last in 25 % of the children more than 8 weeks or recur more than 1 month later.*

Differential Diagnosis, Work-Ups
In case of acute or recurrent abdominal colics without or with loss of blood by the anus, several differential diagnoses of surgical abdomen or melena must be considered, especially acute intussusception. The differential diagnosis is complex because the classic signs of Henoch-Schönlein purpura may commence after the abdominal colics (in about 5 %), may be minimal #, and may lead to intussusception (in about 7 %).

A similar observation is true for the differential diagnosis of scrotal swelling and hematoma with the possibility of testicular torsion #. For exclusion of the quoted differential diagnoses, consultation and follow-up by a pediatric surgeon is necessary. Because abdominal ultrasound is less reliable in ileoileal or jejunoileal **intussusception** that are typical for Henoch-Schönlein purpura, upper GI contrast study, CT with peroral contrast, or diagnostic laparoscopy may be necessary. Plain abdominal x-ray in upright or lateral recumbent position shows signs of obstructive ileus.

Treatment, Prognosis

In case of intussusception, surgical reduction is indicated because hydrostatic reduction may be unsuccessful and dangerous, and segmental resection is often necessary.

Long-term prognosis of Henoch-Schönlein purpura depends on the degree of renal involvement but is otherwise favorable. The prognosis of intussusception is not comparable to idiopathic intussusception due to the possible recurrent bouts of hemorrhage and edema and the relatively frequent necessity of intestinal resection.

23.2.4 Meckel's Diverticulum

Occurrence, Complications

Meckel's diverticulum occurs in about 2 % of the population, and complications develop only in a part of them. Patients with complicated Meckel's diverticulum are mainly infants, toddlers, and schoolchildren up to the age of 10 years. The children with complications and those in whom Meckel's diverticulum is detected by chance at abdominal surgery correspond approximately to half of all children with a Meckel's diverticulum.

The three main **complications** of Meckel's diverticulum are as follows:

- Peptic ulcer with lower gastrointestinal hemorrhage or perforation
- Obstructive ileus
- Meckel's diverticulitis

They occur with the same frequency but to some degree age dependent. Before 5 years, peptic ulcer and obstructive ileus are the most frequent complication and afterward, diverticulitis. Ectopic gastric mucosa as a cause of adjacent peptic ulcer is encountered in one fourth of Meckel's diverticulum with histological examination. It leads more often to bleeding ulcer # than to its perforation.

Clinical Significance

- Meckel's diverticulum becomes clinically only manifest by its complications or is recognized by chance at abdominal surgery or by work-up examinations performed for other reasons, for instance, by a GI contrast study.
- In addition to the quoted main complications, many more specific complications are reported in the literature.
- Clinical presentation depends on the specific type of complications. Therefore, the symptoms and signs are many and diverse, and the preoperative diagnosis is often missed.
- Meckel's diverticulum that is recognized by chance should be resected because of its possibly large morbidity.

Clinical Presentation (Related to Peptic Ulcer)

Without any preceding symptomatology, profuse loss of blood by the anus is observed either as pitch stools followed by masses of clots and fresh blood or from the beginning as fresh blood. Hemoglobin is often unexpectedly low. A history of repeated melena may be ascertained if specifically asked for. The patient is pale and has usually no obvious signs of hemorrhagic shock except for tachycardia; its belly is supple with increased bowel activity on auscultation. Rectal examination yields either traces of denatured or fresh blood on the finger tip.

In case of ulcer perforation #, symptoms and signs of localized or generalized peritonitis are present. Again, the history may discover former episodes of melena.

Differential Diagnosis, Work-Ups

It includes other causes of considerable loss of blood by the anus or of localized or generalized peritonitis (ulcer perforation), for instance, intestinal duplication with peptic ulceration, coagulopathies, Henoch-Schönlein purpura, and other pediatric disorders.

In obstructive ileus or Meckel's diverticulitis, other causes of surgical abdomen with peritonitis or intestinal obstruction must be considered.

A history of gross lower gastrointestinal bleeding combined with low hemoglobin in an otherwise inconspicuous child of preschool age is highly suspicious of a bleeding Meckel's diverticulum. 99 m Technetium scan is a diagnostic with accumulation of the tracer in the stomach, upper and lower urinary tract, and in the gastric mucosa of a Meckel's diverticulum (with <2 % false-negative and <1 % false-positive results in diverticula with gastric mucosa).

Treatment, Prognosis

After confirmation of the diagnosis, elective resection of the Meckel's diverticulum is indicated after a blood transfusion. Resection includes usually a rim of the adjacent, antimesenteric ileum that must be closed with one or two layers of interrupted sutures. The same applies to resection in perforation and other complications that are performed usually as emergency intervention.

In the latter cases, the possibility of perioperative morbidity and obstructive ileus due to adhesions is greater than after a bleeding ulcer. Otherwise, permanent healing is the rule.

23.2.5 Intestinal Duplication

Intestinal duplication may be combined with peptic ulceration similar to Meckel's diverticulum. The reader is referred to Sect. 15.1.6.

23.2.6 Necrotizing Enterocolitis (NEC)

Occurrence, Causes, Pathoanatomy

NEC is a disorder of the premature infant (<34 weeks gestation). It is observed increasingly and mainly in premature infants with a very low birth weight (<1,500 g).

NEC affects 1–5 % of all admissions to a neonatal intensive care unit (NICU) and at least 5–10 % of all premature infants with a very low birth weight. Comparing figures which relate to live births may be misleading because the percentage of premature infants and of their early survival may differ considerably.

NEC is observed in term neonates and small for gestational age newborns in ≥10 %. NEC of the term neonate occurs in <1 % of newborns at term, and most of them enter the NICU for other reason (e.g., congenital heart disease, bacterial septicemia) or have a congenital intestinal malformation such as Hirschsprung's disease or IND #.

An inappropriate inflammatory response of the immature gut to different insults of which some are known (e.g., nosocomial colonization) leads to NEC.

The disease distribution is segmental (focal) in 50 %, multisegmental (multifocal), or panintestinal in one fifth of surgical patients and concerns ileum, colon, or both. In panintestinal disease (NEC totalis), at least 75 % of the intestine is necrotic. At surgery, the bowel is distended with areas of thinning, the serosal surface is red or gray, covered by fibrinous exudate, and subserous gas collections may be present. A black serosal surface and bloody peritoneal fluid correspond to gangrene and a brown and cloudy to perforation.

Clinical Significance

• NEC leads to a surgical abdomen and septicemia, and its clinical course is lethal in at least 15–25 %.
• Nonoperative and surgical treatment may be associated with major morbidity and late intestinal and general sequels.

Clinical Presentation

The lower the birth weight, the higher the risk of NEC. Therefore, the possibility of development of NEC must be considered in the clinical course of every premature infants especially with very or extremely low birth weight. The same attention applies to term infants with NICU admittance.

The tenth day after birth is the preferential time of beginning of NEC although earlier or later onset may be observed (even several weeks or months after birth). The start may be insidious. Vague and unspecific signs such as lethargy, instability of temperature, increasing episodes of apnea, bradycardia, oxygen desaturations, and hypoglycemia may precede more specific signs and symptoms.

These are in descending order of frequency: *distended and tender abdomen with visible intestinal loops, increasing gastric aspirate or vomitus, visible or occult rectal bleeding that is black or purple and of minor degree, and diarrhea.*

The clinical presentation that is of diagnostic relevance is less frequently observed than the symptomatology quoted above. It includes *edema and redness of the abdominal wall and/or a fixed or mobile abdominal mass.*

Although the clinical course takes mostly several days for the development of the overt signs, occasionally a rapidly progressive course may be observed with possibly lethal outcome within 24 h.

The classification of **Bell et al.** is used for staging of the severity of NEC. It uses factors leading to perinatal stress, gastrointestinal and systemic signs, and radiological findings, and stage I corresponds to suspected, stage II to confirmed, and III to advanced NEC:

Stage I: Factors leading to perinatal stress present (as well as in stage II and III)

Poor feeding, increased gastric residue, emesis

Minimal abdominal distension, occult blood in stool

Instability of temperature, bradycardia, apnea, lethargy

Abdominal distension and suggestion of air-fluid levels

Stage II: Marked abdominal distension, persistent occult or visible melena

Significant abdominal distension, air-fluid levels

Specific radiological findings as marked below with an asterisk

Stage III: In addition, deterioration of vital signs, signs of septic shock, lower gastrointestinal hemorrhage

Pneumoperitoneum

Work-Ups, Differential Diagnosis

They include determination of the inflammatory blood signs including serological markers of NEC, serum chemistry, microbiology, specific test of NEC, and radiological imaging.

Neutrocytopenia and thrombocytopenia, and metabolic acidosis are the most common findings. In contrast to the platelet-activating factor and intestinal fatty acid-binding protein, C-reactive protein is not specific as a possible serological marker of NEC. Microbiological examination of blood, peritoneal fluid, and stool may be difficult to interpret, and the role of Clostridium species is unclear. The breath hydrogen test permits exclusion of NEC.

Plain anteroposterior and cross-table lateral abdominal x-ray are in the foreground of diagnostic tools. They have the drawback of radiation exposure in as much as they must be repeated several times. Any, some, or all of the following findings may be encountered in the individual case of NEC and its clinical course:

• Intestinal pneumatosis*

It is *diagnostic of NEC* if the clinical presentation corresponds to NEC because it may also be observed in other disorders, for example, Hirschsprung's disease with enterocolitis. It is a fleeting sign, has a cystic and/or linear pattern depending on the site of gas in the intestinal wall, and its extension does not correlate with the severity of NEC.

• Pneumoperitoneum

It is best depicted in cross-table lateral view or may be recognized in supine view as football or double wall sign (demonstration of the falciform ligament or of the entire wall of an intestinal loop).

Although it is a *sign of intestinal perforation,* free air may be present in one third without pneumoperitoneum. On the other hand, pneumoperitoneum may be caused by alveolar rupture in mechanically ventilated patients. Pneumoperitoneum cannot predict the extent of NEC.

• Persistent dilated loop sign*

It means that the position and shape of a single or several loop(s) remain(s) unchanged for 1–2 days. *It may be a sign of intestinal perforation.*

• Portal vein gas*

It appears as linear lucencies in the area of the liver and is mostly a *sign of poor prognosis,* for example, panintestinal NEC and/or high mortality.

• Bowel distension*

Multiple dilated intestinal loops filled with air and possibly combined with air-fluid levels are an *unspecific* finding but belongs to the *earliest and most frequent findings* in NEC.

• Intraperitoneal fluid

It is recognized by separation of the intestinal loops*, centralization of air-filled loops surrounded by opacity*, and distended gasless abdomen. It may be a *sign of intestinal perforation.*

Although ultrasound may be used for earlier diagnosis of gangrene by recognition of thinning of the bowel wall and lack of perfusion and for delineation of most of the characteristic findings on plain abdominal x-ray (intramural, portal venous, and gas in the peritoneal cavity), its overall use is not yet established because of the considerable expertise needed. Indications of ultrasound are recognition and location of ascites before paracentesis and NEC patient with equivocal clinical findings and normal or unspecific findings on plain abdominal x-ray.

In case of characteristic and/or multiple suspicious clinical and radiological signs, another disorder must not be taken into account. Other disorders must be considered in the prodromal stage of NEC, in term newborns with NEC, or if single clinical and/or radiological signs are present, especially spontaneous gastrointestinal perforation, secondary or primary peritonitis, or omphalitis and cellulitis of the abdominal wall.

Treatment, Prognosis

The nonoperative treatment includes nasogastric tube, parenteral nutrition, systemic antibiotics, probiotic supplements, and if necessary shock therapy and ventilation.

Close surveillance of the clinical course is mandatory. Children in whom medical treatment is successful differ from those who require surgery concerning morbidity and mortality.

Indications for surgery are the following:
- Intestinal perforation (pneumoperitoneum)
- Segmental full-thickness gangrene with imminent perforation
- Risk of or development of panintestinal NEC
- Persistent and progressive septicemia

Clinical, radiological, and laboratory findings are used for the indication and whenever possible in combination. Pneumoperitoneum, portal vein gas, or positive results of paracentesis, and dilated loop sign, erythema, or palpable abdominal mass are very good and good indicators of the quoted indications for surgery. In case of continuous clinical deterioration despite appropriate medical treatment or of less reliable indicators, additional tools should be applied

such as paracentesis (brown and cloudy fluid and positive Gram stain), ultrasound, or laparoscopy with some restrictions.

Preoperative resuscitation is mandatory and must be followed by precautious measures in the operating room appropriate for very sick premature infants.

Surgery: After a transverse incision in the lower abdomen to avoid spontaneous liver hemorrhage, peritoneal fluid is taken for microbiology, the intestine inspected for perforation or full-thickness gangrene, and the length of probably viable intestine measured. The vitality of the involved segments is difficult to evaluate and prognosticate in spite of the impressive findings. Full-thickness necrosis is recognizable by localized dilatation of the intestine that is only covered by serosa or appear as greenish, black, and flabby segments. Resections should be performed only for undoubtedly necrotic segments, should avoid short bowel syndrome, and preserve the ileocecal valve.

Segmental resection and double enterostomy are performed away from or through the original incision if a **single segment** is involved. If involvement of the intestine is exclusively confined to one segment and the child is in a good condition, primary anastomosis may be considered.

In **multisegmental NEC**, multiple resections and enterostomies are performed, a proximal jejunostomy is followed by multiple resections and adaption of the segments together, or after resection of the necrotic segments, the cut ends are closed with staples and after re-laparotomy 2–3 days later, the segments are anastomosed.

In **panintestinal NEC**, intervention is restricted to a proximal enterostomy. Simple peritoneal drainage should be used only as temporary measure in unstable patients with extremely low birth weight and gestation.

After surgery, the same measures are taken as in nonoperative treatment including gastrointestinal rest and antibiotics for two weeks.

Complications include recurrent NEC, development of stricture(s), short bowel syndrome, and sequels of TPN (cholestatic liver disease).

Recurrent NEC is observed in about 5 %, occurs after nonoperative and operative treatment, and at a median time of 6 weeks. Medical treatment is possible in >70 %.

Stricture formation occurs in <10 % up to one third of the patients within weeks to months after medical or operative treatment. 70 % of the strictures concern the colon, 15 % the terminal ileum, and multiple strictures occur much more frequently in surgical NEC.

Stricture formation may lead to *failure to thrive, lower gastrointestinal hemorrhage, obstructive ileus, or no obvious clinical signs are developing*. Resection and primary anastomosis is indicated if clinical (symptomatic strictures) and radiological signs (anterograde contrast study with fluoroscopy) of pathoanatomical and functional obstruction persist. Surgery should be coordinated with enterostomy closure.

The **time of enterostomy closure** depends on complete healing of the acute pathoanatomical findings, exclusion of intestinal stricture(s), excellent general and nutritional condition, and possibly severe long-term side effects of the enterostomy(ies). Therefore, gastrointestinal contrast study is necessary in addition to close clinical observation.

Short bowel syndrome may be observed in >20 % of operated NEC patients. The short small intestine may be combined with hypersecretion of gastric acid, bacterial overgrowth, hypermotility or slow transit time, and B12 and bile salt deficiency.

Prognosis depends on the degree of prematurity, severity of septicemia, and extension of intestinal involvement. Length of intestinal resection and site of anastomosis(es) are more important for the functional prognosis of intestine than the visible pathoanatomical findings in the acute stage of NEC.

If panintestinal NEC is excluded, mortality amounts to <10 %. Panintestinal NEC has a high mortality with 95 % especially in patients with extremely low birth weight.

Intraventricular hemorrhage is unlikely to account mainly for the poor neurodevelopmental outcome.

In the therapeutic category with successful medical treatment, the recovery is usually uneventful and the long-term outcome similar to unaffected infants of matched gestational age. In the therapeutic category that needs surgery, a global mortality of 50 % (in developing) and 30–40 % (in developed countries) is observed early (<30), late (>30 days after surgery), and long term.

23.2.7 Polyps of the Gastrointestinal Tract

Occurrence, Types

Polyps of the gastrointestinal tract occur frequently. Most polyps in children are benign hamartomas and are observed as single or multiple lesions, and much less frequently as different types of polyposis. Polyps with the histological features of adenoma are encountered less frequently #, increase in the second decade, and occur partly in some of the polyposes.

Hereditary colorectal cancers account for 5–10 % of all colorectal cancers and include the following polyposis syndromes as precursors of colorectal cancer that are important in the context of this chapter:

- Familial adenomatous polyposis coli, Gardner and Turcot syndrome, attenuated adenomatous polyposis coli, and flat adenoma syndrome
- Hereditary nonpolyposis colorectal cancer (Lynch syndrome)
- Hamartomatous polyposis syndromes (Peutz-Jeghers syndrome, juvenile polyposis syndrome, and Cowden syndrome)

If a colorectal cancer has been diagnosed in an adult and familiality has been evaluated and molecular genetic testing performed, all potentially affected members are screened depending on the results, and an enhanced surveillance of the patients at risk is recommended that may also include children and measures such as routine colonoscopy and clearing of all polyps. Inherited gastric cancers, for example, the hereditary diffuse gastric cancer may even lead to prophylactic gastrectomy because radiological imaging or endoscopy with biopsy is unreliable.

Clinical Significance

- After exclusion of children with anal fissure or chronic inflammatory diseases of the intestine, ≥25 % of the children with lower gastrointestinal hemorrhage have polyps.
- Multiple polyps may point to one of the polyposis types and forms #.
- In adenomatous polyps and in some of the polyposes quoted above, the possibility of later malignant degeneration must be considered (colorectal cancer), molecular genetic testing be performed, and adequate surveillance carried out.

23.2.7.1 Juvenile Polyp

Clinical Presentation

The juvenile (hamartomatous) polyp occurs in > 70 % in the rectum or sigmoid colon, is in a similar percentage single, and concerns mostly toddlers and preschool children. The less frequently (<30–50 %) multiple polyps are also located proximally to the colon.

The leading sign is passage of mucus intermingled with blood without or with stool.

Less frequently, a mass is visible in the anus (prolapsing polyp #), and recurrent abdominal colic, signs of intussusception (lead point: polyp of colon or small intestine), and anemia are observed.

Differential Diagnosis, Work-Ups

It includes mainly disorders with lower gastrointestinal bleeding, especially idiopathic intussusception or anal fissure. Because childhood polyp is often not considered in the differential diagnosis of small children, its diagnosis may be delayed for months or years.

After exclusion of anal fissure and perineal injury by correct and careful inspection and palpation of perineum, anus, and anorectum, colonoscopy is performed for recognition of possible polyps and endoscopic polypectomy of all polyps (clearing colonoscopy). The pediatric surgeon should be available for resection of anorectal and very large polyps #, respectively; surgery for symptomatic intussusception; and assessment or treatment of complications of polypectomy such as posthemorrhage or perforation (≤0.5 %).

Treatment, Prognosis

After endoscopic or surgical excision, histological examination is indicated in every case. Permanent cure can be expected if the polyp is a hamartoma, less than three polyps are present, and no familiality exists (exclusion of all polyposis syndromes). Posthemorrhage may originate from the site of polypectomy, from another not recognized polyp, or from another site.

23.2.7.2 Familial Polyposis

Depending on the number of encountered polyps (endoscopic and/or radiological findings) and their location and histology, a possible familiality, and additional intestinal and extraintestinal clinical and work-up findings, familial polyposis must be considered and genetic and molecular biological examinations performed.

Clinical Presentation, Follow-Ups, Treatment Strategies

Peutz-Jeghers Syndrome. Two of the three characteristic signs are necessary for the diagnosis: familiality, mucocutaneous hyperpigmentations (they occur before polyposis or may be absent), and hamartomatous polyps (they occur in the whole gastrointestinal tract but preferably in the small intestine).

Recurrent abdominal colics, microhemorrhages, and chronic anemia are in the foreground of clinical presentation, and persistent small intestine intussusceptions and recognizable lower gastrointestinal bleedings are less frequently.

Esophagogastroduodenoscopy, contrast studie of small intestine, and colonoscopy is diagnostic and therapeutic with removal and histological work-up of all encountered polyps. Regular follow-ups are necessary because of possible development of new polyps, malignant colorectal degeneration, and occurrence of extraintestinal polyps and malignancies.

Adenomatous Colon Polyposis. The mainly colorectally localized adenomatous polyposis (>50 polyps) and the multiple adenomatous polyposis with familiality or with characteristic extraintestinal findings (congenital hypertrophy of the retinal pigment epithelium, skin and bone tumors, etc.) are forms of this type of polyposis.

Depending on the location of the responsible gene, *an earlier or later onset (10–14 years of age) of the clinical presentation is observed with diarrhea, abdominal colics, and lower gastrointestinal hemorrhage.*

Familial adenomatous polyposis coli is an autosomal dominant disease in which >100 colorectal adenomas have already developed in 50 % of the patients by 15 years of age. Colorectal cancer develops not later than 40 years of age. Because of the regular malignant degeneration of the "classic" form of adenomatous colon polyposis (early onset, corresponding number of polyps, and specific genetic analysis), proctocolectomy with ileoanal anastomosis and formation of a reservoir (pouch) should be performed in adolescence at latest.

Lynch syndrome is also an autosomal dominant disorder with a penetrance of the mismatched-repaired genes of 70–85 % for colorectal cancer and 50–60 % for endometrial cancer. Colorectal cancer occurs on average no later than 44 years of age. The less numerous polyps and the colorectal carcinoma occur particularly in the proximal colon. The patients need annual clearing colonoscopy and histological work-up that starts before adulthood.

Afterward, in the remainder forms of adenomatous colon polyposis, and in the genetically positive forms, regular follow-ups are mandatory including control of the extracolic and extraintestinal sites of possible manifestation.

Other forms of familial adenomatous polyposis are very rare in contrast to the already quoted. In every suspected case, genetic and molecular biological work-up and follow-ups are necessary.

23.2.8 Incarcerated and Strangulated Inguinal Hernia

In strangulated inguinal, femoral, and umbilical hernia, lower gastrointestinal hemorrhage is not in the foreground of clinical presentation. A painful and hard swelling of the groin and developing signs of obstructive ileus are the characteristic clinical signs #.

Occasionally, *loss of some fresh or denatured blood without or with mucus may be observed in the clinical course of hernia strangulation or after the emergency surgery.*

23.2.9 Hemorrhoids

Occurrence, Pathoanatomy
In contrast to the adults in whom hemorrhoids are a frequent disease, hemorrhoids are infrequent in children.

The inner hemorrhoidal cushion is a part of the continence organ and leads to overt hemorrhoids if the venous vessels extend in the anal channel and are pushed to the outside (stage 1–3).

Clinical Significance
- Hemorrhoids of childhood lead to minor complaints of the anal region and rarely to bleeding or acute thrombosis.
- Hemorrhoids may be sign of portal hypertension. In this case, severe hemorrhage is observed occasionally.

Clinical Presentation
Hemorrhoids are recognize if *the hemorrhoids lead to hemorrhage with blood on the surface of the stool, toilet tissue, or underwear or become visible due to increasing size.* Complaints are *scratching due to itch or stool stains on the underwear.*

Anal inspection performed because of the complaints or a history of lower gastrointestinal hemorrhage demonstrates the hemorrhoids. Phlebectasia concern either the external veins with outflow to the inferior vena cava or the internal veins with outflow to the portal vein. *The internal hemorrhoids prolapse on straining only in grade 1 and spontaneously in grades 2 and 3 #.*

Thrombosis of a variceal node outside of the dentate line is *very painful and manifests as prominent, dark blue, and hard node #.*

Work-Ups, Differential Diagnosis

Work-ups concern additional examinations of a possible cause such as constipation, hard stools, difficult stool evacuation with extensive straining, or portal hypertension. Proctoscopy and colonoscopy may be indicated for differential diagnosis of lower gastrointestinal hemorrhage. It must also consider the possibility of symptomatic hemorrhoids. **Oxyuris vermicularis** is a more frequent cause of anal pruritus in children than hemorrhoids.

Treatment, Prognosis

Surgery is restricted to incision of a painful thrombotic variceal node and blood stanching in case of profuse hemorrhage. Nonoperative treatment includes stool softeners, sitz baths, and anesthetic ointments and concerns the local complaints.

Prognosis depends on the cause of hemorrhoids and on the adherence of parents and child to the local treatment.

23.2.10 Anal Fissure

Occurrence, Causes, Types

A tear of the anal skin in the posterior or anterior midline (=anal fissure) is the most frequent cause of blood on the surface of the stool. It is mostly observed in infants of which up to 80 % will have had an anal fissure by the end of the first year. Older children get less frequently involved.

Possible causes are long-standing diarrhea, hard stools, and constipation. Anal fissure is often combined with a spasm of the internal sphincter muscle and myogenic anal sphincter achalasia.

In contrast to the already quoted primary type, secondary types of anal fissure differ in their specific cause, site, number, shape, and age distribution. Possible causes are Crohn's disease, rigorous transanal interventions, and sexual abuse. Anal fissures of Crohn's disease affect schoolchildren # and have an atypical location, may be multiple, and show signs of chronification.

Clinical Significance

- Anal fissure is a frequent disorder in infancy.
- It may frighten the parents because of fresh blood on the stool.

- Beyond infancy, anal fissure may be a sign of a chronic disorder (secondary anal fissure) including sexual abuse.

Clinical Presentation

Threadlike traces of fresh, clear red blood on the surface of stool or toilet tissue and severe pain at and after defecation are the main symptomatology. The last-mentioned symptom leads to constipation or aggravates it by a spasm of the internal sphincter.

Clinical Skills

Anal inspection should be performed with optimal lighting and by stepwise unfolding of the anal rugae with the fingers of both hands. It shows *a midline tear of the anal channel and in case of chronic fissure, an ulcer in the same extension with raised borders and a cutaneous tag at its distal end.*

Differential Diagnosis, Work-Ups

History and clinical examination confirm the diagnosis and differentiate between **primary and secondary types**. An important differential diagnosis concerns **fistula-in-ano**: It presents with recurrent mucous or purulent discharge from the anus or perianal region, moistening of the anus, lateral perianal abscess, or rarely blood staining on the nappies. Before clinical examination with inspection of the perianal region and anal channel and probing of the sinus tract, the different types of fistulas-in-ano must be considered (Fig. 23.2): Anal fistulas are either congenital or acquired after infection of perianal skin rashes or crypt abscess. They occur mostly subcutaneously in children and present as complete or incomplete form with an opening in the lateral perianal and/ or an opening in the crypt region, a blind end, and radiate course. Transsphincteric fistulas concern either the superficial external sphincter or the deep external sphincter and the internal sphincter muscle. Rectoanal (ischiorectal) fistulas are only observed in Crohn's disease. Subcutaneous types of fistula-in-ano are best treated by incision of the soft tissues over the whole fistula marked with a probe and curettage of the sinus tract, whereas transsphincteric fistulas need a set of setons that

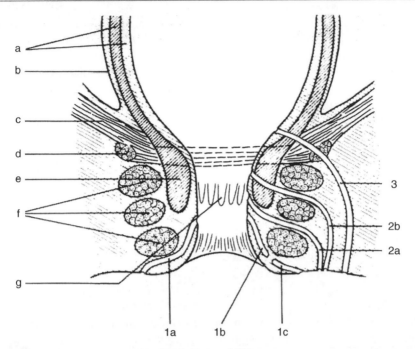

Fig. 23.2 The drawing of M. Bettex illustrates different types of fistulas-in-ano. Except for cases with Crohn's disease (*3*=ischiorectal variant of anorectal fistula), mainly complete and incomplete subcutaneous anal fistulas are observed in children (=*1a–c*) as well as transsphincteric forms (*2a*/*b* which involve only the external sphincter or the external and internal sphincter). Blood on stool may be a leading signs, but a moistening anus and inflammatory perianal and anal findings are usually in the forefront of clinical presentation. *a* and *b* mean parts of the rectal wall; *c* the levator muscle; *d* the puborectalis muscle; *e* the internal sphincter; *f* the deep, superficial, and subcutaneous external sphincter; and *g* the anal crypts

are introduced with a probe in the fistula and tightened stepwise until the soft tissue over the fistula has been slowly divided. Wound care, sitz bath, stool softeners, and possibly antibiotics are important adjuncts.

Work-ups are only needed in case of suspected constipation and for differentiation of suspected secondary types of anal fissure. Constipation and its severity are ascertained by abdominal and gentle rectal examination, and plain abdominal x-ray.

Treatment, Prognosis

In primary anal fissures, cure is possible by non-operative measures such as stool softeners or addition of bulk substances, gently cleansing, sitz baths, anesthetic ointment, etc. In chronic anal fissures, repeated anal dilatation, injection of botulinum toxin into the internal anal sphincter, and lateral internal sphincterotomy combined with excision of the ulcer must be discussed. Secondary types will heal with nonoperative measure if the underlying disorder is treated or interrupted, but secondary scarred **anal stenosis** must be considered on follow-up.

Although 90 % of primary anal fissures disappear with nonoperative measures, recurrences are possible. In Crohn's disease, cure depends on the clinical course of the chronic recurrent intestinal inflammation.

23.2.11 Perineal (Perianal) Injury

Occurrence, Causes

Perineal injury is observed in <10 % of all traumas of the girl between the ages 0–16 years, and boys are involved as well although less attention has been payed to them.

Causes are motor vehicle crashes, falls astride (due to outdoor, playground, and activities related to bicycle or for other reasons), and sometimes rollover accidents (low-velocity motor vehicle).

True impalement injuries with local tissue destruction occur less often (<10 %) than straddle injuries which correspond to a blow to the perineum as result of falling or striking a surface or an object with the force of one's own body weight. They lead mostly to minor abrasion or laceration. Falls astride are more prevalent in the first decade of life, whereas the most frequent motor vehicle accidents occur at any age except for neonates and infants.

Clinical Significance

- Perineal injury may be overlooked, for example, in multisystem organ or rollover injury and underestimated at the first sight in its severity in straddle injury.
- Perineal injury may lead to tears of the female external genitals (<5 %) that are indistinguishable initially and on follow-up from those of sexual assault.
- Perineal injuries need mostly evaluation under general anesthesia because the degree of injuries is underestimated in three fourths in comparison with the preoperative assessment.

Clinical Presentation

Blunt perineal injury leads in 80–90 % to *minor abrasions, grade one lacerations, and contusions* if it is not combined with penetrating mechanism. *Nevertheless, grade 2 lacerations that need sutures and grade 3 with deep tears and possible partial or complete sphincter disruption occur each in about 5 %.*

Even the common perineal injuries are mostly combined with some *anal or genital bleeding. Abrasions and lacerations concern the perineum, anus, and vulva or scrotum and penis.* Those of the female genitals concern mostly the *vulva lateral and anterior to the clitoris with the labia minora as the most frequently involved part and may be followed by grotesque swelling.*

Impalement injuries are anal, perianal, or vaginal located (site of penetration); *extra- or intraperitoneal* (depth of penetration); *combined or not combined with partial or complete destruction of the sphincters; possible injury to the urethra or vagina; and may lead to hypovolemic shock or peritonitis.*

Knowledge of the configuration of the offending object and mechanism of impalement are important for the evaluation of local findings.

Differential Diagnosis, Work-Ups

It encompasses mainly sexual assault or rape. It must be considered if the child is too young for accidental perineal injury and if the quoted history is not convincing.

In addition to cystourethroscopy, colposcopy, anorectoscopy, ultrasound and CT/MRI may be necessary in severe cases of blunt and in true impalement injury.

Treatment, Prognosis

After work-up that includes evaluation in general anesthesia, the therapeutic measures depend on type and severity of the perineal injury. The common lesions need debridement, possibly sutures, and short-term urinary diversion of the bladder by a catheter.

Revision, reconstruction of the destroyed structures, drainage, and protection by a defunctioning colostomy and systemic antibiotic including tetanus prophylaxis are necessary in more severe injuries.

Secondary work-ups are necessary if primary reconstruction has not been possible and include clinical assessment of the degree of possible incontinence (e.g., grading according to the Miller score which considers stool consistency (gas, fluid, and solid stools), the frequency of episodic incontinence, and displays maximum 18 points), dynamic video-contrast enema, and anorectal manometry (low anorectal pressures) and endosonography (lesion of the sphincters and their degree). Reconstructive surgery includes overlapping sphincteroplasty or transposition of the gracilis muscle (Pickrell's gracilis muscle transplantation).

Prognosis depends on the type and degree of injury with possible stool incontinence in impalement injury and fatal outcome if peritonitis or hypovolemic shock is not avoided or treated in time. Prognosis of the common straddle injuries is usually favorable except for not treated injuries of the external genitals with secondary hymenal closure.

23.3 Inflammatory Bowel Diseases (IBD)

Inflammatory bowel diseases are quoted in the chapter "lower intestinal hemorrhage" because chronic diarrhea with or without blood in and on the stool is a characteristic leading sign.

23.3.1 Crohn's Disease

Occurrence, Causes, Pathoanatomy
It is observed in 1:10,000 children and in a cohort of juvenile-onset Crohn's disease, 50 % children <10 years of age may be observed, and one fourth has a history of familial IBD. It is caused by genetic disposition and environmental factors and more frequent in developed countries especially in the northern part of Europe.

Crohn's disease may involve the whole gastrointestinal tract although the distal small intestine and the colon are the preferred sites. It is a transmural inflammation that is partially granulomatous and may involve the regional lymph nodes. The mucous membrane has a cobblestone appearance due to island of normal tissue between the ulcers. The intestinal wall is thickened and may develop segmental strictures or fistulas to other parts of the intestine, bladder, vagina, or skin. Characteristic is the simultaneous involvement of distant segments (skip lesions) and fat encroachment at the mesenteric site of the intestine #. In a cohort of juvenile-onset Crohn's disease, the small and large intestines were involved in 50 %, 10 % had Crohn's colitis, 20 % diffuse involvement of the small intestine, and only 10 % the classic ileocecal form.

Clinical Significance
- The clinical diagnosis is often delayed by several years because Crohn's disease is not considered in childhood and/or the initial presentation as extraintestinal disorder with orthopedic or rheumatic (joint swelling, arthralgia), dermatological or orodental (skin rashes, erythema nodosum, aphthous ulcers, lip and buccal swelling), and ophthalmological findings (conjunctivitis, uveitis) and failure to thrive is treated by different specialists.
- Crohn's disease continues after childhood; treatment during childhood should guarantee physical and sexual development and avoid whenever possible extensive small bowel resection.
- Colorectal Crohn's disease is a risk of carcinoma development.

Clinical Presentation
Vague abdominal pain, diarrhea with/without melena (or constipation), anorexia, loss of weight, and anemia belong to the symptomatology, and unspecific symptoms such as *fatigue, nausea, and subfebrile temperature,* the quoted *extraintestinal signs,* and/or *anorectal disease* (e.g., chronic anal fissure #) may precede the intestinal signs by years. In addition, a *palpable inflammatory mass in the right iliac fossa, delay of physical development* (body weight and length) and *secondary sexual characteristics, gallstones and nephrolithiasis,* and latent pulmonic involvement are observed.

The clinical examination must specifically consider the site of extraintestinal manifestations, mouth and anorectum, and the abdomen. Body weight and length and sexual development should be recorded.

The **complications** "obstructive disease, intestinal perforation, and massive intestinal hemorrhage" are rare, whereas formation of abscesses and fistulas are observed more frequently.

Differential Diagnosis, Work-Ups
It includes mainly ulcerative colitis (IBD that cannot be attributed to either of the two main forms is called IBD type unclassified) or specific infectious enterocolitis, intestinal Bilharziasis, and all disorders dependent on the single signs (e.g., in palpable inflammatory mass in the right iliac fossa, perityphlitic abscess, or torsion of an ovarian cyst or tumor).

The work-ups include colorectoscopy and gastroduodenoscopy (cobblestone appearance, strictures) and biopsy (for histology and bacteriological cultures), gastrointestinal contrast study and contrast enema (abnormal mucosal relief, string sign = intestinal stricture), and laboratory tests (Hb, ESR, C-reactive protein, albumin, and exclusion of Campylobacter jejuni, Yersinia, Entamoeba histolytica, and Salmonella [appropriate tests and cultures of intestinal content and biopsy]). Determination of Hb, thrombocytes, and fecal calprotectin (anemia, thrombocytosis, and increased levels of calprotectin are not disease specific but are signs that evaluation of possible chronic inflammatory bowel is indicated).

The diagnosis of Crohn's disease is composed of clinical, endoscopic, and radiological findings and of the results of histology and laboratory tests.

Endoscopy is useful for follow-up (equivocal clinical course; assessment of complication, e.g., strictures; before treatment with immunosuppressives [exclusion of cytomegalovirus]; carcinoma prophylaxis). On the other hand, abdominal ultrasound that displays exact imaging and measurement of the involved intestinal wall and determination of fecal calprotectin as measure of the degree of intestinal inflammation can also be used as objective measures of the clinical course.

Treatment, Prognosis

Treatment is medical and includes steroids, immunosuppressives, cytostatics, and possibly anti-TNF-antibodies, enteral nutrition (semielemental or elemental diets), and total parenteral nutrition. They are applied according to guidelines of international societies, depending on the stage and complications of the disease, and for treatment, remission, recurrence prophylaxis, and short-term "rescue" management with new drugs.

The **indication of surgery** should neither be too early nor too late except for emergency situations such as massive intestinal hemorrhage, perforation, or obstruction. In juvenile-onset Crohn's disease, surgery is usually needed 3 years after diagnosis and concerns elective intervention in intractable disease especially in early teenage and surgery for persistent complications.

At **surgery**, the child should have optimum conditions (amelioration of general condition, cleaning of intestinal tract, medical and psychological advice of child and parents), excision should include only the most affected part, and guarantee maximum small intestine conservation. Surgery includes the following therapeutic options that depend on the individual patient:

- Excision of the most severely affected area with primary anastomosis is applied mostly in small intestine involvement (ileocecal resection, 70 % of interventions in children) ##.
- Permanent ileostomy in severe colonic disease (only rarely subtotal colectomy and ileorectostomy or proctocolectomy is indicated) and temporary enterostomy in surgery for intestinal perforation or abscess, and as additional measure for anorectal disease.
- Stricturoplasty (longitudinal incision and transverse closure) or segmental resection in strictures (the site of strictures is evaluated by insufflation of the suspected segment).
- Resection of fistulas that persist beyond 3 months and are symptomatic, for example, enterovesical or enterocutaneous forms. It is important that a distal intestinal obstruction is treated as well.

Recurrences occur without surgery and after surgery, but further surgery is not inevitably necessary thereafter. Children with juvenile-onset Crohn's disease require surgery during childhood in 25 to ≥50 % and >80 % within 15 years after beginning of the disease. Mortality is low and normal life can be expected, but lifelong follow-ups are needed, and repeated interruptions of schooling and work must be expected because of relapse, complications of the disease, or treatment.

23.3.2 Ulcerative Colitis

Occurrence, Pathoanatomy

Juvenile-onset ulcerative colitis occurs somewhat less frequently than Crohn's disease, and only <5 % are younger than 10 years of age and <20 % become ill in the second decade. It is probably an autoimmune disease.

The rectum with extension to the colon for a variable distance is involved in >95 %. Pancolitis concerns more patients with juvenile-onset ulcerative colitis than olders.

Crypt abscesses lead to ulceration and undermining of the mucous membrane, whereas the other parts of the wall are secondarily involved. The most severe pathoanatomical changes concern the rectum in its whole circumference.

Clinical Significance

- Ulcerative colitis is a severe chronic disease with diverse possible extracolonic manifestations, livelong relapses of the ulcerative colitis, and possibly life-threatening complications.
- Ulcerative colitis can be cured permanently by proctocolectomy.
- Development of colorectal carcinoma is possible with increasing frequency depending on the length of the diseases (<5 % in the first 10 years).

Clinical Presentation

Less than 20 % of the patients become symptomatic in the second decade, and the beginning is often insidious. *Persistent diarrhea which contains blood, mucus, and pus in the course of time, tenesmus, and lower abdominal colics are followed by possible anorectal involvement, weight loss, anemia, tiredness, apathy, and delay of physical and sexual development.*

The *extracolonic manifestations* are similar to those of Crohn's disease of which arthralgia and other joint symptoms belong to the most common (less than one third of the patients) and may precede the intestinal symptomatology. Although less frequently, chronic skin ulceration (pyoderma gangrenosum, aphthous stomatitis), urolithiasis, chronic sclerosing cholangitis, and osteoporosis need special attention.

The **clinical findings** depend on the stage and treatment of ulcerative colitis, for example, Cushingoid features due to corticosteroids. In general, *paleness etc, and delay in development (weight and length, sexual characteristics), lower abdominal tenderness, and hemorrhoids belong to the chronic stage,* whereas secondary fissures, fistulas, and perianal abscesses are more common in Crohn's disease.

Clinical Course and Complications: Although permanent remission does occur rarely, the majority of patients display a more or less progressive course with shorter periods of remission and increased relapses. 15 % of the patients have a fulminant onset (similar to a peracute surgical abdomen) and a course with fever, profuse diarrhea and hemorrhage, severe abdominal colics, dehydration, and possible septicemia. It corresponds usually to a **pancolitis** that develops in about 5 % into a **toxic megacolon**. Intestinal perforation is rarely observed.

Differential Diagnosis, Work-Ups

The possible differential diagnosis depends on the stage and clinical course. In children with insidious beginning or chronic stage, it is similar to that of Crohn's disease or infectious enterocolitis, whereas in peracute onset (pancolitis), disorders of surgical abdomen or lower intestinal hemorrhage must be considered, for example, intestinal volvulus or bleeding in Meckel's diverticulum.

Work-ups include Hb, inflammatory blood signs, coagulations study including thrombocyte count, electrolytes, albumin, etc. of which all may be abnormal. **Anoproctocolonoscopy** plays an important role including biopsy and cultures for infectious diseases: An edematous and hemorrhagic mucosa is observed that is covered by a hemorrhagic and purulent exudate in the acute stage. Numerous ulcers with serrated borders and so-called pseudopolyps corresponding to remaining islands of intact mucosa are characteristic for ulcerative colitis and concern the whole circumference of the most severely involved rectum. In the chronic stage, intestinal haustration is missing in addition to the quoted irregularities of the inner surface. The contrast enema is used less frequently because extension of the disease is evaluated more precisely by endoscopy and provocation of a relapse may occur thereafter. In chronic stage, the colorectum is narrow, short, and rigid, and haustration is not recognizable anymore.

Treatment, Prognosis

Treatment is medicamentous similar to Crohn's disease and is also performed in peracute onset except for toxic megacolon that needs emergency surgery. Topical application of the drugs is possible in left-sided colorectal disease.

Emergency surgery is **indicated** in fulminant disease that remains resistant to medical therapy, toxic megacolon, extensive lower intestinal hemorrhage, and perforation.

Elective surgery must be considered in every child with severe disease before irreversible sequels of medicamentous treatment including growth arrest occur. It consists either of **permanent proctocolectomy and ileostomy** or **colectomy and mucosal proctectomy with endorectal ileal pull-through with J-shaped pouch and temporary ileostomy**.

The **J-shaped pouch** is created by the ileum that is doubled back and has an opening at its apex for ileoanal anastomosis at the dentate line. Whereas the residual rectum in which the mucosa has been removed as far as the dentate line is 4–5 cm long, the length of the ileal pouch should not exceed 10–12 cm.

Creation of **ileostomy** must consider sufficient length of terminal ileum: mobilization of the mesentery by 3 cm and transference of the ileum beyond the skin level of the abdominal wall by 2–2.5 cm. The seromuscular layer is sutured to the opening in the abdominal wall in two layers, and the free end will fold over spontaneously and create a nipple.

Although both main procedures and specifically the endorectal ileal pull-through with J-shaped pouch display in >95 % and >5 years good results and the mortality is <1 %, **complications** may be observed in one to two thirds. They include mainly **pouchitis** and obstruction of the small intestine: In pouchitis (<10 %), periodic fever and watery diarrhea is observed especially if an outflow obstruction develops and mainly in the first 2 years after surgery. Treatment consists of regular washouts, anorectal dilatation, and metronidazole. Other possible complications include anal stricture (≤ 15 %) and severe incontinence (≤6 %). Most complications can be corrected, and only a few patients need removal of the pouch and permanent ileostomy (e.g., after severe anorectal disease). In expert hands, the following results can be attained in the majority of cases: A residual fecal volume of the pouch of <10 ml that means the patient will have 4–5 stools (volume 150–200 ml), 0.4 soiling episodes per week, withholding of stool after initial urge of >2 h, and micturition or passage of flatus without stool evacuation in >70 %.

23.4   Other Frequent and Rare Causes of Lower Gastrointestinal Bleeding

Examples of other but frequent causes of lower gastrointestinal bleeding are **intestinal parasitoses** in endemic regions of the world (e.g., Bilharziosis with enterocolitis or appendicitis), and rare causes are **angiodysplasia of the intestine**, **postoperative or postinterventional hemorrhage** (e.g., percutaneous endoscopic gastrostomy), **anastomotic ulceration**, and **carcinoid and neuroendocrine tumors**. Anastomotic ulceration may be observed after intestinal resection in NEC and other disorders. Ulceration is very obstinate and may be cured only by revision of the anastomosis.

Intestinal Bilharziasis (schistosomias) presents either as acute enterocolitis with/without melena or appendicitis that clinically cannot be differentiated from simple appendicitis. It is caused by schistosoma mansoni or japonicum that grow in the mesenteric veins. Their eggs lead to localized inflammations of intestinal wall, fallopian tubes etc. and peritoneum and characteristic whitish granular focuses.

Typical eggs in stool, colonic biopsy, removed appendix, and increased serum antibodies are diagnostic and praziquantel and appendectomy are therapeutic. Possible involvement of liver(portal hypertension), lung and other organs must be considered.

Webcodes

The following webcodes can be used on www. psurg.net for further images and data.

2301 Denaturated blood, lower GI bleeding	2313 Numerous polyps, double contrast enema
2302 Mucus intermingled with blood	2314 Prolapsing polyp, hamartomous polyp
2303 Advanced stage, small intestinal volvulus	2315 Large, spherical colonic polyp
2304 Volvulus, anomaly of intestinal rotation	2316 Right strangulated inguinal hernia
2305 Purpura, Henoch-Schönlein purpura	2317 Hemorrhoids, portal hypertension
2306 GI hemorrhage, Henoch-Schönlein purpura	2318 Acute thrombosis, hemorrhoids
2307 Henoch-Schönlein purpura, minimal findings	2319 Chronic anal fissure, Crohn's disease
2308 Scrotal swelling, Henoch-Schönlein purpura	2320 Fat encroachment, Crohn's disease
2309 Peptic ulcer, Meckel's diverticulum	2321 Stenosis from outside, Crohn's disease
2310 Ulcer perforation, Meckel's diverticulum	2323 Ulcerative colitis, pancolitis
2311 Enterocolitis, intestinal neuronal dysplasia	2322 Stenosis from the inside, Crohn's disease
2312 Adenomatous polyp	

Bibliography

General and Differential Diagnosis

Bresalier RS (2002) Screening techniques. In: Feldman M, Friedman LS, Sleisenger MH, Scharschmidt BF (eds) Sleisenger and Fordtran's gastrointestinal and liver disease. Pathophysiology/diagnosis/management, 7th edn. Saunders, Philadelphia

Kaufman SS, Atkinson JB, Bianchi A, Goulet OJ, Grant D, Langnas AN, Mc Diarmid SV, Mittal N, Reyes J, Tzakis AG, American Society of Transplantation (2001) Indications for pediatric intestinal transplantation: a position paper of the American society of transplantation. Pediatr Transplant 5:80–87

Section 23.1

Arensman RM (1998) Gastrointestinal bleeding. In: O'Neill JA Jr et al (eds) Pediatric surgery, vol II, 5th edn. Mosby, St Louis

Section 23.2.1

Ameh EA, Nmadu PT (2000) Intestinal volvulus: aetiology, morbidity, and mortality in Nigerian children. Pediatr Surg Int 16:50–52

Atamanalp SS, Yildirgan MI, Basoglu M, Kantarci M, Yilmaz I (2004) Sigmoid colon volvulus in children: review of 19 cases. Pediatr Surg Int 20:492–395

Larkin JO, Thekiso TB, Waldron R, Barry K, Eustace PW (2009) Recurrent sigmoid volvulus – early resection may obviate later emergency surgery and reduce morbidity and mortality. Ann R Coll Surg Engl 91:205–209

Salas S, Angel CA, Salas N, Murillo C, Swischuk L (2000) Sigmoid volvulus in children and adolescents. J Am Coll Surg 190:717–723

Samuel M, Boddy SA, Nicholls E, Capps S (2000) Large bowel volvulus in childhood. Aust N Z Surg 70:258–262

Section 23.2.2

Young DG (1998) Intussusception. In: O'Neill JA Jr et al (eds) Pediatric surgery, vol II, 5th edn. Mosby, St Louis

Section 23.2.3

Balmelli C, Laux-End R, Di Rocco D, Carvajal-Busslinger MI, Bianchetti MG (1999) Purpura Schoenlein-Henoch: verlauf bei 139 kindern. Schweiz Med Wochenschr 126:293–298

Bless NM, Goti F, Jost R, Decurtins M (2006) Schwere ulzeröse Panduodenitis bei einem 13jährigen Jungen. Schweiz Med Forum 6:831–833

Martinez-Frontanilla LA, Haase GM, Ernster JA, Bailey WC (1984) Surgical complications in Henoch-Schoenlein purpura. J Pediatr Surg 19:434–436

Section 25.2.4

Amoury RA, Snyder CL (1998) Meckel's Diverticulum. In: O'Neill JA Jr et al (eds) Pediatric surgery, vol II, 5th edn. Mosby, St Louis

Burkhardt K, Kaiser RR (1975/76) Komplikationen des meckelschen divertikels. Pädiat Prax 16:401–407

Waldvogel M, Wildi SM, Arn M (2001) Meckel-Divertickel-Szintigraphy. Schweiz Med Forum 43: 1089–1090

Section 23.2.5

Bond SJ, Groff DB (1998) Gastrointestinal duplications. In: O'Neill JA Jr et al (eds) Pediatric surgery, vol II, 5th edn. Mosby, St Louis

Perek A, Perek S, Kaplan M, Goksoy E (2000) Gastric duplication cyst. Dig Surg 17:634–636

Section 23.2.6

Albanese CT, Rowe MI (1995) Necrotizing enterocolitis. Semin Pediatr Surg 4:200–206
Albanese CT, Rowe MI (1998) Necrotizing enterocolitis. In: O'Neill JA Jr et al (eds) Pediatric surgery, vol II, 5th edn. Mosby, St Louis
Al-Hudhaif J, Phillips S, Gholum S, Puligandla PP, Flageole H (2009) The timing of enterostomy reversal after necrotizing enterocolitis. J Pediatr Surg 44: 924–927
Bell MJ, Ternberg JL, Feigin RD, Keating JP, Marshall R, Barton L, Brotherton T (1978) Neonatal necrotizing enterocolitis: therapeutic decisions based upon clinical staging. Ann Surg 187:1–7
Coursey CA, Hollingsworth CL, Gaca AM, Maxfield C, Delong D, Bisset G III (2008) Radiologists' agreement when using a 10-point scale to report abdominal radiographic findings of necrotizing enterocolitis in neonates and infants. AJR Am J Roentgenol 191: 190–197
Deshpande G, Rao S, Patole S, Bulsara M (2010) Updated meta-analysis of probiotics for prevention necrotizing enterocolitis in preterm neonates. Pediatrics 125: 921–930
Epelman M, Daneman A, Navarro OM, Morag I, Moore AM, Kim JH, Faingold R, Taylor G, Gerstle JT (2008) Necrotizing enterocolitis: review of state-of-the-art imaging findings with pathological correlation. Radiographics 28:319–320
Hall NJ, Hiorns M, Tighe H, Peters M, Khoo AK, Eaton S, Pierro A (2009) Is necrotizing enterocolitis associated with development or progression of intraventricular hemorrhage? Am J Perinatol 26:139–143
Hosie S, Loff S, Wirth H, Rapp HJ, von Buch C, Waag KL (2006) Experience of 49 longitudinal lengthening procedures for short bowel syndrome. Eur J Pediatr Surg 16:171–175
Lambert DK, Christensen RD, Besner GE, Baer VL, Wiedmeier SE, Stoddard RA, Miner CA, Burnett J (2007) Necrotizing enterocolitis in term neonates: data from a multihospital health data system. J Perinatol 27:437–443
Rees CM, Pierro A, Eaton S (2007) Neurodevelopmental outcomes of neonates with medically and surgically treated necrotizing enterocolitis. Arch Dis Child Fetal Neonatal Ed 92:F193–198
Ron O, Davenport M, Patel S, Kiely E, Pierro A, Hall NJ, Ade-Ajayi N (2009) Outcomes of the "clip and drop" technique for multifocal necrotizing enterocolitis. J Pediatr Surg 44:749–754
Sola JE, Tepas JJ III, Koniaris LG (2010) Peritoneal drainage versus laparotomy for necrotizing enterocolitis and intestinal perforation: a meta-analysis. J Surg Res 1(161):95–100

Section 23.2.6 Short Bowel Syndrome

Bianchi A (1980) Intestinal loop lengthening – a technique for increasing small intestinal length. J Pediatr Surg 15:145
Duro D, Kamin D, Duggan C (2008) Overview of pediatric short bowel syndrome. J Pediatr Gastroenterol Nutr 47(Suppl 1):S33–36
Goulet O, Sauvat F (2006) Short bowel syndrome and intestinal transplantation in children. Curr Opin Clin Nutr Metab Care 9:304–313
Goulet O, Baglin-Gobet S, Talbotec C, Colomb V, Sauvat F, Jais JP, Michel JL, Jan D, Ricour C (2005) Outcome and long-term growth after extensive small bowel resection in the neonatal period: a survey of 87 children. Eur J Pediatr Surg 15:95–101
Lao OB, Healey PJ, Perkins JD, Horslen S, Reyes JD, Goldin AB (2010) Outcomes in children after intestinal transplant. Pediatrics 125:e550–558
Sala D, Chomto S, Hill S (2010) Long-term outcomes of short bowel syndrome requiring long-term/home intravenous nutrition compared in children with gastroschisis and those with volvulus. Transplant Proc 42:5–8

Section 23.2.7

Behrens R, Seiler A (1990/91) Kolonpolypen im Kindesalter. Pädiat Prax 41:47–51
Chantada GL, Perelli VB, Lombardi MG et al (2005) Colorectal carcinoma in childen, adolescents, and young adults. J Pediatr Hematol Oncol 27:39–41
Emery J, Lucassen A, Murphy M (2001) Common hereditary cancers and implications for primary care. Lancet 358:56–63
Foglia RP (1998) Colorectal tumors. In: O'Neill JA Jr et al (eds) Pediatric surgery, vol II, 5th edn. Mosby, St Louis
Gürses N, Gürses N (1986) Peutz-jeghers syndrome: a clinical study of a large family in two generations. Z Kinderchir 41:364–368
Hampel H, Frankel WL, Martin E et al (2005) Screening for the lynch syndrome (hereditary nonpolyposis colorectal cancer). N Engl J Med 352:1851–1860
Hoffenberg EJ, Sauaia A, Maltzman T et al (1999) Symptomatic colonic polyps in childhood: not so benign. J Pediatr Gastroenterol Nutr 28:175–181
Huntsman DG, Carneiro F, Lewis FR et al (2001) Early gastric cancer in young, asymptomatic carriers of germ-line E-cadherin mutations. N Engl J Med 344: 1904–1909
Kopacova M, Tacheci I, Rejchrt S, Bures J (2009) Peutz-Jeghers syndrome: diagnostic and therapeutic approach. World J Gastroenterol 21(15):5397–5408
Lelli JL, Coran AG (1998) Polypoid disease of the gastrointestinal tract. In: O'Neill JA Jr et al (eds) Pediatric surgery, vol II, 5th edn. Mosby, St Louis

Metzger U, Schnider A (2001) Prophylactic surgery in families with familial adenomatous polyposis (FAP) and colitis. Swiss Surg 7:278–280

Müller HJ, Heinimann K (2002) Kolorektale polypen. Multiple polypen des Dick- und Mastdarmes im Kindes- und Erwachsenenalter – Wann sind Gentests angezeigt? Schweiz Med Forum 4:59–66

Poddar U, Thapa BR, Vaiphei K et al (1998) Colonic polyps: experience of 236 Indian children. Am J Gastroenterol 93:619–622

Van Lier MG, Wagner A, Mathus-Vliegen EM, Kuipers EJ, Steyerberg EW, van Leerdam ME (2010) High cancer risk in Peutz-Jeghers syndrome: a systematic review and surveillance recommendations. Am J Gastroenterol 105:1258–1265

Weitz J, Koch M, Debus J et al (2005) Colorectal cancer. Lancet 365:153–163

Sections 23.2.8–23.2.9

Stafford PW (1998) Other disorders of the anus and rectum, anorectal function. In: O'Neill JA Jr et al (eds) Pediatric surgery, vol II, 5th edn. Mosby, St Louis

Section 23.2.10

Lehner M (1982) Analfistel. In: Bettex M, Genton N, Stockmann M (eds) Kinderchi-rurgie. Diagnostik, indication, therapie, prognose Begründet von M. Grob, 2 aufl. Thieme, Stuttgart

Staffort PW (1998) Other disorders of the anus and rectum, anorectal function. In: O'Neill JA Jr et al (eds) Pediatric surgery, vol II, 5th edn. Mosby, St Louis

Section 23.2.11

Bond RG, Dowd DM, Rimsza M (1995) Unintentional perineal injury in prepubescent girls: a multicenter, prospective report of 56 girls. Pediatrics 95:628–631

Boos SC, Rosas AJ, Boyle C, McCann J (2003) Anogenital injuries in child pedestrians run over by low-speed motor vehicles: four cases with findings that mimic child sexual abuse. Pediatrics 112:e77–e84

Dowd MD, Fitzmaurice L, Knapp JF, Mooney D (1994) The interpretation of urogenital findings in children with straddle injuries. J Pediatr Surg 29:7–10

Felt-Bersma RJF, Cuesta MA, Koorevaar M (1996) Anal sphincter repair improves anorectal function and endosonographic image. A prospective clinical study. Dis Colon Rectum 39:878–885

Jona JZ (1997) Accidental anorectal impalement in children. Pediatr Emerg Care 13:40–43

Jones LW, Bass DH (1991) Perineal injuries in children. Br J Surg 78:1105–1107

Peterli R, Ackermann C, Herzog U, Schuppisser JP, Tondelli P (1997) Results of overlapping sphincteroplasty in fecal incontinence – value of endosonography. Swiss Surg 3:112–116

Kim S, Linden B, Cendron M, Puder M (2006) Pediatric anorectal impalement with **bladder rupture**: case report and review of the literature. J Pediatr Surg 41:E1–3

Scheidler MG, Schultz BL, Schall L, Ford HR (2000) Mechanisms of blunt perineal injury in female pediatric patients. J Pediatr Surg 35:1317–1319

Sterioff S Jr, Izant RJ Jr, Persky L (1969) Perianal injuries in children. J Trauma 9:56–61, discussion 61

Section 23.3

Bunn SK, Bisset WM, Main MJC et al (2001) Fecal calprotectin: validation as a noninvasive measure of bowel inflammation in childhood bowel inflammatory disease. J Pediatr Gastroenterol Nutr 33:14–22

Cabrera-Abreu JC, Davies P, Matek Z et al (2004) Performance of blood tests in diagnosis of inflammatory bowel disease in a specialist clinic. Arch Dis Child 89:69–71

Dignass A, Van Assche G, Lindsay JO, Lemann M, Soderholm J, Colombel JF et al (2010) The second European evidence-based consensus on the diagnosis and management of Crohn's disease: current management. J Crohn's Colitis 4:28–62

Doig CM (1998) Crohn's disease. In: O'Neill JA Jr et al (eds) Pediatric surgery, vol II, 5th edn. Mosby, St Louis

Fagerberg UL, Lööf L, Merzoug RD et al (2003) Fecal calprotectin levels in healthy children studied with an improved assay. J Pediatr Gastroenterol Nutr 37: 468 472

Fonkalsrud EW (1998) Ulcerative colitis. In: O'Neill JA Jr et al (eds) Pediatric surgery, vol II, 5th edn. Mosby, St Louis

Section 23.4

King CH (2009) Global health: toward the elimination of schistosomiasis. N Engl J Med 360:106–109, für Colitis DD

Kucik CJ, Martin GL, Sortor BV (2004) Common intestinal parasites. Am Fam Physician 1(69):1161–1168

Neu B, May A, Schmid E, Riemann JF, Hagenmuller F, Keuchel M et al (2005) Capsule endoscopy versus standard tests influencing management of obscure digestive bleeding: results from a German multicenter trial. Am J Gastroenterol 100:1736–1742

Modlin IM, Sandor A (1997) An analysis of 8505 cases of carcinoid tumors. Cancer 79:813–829

Parashar K, Kyawhla S, Booth IW, Buick RG, Corkery JJ (1988) Ileocolic ulceration: a long-term complication following ileocolic anastomosis. J Pediatr Surg 23: 226–228

Patak MA, Froehlich JM, von Weymarn C et al (2001) Non-invasive distension of the small bowel for magnetic-resonance imaging. Lancet 358:987–988

Richter J (2000) Evolution of schistosomiasis-induced pathology after therapy and interruption of exposure to schistosomes: a review of ultrasonic findings. Acta Trop 23(77):111–131

Sondheimer JM, Sokol RJ, Narkewicz MR (1995) Anastomotic ulceration: a late complication of ileocolonic anastomosis. J Pediatr 127:225–230

Travis SP, Stange EF, Lemann M, Oresland T, Bemelman WA, Chowers Y et al (2008) European evidence-based consensus on the management of ulcerative colitis: current management. J Crohns Colitis 2:24–62

Varnier A, Iona L, Dominutti MC, Deotto E, Bianchi L, Iengo A et al (2006) Percutaneous endoscopic gastrostomy: complications in the short and long-term follow-up and efficacy on nutritional status. Eura Medicophys 42:23–26

Wachter G, Helbling B (2007) Obskure gastrointestinale Blutung und Dünndarm-raumforderung. Schweiz Med Forum 7:261–262

Abdominal Tumor

The term "abdominal tumor" is used for all disorders that lead to a visible and/or palpable enlargement of the abdomen. Although retro- and intra-abdominal neoplastic tumors are in the foreground of clinical interest, malformations, inflammations, traumatic injuries, or parasitoses presenting as solid or cystic mass as well as orga- nomegalies and ascites are quoted here because they may feign a benign or malignant tumor (differential diagnostic significance) and need specific treatment.

Although abdominal tumor is a characteristic presenting sign in childhood, it may manifest as well as **surgical abdomen** or with life-threatening symptoms and signs of the respiratory system due to the urgently needed work-ups, space-occupy- ing effect, or inherent specific complications.

The groups of the quoted disease categories and their individual pathologies are listed in Table 24.1 including **hints of their possible significance as surgical abdomen**. In newborns, two thirds of the patients with the presenting sign "abdominal tumor" have either hydronephrosis or polycystic kidney disease. Urinary retention, renal vein thrombosis, and hydrometrocolpos must also be considered in this age group. Figure 24.1 shows the relative frequencies of the main pediatric malignancies.

24.1 Neoplastic Masses and Cysts

24.1.1 Nephroblastoma (Wilms' Tumor)

Occurrence, Pathoanatomy

Wilms' tumor belongs together with neuroblas- toma and rhabdomyosarcoma to the second most frequent solid malignomas of childhood that have a similarly large percentage of all malignancies (5–7 %, 3–8 %, 4–8.5 %). Every year, 8 children are struck by nephroblastoma in one million below the age of 16 years. The mean age at clini- cal presentation is 3–4 years. Fifteen percent are infants and 70–80 % less than or up to 5 years of age.

The classic Wilms' tumor is composed of three elements in variable amounts. The deriva tives of blastema, tubules, and stroma are possible recapitulations of normal kidney differentiation. Each of these elements may contain anaplas- tic elements leading to the anaplastic type of Wilms' tumor that is more aggressive and less amenable to treatment. Other renal tumors that may be differentiated from nephroblastoma only by histology are **congenital mesoblastic neph- roma** (with only local recurrences), **clear cell sarcoma** (prone to bone metastases), and **renal**

Table 24.1 Differential diagnosis of abdominal tumor

	Manifestation as surgical abdomen
Retro- and intra-abdominal neoplasms	
• Nephroblastoma	Acute hemorrhage, tumor rupture
• Neuroblastoma	Acute retroperitoneal hematoma
o Rhabdomyosarcoma}	Tumor rupture with hemorrhagic
o Teratoma}	Ascites, acute/chronic intestinal obstruction
• Non-Hodgkin's lymphoma	Acute/chronic intestinal obstruction (intussusception, etc.), intestinal perforation
• Ovarian tumor or cysts	Torsion, rupture, hemorrhage
o Hepatic tumors or cysts	Hemorrhage, rupture, torsion
o Pancreas tumors or cysts	
o Adrenal tumors	
Masses or cysts: malformations, inflammations, injuries, or parasitoses	
• Choledochal cyst	Acute obstructive ileus, cholangitis
o Meconium peritonitis	Ileus of the newborn
o Mesenterial or omental cyst	Acute obstructive ileus (compression, volvulus), rupture
o Intestinal duplication	Acute obstructive ileus (volvulus, intussusception), lower GI hemorrhage
• Hydro-(metro-), hemato-(metro-) colpos	Acute obstructive ileus, acute urinary and stool retention
• Obstructive uropathies, intermittent ureteropelvic junction obstruction	Acute abdominal colics
• Abdominal wall, Douglas, and intra-abdominal abscesses	
• Perinephritic abscess, xanthogranulomatous pyelonephritis	
o Hepatic abscess, gallbladder empyema	Acute/chronic septic disorder with abdominal tumor and/or inflammatory findings
o Pseudocyst of pancreas, kidney, spleen	Acute gastrointestinal symptoms, icterus
o Renal vein thrombosis	Acute hematuria
• Echinococcosis	Perforation, anaphylactic shock
Other causes of abdominal enlargement or masses	
• Ascites, meteorism	Surgical abdomen (infection or rapid development)
• Hepatomegaly, splenomegaly	
• Fecaloma, megavesica (different causes)	Acute stool or urinary retention → surgical abdomen

rhabdoid tumor with a bad dignity in comparison to nephroblastoma. Nephroblastomatosis is synonymous with nephrogenic rests and corresponds to focuses of developmental anomalies of the kidney of unknown dignity. They are encountered more frequently in "inherited" than sporadic Wilms' tumor and have a differential diagnostic significance.

Molecular biology becomes increasingly important in Wilms' tumor for differentiation of types with inherited susceptibility to nephroblastoma from sporadic types and of the classic Wilms tumor from other renal tumor as quoted above.

Clinical Significance

• Because nephroblastoma becomes often visible and/or palpable as an asymptomatic abdominal mass by chance, the practitioner must always consider a Wilms' tumor especially in toddlers.

Clinical Presentation

The main sign is a flank mass that expands over the anterior midline without distinct borders in the depths and leads to an abdominal prominence #. Bilateral nephroblastoma (5–10 % of the cases) has a bilateral extension and may appear as a single mass. It occurs more frequently synchronously than metachronously.

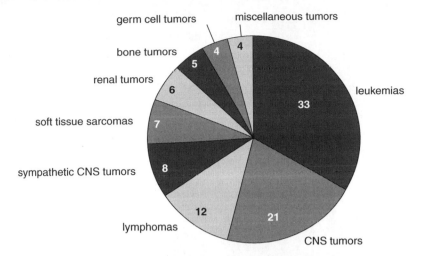

Fig. 24.1 Relative frequency of the main pediatric malignancies. The order of frequency has not changed on the whole in the last 30 years although the absolute figures of single pathologies may have changed: 33 % are leukemias, 21 % CNS tumors, 12 % malignant lymphomas (non-Hodgkin's lymphoma and Hodgkin's disease), 8 % sympathetic CNS tumors (neuroblastoma, etc.), 7 % soft tissue sarcomas (including rhabdomyosarcoma), 6 % renal tumors (nephroblastoma, etc.), 5 % bone tumors, 4 % germ cell tumors, and 4 % miscellaneous tumors (Young and Miller 1975; Pearson and Steward 1969; Bodmer and Grotzer 2005)

An unspecific symptomatology may precede the classic presentation: feeling of uneasiness, weight loss, anemia, and microscopic hematuria. In addition to vague abdominal pain and microscopic or gross hematuria (up to 30 %), arterial hypertension and varicocele on the left side may be occasionally observed.

In <10–15 % of the cases, **associated congenital anomalies** can be found: Urogenital malformations (e.g., hypospadias or cryptorchidism), isolated aniridia or as part of WAGR syndrome [Wilms' tumor, aniridia, genitourinary malformations, mental retardation], EMG (Beckwith-Wiedemann) syndrome [also combined with adrenocortical carcinoma or hepatoblastoma], hamartomas, neurofibromatosis, hemihypertrophy of the limb(s) #, and chromosomal aberrations. *Such patients must be checked specifically for Wilms' tumor by ultrasound screening.*

A surgical abdomen may result from hemorrhage in the tumor without or with retro- or intra-abdominal rupture #. It may occur from a minor trauma to the flank that may also lead to gross hematuria. *If radiological imaging is performed in such cases, nephroblastoma is found unexpectedly.*

Differential Diagnosis, Work-Ups

The clinical and radiological findings must consider other retroperitoneal tumors (neuroblastoma, rhabdomyosarcoma, and teratoma), congenital malformations # (e.g., isolated renal cyst), or acquired disorders especially if the tumor is large and in case of microscopic or gross hematuria, other causes of it such as *Xanthogranulomatous pyelonephritis.* It is a rare disease that is characterized by loin and abdominal pain, signs of urinary tract infection, and possible anorexia or weight loss since several weeks. Anemia, pyuria with positive urine cultures, ultrasound with stones or a space-occupying mass, and contrast CT with diffuse or focal low-density inflammatory areas and reduced cortical uptake are possible findings at work-up. Nephrectomy is mostly necessary.

The work-ups include ultrasound, CT with contrast, and plain chest X-ray for differentiation from other masses, diagnosis of Wilms' tumor (distorted pyelocaliceal system is typical) #, and primary staging (lymph node and bilateral renal involvement, hepatic and pulmonary metastases).

Measurement of blood pressure at the four extremities and urinalysis (microscopic hematuria, bFGF [basis fibroblast growth factor as tumor marker]) are also important. Molecular biological examinations may detect in up to 20 % a tumor suppressor gene. Serum and urine catecholamines are determined for exclusion of neuroblastoma.

Although final staging should be performed at surgery, progress of radiological imaging permits useful preoperative staging. It should also include possible bilateral involvement of the kidneys and tumor extension into the renal vein and cava inferior.

The mostly applied staging according to the NWTS (National Wilms' Tumor Study) is as follows:

Stage I: Tumor limited to one kidney and complete resection with an intact capsule

Stage II: Extension beyond the involved kidney with complete resection (penetration of the capsule, invasion of renal sinus, extension into renal vein # or inferior vena cava, tumor biopsy, or retroperitoneal spillage)

Stage III: Residual tumor present and confined to the abdomen (lymph node involvement, tumor penetration through peritoneum, or implants on its surface; tumor beyond the margins of resection including local infiltration into vital structures; generalized tumor spread not confined to the flank)

Stage IV: Hematogenous metastatic disease to lung, liver, bone, etc or lymph node involvement outside the abdomen and pelvis

Stage V: Bilateral renal involvement

Treatment, Prognosis

Treatment is multimodal with surgery, chemotherapy, and radiotherapy. Whether pre- and/or postoperative chemo- and radiotherapy is performed or not, the selection and combination of cytostatics and mode of radiation depends on the stage and histology of Wilms' tumor (histology with low, moderate, and severe malignancy), age, and the treatment protocol applied. Based on prospective studies, radiation has been eliminated in the last decades in low-risk patients.

Surgery with or without preoperative chemotherapy is the main part of treatment. After introduction of general anesthesia using the upper extremities or neck for the i.v. line, elevation of the involved side, and preparation of abdomen and chest as operating field, a transverse abdominal and transperitoneal incision is performed on the side of the tumor, and the ascending or descending colon is reflected to the other side.

The initial inspection includes the visible part of the involved kidney, liver, and contralateral kidney of which the gerota's fascia is opened for inspection and palpation of the whole organ. The initial part of surgery is used for final staging and occurs according a protocol. Suspicious nodes need biopsy, frozen sections, and their site is marked.

Excision of the tumor starts whenever possible with ligation of renal vein, renal artery and possible pole arteries, and ureter close to the bladder. Preparation of the tumor is performed beyond the renal capsule and laterally beyond Gerota's fascia avoiding strictly any tumor rupture. Preservation of the adrenal gland is often not possible ##, and extension beyond the involved kidney needs en bloc resection, for example, a piece of diaphragm. On the other hand, gross resection of vital organs should not be attempted.

The staging is completed by sampling of suprarenal (above renal vessels), infrarenal, and pelvic (below bifurcation) suspicious or representative lymph nodes after tumor resection. Before abdominal closure, the reflected colon is carefully re-adapted to the abdominal wall to avoid internal hernia, appendectomy is performed, and the small intestine repositioned like a festoon according to Grob. A detailed operative protocol that concerns all oncological important aspects is very important.

Tumor extension into the renal vein and inferior vena cava and bilateral Wilms' tumor need specific consideration: With preoperative treatment, almost all tumor extensions in the inferior cava can be extracted either by suction or an appropriate balloon after occlusion of the vessel; cardiopulmonary bypass is not necessary and embolization is unlikely. In bilateral Wilms' tumor, each kidney is staged separately. It needs rigorous preoperative treatment and possibly staged surgery: nephrectomy of one side and partial nephrectomy or tumor enucleation on the other side # or bilateral partial nephrectomy. Intraoperative ultrasound may be useful in such cases.

Lung metastases are primarily treated with chemotherapy and only radiated or resected in case of resistance to chemotherapy.

Prognosis and outcome must consider the possible sequels of treatment and the outcome of nephroblastoma.

After tumor nephrectomy, an increased number of obstructions of the small intestine may be observed. Most of them are postoperative ileus due to adhesions and few due to intussusception or internal hernia. Whether the adhesions are related to specific factors of tumor surgery (e.g., en bloc resection) and therefore increased in relation to laparotomies for other reasons is not excluded. Important is the observation that most of them occur within the first 3 months. The possibility of development of a second malignant tumor is important for long-term follow-up, and the figures increase with survival of a large number of patients to adulthood (e.g., in about 5 % of patients 25 years after diagnosis). The site and type of secondary malignancies is important as well.

The overall 5-year survival is 90 %. Whereas the 4-year survival is 99.6 % for stage I with favorable histology of whom 92.5 are relapse-free, the same figures for anaplastic nephroblastomas with stage I are 92.3 and 93.8 %, for clear cell carcinomas 88.6 and 66.0 %, and the overall survival for bilateral nehroblastomas is about 70 %.

24.1.2 Neuroblastoma

Occurrence, Pathoanatomy

The incidence of neuroblastoma is 1.1 per 100'000 children <15 years. Children are younger at diagnosis than those of Wilms' tumor (60–70 % <1 year, 20–30 % 1–2 years, and 5–10 % >2 years of age), and the mean age at diagnosis is the second year of age although the majority of patients is observed up to the age of 6, 7, and 8 years (90 %).

Different locations and maturity grade are characteristic for this type of neurogenic tumor;

up to 75 % are retroperitoneal tumors (adrenal medulla > paraspinal (abdominal, thoracic, or cervical grenz ray or paraganglions) > presacral forms) and only 20 % posterior mediastinal or <5 % cervical tumors. The variable course is explained in part by frequent progression and possible regression or maturation in some.

The undifferentiated tumor is a purple to gray mass that has a friable pseudocapsule, is either solid or cystic and highly vascularized, and contains necrotic areas. It is prone to rupture either spontaneously or at surgery with gross bleeding. If the tumor becomes more differentiated, it has a more solid consistency and a fleshy-white color.

Clinical Significance

- Fifty percent of neuroblastomas has already metastases at the time of diagnosis
- General symptoms and local signs due to metastatic disease lead to the diagnosis as often as the primary abdominal tumor that makes early recognition more difficult. The same applies to extraperitoneal sites where the leading symptoms "mediastinal tumor" or "mass of the neck" replace the presenting sign "abdominal tumor."
- Metastases occur in the regional or distant lymph nodes, bone marrow, bone, liver, skin, and CNS.

Clinical Presentation

Suspicious general symptoms are *failure to thrive, weight loss, fever, and paleness (anemia).* Local signs of metastatic tumor are *periorbital swelling, proptosis, and ecchymosis of the eye(s) (metastasis of the orbits and periorbital); refusal to walk and severe pain of the extremities (bone cortex # and marrow metastasis); paraplegia of the newborn (hourglass lesion with intraspinal extension of neuroblastoma #); or disorders of micturition and defecation (presacral tumor location).*

In addition to a *visible and/or palpable abdominal tumor,* unspecific and suspicious abdominal signs may be observed such as *abdominal pain, distension, and tenderness; vomiting; and watery and explosive diarrhea. The abdominal tumor extends more frequently beyond the midline and is nodular on palpation. A presacral tumor may be felt by rectal examination.*

Irritability, sweating, flushing, and arterial hypertension (up to 25 %) are like diarrhea caused by metabolites of the neuroblastoma.

Clinical examination must consider hepatomegaly, subcutaneous skin nodules, enlarged lymph nodes, and occasionally signs of bleeding diathesis.

Differential Diagnosis, Work-Ups

Several differential diagnoses must be considered in view of the numerous and different general, local, abdominal signs and more specifically those of other oncological diseases and abdominal tumor.

The work-ups permit diagnosis of neuroblastoma, its site and extension, and its staging and biological typification.

Preliminary diagnosis is possible by quantification of catecholamines and by-products in 24-h urine with significant increase of homovanillic and vanillylmandelic acid in the majority of cases. LDH and ferritin are unspecific markers, and their elevation can be used for estimation of tumor risk.

Upright plain abdominal X-ray, ultrasound, and MRI or CT with contrast enhancement are the main imaging tools depending on the site of the primary tumor. Plain X-ray may show indirect signs of retroperitoneal or paraspinal mass (bowel displacement and paraspinal widening) and the characteristic numerous punctate calcifications with regular distribution in about 50 % at the site of the tumor. Ultrasound and (angio) MRI or CT reveals a solid or less frequently cystic retroperitoneal mass that pushes the kidney downward without gross deformity of the pyelocaliceal system # or a paraspinal mass in contrast to Wilms' tumor in which the pyelocaliceal system is distorted.

Further work-ups include bone marrow aspirations at different sites, scintiscan (99mTc or 123I-MIBG9 [metaiodobenzylguanidine]) that is used for specific delineation of primary tumor and metastases, skeletal scintiscan, ultrasound, and angio MRI for staging and tumor extension:

bone marrow, skeletal, brain, or liver metastasis and tumor extension into renal vein, inferior cava, and intraspinally. The final diagnosis is performed by tissue histology, immunohistology, and biological typification. The latter is performed for additional treatment stratification and prognostication and encompasses possible amplification of tumor oncogene NMYC and deletion on chromosome 1p.

The International Neuroblastoma Staging System has tried to unify all elements of the former classifications (Evans et al., POG, TNM, and others) and to improve the overall applicability.

International Neuroblastoma Staging System (Brodeur et al.)

Stage 1	Localized tumor (organ of origin); lymph nodes negative; complete resection without/ with microscopic residuals
Stage 2-A	Unilateral tumor with incomplete resection; lymph nodes negative
Stage 2-B	Unilateral tumor with complete/incomplete resection; ipsilateral lymph nodes positive
Stage 3	Tumor infiltrating across midline or without lymph nodes involvement Unilateral tumor and contralateral lymph node involvement Midline tumor and bilateral lymph node involvement
Stage 4	Metastasis to distant lymph nodes #, bone, bone marrow, liver, or other organs
Stage 4-S	Localized primary tumor (stages 1 or 2) with metastasis limited to liver #, skin, or bone marrow

Treatment, Prognosis

It depends on the age of the child, stage, histological classification, adverse biological markers (e.g., Nmyc oncogene, serum ferritin), and the treatment protocol.

Treatment options reach from watch and wait strategy in stage IV-S (4-S) without adverse molecular biological markers, to exclusive surgery, to chemotherapy, and to maximum therapy with high-dose, multiagent chemotherapy; possible local radiation; or high-dose MIGB treatment in high-risk patients and autologous stem cell transplantation. 13-*cis*-retinoic acid (provocation of neuroblastoma differentiation) and monoclonal antibodies are new treatment option in the stage of evaluation.

The role of surgery is different from that of Wilms' tumor. Surgery is applied for biopsy that permits throughout histological and biological work-up and primary resection (stages I and II) or delayed primary resection or second look laparotomy (stage III and IV). Whereas an improved outlook can be expected with complete resection in stage III, this issue is discussed controversially in stage IV. Residual tumor is treated by local radiotherapy.

If **primary, delayed primary, or second look complete # or incomplete (debulking) resection** is intended, the access is similar to Wilms' tumor laparotomy. Anesthesia should be prepared for profuse hemorrhage and sudden onset arterial hypertension. After a transverse, transperitoneal, and supraumbilical abdominal incision or another incision depending on the extension of neuroblastoma, the colon is reflected and the hepatic attachments incised on the right, and spleen and distal pancreas mobilized on the left side. The tumor is carefully resected beyond its pseudocapsule avoiding rupture, gross hemorrhage, en bloc resection of the adjacent organs, injury to the main arteries and veins that may be surrounded by tumor, and heroic debulking. Several suprarenal feeding arteries and the main venous outflow to the inferior vena cave (right) or left renal vein (left side) must be considered. Finally, the margins of the tumor bed should be marked with titanium clips, and surgical staging be completed by asservation of ipsi- and contralateral suspicious and representative lymph nodes.

Prognosis depends on the age, stage, tumor gene Nmyc amplification, depletion on chromosome 1p and other factors. Five-year survival is 95 % in stages I and II, 75 % in stage III, and 30–40 % in stage IV. Nmyc worsens overall survival and event-free survival dramatically.

24.1.3 Rhabdomyosarcoma

Occurrence, Pathoanatomy

Rhabdomyosarcoma is with 50–75 % the most common soft tissue sarcoma in children. Four to seven new cases arise in one million children per year with a similar frequency as Wilms' tumor or neuroblastoma (7–8 % of malignant solid tumors). After a peak at the ages 1–4 years, the rate falls to a lower level between 10 and 14 years and remains steady thereafter. The median age is 5 years.

Diverse sites of origin, histopathological features, and clinical presentations render rhabdomyosarcoma to a complex tumor. It arises from embryonic mesenchyma and differentiates possibly into striated muscles tissue. More than one third occurs in the head or neck region, >20 % in the urogenital tract, and <20 % in the limbs and other sites, respectively. Depending on the site and local extension, and generalization, a diverse symptomatology is observed. The embryonal with 75 % and alveolar subtype with 20 % are mostly encountered in children, the embryonal subtype by preference in small children, and the alveolar subtype in all age groups and at any site.

Less than 5 % have a genetic predisposition, for example, **family cancer (Li-Fraumeni) syndrome**. The disorder with autosomal dominant inheritance displays in addition to childhood rhabdomyosarcomas bone or soft tissue sarcomas, breast and adrenocortical carcinomas, gliomas, and leukemia in other family members less than 45 years of age. CNS or urogenital anomalies, neurofibromatosis, nevoid basal cell carcinoma, and fetal alcohol syndrome or exposure to other intrauterine agents are possible associated disorders.

Clinical Significance

- In contrast to the somewhat more common chest and abdominal wall rhabdomyosarcomas that are recognized early because of a visible mass, the paraspinal, retroperitoneal, or posterior mediastinal rhabdomyosarcoma gets symptomatic often late with advanced involvement of abdominal, pelvic, or vertebral structures.

- Because rhabdomyosarcoma occurs at any site and in any organ, it must be considered in the differential diagnosis of any trunk mass, especially of the chest or abdominal wall and paraspinal, retroperitoneal, or posterior mediastinal space and rarely of the lung (possible association with CCAM) or biliary tree.

Clinical Presentation

Abdominal distension, visible and/or palpable abdominal tumor, and pain are the main symptoms.

Because of locoregional involvement of abdomen, pelvis, or spine in about two thirds at diagnosis, signs of upper urinary tract , intestinal, and venous obstruction (inferior vena cava), or intraspinal extension may be observed. Intraabdominal extension or rupture may lead to hemorrhagic ascites that is recognized by percussion and ultrasound-guided paracentesis.

Differential Diagnosis, Work-Ups

The differential diagnosis includes other abdominal tumors, especially the retroperitoneal ones such as paraspinal neuroblastoma, fibrosarcoma, germ cell tumor, and lymphoma.

In case of suspected or probable rhabdomyosarcoma, work-ups are started with **ultrasound** (yielding a well-defined, slightly hypoechogenic inhomogeneous mass with increased flow). For soft tissue changes as observed in most rhabdomyosarcomas, **MRI** [T1-and T2-W images including gadolinium administration] is the next step (the nonspecific changes "strong enhancement and intermediate and intermediate to high signal intensity" show the compartment(s) of tumor location, its relation to large vessel, possible regional lymph node involvement, and on follow-up after treatment, volume reduction and differentiation between residual tumor and fibrosis are possible).

CT or multidetector CT (MDCT) may be applied instead of MRI especially in case of expected osseous changes at the primary tumor site and possible lung metastases, and 99mTc-MDP scintiscan is used for distant lymph node, bone, and other metastases. Craniospinal MR is indicated if intraspinal or meningeal extension is suspected. PET-CT is a promising tool in the evaluation of pediatric abdominal malignancies, but the delineation of its exact role needs more experience.

In addition, a set of blood, urine, and possibly CSF examinations (depending on the site of the tumor); bone marrow aspirates and trephine; and **surgery for biopsy including frozen tissue and staging** should be performed.

In retroperitoneal rhabdomyosarcoma, the mean size is often 13–16 cm, and locoregional involvement concerns two thirds of the patients (e.g., upper urinary tract, inferior vena cava, lumbosacral plexus involvement, possible intraspinal extension). Involved regional lymph nodes are usually round and have short axis diameter of 1.5–2 cm [in contrast to a normal oval shape and a short axis diameter <1 cm]. Lymphatic mapping with sentinel lymph node biopsy is an additional tool.

The work-ups especially surgery permit clinical group classification (according to the Intergroup Rhabdomyosarcoma Study Group [IRS]):

Group	Residual tumor after resection
I	No gross or microscopic tumor
II a	Microscopic residual tumor at primary site; not involved regional lymph nodes
II b	No residual tumor at primary site; involved regional lymph nodes
II c	Microscopic residual tumor at primary site and involved regional lymph nodes
III	Gross residual tumor
IV	Distant metastases

For risk stratification (treatment and prognosis), the following criteria (International Society of Paediatric Oncology [SIOP]) are used: primary tumor site, postoperative stage (clinical group classification), histology, tumor size (≤5 versus >5 cm), and age <10 versus ≥10 years. The results of adverse biological markers may be used increasingly in the future.

Favorable sites are orbit, nonparamenigeal head/neck, (nonbladder/prostate) paratesticular, and vagina and unfavorable are parameningeal and limbs. Stages with lymph node involvement and mainly III or IV have a worse outcome. The alveolar subtype has a poorer outcome than the embryonal/botryoid. Tumor size >5 cm and age ≥10 years have a worse outcome.

The histological examination including immunohistochemistry uses features of skeletal muscle in the tumor cells and markers of muscle differentiation such as desmin and Myo D1 for the diagnosis of rhabdomyosarcoma and differentiates at least six subtypes. The incidence of anaplasia may be of prognostic significance. The alveolar subtype has two specific translocations with specific fusion transcripts that can be detected by RT-PCR (PAX3- and PAX7-FKHR), and these fusion genes are examples of biological tumor markers related to molecular genetics.

Treatment, Prognosis

In the past, two differing treatment options have been used with aggressive surgery and routine radiotherapy that were followed by prolonged chemotherapy (IRS group) and chemotherapy for attainment of as many complete remissions as possible before using surgery and radiotherapy with a shorter overall chemotherapy (SIOP group). In the last time, extensive cooperation has been evoked between the two groups.

Surgery is used today for biopsy and staging, and possible excision is site- and stage-specific situations. Surgery is more often delayed until the tumor has been reduced by chemotherapy (and possibly radiotherapy) except for paratesticular rhabdomyosarcoma. Complete excision with a margin of noninvolved tissue without mutilation should be intended. Local radiotherapy is usually not indicated in IRS group I (except for nonembryonal subtypes) and indicated for groups II and III. (EFS and OS of stage III are improved by radiotherapy and I and II need further evaluation.)

Overall survival is 70–90 % depending on the site, and the 5-year overall survival is 75 % in localized disease and 24 % in disseminated disease.

The 3-year overall or event-free survivals are between 94 and 89 % (low-risk patients with total excision of the primary tumor at a favorable site) and 66 and 62 % (limb tumors with early dissemination or with alveolar subtype).

Renunciation of radiation, brachytherapy, modulated radiotherapy, or proton treatment is one of the possibilities to avoid late sequelae. They include delayed congestive cardiac failure, high tone deafness and renal tubular acidosis, second primary malignancies, learning difficulties and failure to achieve independence, and anatomic and functional deficiencies. Some are due

to chemotherapy and/or radiotherapy and the last mentioned because of mutilating surgery.

In retroperitoneal rhabdomyo- and fibrosarcomas, complete resection and low histological grade are associated with significantly better disease-specific survival, and major resection can be performed safely in the majority of cases and completely in half of them. Five-year disease-specific survival rate is 62 % (90 % for complete vs. 36 % for incomplete resection). In **trunk rhabdomyosarcoma**, gross tumor excision should be the goal of surgical intervention (in >5 cm 10-year survival after resection at any time is 57 ± 13 %).

24.1.4 Teratoma and Other Germ Cell Tumors

Occurrence, Pathoanatomy

Although mediastinum and retroperitoneum are after the sacrococcygeal location with 10 % the second most common sites of extragonadal germ cell tumors, they are less common in the retroperitoneum than nephro- and neuroblastoma. Three fourths are observed in the first 5 years of life and half of them in infancy.

Teratoma belongs to the family of germ cell tumors and is derived from primitive germ cells. These stem from the yolk sac and are distributed in the embryo in accordance with the germ cell theory. In case of teratoma, a wide diversity of tissues foreign to the anatomical site or organ is encountered where it arises, and these tissues are not necessarily derived from all three germinal layers.

Clinical Significance

- Germ cell tumor of the retroperitoneum and mediastinum are an important differential diagnosis of abdominal and mediastinal tumor and have a variable dignity.

Clinical Presentation

The most common clinical presentation is *an abdominal tumor that is recognized by chance on clinical examination. In advanced cases, an unspecific general symptomatology and signs*

*related to obstruction of the inferior vena cava,
upper urinary tract, or intestine are observed or
hemorrhagic ascites due to tumor rupture or dissemination in the peritoneal cavity.*

On palpation, *the tumor is well delineated and
lobulated with cystic and solid parts and asymmetrical extension in relation to the midline.*

Differential Diagnosis, Work-Ups

It includes mainly other retroperitoneal and
abdominal tumors, especially paraspinal neuroblastoma or rhabdomyosarcoma and cystic ovarian tumors or mesenteric cysts.

The work-ups "ultrasound, contrast CT, and
MRI" show occasionally distinct, coarse, and
irregularly distributed calcifications at the site of
the tumor; an inhomogeneous retroperitoneal
mass possibly with cystic and solid parts, or fat;
and no close relations to the kidney or adrenal
gland. Location and extensions of the tumor display information about the resectability of the
tumor.

Increased levels of tumor markers like α-feto-
protein (AFP) and β-human chorionic gonadotropin (β-HCG) point to a malignant germ cell
tumor.

Treatment, Prognosis

Teratomas and other germ cell tumors are best
completely resected ##. This may be impossible
initially, especially in immature # or malignant
teratomas in which residual germ cell tumor must
be left between the structures of the retroperitoneum. In this situation, surgery is required for
precise staging, biopsy, and possible marking of
tumor extension by titanium clips. Treatment
after initial surgery uses the staging for extragonadal germ cell tumors (according to the
Children's Cancer Study Group and Oncology
Group) including histology, immunochemistry,
and cytogenic characterization for stratified treatment with chemotherapy, radiation, and delayed
tumor excision after shrinkage and devitalization
of the germ cell tumor.

Prognosis depends on the dignity and resectability of the tumor. Complete resection of a mature
teratoma leads to permanent cure without other
measures

24.1.5 Non-Hodgkin's Lymphoma and Hodgkin's Lymphoma

Occurrence, Pathoanatomy

About 9 new cases of non-Hodgkin's lymphoma
(NHL) and 6 new cases of Hodgkin's disease
(HL) with an increasing frequency from 5 to
11 years of age are observed in one million children <16 years of age.

In **NHL**, three main histological subgroups
exist listed with decreasing frequency: diffuse
undifferentiated lymphoma (small noncleaved
cell lymphoma), lymphoblastic lymphoma, and
histiocytoid lymphoma (large cell lymphoma,
15 %). Immunohistological, cytogenetic, and
molecular biological methods lead to refined
classifications, for example, relating to ontogeny
of B and T cells. NHL is a high-grade malignancy
with a diffuse and fast growth and corresponds
mostly to a systemic disease.

Hodgkin's lymphoma has four histological
subtypes with the malignant Reed-Sternberg cell
in common. The Rye classification differentiates
a lymphocyte predominant subtype, a subtype
with mixed cellularity, a lymphocyte depleted,
and nodular sclerotic subtype. The nodular
sclerotic subtype (>50 % and especially adolescent girls) and the mixed cellularity subtype
are the most common (one third). The
histological type may change during the disease course. Except for the lymphocyte-
depleted subtype with a poor outlook, modern
treatment has progressively effaced the different prognoses.

Clinical Significance

- The subtype "small noncleaved cell lymphoma" of non-Hodgkin's lymphoma presents in the majority of cases either as
surgical abdomen or as subacute abdominal
tumor ##.
- Hodgkin's lymphoma has from a pediatric
surgical viewpoint no practical significance
except of staging laparotomy or laparoscopy
in stage I and IIa if treatment with radiation
alone is foreseen. Its significance concerns the
primary neck lymph node and secondary
mediastinal involvement.

Clinical Presentation and Surgical Options

The reader is referred to Sects. 7.7.4, 8.2.1, and 15.2.1.

24.1.6 Tumors and Cysts of the Ovary

Occurrence, Clinical Significance

The annual incidence of new ovarian tumors is 1–2 in one million children <15 years of age. Malignancies are more frequently in the second decade, occur in about 20 % altogether, and concern two thirds of the malignant tumors of the inner genitals.

Clinical Significance

- Prenatal ultrasound has led to an increased number of ovarian cysts and tumors recognized before birth.
- About 20 % of ovarian tumors and cysts are malignant (after exclusion of one third with nonneoplastic disorders) and up to 15 % is hormonally active.
- Up to one fourth of the ovarian cysts and tumors present as surgical abdomen because of torsion, perforation, or intratumoral bleeding.
- Ovarian tumors and cysts differ from those of adulthood in several topics.

Pathoanatomy, Groups and Types

Ovarian tumors and cysts are divided in two large groups "nonneoplastic" ovarian lesions and "neoplastic" ovarian lesions. Different staging systems are used for stromal and germ cell tumors, respectively, and for ovary cancer (FIGO Ovarian Cancer Staging System). In the former staging system (Children's Cancer Group, Pediatric Oncology Group), stage I means tumor limited to ovaries, stage II microscopic residual or positive retroperitoneal lymph nodes ≤2 cm in diameter, stage III gross residual or biopsy only and retroperitoneal lymph nodes ≥2 m, and stage IV distant metastatic disease.

Nonneoplastic Ovarian Lesions. The following nine disorders are classified as nonneoplastic lesions according to the WHO: theca lutein cyst of pregnancy, follicular cyst, simple cyst, corpus luteum cyst, parovarian cyst, endometriosis, inflammatory lesions, polycystic ovaries, and inclusion cysts. The majority of the prenatally or in the first 2 years postnatally recognized ovarian lesion belongs to this group, is caused by different hormonal influences of pregnancy, and confronts the radiologist with the differentiation between simple cyst, complicated cyst, and cyst related to benign or malignant ovarian tumor.

Follicular cysts account for 50 % of nonneoplastic ovarian lesions and are frequent in the 1st two and the following prepubertal years (>80 % and >two thirds of the girls). The majority regresses or resolves spontaneously. They are unilocular, have a thin wall, and contain a clear yellowish fluid. Their size is mostly ≤2 cm in diameter, and some are larger than 2 cm (15–20 %) and may reach a size of 5–10 cm. The simple and the parovarian cyst are related to follicular cyst, cannot be differentiated from each other by ultrasound, and have a similar gross appearance (except for the parovarian cyst that lies between the leaves of the mesosalpinx). Some of the follicular cysts become symptomatic:

- Occasionally, estrogen secretion leads to precocious isosexual development independent of cyst size.
- Large cysts (≥5 cm) and cyst with a long adnexal pedicle may lead to secondary adnexal torsion, cyst rupture, intestinal obstruction, or perforation.
- Cysts may lead to acute severe or chronic recurrent abdominal pain.

Surgery by laparotomy or laparoscopy is indicated if a cyst gets symptomatic, maintains its size, increases to a critical size (≥5 cm), or poses differential diagnostic difficulties, for example, complex cyst on ultrasound in a postpubertal girl.

Large cysts in the neonate and infant correspond often to a prenatal primary adnexal torsion without recognizable ovarian tissue #. The cyst is enucleated and the adnexa only removed if ovary and fallopian tube are not recognizable any more (prenatal primary torsion).

Corpus luteum cysts regress usually. Enucleation is only indicated if the yellowish or hemorrhagic cyst persists and/or leads to chronic abdominopelvic pain or to estrogenization with disorders of menstruation.

Endometrial gland and stromal tissue implantation on the peritoneal surface of the uterus or extrauterine sites (=**endometriosis**) becomes usually clinically manifest at different times after menstruation (and rarely in young girls especially if substantial Müllerian duct remnants are present). It leads to chronic cyclic abdominopelvic pain and dysmenorrhea.

Diagnostic evaluation is carried out by MRI (foci of high T1 signal in their centers due to hemorrhage) or laparoscopy that is superior to MRI in the early stages (small petechial foci or somewhat larger plaques), and medical treatment for endometrial regression (danazol, buserelin). Advanced stages with nodules of 0.5–1.5 cm size and extensive dense adhesions are difficult to treat. Failing medical treatment or advanced stages with dense adhesions need surgical complete excision of the nodules and adhesiolysis to preserve the reproductive potential of the adnexa.

The **group of neoplastic ovarian lesions** differentiates seven types of tumor that are based on the tissue of origin as follows: epithelial tumors, sex cord-stromal tumors, steroid cell tumors, germ cell tumors, small cell carcinoma, unclassified tumors, and metastatic tumors. Neoplastic ovarian tumors may lead to surgical abdomen similar to follicular cysts such as torsion of the ovary # and hemorrhage or perforation of the tumor.

Germ Cell Tumors: They are with 60 % of all ovarian tumors the most common. The gonadal (of which 70 % are ovarian tumors) and the extragonadal sacrococcygeal forms account each for 40 % of all germ cell tumors:

In **germinomas,** no differentiation of the primordial germ cell has taken place. They occur in the ovary (former dysgerminoma) or in the testis (former seminoma). The female germinoma is with 10 % the most common malignancy of the childhood ovary. Its preferential site is dysgenetic gonads. The mostly bulky tumor with massive dimensions has a yellow color, is lobulated, and may be bilateral. **Surgery** includes unilateral adnexectomy, biopsy of the contralateral ovary, and staging. It is followed by multiagent chemotherapy.

Teratomas are mature, immature, or contain malignant components. The **mature or benign teratoma** contains possibly derivates of all three germinal layers and obligatory some embryonic tissue. They are the most common ovarian tumor especially in adolescent girls, mostly composed of solid and cystic components, and present either as a large abdominopelvic tumor with possible obstruction of the urinary and intestinal tract # or less frequently as surgical abdomen because of torsion, hemorrhage, or rupture with development of ascites or severe abdominal adhesions if the last-mentioned complication is not recognized.

For **treatment**, complete resection without intraoperative punction of the cystic parts or injury to the capsule and with preservation of the ovary(ies) is necessary whenever possible. The miliary white and gray nodules of a few millimeters corresponding to intraperitoneal glial implants need histological examination and are left in place if mature tissue is encountered. The resected tumor needs throughout histological work-up.

The **immature teratoma** has also derivates of the germinal layers and contains in addition immature neuroepithelial elements. They are graded from 0 to III dependent on the degree of immaturity and the presence and amount of immature neuroepithelial tissue. The cystic and solid mass has only a thin and transparent capsule and focuses of bleeding. It may coexist with a benign or malignant teratoma.

Stage I and grades 0–I need only adnex resection. Tumors of higher stages and grades are resected in the same way and supplemented by postoperative or pre- and postoperative chemotherapy. Biopsy of the contralateral ovary is unnecessary because immature teratoma is always unilateral and reproductive capacity should be maintained.

Endodermal sinus (yolk sac) tumors and **choriocarcinomas** stem in contrast to teratomas from extraembryonic tissue, and **embryonal carcinomas** from primordial germ cells with some differentiation. **Yolk sac tumor** is the second most common malignant germ cell tumors. The tumor has a rapid and aggressive growth and concerns in newborns and infants mainly the sacrococcygeal region and in older children and adolescents the ovary. *Abdominal pain, increased girth, and tumor becomes manifest within <1 month*. The soft and friable tumor displays often differentiation to vitelline and yolk sac elements or primitive liver or gut tissue on histological examination.

Choriocarcinomas are rare tumors that grow rapidly, present with advanced stages, and display an estrogenic effect (precocious isosexual development, menstrual disorders, and pseudopregnancy).

Whereas in yolk sac tumors unilateral **adnex resection** may be possible in some, **panhysterectomy**, **multiagent chemotherapy**, and possibly **radiation** are mostly necessary in choriocarcinomas.

Embryonal carcinomas are rare and resemble anaplastic carcinomas. All three mentioned tumors occur also as a part of a mixed germinal cell tumor.

Epithelial tumors come to about 15 % of all ovarian tumors. >10 % and <20 % are **malignant** and one third of these belong to a group with **low malignant potential**. The occurrence of bilaterality and malignity is different for the serous and mucinous subtypes with more bilaterality and minimal malignancy of the former and the reverse for the latter.

The **ovarian carcinoma** differs in several aspects from that of adulthood. If an epithelial tumor is suspected, **surgery** is performed for staging and resection. Unilateral adnex resection with bivalved biopsy of the contralateral ovary (stage I a), bilateral gonadectomy with preservation of the uterus (stage I b), and abdominal hysterectomy; bilateral adnex resection; and resection of intra-abdominal tumor including omentectomy (advanced stages) are performed depending on the stage. Advanced stages are treated with biagent chemotherapy and depending on the clinical course, radiation and/or second look surgery. In the group with low malignant potential, treatment is less aggressive.

Sex cord-stromal tumors are called functioning ovarian tumors with hormonal activity and account for about 15 % of childhood tumors of the ovary. The most frequent types are the juvenile granulosa cell and Sertoli-Leydig cell tumor.

Granulosa-theca cell tumor produces estrogen in excess and is observed in childhood as subtype named **juvenile granulosa cell tumor** that is the most frequent functioning ovarian tumor.

The clinical presentation depends on the time before (>40 % is observed in the first decade of life) or after puberty: *isosexual precocious pseudopuberty with all features in the former and menstrual disorders or amenorrhea and signs of lower abdominal tumor in the latter (hypertrophy of the clitoris does not belong to the presentation)*. Complications include rapid development of pleural effusion and ascites leading to respiratory signs and abdominal distension, and rupture of the tumor with hemorrhagic ascites (<10 %).

Work-ups include determination of estrogen in blood and urine, gonadotropin (decreased), and inhibin as possible tumor marker and ultrasound and CT or MRI for confirmation of the diagnosis and tumor staging. Isosexual precocious true puberty, feminizing adrenocortical tumor, and gonadotropin-secreting disorders must be considered in the differential diagnosis.

The tumors are usually large, unilateral (<98 %), and of stage I. Therefore, unilateral adnex resection or ovariectomy is mostly possible. Bilateral and extensive surgery becomes necessary in higher stages (<10–15 %) as part of multimodal treatment. Survival is >90 % in a cohort of such tumors (95–80 % in stages Ia–Ic).

The **Sertoli-Leydig cell tumors** (arrhenoblastoma) account for ≤30 % of all functioning ovarian tumors, secrete testosterone in excess, and somewhat more than juvenile granulosa cell tumors are malignant (>10–20 %).

In prepubertal girls, *precocious masculinization and acceleration of growth occurs, whereas postpubertal girls lose first their female sex characteristics (disorders of menstruation, loss of female habitus) and develop later masculinization (clitoris hypertrophy, hirsutism, deepening of the voice)*.

Juvenile granulosa and Sertoli-Leydig cell tumors may be associated with multiple enchondromatosis.

The work-ups include determination of testosterone, gonadotropin (decreased), α-fetoprotein as possible tumor marker, and urine 17-ketosteroids and pregnanetriol, and radiological imaging for confirmation of diagnosis and staging. The differential diagnosis must consider masculinizing adrenocortical tumor, exogenous androgens, and true hermaphroditism.

Treatment is similar to juvenile granulosa cell tumor. The usually smaller Sertoli-Leydig tumors are often of stage I although malignancy occurs somewhat more frequently, and aggressive and multimodal treatment must be applied more frequently. Prognosis depends on the stage and the histology that includes five subtypes.

The **rare functional ovarian tumors** encompass fibromas, calcified or luteinizing type of thecomas, sclerosing stromal tumor, sex cord tumors with annular tubules, and the otherwise not specified steroid cell tumor. Fibromas may be associated with basal cell nevus syndrome and sex cord tumors with annular tubules with Peutz-Jeghers syndrome. Their hormonal effects are different with preference of androgen (such as steroid tumor and thecomas) and occasionally estrogen secretion. The treatment is the same as in juvenile granular cell tumor or gross tumor resection (fibromas, bilateral thecomas, sclerosing stromal tumor).

24.1.7 Liver Tumors

Occurrence, Pathoanatomy

Three fourths of all hepatic mass lesions are malignant tumors in childhood. The two most common malignancies "**hepatoblastoma**" (with 65 %) and "**hepatocellular carcinoma**" (with 25 % of the malignant tumors) occur in 1–2 of one million children <16 years of age per year.

The hepatocellular carcinoma is increased in chronic inflammatory, infectious, and metabolic liver disorders and congenital anomalies such as biliary atresia and hepatitis B or EMG (Beckwith-Wiedemann) syndrome and familial adenomatous polyposis. Endemic hepatitis B is responsible for predominance of hepatocellular carcinoma in some regions of Africa and Asia.

Clinical Significance

- Hepatoblastoma is resectable in the majority of cases, whereas this is not the case for hepatocellular carcinoma at the time of diagnosis.
- Resection needs large surgery and survival is possible for two thirds of hepatoblastoma and only for one third of hepatocellular carcinoma when complete resection has been possible.
- The possibility of development of a hepatocellular carcinoma must always be considered in children with chronic liver disorder.

Clinical Presentation

Hepatoblastoma is observed mainly at 1–3 years of age, whereas hepatocellular carcinoma is a preferred malignancy of schoolchildren. Ultrasound permits occasionally recognition of a developing hepatoblastoma.

In more than 90 %, an abdominal mass # and/or abdominal distension is observed, and substantial weight loss, abdominal pain, and vomiting are less common. The mass is more frequently confined to the right and less frequently to the left liver #, and enlargement is either diffuse or nodulus.

Differential Diagnosis, Work-Ups

The differential diagnosis includes the majority of the other abdominal tumors, other causes of hepatic mass lesions, and hepatomegaly. More specifically, a benign vascular tumor #, sarcoma, mesenchymal hamartoma, and other mass lesions of the liver including both forms of echinococcosis and bilateral Wilms' tumor # or stage IV-S neuroblastoma of infancy with hepatomegaly #.

The aim of radiological imaging is assignment of the abdominal tumor to the liver. Determination of the extension, composition, resectability, and finally of dignity and specific diagnosis of the tumor is possible as well. Ultrasound, MRI, and (spiral) CT are the most useful tools that permit also evaluation of the integrity of the major blood vessels and their relation to the tumor, exclusion of lung metastases, and tumor persistence and recurrence on follow-up.

Complete blood and platelet count, coagulation profile, and liver parameters are important for exclusion of general and hepatic functional disorders. Anemia and thrombocytosis or thrombocytopenia is encountered more frequently than hyperbilirubinemia. AFP (α-fetoprotein) is increased in >90 %. This unspecific tumor marker is mainly used for follow-up (persistence or recurrence of tumor) and less for initial diagnosis or prognosis.

Because radiological imaging is not 100 % reliable for the specific diagnosis and to a lesser degree for the respectability, diagnostic laparotomy or at least surgical biopsy from a metastatic site has been recommended.

Different staging systems exist worldwide. The intergoup (CCG/POG) staging system of both malignancies is based on the findings at surgery, outcome of the initial operative procedure, and the histopathological result. At surgery, hepatoblastoma presents as a bulky, nodular, and encapsulated mass # that is even in case of bilobar involvement mostly resectable. In contrast, hepatocellular carcinoma displays either a bilobar multicentric nodular mass or diffuse intrahepatic spread, and complete resection appears often impossible at the time of diagnostic laparotomy. In hepatoblastoma, six subtypes are differentiated of whom the fetal subtype has possibly a favorable effect on outcome if complete resection is possible.

Treatment, Prognosis

Treatment options are guided by the experience that the best outcomes have been achieved by initial complete resection but that this is not always possible, is combined with major surgery, and may be associated with major morbidity and possible mortality. In addition, by the experience that hepatoblastoma differs from hepatocellular carcinoma relating to the response rate to multiagent chemotherapy (80 % vs. 20 %); complete primary, delayed primary, or secondary resectability (80 % vs. ≥ 30 %); and radiosensitivity (sensitivity vs. resistance).

Therefore, either initial surgery with possibly complete resection # is followed by multiagent chemotherapy or with delayed primary or secondary resection (CCG/POG and German Cooperative Pediatric Liver Study), or primary multiagent chemotherapy is followed by complete resection if possible (SIOP).

The different multiagent regimes have different response rates and toxicities. Depending on the resectability, response to chemotherapy, and stage, arterial transcatheter chemoembolization, hepatic arterial infusion, or radiation of limited tissue fields are applied or selective hepatic transplantation for both malignancies if the children are free of extrahepatic tumor and not completely resectable after chemotherapy.

Today, disease-free 3.5-year survival amounts to >80 % for hepatoblastoma and 30 % for hepatocellular carcinoma (1.6-year survival >70 % and >15 % in SIOPL-1).

24.1.8 Pancreatic and Adrenal Gland Tumors

24.1.8.1 Tumor-like Disorders and Tumors of the Pancreas

Occurrence, Pathology

Hyperinsulinism especially in the neonate and infant plays an important role among the actually rare tumors of the pancreas. It is defined as elevation of insulin level which is associated with hypoglycemia and is observed as autosomal recessive inherited disorder with dysregulation of insulin storage and release in the neonate and infant or as islet cell adenoma (insulinoma) in toddlers.

Clinical Significance

- Neonatal and infantile hyperinsulinism is the most common cause of persistent hypoglycemia in the first month of life and in 50 % thereafter.
- Persistent or episodic hypoglycemia leads to cerebral damage and mental retardation if it is not recognized and treated immediately.
- Insulinoma becomes usually symptomatic after infancy.
- Different cystic and solid tumors occur in the pancreas albeit very rarely.

Clinical Presentation

Severe forms of neonatal hyperinsulinism lead to *irritability and seizures shortly after birth*. The other forms display earlier or later episodic hypoglycemia or become symptomatic under stress. The symptomatology of hypoglycemia is often less dramatic and includes *neurological and neurovegetative signs*, for example, hypotonia, abnormal reflexes and pallor, and sweating although severe manifestations may be observed as well. The familial hyperinsulinism may be associated with multiple endocrine adenomatosis.

Differential Diagnosis, Work-Ups

It encompasses disorders with the described neurovegetative and neurological signs up to convulsions and coma. History, clinical examination, and work-ups must consider specifically disorders that lead to permanent or episodic hypoglycemia: endocrine deficiencies, inborn errors of metabolism, and hyperinsulinism. The ketotic hypoglycemia is the most frequent disorder with hypoglycemia beyond infancy and Beckwith-Wiedemann syndrome associated with omphalocele is an inborn error of metabolism, displays spontaneous recovery with time, and is well known to the pediatric surgeon.

Hyperinsulinism is confirmed by the following test results: (1) Insulin is increased (>10 uU/ml) and glucose decreased (<50 mg/dl) under different conditions, (2) glucose infusion rate >10 mg/kg/min is necessary for maintenance of glucose levels >35 mg/dl without glucosuria, (3) low levels of free fatty acid and ketone bodies occur at hypoglycemia, and (4) glycemic response to glucagon is observed despite hypoglycemia. In addition, the C peptide is usually increased. Radiological imaging is used for exclusion of localized tumors.

Treatment, Prognosis

Treatment of hypoglycemia needs a central venous line and includes an infusion of 15–20 % glucose and frequent feedings as primary measures. It is followed by short- and long-term medicaments (octreotide and diazoxide) with a success rate of <50–75 % depending on the severity of the hyperinsulinism.

Early surgery is **indicated** in failure of medicamentous therapy, insulinoma, and if long-term medication is not desired or unreliable.

Surgery encompasses exposition of the entire pancreas; inspection, palpation, and intraoperative ultrasound for exclusion of islet cell adenoma(s) and biopsies of the pancreas; and resection of ≥95 % of the pancreas with preservation of pancreas tissue adjacent to the choledochus. The plasma level of glucose should be checked intra- and postoperatively.

About 5 % need a second operation, 10 % diazoxide supplementation, and <10 % insulin. Reported percentage of mental retardation, for example 12.5 %, depends largely on the recognition of hyperinsulinism in time and its effective and continued treatment.

Pancreatic tumors are rare and include different types of cystadenoma, teratomatous cyst, different types of pancreas carcinoma, and endocrine adenomas such as insuloma, gastrinoma, and vipoma.

Insulinomas may be present already in infancy, but they become usually symptomatic in preschool age or later. A plasma insulin-to-glucose ratio >1.0 (normal value <0.4) and increased C peptide levels are diagnostic. Although 90 % are benign and 80 % occur as single lesion, pre- and intraoperative location of insuloma is difficult despite work-up with ultrasound, angio CT, selective celiac arteriography, or venous sampling of insulin by transhepatic access (small and/or multiple tumors distributed throughout the entire pancreas and possibly combined with nesidioblastosis). Therefore, insulinomas are enucleated if possible or treated with 80–90 % resection of the pancreas.

Gastrinomas are associated with Zollinger-Ellison syndrome and a part of multiple endocrine neoplasms (type I). Hypergastrinemia is treated with gastric acid blockers, and the insulinoma is resected if a solitary tumor is present without metastatic disease. Total gastrectomy is only performed if the medicamentous treatment fails or in case of advanced gastrinoma.

The very rare **vipoma** is often related to neurogenic tumors and leads to severe diarrhea due to the vasoactive intestinal polypeptide (=VIP). Surgical resection of the tumor is recommended whenever possible because half of them are malignant.

Treatment of the pancreatic tumors depends on the type and dignity of the individual neoplasm, and surgical resection plays a major role.

24.1.8.2 Adrenal Gland Tumors

24.1.8.2.1 Cushing's Syndrome
Pathophysiology and Pathoanatomy, Occurrence

Cushing's syndrome is caused by hyperactivity of the adrenal cortex and leads to hyperinsulinemia. It has a comparable clinical significance with that of pheochromocytoma of the adrenal medulla. The **corticotrophin-dependent form** is characterized by stimulation of the adrenal cortex due to high levels of corticotrophin, whereas excessive production of cortisol by adrenocortical abnormal tissue leads to the same clinical picture in **corticotrophin-independent Cushing's syndrome**. **Cushing's disease** is caused by a pituitary corticotroph tumor and is the most common cause of Cushing's syndrome. **Therapeutic Cushing's syndrome** is in the foreground of children, and the less frequent **Cushing's disease** is observed in 85 %, adrenocortical adenoma or carcinoma in 15 %, and extra-adrenal or adrenal medullary corticotroph tumor in 5 % of childhood neoplastic Cushing's syndrome. Adrenocortical adenoma or carcinoma is relatively frequent in infancy. Carcinomas account for one third up to >50 %, are usually large tumors, and possibly associated with related disorders. Corticotrophin plasma levels are low and dexamethasone fails to suppress cortisol secretion in adenomas and carcinomas.

Clinical Significance

- Cushing's syndrome is an indication of anterior pituitary, adrenocortical, or extra-adrenal corticotroph neoplasm after exclusion of the more frequent medicamentous form.
- Location of the cause may be a challenging task after laboratory confirmation of Cushing's syndrome.

Clinical Presentation

The characteristic appearance is mainly observed in older children and includes *truncal and facial obesity that contrasts to thin limbs, abdominal striae and peripheral edema, arterial hypertension, growth retardation of the skeleton, and fragile skin and bones with possible pathological fractures. It leads to virilization of the boys and to acne, hirsutism, and amenorrhea in female teenagers.* In younger children, *obesity is more generalized and combined with muscular atrophy and growth retardation.*

Work-Ups, Differential Diagnosis

They are used for confirmation and location of the causes of Cushing's syndrome. Twenty-four hour urinary free cortisol ($\geq$100 µg/day), plasma cortisol, and urinary 17-hydroxycorticosteroid determination belong to the basic examinations. Low-dose dexamethasone suppression test and corticotrophin-releasing hormone stimulation test are additional examinations. An algorhithm of laboratory tests and radiological imaging is used for location.

Treatment, Prognosis

The tumor of **Cushing's disease** is completely resected under microscopic control by transsphenoidal approach. Eighty-five to ninety percent resection of the anterior pituitary is performed if no localized mass can depicted. Complete tumor resection leads to endocrinological deficit in one seventh. Bilateral adrenal resection is discussed if multimodal treatment of Cushing's disease fails. Cushing's syndrome caused by **adrenocortical adenoma** needs unilateral adrenalectomy and contralateral biopsy. Cortisol replacement is indicated if the contralateral adrenal cortex is atrophic or both adrenal glands have been removed. In **adrenocortical carcinoma**, transabdominal complete excision or debulking is performed that includes local metastases and ipsilateral nephrectomy and later resection of the functioning metastases.

Resection is also indicated in **corticotrophic tumors** of the bronchus, thyroid gland, or other locations including the adrenal medulla.

Prognosis of survival depends on the dignity and stage of the tumors and the possibility of complete resection. Sequels of the disease and possibly multimodal treatment (e.g., radiotherapy of Cushing's disease) are possible in every case.

24.1.8.2.2 Pheochromocytoma
Occurrence, Pathoanatomy and Pathophysiology

Pheochromocytoma belongs to the most important adrenal medullary tumors although only 10 % of them are observed in childhood. The mean age of presentation is 9–10 years of age and about 10 % are familial cases. The tumor is bilateral in 25–50 % and has an extramedullary site in 25–30 % (extra- and intra-adrenal paraganglia along the sympathetic paraganglia of the aorta).

The catecholamines (with a higher proportion of norepinephrine than epinephrine) are secreted by the pheochromocytoma and lead to arterial hypertension that is mostly sustained in children although episodic crises with very high values are also observed in children.

Clinical Significance

- Numerous and colorful signs mimic several disorders of childhood that lead to erroneous measures especially in seeming emergency conditions and delay the correct diagnosis.
- Rapid recognition and treatment of pheochromocytoma avoids life-threatening complications and sequels of arterial hypertension.

Clinical Presentation

Sustained arterial hypertension develops rapidly. It is accompanied with *neurovegetative signs in more than half of the patients such as headache, nausea, pallor, intermittent fever, sweating, and weight loss.* In addition, numerous symptoms and signs may be recorded which mimic other disorders, for example, diabetes mellitus, hyperthyroidism, cerebrovascular and psychiatric disorders, and emergency conditions such as gastrointestinal hemorrhage or surgical abdomen (e.g., due to acute abdominal pain or lumbago). Depending on the preponderance of norepinephrine or epinephrine, diastolic hypertension and bradycardia or systolic hypertension, arrhythmia, and tachycardia are in the foregrounds.

Episodic hypertension with possible heart failure, encephalopathy, and death occurs relatively rarely in childhood. On the other hand, pheochromocytoma may be associated with neurological disorders, for example, neurofibromatosis or multiple endocrine adenomatosis or neoplasms (type II).

Differential Diagnosis, Work-Ups

It includes other causes of arterial hypertension and several disorders that are mimicked by the numerous and colorful symptomatology.

The work-ups concern confirmation of the clinically suspected pheochromocytoma and its location.

Twenty-four-hour urine secretion of the norepinephrine and epinephrine metabolites free catecholamines, vanillylmandelic acid (VMA), and metanephrine (MN) are diagnostic if they exceed 100, 7, and 1.3 mg. In addition, plasma catecholamines are determined by radioenzyme assay. Increased levels of homovanillic acid (HVA) are encountered in malignant pheochromocytoma. CT allows location of the tumor in >95 %. Small, extrarenal, recurrent, or residual tumor is recognized better by MRI. Location by blood sampling at various levels of the inferior vena cava is used if it is impossible by radiological imaging.

Treatment, Prognosis

Tumor resection is the golden standard of treatment though only successful if several pre-, intra-, and postoperative measures are taken. The children need preoperatively α-adrenergic blockers to reduce the elevated arterial pressure and to avoid crises of hypertension, re-expansion of the vascular system (because of hypovolemia), and possibly nutritional support. During surgery, β-adrenergic blockers are added and blood pressure must be kept low initially and after devascularization of the tumor high. Continuous recording of electrocardiogram, arterial, and central venous pressure, and urinary output are indispensable. Arterial hypertension may persist after surgery for maximum 2–3 weeks and requires α-adrenergic blockers, or persistent hypotonia needs norepinephrine for several days.

Surgery: Because >95 % of the pheochromocytomas concern the abdomen (adrenal medulla or paraganglioma of one or both sides), the transabdominal access must visualize both adrenal glands completely, the para-aortic sympathetic paraganglions, mesentery, and pelvis. The right adrenal gland is more frequently involved and holds the danger of the injury to the short main vein. After division of the veins, the arteries are ligated and the adrenal gland(s) dissected free and removed.

The operative mortality is quoted with <2 %. Persistent or recurrent hypertension corresponds to second pheochromocytoma, that has not been removed or has grown since the first operation, or recurrence of a malignant form.

Regular follow-ups with measurement of the arterial pressure and urine catecholamines are recommended for at least 5 years. Malignant pheochromocytoma with nonfunctioning metastases occurs in children in <6 %. MBIG is used for detection of metastasis in the skeleton or other organs and possibly for their treatment.

Other neoplasms of the adrenal gland are rare and include virilizing (boys and girls) and feminizing tumors (usually boys and malignancies), and hyperaldosteronism due to bilateral hyperfunction with or without hyperplasia or adenoma. The former is mainly observed in children and needs medicamentous treatment.

Small cysts may be an incidental finding at surgery or radiological imaging that bear the sequel of perinatal adrenal hemorrhage due to anoxia. Large cysts of the same origin feign a tumor and are resected by adrenalectomy.

24.1.9 Rare Tumors

The reader is referred to the quoted literature.

24.2 Masses or Cysts Caused by Anomalies, Inflammations, and Injuries

24.2.1 Mesenteric and Omental Cysts

Occurrence, Pathoanatomy

Although the rare mesenteric and omental cysts are observed at any age, most of those that occur in childhood are brought to attention before 10 years of age.

Whereas **lymphangiomas** are confined to the retroperitoneum or mesentery and display a cyst wall with several layers, **mesenterial and omental cysts** have a simple wall and concern mainly mesentery or omentum. The mesenterial cysts occur along the whole gastrointestinal tract (small bowel>large bowel>retroperitoneum), most commonly in the ileal mesentery, and more frequently than omental cysts. Single and/or multilocular cysts are encountered more frequently than multiple and/or unilocular forms. Their sizes vary from a few centimeters to 10–40 cm in the three dimensions and contain a clear, chylous, or hemorrhagic fluid.

Clinical Significance

- In children of any age with a subacute or chronic symptomatology and a palpable and freely movable abdominal mass, a mesenteric or omental cyst must be considered in the differential diagnosis

Clinical Presentation

In more than half of the cases, *a chronic or subacute abdominal symptomatology combined with a visible and/or palpable mass is encountered,* and one fourth is symptomless; *the abdominal distension and/or mass is an incidental finding or is detected by chance* on prenatal ultrasound, postnatal work-ups, or at surgery performed for other reasons. In less than one fourth, a *surgical abdomen develops because of compression or stretching of the intestine by the cyst.*

On clinical examination, *mostly a mass is palpable that feels soft or cystic, mobile, and may be difficult to delineate* dependent on location and size. Very large cysts *may simulate ascites* and display dullness and a fluid wave on percussion. Occasionally, the clinical findings may be modified by the inherent cyst complications.

Cyst complications include rapid enlargement by hemorrhage, cyst torsion or rupture, intestinal volvulus, cyst infection (with possible peritonitis and septicemia), and rarely obstruction of the biliary or upper urinary tract.

Differential Diagnosis, Work-Ups

It includes disorders with abdominal tumor or surgical abdomen, and more specifically intestinal duplication cyst; choledochal cyst; congenital or acquired cysts of spleen, pancreas, or kidney; gross hydronephrosis; ovarian cyst; cystic teratoma or dermoid cyst; hydatid cyst; or ascites.

Plain abdominal X-ray, ultrasound, and CT with GI contrast display different information: A homogeneous mass displaces the intestine to either side on the plain X-ray, the cysts have a thin wall, are filled with fluid and contain septa, and are combined with internal echos on ultrasound. Gastrointestinal contrast study # or CT with p.o. contrast demonstrates mostly the origin of the cyst(s) and the pathoantomical relation of the bowel to the cyst.

Treatment, Prognosis
Complete cyst resection should be accomplished whenever possible. Whereas cyst enucleation or resection is possible in omental cysts, mesenteric cysts need in >50 % additional segmental intestinal resection and primary anastomosis due to the close relation of the cyst with the intestine #.

Rarely, resection remains incomplete especially in retroperitoneal cyst location. The residual part should be marsupialized and sclerosed or electrocauterized.

In most cases, permanent cure can be expected. The recurrence rate of >5 % in relatively large populations concern incomplete resections without additional measures and retroperitoneal site.

24.2.2 Other Malformative Abdominal Masses and Cysts

Other malformative masses and cysts include choledochal cyst, intestinal duplication, hydro-(metro-) colpos and hemato-(metro-) colpos, and upper obstructive uropathies. The reader is referred to the corresponding Sects. 25.2, 23.6, 33.3, and 26.1.1.

24.2.3 Abdominal Masses and Cysts Related to Inflammation

Abdominal wall abscess, perityphlitic and other intra-abdominal abscesses, paranephritic abscess including xanthogranulomatous pyelonephritis, empyema of the gall bladder, and liver abscess belong to this group. The reader is referred to the Index.

24.2.4 Abdominal Masses and Cysts Related to Trauma and Other Causes

This group includes posttraumatic pseudocyst of kidney, spleen, and pancreas and renal vein thrombosis. The reader is referred to Sects. 16.1 and 26.6.

24.3   Abdominal Masses and Cysts due to Parasitoses

24.3.1 Echinococcosis (Hydatid Disease)

Occurrence, Forms
Echinococcosis is a relatively rare parasitosis in western countries but is increasingly observed due to migration and travel activities. Endemic regions are the Mediterranean countries, Middle East, and Australia.

Echinococcus granulosus is the responsible parasite of the cystic form (echinococcal abscess) and is observed in three fourths of hydatid disease in Middle Europe. It is caused by the larval stage of the dog tapeworm for which the sheep is also a host. *Echinococcus multilocularis* causes the alveolar form and accounts for one fourth of hydatid disease. The main hosts of *Echinococcus alveolaris* are dogs and foxes, and occasionally man as intermediate host, and the ova are transmitted by direct contact, water, and unwashed food such as berries and mushrooms.

Clinical Significance
• Hydatid disease is mostly unexpectedly recognized if it is not epidemic as in most western countries. A history of migration or travel activities needs special consideration in respect to echinococcosis.

- Rarely, hydatid disease manifests as surgical abdomen, acute respiratory disorder, or anaphylactic shock because of spontaneous cyst rupture.

Clinical Presentation

The observation that children develop delayed symptoms and signs is explained by a long incubation time combined with a slow growth of the cyst(s). This applies even more to the alveolar form that occurs in western Europe in several circumscribed endemic places and lasts 10–15 years till clinical manifestation.

The cysts of *Echinococcus granularis* occur in up to 90 % as single cyst in one organ (such as liver, lung, and spleen) and less frequently in ≥2 organs and composed of two or more cysts. The liver is in ≥60 % and the lung in ≤30 % involved.

They cause vague or distinct intermittent abdominal pain and lead to hepatomegaly or a circumscribed liver enlargement simulating abdominal tumor, or to a respiratory symptomatology.

The alveolar form manifests often as *liver tumor* in early adulthood.

Differential Diagnosis, Work-Ups

Differential diagnosis includes disorders with chronic (vague) abdominal pain, hepatomegaly, or abdominal tumor and rarely surgical abdomen. In radiological imaging, other cystic lesions of liver or lung must be considered, for example, amebic abscesses or lung cyst and CCAM.

Ultrasound and contrast CT yield a round or oval homogeneous mass with diminished translucency. The cyst may display an air-fluid level or calcified rim, or multiple cysts of different size are present, or a characteristic daughter cyst within a cyst is visible. In the alveolar form, preoperative delineation of the mass including its extension and relation to the large vessels by MRI is mandatory.

For specific diagnosis, indirect hemagglutinin assay, complement fixation test, or immunoelectrophoretic assay should be applied in combination.

Treatment, Prognosis

If possible, cystectomy after disinfection of the content with a special funnel and 20 % NaCl solution should be performed. Enucleation within the host capsule of connective tissue is possible in 80 %. Otherwise, atypical or segmental resections are performed. Albendazole medication for 1–2 months should avoid recurrences.

The alveolar form needs albendazole combined with complete resection identical to tumor surgery.

The alveolar form leads untreated within 10–15 years to death in >90 % and predisposes to recurrence if treated by resection. Recurrences after the cystic form are caused by spontaneous or intraoperative cyst rupture with spillage of scolices or due to multiple cysts that have not been recognized or were not recognizable before surgery.

24.4 Abdominal Tumors Related to Other Causes

24.4.1 Ascites

Occurrence, Causes

Abnormal accumulation of fluid in the peritoneal cavity occurs in any age group and for numerous causes.

Six groups of ascites are in the fore of clinical consideration in pediatric surgery after exclusion of cardiovascular, gastrointestinal, and renal disorders:

1. Ascites in chronic inflammatory, infectious, or metabolic liver disorders, for example, biliary atresia or cirrhosis; in portal hypertension, for example, suprahepatic and intrahepatic obstruction; and in liver tumors
2. Bilious ascites because of disorders of the biliary tree, for example, spontaneous perforation of the common bile duct in neonates, hepatic and biliary tree injury in older children, or after injury during surgery
3. Chylous ascites because of malformations or acquired disorders of the lymphatic system in newborns and older children

4. Urinary ascites because of urinary tract malformations in newborns, for example, urethral valves
5. Ascites because of spontaneous or traumatic rupture of cysts, cystic disorders, hollow organs, and benign or malignant tumors
6. Ascites combined with synthetic implants, for example, peritoneal dialysis catheter or ventriculoperitoneal shunt

Clinical Significance

• Ascites is usually a sign of a specific underlying disorder.
• Ascites may simulate an abdominal tumor or a surgical abdomen and lead to a secondary respiratory distress syndrome or respiratory symptomatology.
• Ascites becomes symptomatic because of infection or dysfunction of the implanted system.

Clinical Presentation

Abdominal distension caused by ascites displays the following characteristics: *The prominent abdomen extends to the flanks, the navel is either effaced or prolapsing, and the abdominal veins become visible.*

The dullness on percussion is displaced by change of the trunk position, and a fluid wave may be felt by contralateral percussion.

These characteristics become more pronounced dependent on the amount and velocity of development of ascites, the age group, cause of ascites, and the absence or presence of infection. *A scrotal and/or testicular swelling is observed occasionally with possible discoloration according to the type of ascites.*

Differential Diagnosis, Work-Ups

Ascites must be differentiated from abdominal tumor, for example, mesenteric and omental cyst and surgical abdomen, especially from primary and secondary peritonitis, and from meteorism.

Work-ups are performed for confirmation of the clinical diagnosis of ascites and for evaluation of its characteristics and specific cause.

Plain abdominal X-ray in supine position shows a diffuse opacity with minimal intestinal gas or an increased distance between the intestinal loops and between colon and lateral abdominal wall. Ultrasound permits recognition of ascites (even in case of small amounts of fluid if looked at specific sites), its possible shifting (freely movable vs. encapsulated ascites), and its content (clear vs. turbid ascites). CT may be used for delineation of the cause of ascites, its location, and extension.

Depending on the suspected cause according to history (the probable cause of ascites is often known) and clinical examination, radiological imaging is not necessary or only used for ultrasound-guided paracentesis. Gross examination of ascites and determination of its components including Gram stain and cultures are essential for the specific diagnosis. The main possible components are protein and albumin, total and direct bilirubin, lipids and lymphocytes, urea and creatinine, and inflammatory and other cells. See also Chap. 14.2.6.

Treatment, Prognosis

Both depend on the cause of ascites and the possibility of effective treatment.

Group 1: Repeated paracenteses, external drainage with or without an implanted device, or porto- or peritoneovenous shunts must be considered if medical treatment is ineffective or the underlying disorder can be treated only with supportive measures. Medical treatment consists of NaCl and fluid restriction, albumin replacement, and diuretics. Regular cultures of ascites should be performed.

Group 2: Laparotomy and continuous drainage of bile combined with antibiotics are necessary in spontaneous perforation that is usually followed by closure of the perforation site. In abdominal trauma, intervention depends on the type of injury to liver and biliary tree.

Group 3: The primary procedure depends on the age group and cause of chylous ascites – parenteral nutrition followed by MCT feeding till spontaneous recovery in neonatal chylous ascites and laparotomy in acquired forms. For persistent chylous ascites without recognizable leak, a peritoneovenous shunt may be an option.

Group 4: Newborns with obstructive uropathy are usually involved (e.g., posterior urethral valves or hydronephrosis) in urinary ascites in which the minor leak of bladder or upper urinary tract should not be revised. Instead, continuous drainage of the bladder or pelvis is necessary by bladder catheter or percutaneous nephrostomy combined with antibiotics. After spontaneous closure of the leak, further work-up and treatment of the malformation is necessary.

Group 5: Emergency or delayed laparotomies are necessary for cyst or tumor resection (rupture of malignancies causes change to higher stages) and for resection or reconstructive surgery of the involved organs.

Group 6: Different therapeutic approaches are applied. Shunt infection needs removal of the whole shunt followed by external ventricular drainage and re-shunting as soon as the infection is cured. In infected peritoneal dialysis, repeated medication of antibiotics permits maintenance of the peritoneal dialysis. Nevertheless, removal of catheter may become necessary followed by reinsertion after clearing of peritoneal infection.

2405 Distortion pyelocaliceal system	2421 Perinatal torsion ovarian cyst
2406 Tumor extension renal vein	2422 Torsion ovarian tumor
2407 Wilms' tumor, total involvement kidney	2423 Teratoma ovary
2408 Wilms' tumor, partial involvement kidney	2424 Visible/palpable hepatic tumor
2409 Lower pole resection, bilateral Wilms' tumor	2425 Hepatoblastoma
2410 Fibula metastasis neuroblastoma	2426 Hemangioendothelioma liver
2411 Spinal extension neuroblastoma	2427 Bilateral Wilms' tumor
2412 Displacement pyelocaliceal system	2428 Liver metastases neuroblastoma
2413 Lymph node metastasis neck	2429 Hepatoblastoma
2414 Liver metastasis neuroblastoma 4-S	2430 GI contrast study, mesenteric cyst
2415 Primary resection neuroblastoma	2431 Trilocular mesenteric cyst
2416 Retroperitoneal mature teratoma	

24.4.2 Other Causes Simulating Abdominal Tumor

Meteorism, hepatomegaly and splenomegaly, fecaloma, or megavesica of different origin give occasionally the impression of abdominal tumor and must therefore always be considered in the differential diagnosis of abdominal tumor.

Webcodes

The following webcodes can be used on www.psurg.net for further images and data.

2401 Visible/palpable nephroblastoma	2417 Retroperitoneal mature teratoma
2402 Left leg hypertrophy	2418 Retroperitoneal immature teratoma
2403 Hematoma/rupture nephroblastoma	2419 Abdominal non-Hodgkin's lymphoma, operable
2404 Simple renal cyst	2420 Abdominal non-Hodgkin's lymphoma, nonoperable

Bibliography

General and Differential Diagnosis

Andreou D, Tunn PU (2009) Sentinel node biopsy in soft tissue sarcoma. Recent Results Cancer Res 179:25–36

Hussein N, Osman Y, Sarhan O, el-Diasty T, Dawaba M (2009) *Xanthogranulomatous pyelonephritis* in pediatric patients: effect of surgical approach. Urology 73:1247–1250

Kaatsch P (2010) Epidemiology of childhood cancer. Cancer Treat Rev 36:277–285

Kolesnikov-Gauthier H, Leblond P, Rocourt N, Carpentier P (2011) Contribution of FDG-PET in the management of pediatric sarcomas in 2011. Bull Cancer 98:501–514

Moore SW, Satgé D, Sasco AJ, Zimmermann A, Plaschkes J (2003) The epidemiology of neonatal tumours. Report of an international working group. Pediatr Surg Int 19:509–519

Pearson D, Steward J-K (1969) Malignant disease in juveniles. Proc R Soc Med 62(62):685–688

Rohr A et al (2002) Radiological assessment of small bowel obstruction. Value of conventional enteroclysis and dynamic MR-enteroclysis. Rofo 174:1158–1164

Young JL Jr, Miller RW (1975) Incidence of malignant tumors in U.S. children. J Pediatr 86:254–258

Section 24.1.1

Biemann Othersen H Jr, Tagge EP, Garvin AJ (1998) Wilms' tumor. In: O'Neill JA Jr et al (eds) Pediatric surgery, vol I, 5th edn. Mosby, St. Louis

Breslow NE (2010) Pregnancy outcome after treatment for Wilms' tumor: a report from the national Wilms tumor long-term follow-up study. J Clin Oncol 28:2824–2830

Cooke A, Deshpande AV, La Hei ER, Kellie S, Arbuckle S, Cummins G (2009) Ectopic nephrogenic rests in children: the clinicosurgical implications. J Pediatr Surg 44:e13–e16

Davidoff AM (2009) Wilms' tumor. Curr Opin Pediatr 21:357–364

Graf N, Semler O, Reinhard H (2004) Prognosis of Wilm's tumor in the course of the SIOP trials and studies. Urologe A 43:421–428

Green DM, Lange JM, Peabody EM, Grigorieva NN, Peterson SM, Kalapurakal JA, Breslow NE (2010) Pregnancy outcome after treatment for Wilms tumor: a report from the national Wilms tumor long-term follow-up study. J Clin Oncol 28:2824–2830

Gupta S, Araya CE, Dharnidharka VR (2010) Xanthogranulomatous pyelonephritis in pediatric patients; case report and review of literature. J Pediatr Urol 6: 355–358

Paya K, Horcher E, Lawrenz K, Rebhandl W, Zoubek A (2001) Bilateral Wilms' tumor – surgical aspects. Eur J Pediatr Surg 11:99–104

Sarhan OM, El-Baz M, Sarhan MM, Ghali AM, Ghoneim MA (2010) Bilateral Wilms' tumors: single-center experience with 22 cases and literature review. Urology 76:946–951

Spreafico F, Pritchard Jones K, Malogowkin MH, Bergeron C, Hale J, de Kraker J, Dallorso S, Acha T, de Camargo B, Dome JS, Graf N (2009) Treatment of relapsed Wilms tumors: lessons learned. Expert Rev Anticancer Ther 9:1807–1815

Vujanic GM, Sandstedt B (2010) The pathology of Wilms' tumour (nephroblastoma): the International Society of Paediatric Oncology approach. J Clin Pathol 63:102–109

Vujanic GM, Harms D, Sandstedt B, Weirich A, de Kraker J, Delemarre JF (1999) New definitions of focal and diffuse aplasia in Wilms tumor: the International Society of Paediatric Oncology (SIOP) experience. Med Pediatr Oncol 32:317–323

Wilde JC, Lameris W, van Hasselt EH, Molyneux EM, Heij HA, Borgstein EG (2010) Challenges and outcome of Wilms' tumour management in a resource-constrained setting. Afr J Paediatr Surg 7:159–162

Wright KD, Green DM, Daw NC (2009) Late effects of treatment for Wilms tumor. Pediatr Hematol Oncol 26:407–413

Section 24.1.2

Berthold F, Hero B (2000) Neuroblastoma: current drug therapy recommendations as part of the total treatment approach. Drugs 59:1261–1277

Bodmer N, Grotzer M (2005) Solide Tumoren bei Kindern. Neuroblastome, Wilms-Tumoren, Medulloblastome. Onkologie 2:14–20

Brodeur GM, Seeger RC, Barrett A et al (1988) International criteria for diagnosis, staging, and response to treatment in patients with neuroblastoma. J Clin Oncol 6:1874–1881

Escobar MA, Grosfeld JL, Powell RL, West KW, Scherer LR 3rd, Fallon RJ, Rescorla FJ (2006) Long-term outcomes in patients with stage IV neuroblastoma. J Pediatr Surg 41:377–381

Green DM, Lange JM, Peabody EM, Grigorieva NN, Peterson SM, Kalapurakal JA, Grosfeld JL (1998) Neuroblastoma. In: O'Neill JA Jr et al (eds) Pediatric surgery, vol I, 5th edn. Mosby, St. Louis

Moon SB, Park KW, Jung SE, Youn WJ (2009) Neuroblastoma: treatment outcome after incomplete resection of primary tumors. Pediatr Surg Int 25: 789–793

Section 24.1.3

Blakely ML, Andrassy RJ, Raney RB, Anderson JR, Wiener ES, Rodeberg DA, Paidas CN, Lobe TE, Crist WM, Intergroup Rhabdomyosarcoma Studies I through IV (2003) Prognostic factors and surgical treatment guidelines for children with rhabdomyosarcoma of the perineum and anus: a report of Intergroup Rhabdomyosarcoma Studies I through IV, 1972 through1997. J Pediatr Surg 38:347–353

Crist WM, Anderson JR, Meza JL, Fryer C, Raney RB, Ruymann FB, Breneman J, Qualman SJ, Wiener E, Wharam M, Lobe T, Webber B, Maurer HM, Donaldson SS (2001) Intergroup rhabdomyosarcoma study-IV: results for patients with nonmeat-static disease. J Clin Oncol 19:3091–3102

Hayes-Jordan A, Andrassy R (2009) Rhabdomyosarcoma in children. Curr Opin Pediatr 21:373–378

McDowell HP (2003) Update on childhood rhabdomyosarcoma. Arch Dis Child 88:354–357

Pham TH, Iqbal CW, Zarroug AE, Donohue JH, Moir C (2007) Retroperitoneal sarcomas in children: outcome from an institution. J Pediatr Surg 42:829–833

Qualman S, Lynch J, Bridge J, Parham D, Teot L, Meyer W, Pappo A (2008) Prevalence and clinical impact of anaplasia in childhood rhabdomyosarcoma: a report from the Soft Tissue Sarcoma Committee of the Children's Oncology Group. Cancer 113:3242–3247

Wiener ES (1998) Rhabdomyosarcoma. In: O'Neill JA Jr et al (eds) Pediatric surgery, vol I, 5th edn. Mosby, St. Louis

Section 24.1.4

Barksdale EM Jr, Obokhare I (2009) Teratomas in infants and children. Curr Opin Pediatr 21:344–349

Billmire DF (2006) Malignant germ cell tumors in child-hood. Semin Pediatr Surg 15:30–36

Sheil AT, Collins KA (2007) Fatal birth trauma due to an undiagnosed abdominal teratoma: case report and review of the literature. Am J Forensic Med Pathol 28:121–127

Tapper T, Sawin R (1998) Teratomas and other germ cell tumors. In: O'Neill JA Jr et al (eds) Pediatric surgery, vol I, 5th edn. Mosby, St. Louis

Section 24.1.5

Abbasoglu L, Gün F, Salman FT, Celik A, Uenüvar A, Oe G (2003) The role of surgery in intraabdominal Burkitt's lymphoma in children. Eur J Pediatr Surg 13:236–239

La Quaglia MP (1998) Non-Hodgkin's lymphoma and Hodgkin's disease in childhood and adolescence. In: O'Neill JA Jr et al (eds) Pediatric surgery, vol I, 5th edn. Mosby, St. Louis

Section 24.1.6

Haase GM, Vinocur CD (1998) Ovarian tumors. In: O'Neill JA Jr et al (eds) Pediatric surgery, vol I, 5th edn. Mosby, St. Louis

Martelli H, Patte C (2003) Gonadal tumours in children. Arch Pediatr 10:246–250

Tanaka N, Yoneda A, Fukuzawa M (2009) Mature tera-toma arising from an intra-abdominal testis in a 2-month-old boy: case report and review of intraab-dominal testicular tumors in children. J Pediatr Surg 44:E15–E18

Till H, Schmidt H (2005) Juvenile granulosa cell tumour (JGCT) of the ovary in a 6-year-old girl: laparoscopic resection achieves long-term oncological success. Eur J Pediatr Surg 15:292–294

Yazici M, Etensel B, Gürsoy H, Erkus M (2002) Mucinous cystadenoma: a rare abdominal mass in childhood. Eur J Pediatr Surg 12:330–332

Section 24.1.7

Brouwers MA, Peeters PM, de Jong KP, Haagsma EB, Klompmaker IJ, Bijleveld CM, Zwavelling JH, Sloof MJ (1997) Surgical treatment of giant haemangioma of the liver. Br J Surg 84:314–316

Chan CY, Tan CHJ, Chew SP, Teh CH (2001) The laparo-scopic fenestration of a simple hepatic cyst. Singapore Med J 42:268–270

Chung EM, Cube R, Lewis RB, Conran RM (2010) From the archives of the AFIP: pediatric liver masses: radio-logic-pathologic correlation part 1. Benign tumors. Radiographics 30:801–826

Henne-Bruns D, Klomb JH, Kremer B (1993) Non-parasitic liver cyst and polycystic liver disease: result of surgical treatment. Hepatogastroenterology 4:1–5

Holzinger F, Baer HU, Krähenbühl L, Büchler MW (1999) Solitare Leberzysten und polyzystische Lebererkrankung. Kongenitale Leberleiden mit unter-schiedlicher chirurgischer Behandlunsstrategie (Solitary liver cysts and polycystic liver disease: aspect of surgical management of congenital cystic liver dis-ease). Swiss Surg 5:136–142

Kabbej M, Sauvanet A, Chauveau D, Farges O, Belghiti J (1996) Laparoscopic fenestration in polycystic liver disease. Br J Surg 83:1697–1701

King DR (1998) Liver tumors. In: O'Neill JA Jr et al (eds) Pediatric surgery, vol I, 5th edn. Mosby, St. Louis

Sanchez H, Gagner M, Rossi RL, Jenkins RL, Lewis WD, Munson JL, Braasch J (1991) Surgical management of nonparasitic cystic liver disease. Am J Surg 161:1138

Schilling MK, Redaelli C, Baer HU, Büchler MW (1999) Chirurgische Therapie heap-tischer Riesenhämangiome (Surgical treatment of giant hemangiomas). Swiss Surg 5:133–135

Section 24.1.8

Fonkalsrud EW, Dunn J (1998) Adrenal glands. In: O'Neill JA Jr et al (eds) Pediatric surgery, vol II, 5th edn. Mosby, St. Louis

McHugh K (2007) Renal and adrenal tumours in children. Cancer Imaging 7:41–51

Miyano T (1998) The pancreas. In: O'Neill JA Jr et al (eds) Pediatric surgery, vol II, 5th edn. Mosby, St. Louis

Snajdauf J, Rygl M, Petru O, Kalousova J, Kuklova P, Mixa V, Keil R, Hribal Z (2009) Duodenum-Sparing technique of head resection in solid pseudopapillary tumor of the pancreas in children. Eur J Pediatr Surg 19:354–357

Wagner AS, Fleitz JM, Kleinschmidt-Demasters BK (2005) Pediatrc adrenal cortical carcinoma: brain metastases and relationship to NF-1, case reports and review of the literature. J Neurooncol 75:127–133

Section 24.1.9

Intenzo CM, Jabbour S, Lin HC, Miller JL, Kim SM, Capuzzi DM et al (2007) Scintigraphic imaging of body neuroendocrine tumors. Radiographics 17: 1355–1369

Juergens KU, Weckesser M, Bettendorf O, Wormanns D (2006) Duodenal somatostatinoma and gastrointes-tinal stromal tumor associated with neurofibroma-tosis type 1: diagnosis with PET/CT. AJR Am J Roentgenol 187:W233–W234

Müller-Brand J, Forrer F (2008) Octreotide-Szintigraphie zur molekularen Bildgebung neuroendokriner Tumoren. Schweiz Med Forum 8:757–758

Saab R, Khoury JD, Krasin M, Davidoff AM, Navid F
(2007) Desmoplastic small round cell tumor in childhood: the St. Jude Children's Research Hospital experience. Pediatr Blood Cancer 49:274–279

Schäfer HH, Appelt M, Pfeiffer D, Lerf B (2008)
Duodenales Somatostatinom – milde Klinik bei
malignem Tumor (Duodenal somatostatinoma – a clinically subtle malignant tumour). Schweiz Med Forum
8:63–65

Section 24.2.1

Muramori K, Zaizen Y, Noguchi S (2009) Abdominal
lymphangioma in children: report of three cases. Surg
Today 39:414–417

Section 24.2

Hornick JL, Fletcher CD (2005) Intraabdominal cystic
lymphangiomas obscured by marked superimposed
reactive changes: clinicopathological analysis of a
series. Hum Pathol 36:426–432

Prakash A, Agrawal A, Gupta RK, Sanghvi B, Parelkar S
(2010) Early management of mesenteric cyst prevents
catastrophes: a single center analysis of 17 cases. Afr
J Paediatr Surg 7:140–143

Ricketts RR (1998) Mesenteric and omental cysts. In:
O'Neill JA Jr et al (eds) Pediatric surgery, vol II, 5th
edn. Mosby, St. Louis

Section 24.3

Eckert J, Ewald D, Siegenthaler M, Brossard M, Zanoni
RG, Kappeler A (1993) Der "Kleine Fuchsbandwurm"
(*Echinococcus multilocularis*) in der Schweiz:
Epidemiologische Situation bei Füchsen und
Bedeutung für den Menschen. Bull BAG 25:468–476

Eckert J, Jacquier P, Baumann D, Raeber PA (1995)
Echinokokkose in der Schweiz, 1984–1992. Schweiz
Med Wochenschr 125:1984–1992

Nationales Zentrum für Echinokokkose, Institut für
Parasitologie der Universität Zürich (1995)
Echinokokkose beim Menschen, Schweiz 1984–1992.
Bundesamt für Gesundheitswesen. Epidemiologie und
Infektionskrankheiten. Bull BAG 43:4–5

Uelkü R, Onen A, Onat S (2004) Surgical treatment of
pulmonary hydatid cysts in children: report of 66
cases. Eur J Pediatr Surg 14:255–259

Uhl W, Löffler H, Zimmermann A, Tcholakov O, Gloor
B, Büchler MW (1999) Chirurgische Therapie der
Leber-Echinokokkose. Swiss Surg 5:126–132

Section 24.4

Smith SD, Vazques D (1998) Ascites. In: O'Neill JA Jr
et al (eds) Pediatric surgery, vol II, 5th edn. Mosby, St.
Louis

Jaundice (Icterus)

25

Jaundice is a frequent sign in newborns and young infants and much less frequently later in life. The causal hyperbilirubinemia (>100 μmol/l total bilirubin needed) is a result of decreased hepatic uptake, conjugation of bilirubin, biliary excretion, or increased degradation of hemoglobin.

Hyperbilirubinemia is divided for practical purposes into two forms: **indirect hyperbilirubinemia** in which the unconjugated bilirubin is increased and **direct hyperbilirubinemia** with increased direct or conjugated bilirubin (direct bilirubin >15 % of total bilirubin/direct bilirubin >35 μmol/l).

Direct hyperbilirubinemia includes disorders with biliary obstruction, infection (e.g., septicemia, urinary tract infection, and cholangitis), metabolic disorders (e.g., cystic fibrosis), chromosomal aberrations (e.g., Turner syndrome), drugs (e.g., antibiotics, cytostatics), and miscellaneous disorders (e.g., neonatal hepatitis syndrome, TPN = total parenteral nutrition), and is of special interest to pediatric surgery.

In contrast to the other groups, **obstructive jaundice** is combined with pale or clay-colored stools # and dark-brown urine if obstruction is complete and permanent. Initially, mainly the conjugated serum bilirubin (normal indirect bilirubin <35 μmol/beyond the neonatal period) is increased together with alkaline phosphatase, γ-GT, LAP, and GLDH.

Enterohepatic recirculation, hemolytic disorders, and transitory neonatal icterus are examples of groups of disorders that lead to **indirect hyperbilirubinemia**. Examples of the first two groups are **hypertrophic pyloric stenosis, small intestine atresia, and Hirschsprung's disease** or hemolytic disorders in which indirect hyperbilirubinemia may be or are observed. But only hereditary spherocytosis leads to jaundice in the neonate in contrast to thalassemia major (β-thalassemia) and homogenous sickle cell anemia with later episodic jaundice.

Transitory neonatal icterus is observed as physiological icterus (more frequently in preterm than in term neonates), in breast feeding, and resorption of large hematomas (e.g., **cephalhematoma** with excess of bile pigments and urobilinogen that are visible in stool and urine). Icterus in the neonate is pathological if it occurs at or within 24 h of birth, persists beyond the second week, the total bilirubin is >350 μ/l, and and direct hyperbilirubinemia is present (first 2 weeks: >35 μmol/l or >10 % of total bilirubin, after it >10 μmol/l). Sometimes direct and indirect hyperbilirubinemia occur together (e.g., septicemia, drugs).

In Table 25.1, the differential diagnosis of jaundice is listed from a pediatric surgical viewpoint. It includes disorders with direct hyperbilirubinemia. This form of jaundice is less frequent beyond infancy and includes mainly biliary obstruction caused by **injuries, neoplasms, gallstones, and parasites**. Occasionally, disorders with indirect hyperbilirubinemia may play a differential diagnostic role, for example, hemolytic disorders and septicemia. The disorders that play an important role in the differential diagnosis are different depending on the age (neonatal period and infancy vs. older children).

G.L. Kaiser, *Symptoms and Signs in Pediatric Surgery*,
DOI 10.1007/978-3-642-31161-1_25, © Springer-Verlag Berlin Heidelberg 2012

Table 25.1 Differential diagnosis of jaundice in newborns and infants or later from a pediatric surgical viewpoint

- Biliary atresia
- Choledochal cyst
- o Interlobular biliary atresia (Alagille syndrome, nonsyndromic type)
- Inspissated bile syndrome
- Cholelithiasis and sludge
- o Spontaneous perforation of the extrabiliary system
- Pediatric disorders with direct and indirect hyperbilirubinemia

25.1   Biliary Atresia

Occurrence, Types

Biliary atresia is observed worldwide in 1 of 10,000–15,000 live births and in Europe somewhat less frequently (in 1 of 18,000 live births). Although atresia of the biliary tree is congenital, it is probably an acquired disorder with further postnatal progression. It is often an isolated disorder except for occasional congenital heart failure and polysplenia syndrome.

In contrast to the less frequent intrahepatic hypoplasia or aplasia of the biliary tree, extrahepatic biliary atresia occurs nine times more frequently. It can be divided into three types (main sites of atresia), four subtypes (patterns of common bile duct), and several subgroups (patterns of hepatic duct radicles at the porta hepatis) and is described by a Roman number, small letter, and Greek letter.

The main types are in order of decreasing frequency and atresia at or of the porta hepatis (III), common bile duct (I), or hepatic duct (II). In the subtypes, fibrous, patent, or aplastic common bile duct (b, a, or c) are the most common. 95 % of the subgroups have no normal ductal structures at the porta hepatis (noncorrectable types), and only subgroup alpha has open radicles (Fig. 25.1).

Clinical Significance

- Untreated, the majority of children with biliary atresia will die within a mean time of 1.6 years.
- Diagnosis and treatment should be finished by the age of 2 months because of postnatal progression of biliary atresia.

- Biliary atresia remains a chronic disease with possible progression of biliary cirrhosis and portal hypertension (in at least 10 %) although it can be operated in the majority of children.
- Substantial part of the children needs earlier or later liver transplantation with or without the necessity of intervening treatment of portal hypertension.

Clinical Presentation

Jaundice develops either after the period of physiological icterus for term and preterm newborns in two thirds or is present already at birth in one third. Discoloration of skin and mucous membranes is yellowish with green tinge and may change in its intensity according to the changing bilirubin blood levels.

After passage of normal meconium in the majority of cases, the feces becomes yellow, light yellow, and/or clay colored in >95 % and the urine dark brown.

The third sign of the classic triad is hepatomegaly #.

Anemia, malnutrition, and underdevelopment combined with increasing liver stiffness and splenomegaly develop after the first few months. The natural history leads to death in the majority of cases below the age of 3 years.

Differential Diagnosis, Work-Ups

It includes all surgical and pediatric disorders with direct hyperbilirubinemia and more specifically those with biliary obstruction, for example, neonatal hepatitis syndrome.

Initially, mainly the conjugated (direct) serum bilirubin is increased together with alkaline phosphatase, γ-GT, LAP, and GLDH. Increased levels of bilirubin, direct bilirubin, γ-GTP (γ-glutamyl transpeptidase), lipoprotein-X, alkaline phosphatase, cholic acid, and possibly increased liver cirrhosis parameters including abnormal coagulation profile confirm the diagnosis of obstructive jaundice and possible liver damage.

Treatment, Prognosis

After confirmation of the diagnosis, portoenterostomy should be performed within the first 6 weeks of life. The early recognition of biliary

Fig. 25.1 Main types of biliary atresia, subtypes according to the patterns of the distal ducts, and subgroups according to the patterns of hepatic radicles. The drawing at the top shows the most common main type III (atresia at the porta hepatis in 88%). Remove the rest of the sentence 'and type I (atresia of the common bilde duct in 10%).' The three drawings in the *middle row* show from the *left* to the *right side* the most common subtypes b (fibrous common duct in 62 %), a (patent common bile duct in 20 %), and c (aplasia of the common bile duct in 10 %). The three drawings at the *bottom* show from the *left* to *right side* in the row the two most common subgroups v (with a fibrous mass at the porta hepatic in 56 %) and μ (with fibrous hepatic ducts in 19 %) and the interesting subgroup α (dilated hepatic ducts in 5 %) (Redrawn according to Ohi and Nio (1998))

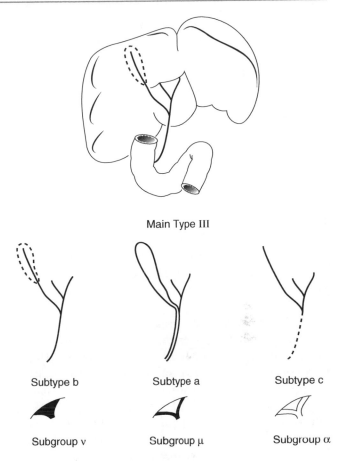

Main Type III

Subtype b   Subtype a   Subtype c

Subgroup v   Subgroup μ   Subgroup α

atresia can be achieved by infant stool color card that is handled to the parents at birth. The results of the observations are communicated to the family doctor at the 1-month follow-up at latest. Timely surgery increases the chance of survival with the own liver, diminishes the need of an early transplantation, and increases total survival.

Surgery is performed in supine position with the back somewhat elevated. After a right subcostal abdominal incision, cholangiography is performed in case of a patent gallbladder, the extrahepatic biliary tracts are inspected, and a liver biopsy carried out. Prior portoenterostomy, additional information are gathered by dissection of the gallbladder and the remnants of its duct, the common bile duct, and the hepatic duct from the underlying structure. The former common bile duct is divided in its distal part. Afterward, the cone-shaped portal bile duct

-remnant is dissected in its anterior and posterior aspect from the surrounding connective tissue and underlying hepatic artery and portal vein advancing on the right side to the proximal anterior branch of the right hepatic artery by 5 mm and on the left side to the umbilical part of the left portal vein.

The portal bile duct remnant is now transected at a level posteriorly of the portal vein leaving an oval area of liver tissue that is elongated in the transverse direction, shows minute bile ducts, and possibly some bile flow. In **hepatic portoenterostomy (Kasai's procedure)**, the open end of the Roux-en-Y limb is now anastomosed with the edges of the exposed liver area. In case of an open and dilated hepatic duct remnant, the already quoted portal dissection is less wide and deep, the hepatic duct is transected at the level of the porta hepatis, and a **hepaticoenterostomy** is carried out. To avoid ascending cholangitis, a Roux-en-Y limb of 50–70 cm is chosen without or combined with an intussuscepted valve above the end-to-side jejunostomy.

Diversion of the bile conduit or the use of the gallbladder in case of open distal ducts is an alternative technique that has several drawbacks.

Medical treatment consists of antibiotics, ursodeoxycholic acid, fat-soluble vitamin supplementation, and nutritional support.

Liver transplantation is not the first choice because adequate liver function is achieved today in about 50 % in the first 1–5 years of life. Indications are absent regression of cholestasis and/or progressive cirrhosis with associated complications. Although about 80 % of the children need afterward some time or another a liver transplantation, overall survival is 90 % (in Europe at age 4–5 years).

Complications include cessation of bile flow, cholangitis, portal hypertension, and persistence of hepatic dysfunction. If re-portoenterostomy is considered in case of **cessation of bile flow**, surgery is only indicated if proper bile flow has been observed immediately after the primary intervention. **Cholangitis** occurs in 2–3 fifths of patients and is especially undesirable in the first few months after portoenterostomy because it is often followed by interruption of bile flow. *Fever, decreased bile flow, increased bilirubin serum levels, and inflammatory blood signs* permit the diagnosis and the corresponding treatment with nonhepatotoxic antibiotics and fluid replacement. **Portal hypertension** occurs in one third to three fourths of the cases and is observed in icteric and anicteric patients. It may lead to *variceal bleeding* in up to three fifths. Initially, a nonoperative treatment is indicated. *Hypersplenism* occurs in up to one third. Treatment is indicated with endoscopic sclerotherapy or banding of the esophageal varicose veins and possibly partial splenic embolization, if prophylactic endoscopy displays gross varicosis or gastrointestinal bleeding occurs and the platelets become <5,000 per mm³.

Age below 8 weeks of life, precise dissection and transection at the porta hepatis (experience of the involved surgeon), minimal involvement of the liver evaluated by liver biopsy, and immediate postoperative course with proper bile flow are prognostic signs for a good outcome. The reported results after portoenterostomy were different in Japan from that of the rest of the world in the 1990s: overall 10-year cumulative survival rate of 65 % (with 85 % in anicteric and 10 % in icteric patients) in contrast to 30 % with one fourth with normal liver function and no detectable signs of portal hypertension.

Today, in the western part of the world, survival has improved to over 90 % with more than half who clear the jaundice and have a greater than 80 % chance of good quality of life. Nevertheless, a substantial part has many health problems related to recurrent cholangitis, portal hypertension, nutrition and growth, and psychosocial problems.

25.2   Choledochal Cyst

Occurrence, Types

Choledochal cyst is observed less frequently than biliary atresia. The following five pathoanatomical types are recognizable (Fig. 25.2) of which **type I** with saccular or diffuse and fusiform dilatation of the extrahepatic bile duct is encountered in >90 % of choledochal cyst. Gallbladder, cystic, and both hepatic ducts are not dilated in this type. **Type II** consists of a diverticulum closely beside the extrahepatic bile duct that is of normal size and communicates with the diverticulum, **type III** consists of an intraduodenal (or rarely intrapancreatic) choledochocele. The more frequent choledochocele subtype 1 corresponds to a protrusion of the papilla of Vater. A protrusion originates from the common route after fusion of choledochus and pancreatic duct in subtype 2 (Fig. 25.2). The duodenal orifice is narrow in both subtypes.

In **type IV,** multiple intrahepatic, extrahepatic, or combined cystic dilatations of the biliary tree are present. Type III and IV occur sometimes at the same time. Cystic dilatations of the intrahepatic biliary tree (**type V**) in which the extrahepatic biliary tract is normal correspond to the Caroli's disease (Fig. 25.2). **Caroli's disease** has two variant forms: one spontaneous form without a genetic cause or primary fibrosis in which the

Fig. 25.2 The drawing of
the five main types of
choledochal cyst and the two
main types of choledo-
chocele. The drawings from
top on the *left* side to the
bottom on the *right* side show
the most common saccular
or fusiform type I with gross
dilatation of the common bile
and hepatic duct, type II
corresponding to a diverticulum of the common bile duct,
type III as choledochocele of
the distal common duct (with
magnification of the more
common type I on the left and
the less frequent type II of
choledochocele on the *right
side*), type IV with multiple
cysts of the intrahepatic
and/or extrahepatic ducts, and
type V with single or multiple
intrahepatic cysts (with
appearance in the MRI)
(added to and redrawn
according to O'Neill (1998))

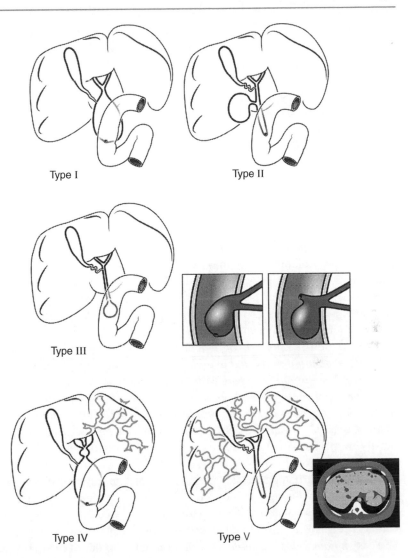

Type I

Type II

Type III

Type IV

Type V

dilatations have often a segmental distribution
and one genetic form in which a frequent diffuse
distribution of the dilatations is combined with
congenital hepatic fibrosis and combination with
the polycystic renal disease is possible.

Clinical Significance

- The infantile type should be operated whenever possible in the neonatal period with the
  aim to prevent from further damage to the
  liver.
- Early recognition of the adult type may be a
  challenge to the clinician and is even more
  indispensable for the same reason as in the
  infantile type.

- The majority of type I choledochal cysts have
  a malunion of choledochus and pancreatic
  duct that is a fusion proximal to the circular
  muscle of Vater. A possible pancreaticobiliary
  reflux must be avoided by the chosen surgical
  technique.
- In adulthood and rarely in children, an ade-
  nosquamous or small-cell carcinoma may originate from the wall of the choledochal cyst that
  should be avoided by the surgical technique.

Clinical Presentation

Prenatal diagnosis is possible in the second to
third trimester by demonstration of a cystic structure with communication in both hepatic ducts.

Depending on the time of clinical manifestation and symptomatology, an infantile and an adult type of choledochal cyst can be differentiated.

In the **infantile type** with *manifestation in the first trimenon (first to third month of life), the symptomatology is similar to biliary atresia with obstructive jaundice (acholic stools and dark-brown urine) and hepatomegale #*. Possibly, low-grade fever and signs of cirrhosis may be present, and obstructive jaundice occurs after prenatal diagnosis in the same time frame as those newborns with a clinical diagnosis.

The **adult type** does not manifest before age two, and the symptomatology may be vague and intermittent so that diagnosis may be delayed till school age, adolescence, or adulthood when the disease is already advanced with signs of portal hypertension or recurrent cholangitis.

The classic triad consists of abdominal pain, palpable abdominal mass, and jaundice.

The abdominal pain is vague with location in the right upper abdomen and possible radiation to the back and the jaundice is intermittent #.

In **Caroli's disease**, manifestation occurs mostly in the first three decades by the possible complications: recurrent cholangitis, septicemia, liver abscess, gall sludge or gallstones, signs of liver cirrhosis including portal hypertension, and rarely in adulthood carcinoma of the biliary tree. Cholangitis leads to a *slight or moderate cholestatic symptomatology combined with signs of infection*.

Work-Ups, Differential Diagnosis

Ultrasound allows as screening method to recognize the pathoanatomy of the extrahepatic, intrahepatic biliary tree, and portal fields (site and type of dilatations, fibrosis). A better surview and differentiation is possible by (cholangio) MRI or ERCP. Other possible tools are peroral cholecystography, i.v. cholangiography, (cholangio) CT, and scintiscan (DISIDA). The latter may be used together with ultrasound for postoperative follow-up.

In Caroli's disease, sonography, CT, and MRI are diagnostic: multiple oval or roundish cystic lesions of different size that continue into tubular structures with possible signs of fibrosis.

Increased levels of bilirubin, direct bilirubin, γ-GTP (γ-glutamyl transpeptidase), lipoprotein-X, alkaline phosphatase, cholic acid, and possibly increased liver cirrhosis parameters including abnormal coagulation profile confirm the diagnosis of obstructive jaundice and possible liver damage. In Carolis's disease with cholangitis, some cholestatic and inflammatory parameters may be increased, whereas bilirubin is not necessarily increased.

The differential diagnosis must consider the possible diseases leading to obstructive jaundice, especially the surgical ones (choledochal cyst may be associated also with biliary atresia), those leading to portal hypertension, and cholangitis.

Primary sclerosing cholangitis and congenital stricture of extrahepatic biliary duct are examples of rare specific disorders.

Treatment, Prognosis

Surgery is indicated in the infantile type at the moment of diagnosis and after prenatal diagnosis, already in the neonatal period. In the types I, II, and IV and in infantile and many of the adult type, respectively, total cystectomy should be performed.

Surgery: After a transverse upper abdominal incision, cholecystography (if no precise preoperative radiological imaging is available) and wedge liver biopsy is performed. Afterward, a total cyst excision is performed from the upper border of the duodenum close to the bifurcation of the hepatic duct taking care to avoid injury to the hepatic artery, its branches, and the portal vein while dissecting the posterior cyst wall. After ligation of the choledochus above and somewhat behind the duodenum, a hepaticojejunostomy with the limb of the Roux-en-Y jejunostomy end to end or end to side is performed in front and above pars I of the duodenum with a single layer of interrupted sutures.

In **long-standing adult forms** with recurrent cholangitis leading to severe adhesions between posterior cyst wall and portal vessels, **intramural excision of the cyst** according to Lilly is indicated: After a transverse anteromedial and – lateral incision in the middle part of the cyst – the inner layer is peeled off in a caudal and cranial direction and completely resected. Thereafter, the external layer of the cyst is resected except for the area over the portal vessels that are left in place.

For **type III**, a longitudinal duodenotomy is performed, and after that the choledochocele is unroofed starting from the tiny opening of choledochus. Adaption of the mucosa and sphincteroplasty of the mostly stenotic orifices of choledochus and pancreatic duct are performed before closure of the duodenum. In the intrapancreatic form, either a similar internal drainage or rarely a pancreaticoduodenectomy is necessary.

Treatment for **Caroli's disease** is mostly symptomatic. It includes adequate antibiotics and in case of sludge or cholelithiasis, ursodeoxycholic acid treatment or ECRP extraction. Only in advanced cases with diffuse involvement, liver transplantation becomes necessary. In localized variants or proximal ductal obstruction, segmental hepatic resection or unroofing with jejunostomy may be discussed.

Patients with operated choledochocele need lifelong clinical follow-ups combined with determination of liver and cholestasis parameters and sonography. A precise and always available protocol of the former surgical intervention is indispensable for the follow-up.

Depending on the chosen technique and the degree of liver involvement, **recurrent cholangitis**, **cholelithiasis** of the intrahepatic biliary ductal system, progressive **cirrhosis**, and **adenocarcinoma** originating from remnants of the choledochal cyst can be expected. Adenocarcinoma occurs mostly in adulthood. The quoted complications need reevaluation of the intrahepatic biliary tree and anastomosis for possible stenoses, and in case of surgery with cyst drainage, re-operation with cyst resection should be evaluated. In cyst resection with hepaticojejunostomy, cholangitis and/or intrahepatic lithiasis occurs in <2.5 % of the cases during >10-year follow-up.

25.3   Interlobular Biliary Hypoplasia

Occurrence, Types

This rare entity is characterized by a tiny extrahepatic biliary ductal system combined with a diminished number of intrahepatic bile ducts (reduced number in relation to the number of the portal tracts).

Alagille syndrome consists of chronic cholestasis (decreased bile flow associated with the above quoted morphological features), pulmonary artery hypoplasia or aplasia, butterfly-like vertebral arch defect, and characteristic physiognomy. This disorder with autosomal dominant inheritance leads to cirrhosis in about one fourth.

The **nonsyndromic type** has several causes, is not associated with the different disorders of Alagille syndrome, and has a worse prognosis with cirrhosis in about 50 % and death within the first year of life.

Clinical Significance

- Both types of interlobular biliary hypoplasia are important differential diagnoses of obstructive jaundice in the first year of life and neonatal period.

Clinical Presentation

Whereas the Alagille syndrome leads to obstructive jaundice combined with pruritus in the first year of life, jaundice of the nonsyndromic type becomes manifest already in the neonatal period with similar signs as in biliary atresia. In Alagille syndrome, the quoted associated disorders together with the time frame of cholestasis point to it.

Work-Ups, Differential Diagnosis

The suspected diagnosis is confirmed by intraoperative cholangiography and biopsy of a hepatic wedge. Alternatively, liver needle biopsy and MRI cholangiography may be performed, especially in suspected Alagille syndrome. In addition to the increased cholestatic parameters, the levels of total bile acid, cholesterol, and triglyceride are elevated.

The differential diagnoses are mainly those of obstructive jaundice.

Treatment, Prognosis

It is only symptomatic and includes medium-chain triglyceride, supplementation with fat-soluble vitamins, and medication with phenobarbital and cholestyramine. Liver transplantation may be an option in some patients.

25.4   Inspissated Bile Syndrome

Occurrence, Causes
In the increasingly observed inspissated bile syndrome, the extrahepatic biliary ductal system of newborns is obstructed by thick bile or sludge in its distal part that is slightly dilated in its proximal part.

The disorder is observed in disorders with hemolysis, diuretics, parenteral nutrition, exsiccosis, or decreased bile production.

Clinical Significance
• Inspissated bile syndrome mimics other disorders with obstructive jaundice and may lead to cholelithiasis.

Clinical Presentation
It is identical with that of biliary atresia and other disorder with obstructive jaundice. The conspicuous history and missing hepatomegaly may lead to the suspicion of inspissated bile syndrome.

Work-Ups, Differential Diagnosis
Ultrasound with recognizable extrahepatic biliary ducts and normal or slightly dilated proximal part and sludge in the distal part confirm the suspected diagnosis.

The differential diagnoses are those of obstructive jaundice.

Treatment, Prognosis
It concerns mainly treatment of the underlying cause because spontaneous resolution is possible. If resolution does not occur or the differential diagnosis is uncertain, intraoperative cholangiography is often therapeutic. Permanent cure can be expected.

25.5   Cholelithiasis, Cholecystitis

See Sect. 14.2.3.

25.6   Spontaneous Perforation of the Extrahepatic Biliary System

Occurrence, Pathoanatomy
Spontaneous perforation of the extrahepatic biliary system is a rare disorder and concerns in the majority of children early infancy with an age between 1 and 3 months. The site of a minute perforation is usually the union between cystic duct and choledochus. The leaking gall leads to bilious peritonitis with ascites or formation of a subhepatic, dark-green discolored, and fibrinous pseudocyst in up to 50 % that may be mixed up at surgery with a choledochal cyst.

Clinical Significance
• The mostly inconspicuous beginning is insidious because the biliary peritonitis may be recognized only in an advanced stage and is associated with failure to thrive.

Clinical Presentation
An inconspicuous beginning of the disorder is mostly observed with a slowly increasing and painless abdominal distension like a balloon, occasional vomiting and irritability, failure to thrive, and a slight to moderate obstructive jaundice of variable intensity after an uneventful neonatal period. It may be accompanied by manifestation of an inguinal or umbilical hernia. *Much less frequently, a peracute onset occurs with vomiting, crying, and signs of biliary peritonitis.*

On clinical examination, *ascites, cystic mass, or signs of peritonitis* may be recognized as a cause of abdominal distension.

Work-Ups, Differential Diagnosis
Plain X-rays performed in cases with peracute onset show free abdominal fluid. The same is true with the classic clinical presentation, or a space-occupying process in the right upper abdomen is recognizable.

Ultrasound displays either signs of diffusely distributed intraperitoneal fluid or a pseudocyst in vicinity of the gallbladder and porta hepatis combined with a normal extrahepatic biliary tree.

The conjugated bilirubin is only slightly increased and the cholestatic parameters not at all. Paracentesis (ascites with bilirubin levels higher than in the serum) and scintiscan (excretion of the tracer in the abdominal cavity or pseudocyst) are diagnostic.

In the differential diagnosis, disorders with obstructive jaundice are not in the foreground due to the only slight hyperbilirubinemia. More likely, disorders with abdominal distension, for example, ascites due to cirrhosis or abdominal tumor, or delayed disorders of surgical abdomen must be considered.

Treatment, Prognosis

Most infants need preoperative resuscitation of exsiccosis and electrolyte imbalance. Immediate antibiotic treatment is appropriate either to treat a superinfection or to avoid it.

Surgery is indicated for intraoperative evaluation of a possible cause by cholangiography and inspection (papillary stenosis, biliopancreatic malunion, extrabiliary space-occupying mass), drainage of ascites or pseudocyst including fenestration, inspection and suture of the leaking site, and insertion of a cholecystostomy or T-tube (in case of wall necrosis or distal obstruction).

Drainage and tube are left in place till cessation of bile flow and absence of extravasation and free flow in the duodenum on contrast study. Depending on an underlying anomaly, papillotomy by ECRP in papillary stenosis or hepaticojejunostomy after choledochus resection must be performed in biliopancreatic malunion as second look procedures.

Prognosis is usually favorable if no cause is present except for possible postoperative ileus due to adhesions. Otherwise, prognosis depends on the possibility of complete and permanent alleviation of the underlying disorder.

Webcodes

The following webcodes can be used on www.psurg.net for further images and data.

| 2501 Pale/clay-colored stool | 2503 Infantile type, choledochal cyst |
| 2502 Infant, biliary atresia | 2504 Adult type, choledochal cyst |

Bibliography

General and Differential Diagnosis Jaundice

Ling SC (2007) Congenital cholestatic syndromes: what happens when children grow up? Can J Gastroenterol 21:743–751

Mazigh MS, Aloui N, Fetni I, Boukthir S, Aissa K, Sellami N, Bellagha I, Bousnina S, Barsaoui S (2006) Congenital hepatic fibrosis in children. Report of 9 cases and review of the literature. Tunis Med 84: 182–188

Medeiros FS, Tavares-Neto J, D'Oliveira A Jr, Parana R (2007) Liver injury in visceral leishmaniasis in children: systematic review. Acta Gastroenterol Latinoam 37:150–157

Pariente D, Franchi-Abella S (2010) Paediatric chronic liver disease: how to investigate and follow up? Pediatr Radiol 40:906–919

Shneider BL, Magid MS (2005) Liver disease in autosomal recessive polycystic kidney disease. Pediatr Transplant 9:634–639

Section 25.1

Duché M, Ducot B, Tournay E, Fabre M, Cohen J, Jacquemin E, Bernard O (2010) Prognostic value of endoscopy in children with biliary atresia at risk for early development of varices and bleeding. Gastroenterology 139:1952–1960

Erlichman J, Hohlweg K, Haber BA (2009) Biliary atresia: how medical complications and therapies impact outcome. Expert Rev Gastroenterol Hepatol 3: 425–434

Hsiao CH, Chang MH, Chen HL, Lee HC, Wu TC, Lin CC et al (2008) Universal screening for biliary atresia using an infant stool color card in Taiwan. Hepatology 47:1233–1240

Kelly DA, Davenport M (2007) Current management of biliary atresia. Arch Dis Child 92:1132–1135

Lai MW, Chang MH, Hsu SC, Hsu HC, Su CT, Kao CL, Lee CY (1994) Differential diagnosis of extrahepatic biliary atresia from neonatal hepatitis: a prospective study. J Pediatr Gastroenterol Nutr 18:121–127

Le Coultre C, Battaglin C, Bugmann P, Genin B, Bachmann R, McLin V, Mentha G, Belli D (2001) Biliary atresia and orthotopic liver transplantation. 11 years of experience in Geneva. Swiss Surg 7:199–204

Ohi R, Nio M (1998) The jaundiced infant: biliary atresia and other obstructions. In: O'Neill JA Jr et al (eds) Pediatric surgery, vol II, 5th edn. Mosby, St. Louis

Sinha CK, Davenport M (2008) Biliary atresia. J Indian Assoc Pediatr Surg 13:49–56

Wildhaber BE, Majno P, Mayr J, Zachariou Z, Hohlfeld J, Schwoebel M et al (2008) Biliary atresia: Swiss national study, 1994–2004. J Pediatr Gastroenterol Nutr 46:299–307

Wildhaber BE, McLin VA (2010) Schweizerisches Screeningprogramm für Gallen-atresie. Schweiz Med Forum 10:480–482

Section 25.2

Altman RP, Hicks BA (1995) Choledochal cyst. In: Spitz L, Coran AG (eds) Rob & Smith operative surgery. Chapman & Hall, London

Arda IS, Tuzun M, Aliefendioglu D, Hicsonmez A (2005) Spontaneous rupture of extrahepatic choledochal cyst: two pediatric cases and literature review. Eur J Pediatr Surg 15:361–363

Blockhorn M, Malago M, Lang H, Nadalin S, Paul A, Saner F et al (2006) The role of surgery in Caroli's disease. J Am Coll Surg 202:928–932

Caroli J, Soupault R, Kossakowski J, Plocker L, Para-dowska M (1958) La dilatation polycystic congénitale des voies biliaires intrahéepatique. Sem Hop 34:488–495

Lipsett PA, Pitt HA (2003) Surgical treatment of chole-dochal cysts. J Hepatobiliary Pancreat Surg 10:352–359

Miller WJ, Sechtin AG, Campbell WL, Pieters PC (1995) Imaging findings in Caroli's disease. Am J Roentgenol 165:333–337

O'Neill JA Jr (1998) Choledochal cyst. In: O'Neill JA Jr et al (eds) Pediatric surgery, vol II, 5th edn. Mosby, St. Louis

Stalder PA, Desbiolles AM, Neff U (1996) Choledochuskarzinom in Choledochuszy-ste – eine Rarität. Präsentation des Krankheitsbildes anhand eines Fallbeispieles. (Carcinoma within a choledochal cyst. A case report). Swiss Surg 5:123–126

Takahashi T, Shimotakahara A, Okazaki T, Koga H, Miyano G, Lane GJ, Yamataka A (2010) Intraoperative

endoscopy during choledochal cyst excision: extended long-term follow-up compared with recent cases. J Pediatr Surg 45:379–382

Todani T, Watanabe W, Toki A et al (1987) Carcinoma related to choledochal cyst with internal drainage operations. Surg Gynecol Obstet 164:61–64

Section 25.3

Wang JS, Wang XH, Zhu QR, Wang ZL, Hu XQ, Zheng S (2008) Clinical and pathological characteristics of Alagille syndrome in Chinese children. World J Pediatr 4:283–288

Section 25.4

Davenport M, Betalli P, D'Antiga L, Cheeseman P, Mieli-Vergani G, Howard ER (2003) The spectrum of surgi-cal jaundice. J Pediatr Surg 38:1471–1479

Yeh ML, Chang PC (2012) Laparoscopic cholecystos-tomy and bile duct lavage for treatment of inspissated bile syndrome: a single-centre experience. World J Pediatr 8:88, author replay 88

Section 25.5

Holcomb GE III, Pietsch JB (1998) Gallbladder disease and hepatic infections. In: O'Neill JA Jr et al (eds) Pediatric surgery, vol II, 5th edn. Mosby, St. Louis

Section 25.6

Ozdemir T, Akgül AK, Arpaz Y, Arikan A (2008) Spon-taneous bile duct perforation: a rare cause of acute abdominal pain during childhood. Ulus Travma Acil Cerrahi Derg 14:211–215

Part V

Urogenital System

Hematuria

Every discoloration of urine is worrying the parents and involved schoolchildren because imagination of hemorrhage is connected with it, and the family doctor is contacted quickly.

Confusion may occur if the discolored fluid corresponds to a lower gastrointestinal hemorrhage, a perigenital or perianal injury, or a genital bleeding in girls. It concerns specifically infants and small children in whom discolored nappies (diapers) and panties may be the only source of informations.

If urine is discolored, the question arises whether change in color is caused by components of food, drugs, etc., hemo- or myoglobinuria, or true hematuria. Because the stripe test cannot differentiate between the last two categories and in case of hematuria, false-positive as well as false-negative results may be obtained, evaluation of urine sediment is indispensable: <3 erythrocytes (ec) per visual field or mm³ are normal, and >10 ec per mm³ are pathological and called **microscopic hematuria** if hematuria is not recognizable by the naked eye.

The differential diagnosis of gross hematuria # and microscopic hematuria may be carried out according to the following four criteria:

- The most common causes of hematuria are **in accordance with the pediatric nephrologists**: glomerulonephritis, urinary tract infection, injury of kidneys and urinary tract system, and idiopathic hematuria.
- **According to the following subgroups** of hematuria: (a) unconfirmed hematuria, (b) isolated hematuria, (c) hematuria combined with bacteriuria, and (d) hematuria combined with proteinuria.
- Examples of unconfirmed hematuria are the following: uraturia of the newborn (discoloration by urine and crumbles in the diapers due to uric acid excretion, so-called brick dust deposit), carmine red discoloration by ingestion of beets (beetroots), and contamination of urine by povidone-iodine (Betadine®). In addition, hemoglobinuria is observed in burns, incompatibility to blood transfusions, or snakebites. Myoglobinuria occurs by muscle necroses due to severe crush injuries, surgical infections, and disorders of peripheral blood supply.
- In pediatric urological disorders, mostly isolated hematuria is encountered, occasionally combined with bacteriuria, and rarely with proteinuria (e.g., ureteropelvic junction obstruction with advanced damage to the kidney).
- **According to the organs of origin of hematuria**: The methods of determination of the origin of erythrocyturia by the distribution of the ec volumes and occurrence of dysmorphic ec are of minor significance in pediatric urology and surgery.
- The differential diagnosis **according to pathoanatomical criteria** is the most appropriate for pediatric urology and surgery. If the pathoanatomical criteria are used as quoted in Table 26.1, it must be remembered that hematuria or microscopic hematuria may be a leading sign in all, but depending on the individual case, for example,

Table 26.1 Differential diagnosis of hematuria and microscopic hematuria from a pediatric urological or surgical point of view

Urinary tract malformations

- Pelvicureteric junction anomalies (obstruction)
o Retrocaval ureter
- Obstructive megaureter
- Ureterocele
- Diverticulum (renal pelvis, bladder, urethra)
- Ureteral duplications
o Renal fusion
- Vesicoureteral reflux
- Neurogenic bladder
- Lower urinary tract obstructions

Tumors

- Nephroblastoma and other renal tumors
- Rhabdomyosarcoma (bladder trigonum, prostate)
- Polyp (pelvicureteric junction, ureter, bladder, urethra)
o Hemangioma, neurofibroma, etc.

Injuries

- Renal injury
- Bladder, urethral, and ureteral rupture
- Other types of renal trauma and injuries to external genitals and urethra
- Postinterventional and operative hematuria
o Penis manipulations

Urinary lithiasis, foreign bodies

- Urolithiasis
o Foreign Bodies of bladder and urethra

Urinary tract infections

o Urogenital schistosomiasis (bilharziosis)

Pediatric disorders of pediatric urological relevance

- Renal vein thrombosis
o Shunt nephritis
- Hemolytic-uremic syndrome

age group, other leading symptoms and signs may be in the foreground, for instance, urinary tract infection. The important and relatively frequent disorders are emphasized in the table.

26.1 Urinary Tract Malformations

Anomalies of the urinary tract are an important pathoanatomical group in children and occur in >1 of 1,000 pregnancies. Although they are increasingly recognized or suspected by prenatal ultrasound, leading symptoms and signs such as urinary

tract infection, abdominal tumor, or disorders of micturition are still in the foreground. Nevertheless, microscopic hematuria and hematuria may be a presenting sign again and again specifically in pelvicureteric junction obstruction or retrocaval ureter and especially if combined with urinary tract infection or minor trauma of schoolchildren.

26.1.1 Pelvicureteral Junction Anomalies (Obstruction)

Occurrence, Types, Pathoanatomy

Pelvicureteric junction obstruction (PUJ obstruction) is the most common cause of upper urinary tract obstruction, and hydronephrosis has been encountered in 50 % of neonates and infants with a palpable abdominal mass.

The following three types of congenital and acquired PUJ obstruction that also occur in combination are observed and arranged in decreasing order of frequency:

- Pelvicureteric junction obstruction in a restricted sense is also called the parietal type because the wall of the junction is macroscopically and histologically abnormal (abnormal distribution and arrangement of the muscular and collagen fibers). Other terms are subpelvic ureteral or ureteric outlet stenosis #.
- The extraluminal type is caused by aberrant renal arteries and combined with kinking and adhesions of the ureteric outlet #.
- The intraluminal type is due to intraluminal anomalies, benign polyps, or other tumors #.

Clinical Significance

- Prenatal hydronephrosis is a frequent ultrasound finding that needs further follow-ups and possibly postnatal work-up (precursor of PUJ obstruction).
- PUJ anomalies may lead to significant morbidity and if they are of advanced stage or bilateral, loss of one kidney or impaired renal function.
- Intermittent PUJ stenosis is a possible cause of suspected surgical abdomen or chronic abdominal pain and often misinterpreted.

Clinical Presentation

Prenatal hydronephroses # which are not a transitory phenomenon and persist in the second half of pregnancy need postnatal work-up and follow-up up to 1 year of age for exclusion of PUJ anomaly, megaureter, vesicoureteral reflux, infravesical obstruction, and multicystic dysplastic kidney.

In young children, recurrent urinary tract infection or a palpable abdominal mass is the most common presenting sign, whereas older children present more frequently with abdominal and/or flank pain, microhematuria, or macrohematuria after minor abdominal trauma. Hematuria may be the first manifestation of an advanced PUJ obstruction.

Less frequently are *symptoms and signs of urolithiasis* (in up to one of five infants with PUJ obstruction), *recurrent attacks of severe abdominal colics in which the children are lying down bent double and drawing up the knees,* **intermittent PUJ obstruction** and *arterial hypertension.* Occasionally, hydronephrosis due to different degrees of a PUJ obstruction is detected by chance on work-ups performed for other reasons.

PUJ anomalies occur frequently bilaterally (up to 40 %) and may be associated with other urological anomalies, of which vesicoureteral reflux, multicystic dysplastic kidney, and disorders of fusion and ectopia are of special interest, and with extraurological malformations.

Differential Diagnosis, Work-Ups

Prenatal hydronephrosis has several differential diagnoses as already quoted above.

At clinical presentation, other causes of urinary tract infection, abdominal tumor, recurrent abdominal and/or flank pain, hematuria, and urolithiasis must be considered.

Rarely, **uni- or bilateral megacalicosis** may be mixed up with pelvicureteric junction obstruction. The calices are dilated due to a maldevelopment of the renal papilla. The renal size may be normal or enlarged, and number of calices is increased that drain poorly. Urinary tract infection and urolithiasis are possible sequels.

Work-up consists of ultrasound, IVU, and functional studies. Diuresis renography combined with forced hydration #, VCU, CT, or MRI are indicated for specific questions, for example, for confirmation of intermittent PUJ obstruction, for differentiation of primary versus secondary PUJ obstruction in bladder reflux, or for delineation of PUJ obstruction in horseshoe kidney or ureteral duplication.

Ultrasound displays pyelocaliceal dilatation and its degree, morphology of renal parenchyma, size and morphology of the contralateral kidney, and other urological anomalies. Grading of pelvic dilatation by measurement of its anteroposterior or other diameters permits differentiation between minimal, moderate, and severe dilatation and is useful for follow-up. **IVU** yields in addition to overview imaging some informations about the function such as delayed secretion and passage of contrast. **Functional studies** with isotopes are very important for indication for surgery, prognostication, and follow-up.

Treatment, Prognosis

Open or minimally invasive surgery is **indicated** in symptomatic PUJ obstruction, if the pelvic dilatation is in- and the ipsilateral renal function is decreasing, in bilateral PUJ obstruction, and in advanced cases with sufficient renal function. Compensatory hypertrophy of the contralateral kidney may be an additional criterion of surgery.

Surgery is performed for reconstruction of the abnormal pelvis and pelvicureteral junction, alleviation of symptoms, and recovery or maintenance of renal function. If the involved kidney has a relative function of <10 %, **nephrectomy** is indicated without or with preliminary percutaneous nephrostomy and repeated functional assessment depending on the age of the child. Although **nonoperative approach** is recommended by some during infancy in asymptomatic cases with stable dilatation and/or function, the excellent outcomes of patients with slightly or moderately impaired function (possibility of recovery of renal function), expenditure of follow-ups, and parental anxiety about an unresolved disorder need special

Fig. 26.1 The steps of Anderson-Hynes pyeloplasty in ureteropelvic junction obstruction are depicted from the *left* to the *right side*. The surplus pelvis is resected, the ureter incised below the obstruction in an oblique plane, the pelvis closed, and anastomosed at its deepest point with the ureter

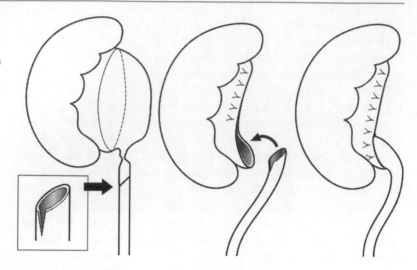

attention. **Fetal urinary diversions** (vesicoamniotic or bilateral pelvicamniotic shunts) may be useful for lung development but carry risks for the unborn patient and development of its bladder and urethra #.

For open **surgery** (Fig. 26.1), the involved flank is somewhat elevated, an anterior abdominal incision is performed with peeling off the peritoneum, and the pelvis, pelvicureteral junction, and uppermost part of the proximal ureter are prepared. After marking the foreseen incision of the pelvis and uppermost part of normal ureter with stay sutures, the bulging pelvis and the pyelouretic junction are resected, the pelvis closed and anastomosed with the obliquely cut proximal ureter with interrupted sutures, and a stent is left in place that includes ureter, anastomosis, and renal pelvis and leaves the body through a minimal nephrotomy site.

Global **prognostic statements** are difficult because no case is identical with the other: Symptoms and signs disappear or do not recur any more after an appropriate Anderson-Hynes pyeloplasty (except for arterial hypertension that may persist). Relating to renal function, unilateral PUJ obstruction with slightly or moderately impaired function especially in infants and intermittent PUJ obstruction have good outcomes. Unfavorable cases are bilateral PUJ obstructions with severely impaired function and/or signs of renal dysplasia.

26.1.2 Retrocaval Ureter

Occurrence, Pathoanatomy

Retrocaval and retroiliac ureter are two very rare obstructive uropathies in which the ureter runs either in its proximal part with an S-like sling behind the inferior vena cava or in its more distal part behind the iliac vessels.

Clinical Presentation

The uni- or bilateral obstructive hydroureter leads to *urinary tract infections, hematuria, or ureteral colics*. It may be recognized also by chance.

Differential Diagnosis, Work-Ups

In addition to other causes of urinary tract infections or hematuria, nephroureterolithiasis, ureteral polyp, or another tumor and congenital or acquired strictures must be considered specifically.

Ultrasound shows pelvic and proximal ureteral dilatation. IVU or retrograde pyelography with video recording demonstrates the abnormal course and relation to the quoted vessels and is diagnostic.

Treatment, Prognosis

After preparation of the retrovascular ureter with preservation of its blood supply, the superfluous and injured ureteral segment is resected and a tension-free anastomosis performed in front of the vessels. Permanent cure can be expected.

26.2 Tumors

Nephroblastoma is the most common of the listed tumors. In contrast to renal cell carcinoma of adulthood, *a visible and/or palpable abdominal tumor* and not painless hematuria is the most frequent presenting sign. Rhabdomyosarcoma of bladder or urethra that is observed mainly in small children manifests with *disorders of micturition and abdominal pain*, and hematuria is less in the foreground. On the other hand, hematuria is frequent in polyps and hemangiomas of the urinary tract.

26.2.1 Polyps of the Urinary Tract

Occurrence, Pathoanatomy
Polyps of the urinary tract are rare and benign fibroepithelial tumors in childhood. Although they may occur anywhere along the urinary tract, **preferred sites** are the pyeloureteric junction, bladder trigonum, and posterior urethra. They may be composed of several relatively long tentacles. Therefore, it may be difficult to localize its precise site of origin at surgery #.

Clinical Significance
- In case of recurrent hematuria, intermittent abdominal and/or flank colics, or disorders of micturition, the possibility of urinary tract polyps must be considered

Clinical Presentation
Pelvicureteral junction polyps lead to a *symptomatology of intermittent or constant PUJ obstruction*, whereas in polyps of the trigonum or posterior urethra, disorders of micturition up to *recurrent urinary retention* are in the foreground. *Hematuria and microscopic hematuria* are a frequent sign in all polyps.

Differential Diagnosis, Work-Ups
The rare hemangioma # of the urinary tract presents exclusively with hematuria in contrast to the polyps. The clinical presentation of polyps resembles urolithiasis. At endoscopy, other tumors including rhabdomyosarcoma must be considered.

Diagnostics are IVU or retrograde pyelography for polyps of the pyeloureteric junction (irregular filling defects at the site of polyp #) and VCU and cystoscopy for more distal polyps (urethral filling defect, direct visualization #).

Treatment, Prognosis
PUJ polyps need open segmental resection with ureteropyeloplasty, and bladder or urethral polyps are treated by endoscopic electroresection. In children, usually permanent cure is obtained.

26.3 Traumatic Injuries

26.3.1 Bladder, Urethral, and Ureteral Injuries

Occurrence, Pathoanatomy, Types
Although these injuries are relatively rare in children, they must always be considered in blunt or penetrating abdominal injury (especially in motor vehicle-related injury and/or trauma to the lower abdomen), multisystemic organ injury, straddle, or impalement trauma, and if a pelvic fracture is present. In pelvic fracture, urethral injuries are observed in 5 % and up to one fifth of them are combined with bladder injury.

Bladder injuries occur due to pelvic fracture, shearing forces, or direct blow. Eighty percent are extraperitoneal ruptures and the remaining of the intraperitoneal type. The former type is related to pelvic fracture and associated in up to 20 % with urethral injury. The intraperitoneal rupture often concerns the dome, is due to a direct blow, and is more common in small children.

Urethral injuries need evaluation of their severity and site: Grade I=contusion, II=urethral elongation, III=partial, and IV=total disruption. Most injuries concern the posterior urethra at three possible sites (shearing injury between prostatic and membranous urethra, direct force to the prostatic urethra without/with bladder neck, or external sphincter involvement) and less frequently the anterior urethra (Fig. 26.2). Urethral injuries in girls are less frequent, are either a distal avulsion or a proximal disruption without/with bladder neck or vaginal involvement, and are often missed.

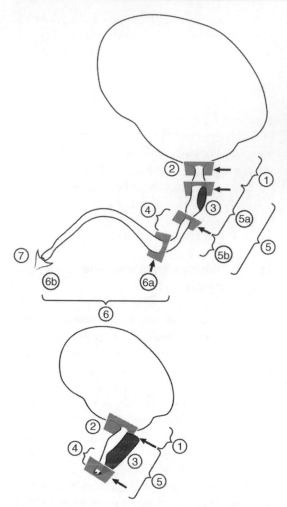

Fig. 26.2 Traumatic injury to the male and female urethra in children. At the *top* bladder and urethra according to the voiding cystourethrogram in the boy: *gray rectangle* = possible sites of urethral injury. *1* Trigonum of the bladder; *2* bladder neck; *3* verumontanum; *4* external sphincter; *5* posterior urethra; *5a* prostatic urethra; *5b* membranaceous urethra; *6* anterior urethra; *6a* bulbous urethra; *6b* navicular fossa; *7* preputial sac. At the *bottom* bladder and urethra according to the voiding cystourethrogram in the girl: *gray rectangle* = possible sites of urethral injury. *1* Trigonum of the bladder; *2* bladder neck; *3* vagina (spontaneous retrograde contrast filling); *4* external sphincter; *5* urethra with urethral meatus

Ureteral injuries are rare. Five grades may be differentiated, of which grades II–V include partial (< or >50 % transection) or complete rupture with < or >2 cm of devascularized adjacent ureter. The ureteropelvic junction is a preferential site and obstructive megaureter or some interventions

(e.g., percutaneous endourological procedures, surgery for abdominal tumor, or colectomy) a specific risk.

The possible complications of unrecognized ureteral injury are similar to bladder rupture (cellulitis, peritonitis, etc.) but in addition, delayed ureteral obstruction or even ipsilateral renal loss may occur. Ureteral injuries must be suspected and looked for in specific traumatic settings (e.g., multisystemic organ injury, penetrating trauma) because the clinical findings may be minimal (e.g., flank tenderness, soft tissue signs of truncal impact) and hematuria is absent in ≥ one third. Because IVU and CT may be unreliable, the suspected ureteral injury must often be confirmed and localized by retrograde ureterography.

Surgical options are PUJ junction reconstruction or ureterocalicostomy, spatulated end-to-end anastomosis, or ureteral reimplantation depending on the site of injury. On the other hand, occasionally, only preliminary measures may be meaningful such as anterograde ureteral stenting or ureteral ligation combined with nephrostomy (e.g., multisystemic organ injury, serious infectious complications, and/or long-segment injury). Mobilization of the ipsilateral kidney is one option for secondary ureteral plasty.

Clinical Significance

- Bladder rupture leads to a considerable urine extravasation and if not recognized early, to major morbidity (cellulitis, abscess, peritonitis) up to septicemia.
- Serious urethral injury may be followed by a considerable percentage of impotence, urethral stricture, and incontinence depending on its site and treatment.

Clinical Presentation

Bladder rupture may be missed by clinical examination. *Therefore, its possible diagnosis must be taken into account depending on the trauma history and local findings. Intraperitoneal bladder rupture leads to urinary ascites, to possible urinary retention, and hematuria. The latter signs may also be present in extraperitoneal rupture. Clinical examination reveals possibly a full bladder, ascites, peritonitis, or pelvitis due to the urine, hematoma, or infection and a bulging Douglas' pouch on rectal examination.*

In urethral injury, *blood at the external urethral meatus, hematuria, urinary retention, and unsuccessful urge to void are possible clinical signs. They are usually combined with pelvic contusional marks, swellings, and ecchymoses of the external genitals and perineum on clinical examination. On rectal examination, the prostate may be displaced in a more superior direction, or a hematoma may be felt at this site. In girls with straddle injuries, blood in the panties or external genitals and vulvar lacerations or edemas # need specific consideration of possible urethral injury by endoscopy.*

Differential Diagnosis, Work-Ups

The single quoted signs and symptoms may have another explanation, for example, urinary retention due a large pelvic hematoma or contrast stop at retrograde urethrography due to a spasm of the external sphincter muscle.

Work-ups start with plain abdominal X-ray that should always include the whole pelvis. Evaluation of the bladder by cystography must first exclude an injury of the urethra by retrograde urethrography under fluoroscopic control. It shows grade and site of injury with contrast extravasation in grade III and IV. Grade III is recognized by possible backflow of contrast in the bladder and a disruption of <2 m distance #, whereas the distance is >2 cm in total disruption. Evaluation of possible urethral rupture in girls is best performed by urethroscopy and supplemented by colposcopy. After exclusion of a severe urethral rupture, the examination is completed by cystography that may also be performed by suprapubic puncture. It shows either extra- or intraperitoneal contrast accumulation.

Treatment, Prognosis

Intraperitoneal **bladder rupture** needs immediate debridement, two-layer closure, and drainage of bladder and peritoneum, whereas extraperitoneal bladder rupture may be treated by continuous transurethral or suprapubic catheter drainage and antibiotics like the additional therapy of the intraperitoneal type. If the extraperitoneal

bladder rupture persists beyond 2–3 weeks or is encountered at laparotomy for other reasons, the rupture is closed from the inside after intraperitoneal bladder incision.

In **urethral injury** grade I to III, treatment is expectantly with antibiotics combined with transurethral or suprapubic catheter if micturition is impaired and in grade III. This regime may also be applied in anterior urethral injury with late urethroplasty in case of severe stricture formation.

In grade IV injury, time and type of early surgery depends on the site of injury. Disruption at the prostatomembranous junction is treated by delayed (7–10 days after injury) realignment with evacuation of the hematoma, introduction of a foley catheter with the aid of an antero- and retrograde catheter, and traction sutures around the prostate that are exteriorized to the perineum. In contrast, disruption of the prostatic urethra or the bladder neck needs immediate primary suture repair. Both interventions are performed after a suprapubic midline incision. In girls, the distal avulsion and especially the proximal disruption need repair and in the latter condition with reapproximation of bladder neck to the urethra and possibly repair of associated vaginal rupture.

Prognosis. Whereas rupture of the prostatomembranous junction is associated with a good outcome in ≤60 %, 0 % incontinence, and impotence <15 % after early surgery 1 week following trauma, early surgery of rupture of the prostatic urethra achieves good results in 0–50 % and is associated with impotence in 50–100 % and 0–50 % incontinence depending on the level of disruption.

26.3.2 Other Forms of Injuries to Kidney, Urinary Tract, and External Genitals

Occurrence, Forms of Injuries, Clinical Significance, Proceedings

Hematurias of different degree may be observed after physical activity of which **long-distance running** is a typical example. In case of *gross or microscopic hematuria*, this explanation must be excluded by a corresponding history especially in athletic-looking teenagers.

Falls astride of a beam or fence, similar blows by cycling, for example, **mountain biking**, and **other straddling injuries** are examples of the increasing playing and sporting activities of small children, schoolchildren, and adolescents. They lead to trauma to the bulbous urethra and other parts of the urethra of different degree that have not been considered furthermore up to now. *Acute or chronic voiding disorders, symptoms and signs of cystourethritis, and hematuria* may point to the possibility of such injuries and their sequels (e.g., urethral stricture). In girls, impalement injuries are quite frequently observed, and the parents may become aware of them by *hematuria and/or blood in the panties*.

For different reasons (among other things, for psychological and ethnic reasons, because of the frequent underestimation of severity of trauma, the possible combination of injury to vulva, perineum, vagina, urethra, and anorectum and the necessity of endoscopy), clinical examination, endoscopic evaluation (urethroscopy, colposcopy, anorectoscopy), and treatment should be performed in general anesthesia. In boys, the injuries of the corpora cavernosa need emergency surgery if gross bleeding, a large hematoma, or a palpable defect is present.

26.3.3 Peri-interventional and Perioperative Hemorrhage

Occurrence, Forms of Injuries, Clinical Significance, Procedure
Bladder catheterization, percutaneous suprapubic cystostomy, cystourethroscopy without/with ureteral catheterization, and urethral bougienage may lead to hematuria. The same applies to percutaneous renal biopsy or nephrostomy, minimally invasive or open surgery, in which kidney and/or urinary tract are involved.

The clinical significance of hematuria and related procedures are as follows:
- Responsible physicians or surgeons must ascertain that *hematuria* is not a sign of significant or severe injury, for instance,

urethral perforation by endoscopy or catheterization, and that the bleeding does not *obstruct the urinary flow* with formation of clots, for instance, following pyeloplasty in PUJ obstruction with hematuria and ureteric colics similar to nephroureterolithiasis. Injury to the urethra because of unprofessional catheterization may lead to delayed *urethral stenosis*.
- Good guidance of parents and older children by surgeons requires preoperative information about the possibility of *postoperative hematuria* for several days and good explanations of *hematuria* and its consequences if an unexpected intraoperative injury has occurred.

26.3.4 Manipulation of the Penis

Occurrence, Forms of Injury, Clinical Significance, Procedure
Manipulation of the penis by transurethral introduction of objects at masturbation and sexual intercourse may lead to injury of penis and urethra. If overt signs are not visible from the outside, it is only rarely possible to get informations by history about the cause of following findings: **foreign bodies in bladder or urethra**, **localized fibrinous urethritis, or urethral stricture**.

If *disorders of bladder voiding (thin urinary jet or dripping micturition that occurs with strength) and symptoms and signs of lower urinary tract inflammation (burning pain at micturition)* are present, the already quoted injuries must be considered. At the same time, initial hematuria at each micturition and mainly recurrent microscopic hematuria may be a sign that bothers the family doctor if the history is not known.

After examination of the urinary sediment including Gram stain and cultures, the so-called three-glass test may be performed in older children. Microscopic hematuria in the first or third glass points to a bleeding source in the urethra or posterior urethra and bladder trigone and hematuria in all three glasses to a more proximal bleeding source. Referral for uroflowmetry, VCU or retrograde urethrography, and cystoscopy are the next step. Long-term follow-ups by uroflowmetry are necessary to exclude delayed urethral stricture.

26.4   Urolithiasis and Foreign Bodies of the Urinary Tract

26.4.1   Urinary Lithiasis

Occurrence, Formal Genesis

Although only <10 % of all urolithiasis cases occur in children <16 years of age, urinary lithiasis is not an infrequent disorder in children and is observed in all age groups. 1.4–2.2 new cases in 100,000 children or 2 in one Wilms' tumor suffer from urolithiasis in Europe.

Several factors are involved in formation of stones, and the implications of these factors differ depending on the stone type, its overall composition, and the individual patient. Such factors are the appearance of substances that form stones and/or their degree of saturation (supersaturation), pH at the site of stone formation, concentration of promotors and inhibitors of crystallization, urinary flow per unit of time, urinary tract infection with urease-producing organisms.

Forms, Classification

Urinary stones occur single or multiple (up to 40 % #), uni- or bilateral (up to 10–20 %), and achieve different sizes (grain of sand to several cm) and shape depending on the site of origin or final location. The staghorn calculus corresponds to the shape of the calicopelvic system and increases to a dimension larger than the normal original collecting system #. Two thirds of all stones concern the kidney(s), one fourth the ureter(s), and the remaining are either bladder (including diverticular stones) or urethral stones (posterior urethra, urethral diverticulum, fossa navicularis) at initial diagnosis.

Few stones have an organic composition (matrix strones), and >40 % have multiple components. Ammonium, magnesium, or calcium **phosphate-containing stones** (struvite #) (about one third) grow quickly, have a laminar structure, are soft, and surrounded by crumbly masses. **Oxalate stones** (about 15 %) are hard with a jagged surface and calcium oxalate dihydrate # (weddellit) predominates in children. Ammonium and calcium **urate and uric acid stones** are hard with a

smooth surface, and **cystine stones** # are smooth and feel like wax.

Depending on the cause, urinary stones may be classified as follows:

- Metabolic stones
- Infectious stones with or without urinary stasis (stasis stones)
- Idiopathic stones

The percentage of these stone types depends on the time of observation, geographic region, draining area, and completeness and thoroughness of work-ups. Whereas the **metabolic type** is probably the largest group, the **idiopathic type** occurs only in one fourth to <15 %. The main disorders of metabolic stones are as follows:

- Hypercalcemic or hypercalciuric states with the main disorders "corticosteroid excess, immobilization, and primary hyperparathyroidism"
- Cystinuria, primary hyperoxaluria
- Chronic inflammatory bowel diseases (IBD), enterostomies
- Idiopathic hypercalciuria, hyperoxaluria, and uricosuria

Infectious stones without urinary stasis in Europe and to a lesser degree the endemic stones (due to unbalanced nutrition with low milk and animal protein intake) in the Mediterranean countries and Far East occur less frequently. The incidence of immobilization or foreign body stones is also decreasing in developed countries.

On the other hand, **the infectious stone type with urinary stasis** is observed constantly with about one third of the cases. It includes mainly urinary lithiasis related to congenital urological malformations and their treatment by bladder reconstruction and urinary diversions. The main disorders associated with urinary lithiasis are the following:

- Obstructive uropathies: PUJ obstruction, obstructive megaureter, horseshoe kidney, ureterocele, and posterior urethral valves
- Vesicoureteral reflux, ureteral duplication #
- Neurogenic bladder, bladder exstrophy after reconstruction, urinary diversions, and urethral stricture

Maximum incidence is one urinary lithiasis case in 4–6 PUJ obstructions and horseshoe kidneys. The term "stasis stones" takes into account that some of these stones are not associated with infection but with a metabolic disorder.

Clinical Significance
- Urinary lithiasis in children differs from that of adulthood in relation of the distribution of the causal groups and clinical presentation.
- Depending on the age group, history, and clinical presentation, urolithiasis must always be considered in the differential diagnosis of a pediatric urological symptomatology.
- Urinary lithiasis may be a lifelong disease especially in familial cases (about one third of involved children).

Clinical Presentation
The clinical presentation is determined by the age of the child, cause, site, and size of urinary stones, and their possible complications.

In **infancy and small children**, *recurrent urinary tract infections including their clinical equivalents (e.g., gastroenteritis) and incidental radiological findings belong to the most frequent clinical presentation*, and microscopic or gross hematuria and abdominal pain are less in the foreground. On the other hand, *flank and abdominal pain followed by hematuria is predominant in* **teenagers** in whom infections and incidental findings become infrequent. **Children between 6 and 11 years** *display a nearly equal distribution of the main clinical presentations "urinary tract infection or incidental finding, pain, and hematuria."*

Episodes of unexplained crying, vague stomachache, or attacks of abdominal pain, and typical colic belong to the variations of abdominal and flank pain in urolithiasis. In typical colic ##, the pain is of never experienced severity before and starts from the flank in direction of bladder with radiation to the urethra or along the groin to the scrotum or inner side of the thigh. Such colic may be accompanied with collapse (tachycardia, vomiting, sweating, and paleness). Uni- and bilateral stone incarceration may rarely lead to reflectory anuria that may last several days.

Prevesical concrements lead to urge, pollakiuria, and pain on micturition. Dysuria and disorders of micturition occur also in bladder and urethral stones. In contrast to the painful stones travelling from the pelvis to bladder, bladder and urethral concrements may interrupt the urinary jet, cause urinary retention, and/or lead to incarceration with scrotal cellulitis. Small stones in the calicopelvic system, ureter, bladder, and urethra may remain symptomless.

Differential Diagnosis, Work-Ups
It includes disorders with urinary tract infection, surgical abdomen, hematuria with or without abdominal and flank pain, disorders of micturition, and abdominal tumor. Passage of blood clots through the urinary tract and pelvic appendicitis may specifically simulate nephroureterolithiasis.

The work-ups for urinary lithiasis must also consider the possible causes of urolithiasis and the differential diagnosis. It includes supine plain abdominal X-ray, **ultrasound** #, IVU, and **CT without or with contrast**. These imaging tools recognize site and size of concrement(s) with increasing sensitivity and specificity, site and degree of obstruction of the urinary tract, and possibly the underlying cause. Opaqueness is good in calcium-containing oxalate and phosphate stones, weak in cystine, and absent in urate, uric acid, and xanthine stones. The latter stone types appear as filling defect if contrast is applied.

Urinalysis is very important for exclusion of urinary tract infection (urine cultures, leukocyte count), microscopic hematuria, and crystals (e.g., hexagonal cystine crystals).

In addition, renal and inflammatory parameters and electrolytes including calcium, phosphorus, and magnesium should be determined. Exclusion of specific metabolic stones needs specific work-ups including stone analysis.

Treatment, Prognosis
Treatment options are extracorporeal shock wave lithotripsy (ESWL), ureteroscopic stone extraction, cystolithopaxy, percutaneous nephrostolithotomy, open surgery, and expectant noninterventional approach. Complete stone removal should be attained by either method to prevent recurrence, and associated urinary tract infection needs preliminary antibiotic treatment before any intervention.

In asymptomatic very small stones, observation is possible. In small stones, (diameter ≤third of the patient's age in mm) **noninterventional treatment** with hydration and being in motion may be performed for maximum of 3 weeks if no urinary tract infection is present.

ESWL is used for caliceal and pelvic renal and upper and lower ureteric stones of ≤2.5 cm in diameter and children of ≥10 kg body weight. ESWL may be difficult in lower ureteric stones (due to difficult positioning) and should be avoided in girls (unknown effects to the ovary).

Open surgery is indicated in obstructive uropathies such as PUJ obstruction and obstructive megaureter and may be combined with stone removal, in staghorn calculi, and in very large bladder stones.

For the remaining stones, **ureteroscopic "stone extraction"** by electrohydraulic or laser lithotripsy (lower ureteral stones), **cystolithopaxy** by electrohydraulic lithotripsy (bladder stones), **endoscopic extraction** (in small bladder and urethral stones), and **percutaneous nephrostolithotomy** (ultrasonic or electrohydrostatic lithotripsy for hard or large stones (≥2.5 cm in diameter) or as preliminary measure before ESWL or for dissolution of struvite stones is performed).

Severe **complication** of urolithiasis such as pyonephrosis, hydronephrosis or caliceal diverticulum, renal shrinkage, ureteral stricture, bladder shrinkage, and purulent urethritis with periurethral urinary cellulitis # are rare in developed countries in contrast to former times (with 8 % pyonephrosis and 3 % renal shrinkage).

The **recurrence rates** depend on the cause of urinary lithiasis and its treatment. Recurrence is unusual in stasis stones with permanent correction of the underlying anomaly (obstructive uropathies and reflux disease) and exclusion of a combined metabolic disorder; recurrence is decreasing in immobilization, foreign body, and possibly in endemic stones. For metabolic stones, recurrence rates depend on the individual disorder, effectiveness of its treatment, and possible prophylaxis. Familial urolithiasis may be a lifelong disorder.

The percentages of stone-free patients after treatment are for ESWL up to 85 % in pelvic and <85 % in ureteral stones, for ureteroscopic stone extraction >95 %, for repeated nephrostolithotomy about 85 %. ESWL may lead to perirenal hematoma, trunk ecchymoses, abdominal colics, and fever. In ureteroscopic stone extraction, ureteral perforation, reflux, or stricture, proximal stone migration or extravasation may occur and after nephrostolithotomy, perforation of collecting system, hemorrhage, extravasation of rinsing liquid, and injury to colon or duodenum or pneumothorax are possible complications.

26.4.2 Foreign Bodies of Bladder and Urethra

They occur after manipulations of the penis in which objects are introduced into the urethra and bladder by the patient and remain there completely or in parts. The same applies to catheters that break off and nonabsorbable and braided threads used for urological interventions and surgery of the urinary tract. The foreign bodies become usually calcified (foreign body stone #), lead to urinary tract infection, and occasionally to disorders of micturition. They must be completely removed for relieve of the symptomatology.

26.5 Urinary Tract Infection

Urinary tract infection is an important differential diagnosis of hematuria. **Symptomatic and idiopathic granular cystitis** belong to this category. They lead to urge, pollakiuria, and burning and painful micturition. Idiopathic granular cystitis and the hemorrhagic variant are associated with urinary tract infection in 50 %, and hematuria may also be observed independent of it.

26.5.1 Bilharzial Cystitis and Urogenital Schistosomiasis

Causes, Occurrence
Bilharzial cystitis and urogenital schistosomiasis is caused by Schistosoma haematobium which is

one of the five species leading to human schistosomiasis. It is endemic in Africa (sub-Saharan regions), Asia (Middle East), and South America. The parasites enter the lymphatic vessels through the skin (during a bath in running waters or after drinking contaminated water), reach from there the mesenteric and portal veins or the venous plexuses of the bladder (*S. haematobium*), and develop in the body organs into worms. The worms have a length of 2 mm, survive in the involved organs for >30 years, and secrete eggs by the urine or stool which enter again the running waters, and there are the leeches as temporary intermediate host.

Clinical Presentation

Bladder or urogenital Bilharziosis manifests months to years after the infection. It leads to *terminal or intermittent hematuria and possible disorders of micturition,* to *ureteritis and pyelonephritis* with secondary ureteral stricture, hydronephrosis, and renal insufficiency, or to *genital tract involvement in females* with possible extrauterine pregnancy and infertility, and *epididymoorchitis* with infertility *in men.*

Work-Ups, Differential Diagnosis

Demonstration of the eggs in urine or stool, biopsy of involved bladder mucosa, or intestinal mucosa is diagnostic (the eggs are surrounded by lymphocytes and display a thorn). Cystoscopy shows granulomatous findings with papillomatous bladder mucosa surrounded by whitish nodules in the submucosa. The immunodiagnosis may be false positive because of other helminthiases but Bilharziosis is excluded if no antibodies are demonstrated. Secondary sequels of the urinary or genital tract should be excluded by ultrasound.

Schistosomiasis should be considered and looked for in children with family Migrationshintergrung combined with the quoted symptomatology.

Treatment

It consists of medication of praziquantel that leads mostly to cure. Resistance to praziquantel may occur.

26.6 Pediatric Nephrological Disorders

The reader is referred to the relevant literature. Renal vein thrombosis, shunt nephritis, and hemolytic-uremic syndrome have some relevance to the pediatric surgeon as cause of hematuria.

Thrombosis of the extra- and intrarenal veins occurs in neonates after perinatal asphyxia, hypovolemic shock, and cyanotic heart failure and in older children related to nephrosis. *Hematuria, palpable kidney(s), and IVU without contrast excretion* are the main signs. Ultrasound with Doppler is diagnostic. Treatment includes early fibrinolysis, later heparinization, and possible dialysis. Gross vena cava and renal vein thrombosis needs surgical thrombectomy. Nephrectomy is rarely indicated. Complete recovery of renal function occurs rarely although survival is mostly possible (mortality 10 %).

Shunt nephritis has lost its significance because vascular shunts are used today only as an exception. The endo- and extracapillary or membranous proliferative glomerulonephritis leads to hematuria and is reversible after shunt replacement by a ventriculoperitoneal shunt.

In the differential diagnosis of surgical abdomen of infants and toddlers, **the hemolytic-uremic syndrome** may play again and again a role because it may be mixed up with intussusception and other surgical disorders. *After several days with vomiting, abdominal colics, and hemorrhagic diarrhea or respiratory tract syndrome, increasing paleness and decreasing urinary production is* observed. The disorder is characterized by hemolytic anemia, thrombocytopenia, and acute renal insufficiency. Its mortality rate is about 5 %.

Webcodes

The following webcodes can be used on www. psurg.net for further images and data.

2601 Hematuria, kidney injury	2613 Grade III urethral injury
2602 PUJ obstruction, intrarenal pyelocalicectasy	2614 Multiple kidney stones, PUJ obstruction

Bibliography

General, Differential Diagnosis, and Treatment

Baker MD, Baldassano RN (1989) Povidone Iodine as a cause of factitious hematuria and abnormal urine coloration in the Pediatric Emergency Department. Pediatr Emerg Care 5:240–241

Feld LG, Stapleton FB, Duffy L (1993) Renal biopsy in children with asymptomatic hematuria or proteinuria: survey of pediatric nephrologists. Pediatr Nephrol 7: 441–443

Greenfield SP, Williot P, Kaplan D (2007) Gross hematuria in children: a ten-year review. Urology 69:166–169

Steyaert H, Valla JS (2005) Minimally invasive urologic surgery in children: an overview of what can be done. Eur J Pediatr Surg 15:307–313

Ward JF, Kaplan GW, Mevorach R et al (1998) Refined microscopic urinalysis for red blood cell morphology in the evaluation of asymptomatic microscopic hematuria in a pediatric population. J Urol 160:1492–1495

Section 26.1

Biewald W, Scigalla P, Duda SH (1987) Die Megakaliose im Kindesalter (Megacalycosis in childhood). Z Kinderchir 43:427–429

Mourigant P (1998) Congenital anomalies of the pyelopelvic junction and the ureter. In: O'Neill JA Jr et al (eds) Pediatric surgery, vol II, 5th edn. Mosby, St. Louis

Section 26.2

Ellis DG, Mann CM Jr et al (1998) Abnormalities of the urethra, penis, and scrotum. In: O'Neill JA Jr (ed) Pediatric surgery, vol II, 5th edn. Mosby, St. Louis

Section 26.3

Biserte J, Nivet J (2006) Trauma to the anterior urethra: diagnosis and management. Ann Urol (Paris) 40:220–232

Garcia VF, Sheldon C (1998) Genitourinary tract trauma. In: O'Neill JA Jr et al (eds) Pediatric surgery, vol I, 5th edn. Mosby, St. Louis

Hussein N, Osman Y, Sarhan O, el-Diasty T, Dawaba M (2009) Xanthogranulomatous pyelonephritis in pediatric patients: effect of surgical approach. Urology 73:1247–1250

Jordan GH, Virasoro R, Eltahawy EA (2006) Reconstruction and management of posterior urethral and straddle injuries of the urethra. Urol Clin North Am 33: 97–109, vii

Leibovitch I, Mor Y (2005) The vicious cycling: bicycling related urogenital disorders. Eur Urol 47:277–286, discussion 286–287

Section 26.4

Barbancho DC, Fraile AG, Sanchez RT, Diaz ML, Otero JR, Vazquez FL, Bramtot AA (2008) Minimally invasive endourological management of urinary tract calculi in children. Cir Pediatr 21:15–18

Ewalt DH (1998) Renal infection, abscess, vesicoureteral reflux, urinary lithiasis, and renal vein thrombosis. In: O'Neill JA Jr et al (eds) Pediatric surgery, vol II, 5th edn. Mosby, St. Louis

Kleta R, Bernardini I, Udea M et al (2004) Long-term follow-up of well-treated nephropathic cystinosis patients. J Pediatr 145:555–560

Perrone HC et al (1992) Urolithiasis in childhood: metabolic evaluation. Pediatr Nephrol 6:54

Stapleton FB, the Southwest Pediatric Nephrology Study Group (Baylor Univ Med Ctr, Dallas) (1990) Idiopathic hypercalciuria: association with isolated hematuria and risk for urolithiasis in children. Kidney Int 37:807–811

Thomas R, Frentz JM, Harmon E, Frentz GD et al (1992) Effect of extracorporeal shock wave lithotripsy on renal function and body height in pediatric patients. J Urol 148:1064–1066

Section 26.5

Gerber S, Holliger S (2011) Bilharziose der Harnblase. Schweiz Med Forum 11(10):181–183

Gryseels B, Polman K, Clerinx J, Kestens I (2006) Human schistosomiasis. Lancet 368(9541):1106–1118

Section 26.6

Ricci MA, Lloyd DA (1990) Renal thrombosis in infants and children. Arch Surg 125:1195–1199

Urinary Tract Infection

Urinary tract infection belongs to the most common bacterial infections in childhood: 3–5 % of girls and 1–2 % of boys suffer from it until puberty. In infancy, boys are preferably involved and later girls with a reinfection rate of two thirds. Five percent of infants with fever (≥38°C) have a urinary tract infection.

Numerous urogenital malformations and other disorders manifest uniformly and nearly exclusively by a urinary tract infection if they are not recognized incidentally by prenatal ultrasound or on the occasion of a medical check-up postnatally.

It makes matter worse that the clinical presentation of urinary tract infection is the more unspecific, the younger the child. Burning and pain at micturition (dysuria), pollakiuria, secondary enuresis, and suprapubic, upper abdominal, or flank pain are not recognized as such and reported by the patient until beginning **school age**.

In **newborns and infants**, the spectrum of symptoms and signs extends from hypo- to hyperthermia and increased temperature to paleness, gray-cyanotic skin, or jaundice; to irritability, apathy, and seizures; to abdominal symptomatology (meteorism, vomitus, diarrhea, frowning, and crying because of pain, and failure to thrive); and to tachypnea, tachycardia, and signs of shock. Attentive parents report a conspicuous odor or appearance of urine.

Urinary tract infection is defined as significant leukocyt- and bacteriuria with/without clinical symptoms and signs. Cystourethritis is also called **simple or lower** and pyelonephritis **complicated or upper urinary tract infection**.

The **definition** of urinary tract infection as well as its differentiation between its lower and upper form is clinically only partly and not with certainty possible. High fever (≥38.5 °C) and upper abdominal and flank pain speak in favor of pyelonephritis and some of the quoted symptoms and signs of very young patients of urosepsis. In this age group, urinary tract infection is rather a hematogenous process and thereafter rather a canalicular ascending process.

Even laboratory examinations remain open to the question of definition of urinary tract infection. At the same time, it is crucial that urine is collected correctly and examined quickly: recovery by percutaneous bladder punction, intraoperatively, bladder catheterism, midstream urine, or collecting bag after appropriate preparation.

Because the clinical data, urine inspection, and dip tests are only screening methods and cannot exclude urinary tract infection by 100 %, confirmation of urinary tract infection is only possible safely by determination of the leukocytes in the sediment (pyuria) and cultivation of bacteria (bacteriuria):

>50 Lc/µl urine (≥25 Lc/µl in boys) or ≥5 Lc/visual field and ≥100,000 germs/ml urine. The urine recovered by bladder puncture is normally sterile and should contain <10 Lc/µl urine.

There is a tendency to put the permitted number of bacteria to a lower level if clinical signs and symptoms are present. At the same time, microscopic hematuria is often present and less frequently gross hematuria.

For differentiation between lower and upper urinary tract infection, ESR, C-reactive protein, and the proof of granular casts are used (that should amount to >25 mm/h, >8 mg/l and be present in case of pyelonephritis). In addition, positive blood cultures and characteristic focuses in the dimercaptosuccinic-(DMSA-) scintiscan are used for confirmation of complicated urinary tract infection.

All children <5 years of age with a **febrile urinary tract infection** need radiological work-up with ultrasound and possibly VCUG, whereas work-up in older children depends on the symptomatology (simple vs. complicated UTI). Less than 10 % of the children with a febrile urinary tract infection have normal radiological findings.

The recurrence rate is one third and concerns mostly girls (except for boys in infancy), and their age is not predictive for recurrence; beyond 5 years of age, **dysfunctional voiding** must be considered as possible cause. After a febrile urinary tract infection, scarring of the kidneys must be excluded by a (99 m) Tc-dimercaptosuccinic acid (DMSA) scan, and if present, the parents must be informed about the possibility of hypertension, progressive nephropathy, and risk for complicated pregnancies.

Febrile UTI needs immediate antibiotic **treatment** for 1½–2 weeks that must be applied by i.v. infusion in young children and changed according to the evaluation of resistance.

Work-ups for urological malformations or disorders should be performed, especially in upper urinary tract infection, in infants, and in general, after the first simple urinary tract infection in boys and recurrent urinary tract infections in girls.

It is crucial to consider always the possibility of **urological malformation** and **disorders** as quoted in Table 27.1 and to recognize by ultrasound and after alleviation of the infection by VCU, cystoscopy, and if necessary also by MRI/CT and other additional examinations.

Because complicated urinary tract infection (pyelonephritis) leads to formation of scars in a

Table 27.1 Differential diagnosis of urinary tract infection in pediatric urology

Obstructive uropathies upper urinary tract (about 40 %)[a]
- Ureteropelvic junction obstructions
- Obstructive megaureter
o Retrocaval ureter
o Prune-belly syndrome
- Ureteroceles
o Polyps in urinary tract, nephrolithiasis
o Extrinsic obstructions

Ureteral duplications (about 1 %)
- Complete ureteral duplication
o Incomplete ureteral duplications

Renal fusions, ectopia, and a-, hypo-, and dysplasia (about 2.5 %)
o Horseshoe kidney
o Renal ectopia
- Renal agenesis, a-, hypo-, dysplasia (**about 35 %**)

Cystic renal diseases (about 14 %)
- Multicystic renal dysplasia
o Solitary renal cyst
o Other cystic renal diseases, megacalycosis

Vesicoureteral reflux

Bladder diverticula

Cystitis
- Granular cystitis

Neurogenic bladder, functional voiding disorders, obstructive uropathies lower urinary tract
- Phimosis
- Other disorders

[a]Percentage of renal disorders that have been recorded by screening ultrasound in a large cohort of schoolchildren. 0.5 % of this population or about 1:200 has a renal abnormality excluding reflux, diverticula, and the other disorders at the bottom of Table 27.1

significant percentage independent of age, it is of special importance to recognize the possible anomalies and disorders and to correct them before reinfections.

27.1   Obstructive Uropathies of the Upper Urinary Tract

Ureteropelvic junction obstructions, retrocaval ureter, and polyps of the urinary tract have been dealt with under the leading sign "hematuria" because these disorders may manifest with bloody

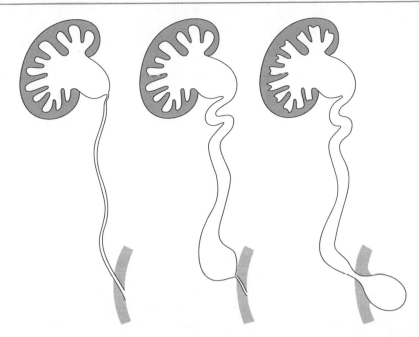

Fig. 27.1 Drawing of the three main congenital malformations leading to obstruction of upper urinary tract. On the *left side* an ureteropelvic junction obstruction is visible; pelvis and calices are dilated. In the *middle*, there is a juxtavesical ureteral stenosis; in addition to the pelvis, nearly the whole ureter is dilated; this anomaly occurs somewhat less frequently. On the *right side*, a ureterocele can be seen; the ureterocele lies in the bladder cavity like a balloon, or in the bladder neck or urethra in case of ectopically situated ureterocele. The orifice lies mostly at the lower end of the ureter and is competent or combined with reflux

urine with increasing frequency. Of course, urinary tract infection is in the foreground of clinical presentation in PUJ obstructions like in the following disorders with obstructive uropathies. Vice versa, these disorders may display hematuria as well (Fig. 27.1).

27.1.1 Obstructive Megaureter

Occurrence, Grading, Forms
Obstructive megaureter is – after ureteropelvic junction obstructions – the second most common obstructive uropathy of the ureter. Instead of regularly distributed and arranged musculature, collagenic connective tissue is found on histological examination of the distal ureter (Fig. 27.1 in the middle of the picture).

It leads to dilatation of the juxtavesical ureter, the whole ureter, or the whole upper collecting system (corresponding to grades I, II, or III). Obstructive megaureter is bilateral in about 25 %.

Megaureter may be divided into the following categories:
- Megaureter without obstruction or reflux
- Obstructive megaureter #
- Megaureter due to reflux
- Obstructive megaureter combined with reflux
  Neurogenic bladder and infravesical obstruction leads to **secondary megaureter** by different mechanisms that may resolve after alleviation of these disorders. Ureteroceles and posterior urethral valves are typical examples of infravesical obstruction leading to secondary megaureter.

Clinical Significance
- Megaureter in general and the obstructive category in particular are prone to recurrent urinary tract infection and possibly to localized or generalized renal damage, arterial hypertension, and renal insufficiency.
- Differentiation of the four categories and the secondary megaureter is very important

because the therapeutic approach and prognostic outlook differs considerably.

Clinical Presentation

Prenatal ultrasound yields hydronephrosis and possibly megaureter and its radiological course. **Differential diagnosis of hydronephrosis** that includes upper or lower obstructive uropathy, megaureter without obstruction or reflux, vesicoureteral reflux, secondary megaureter, and polycystic renal dysplasia is **often only possible after birth**.

Obstructive megaureter manifests *already in infancy with urinary tract infection (70–90 %), hematuria (10–15 %), or less frequently with abdominal pain and abdominal tumors like PUJ obstructions or even with signs of renal insufficiency.*

In nonobstructive and nonrefluxing megaureter, *recurrent urinary tract infections are in the foreground.*

Differential Diagnosis, Work-Ups

It includes disorders with urinary tract infection, hematuria, chronic recurrent abdominal pain, abdominal tumor, and surgical abdomen. For the differential diagnosis of the radiological sign "megaureter," the reader is referred to the already quoted categories.

The work-ups with ultrasound, VCUG, cystoscopy, IVU combined with fluoroscopy demonstrates combined with history, clinical findings, and urodynamic studies the megaureter, differentiation between primary and secondary megaureter, and its categories.

Delineation of obstructive from nonobstructive megaureter is more difficult and possible in only 85 % at most because technetium-99 m-diethylenetriaminepentaacetic acid =DTPA-furosemide scintiscan for evaluation of outflow in the bladder (and the rarely applied Whitaker test [pressure gradient between renal pelvis and bladder is abnormal if ≥20 mmHg]) display not always clearly usable results.

The following findings speak in favor of obstructive megaureter (**indications of obstructive megaureter**):

- Configuration of the distal ureter like the head of a snake that continues in an extremely narrow intramural ureter #

- Ineffective for- and backward peristalsis of the dilated distal ureter visualized by contrast ureterography #
- Retention of contrast in the distal ureter by >6 h
- Flood-like evacuation of urine after retrograde introduction of a ureteral catheter
- Decreased function of the involved kidney on scintiscan

Treatment, Prognosis

The indication of surgery is controversial: (1) Because spontaneous resolution of megaureter is observed in many cases within several months to years #, meticulous differentiation between obstructive and nonobstructive megaureter is pointless, an expectant approach with long-term regular follow-ups and prophylactic antibiotic treatment is indicated, and surgery is only performed in breakthrough infection and worsening renal function. (2) Surgery is indicated in case of proven obstruction independent on renal function.

Whereas the first option avoids possibly unnecessary surgery, the second option performs unnecessary interventions if not reliable criteria of obstruction are applied. On the other hand, the first option needs continuous antibiotic treatment and work-ups over several months to years, and if renal deterioration is recognized, its remains open if recovery does occur, whereas the second option resolves a problem straight away and possibly avoids deterioration of renal function in period of considerable renal growth and vulnerability.

Surgery is indicated in obstructive megaureter without/with reflux and primarily not in nonobstructive and secondary megaureter.

It includes resection of the fibrotic segment and often modelling of the dilated distal ureter. The approach is either a suprapubic incision in a skin fold with extraperitoneal midline incision of fascia and bladder wall (that may be extended by a paracolic approach) or a transperitoneal midline incision with reflection of the ipsilateral colon.

After introduction of a smooth catheter and a stay suture at the orifice, the ureteral orifice is circumcised and the intramural ureter dissected and pulled through the vesicoureteral tunnel in the paravesical space. Further dissection of the distal and possibly middle ureter takes care to the ureteral blood supply by far division of the periureteral tissue, divides the lateral umbilical ligament, and preserves the paravesical nerves, vas, and hypogastric vessels. After division of periureteral tissue in front of the ureter, the ureter is trimmed for a distance of several cm and a part of its diameter corresponding to its size. Reconstruction of the ureter is performed either by interrupted sutures in its whole length or only in its most distal part combined with a proximal running, locking suture. The line of sutures is covered by the periureteral tissue.

After formation of a new bladder opening cranial and paramedian of the old one and incision of its caudal rim, the bladder mucosa is incised along the foreseen new tunnel (length > 3 times the diameter of the reconstructed ureter), the old opening closed, a possible diverticulum repaired, and the new ureteric end anchored to the muscles of the trigonum after resection of its stenotic part. After closure of the mucosa over the new tunnel, a smooth catheter is left in the ipsilateral ureter and a suprapubic or transurethral catheter in the bladder for <14 days, and the wound is stepwise closed.

Modellage of the proximal ureter is not performed at the first intervention and only considered for secondary intervention, if spontaneous recovery does not take place after several months: persistent functional obstruction by tortuosity, elongation, and kinking especially close to the pyeloureteric junction.

Surgery performed by experienced hands corrects obstructive megaureter in >90 %, and the success rate is better in otherwise normal bladders than in valve bladder, ureteroceles, prune-belly syndrome, bladder exstrophy, or neurogenic bladder that need possibly a second intervention. Residual ureteral dilatation resolves within 1–3 years, and growth of the ipsilateral kidney corresponds to that of the normal contralateral kidney. **Complications** include postoperative reflux because of a short tunnel, lateral orifice, ureteral fistula at the bladder entrance,

or postoperative obstruction due to angulation of the ureter, a large postoperative diverticulum obstructing the ureter at the bladder entrance site, or fibrosis of the reimplanted ureter.

27.1.2 Prune-Belly Syndrome (Eagle-Barrett or Triad Syndrome)

Occurrence, Definition, Pathoanatomy

It is a rare disorder (1:30–40,000 male live births) that occurs mostly in boys (>95 %) and consists of different degrees of deficiency of abdominal wall muscles, hydroureteronephrosis, and cryptorchidism.

1. The **deficiency of abdominal wall muscles** is responsible for the characteristic skin appearance of prune-belly syndrome #. In mild cases, wrinkling skin is missing, but consistence and contour of the abdomen are rather conspicuous with a lax protruding abdominal wall. It may be combined with flaring rib margins, funnel chest, and kyphoscoliosis like in severe cases.

2. **Kidneys and Urinary Tract**. The collecting system of the kidneys is either dilated or dysmorphic, and the ureters reveal extreme dilatation, elongation, and tortuosity. Their walls have a defective architecture of different degrees and variable distribution, and their peristalsis is weak or ineffective. The renal parenchyma varies between normality and dysplasia. The tortuous proximal ureter corresponds not always to a real PUJ obstruction.

The **bladder** has a thick and smooth wall. It is mostly large and may display an elongated shape with a dome similar to a large diverticulum, a patent urachus with a wetting navel, and gaping ureteral orifices that are displaced out of the trigonum and responsible for gross reflux.

The **wide bladder neck continues in a dilated prostatic urethra** that yields a characteristic shape in the VCUG like a heart. At the level of verumontanum, **valve-like narrowing** (in up to 50 %) and **posterior urethral valves** (>10 %) at its caudal end may be present. Other possible abnormalities are **urethral atresia, stenosis, or megaurethra.**

3. The usually **undescended and small testicles** lie close to the internal inguinal ring. Their vessels are short and testis-epididymis dissociation or tortuous vasa with atresia may be observed.

Clinical Significance

- Prune-belly syndrome may be misdiagnosed as posterior urethral valves by prenatal ultrasound.
- Incomplete and/or forms with slight external signs of the triad may not be recognized as prune-belly syndrome.
- Immediate and long-term treatment is demanding and must be adapted to the individual case because the ubiquitous disorder of urine transport is based on a true obstruction only in a minority of cases.

Clinical Presentation

Prune-belly syndrome may be recognized by prenatal ultrasound in the second trimester (abnormally distended bladder and abdomen, absence of keyhole sign). After birth, the *characteristic irregular wrinkling of the whole abdominal skin or parts of the extremely lax skin, the protrusion of the flanks or of the belly in an anterior direction in upright position, and the visible and palpable intestinal loops and even ureters or bladder that are recognizable by their shapes and peristaltic waves* permit the diagnosis together with *nonpalpable testes*.

Differential Diagnosis, Work-Ups

The differential diagnosis may be difficult in abortive (incomplete) cases or patients with slight degrees of the syndrome. It includes disorders of micturition, with cryptorchidism, and recurrent urinary tract infections. If only the lax skin is considered, several disorders may be considered. Ultrasound, VCUG (after retro- or anterograde filling), urine (sediment, cultures), and serum analyses (creatinine, urea, electrolytes, etc.) belong to the first examinations: They display dilated bladder with thickened wall, dilated and tortuous ureters, hydronephrosis and/or dysplasia, reflux (up to 85 %), and possible patent urachus. In addition, IVU; MRI; scintiscan for evaluation of renal function, possible site of obstruction, and quantification of urine transport; and urethrocystoscopy for evaluation of the urethral pathoanatomy may be performed.

Finally, depending on the clinical examination, possible **associated anomalies** must be excluded that occur in three fourth of the cases: pulmonary hypoplasia secondary to oligohydramnios and congenital heart disease, gastrointestinal (anorectal and cloacal malformations, malrotation, Hirschsprung's disease, gastroschisis and omphalocele), and orthopedic anomalies (pectus excavatum, scoliosis, torticollis, hip dislocation, and talipes equinovarus).

Treatment, Prognosis

In one fourth to two thirds of prune-belly syndrome and other malformations recognizable by ultrasound, the pregnancy is terminated in developed countries. The indication of vesicoamniotic shunt may be normal karyotype, renal function, and exclusion of major associated anomalies, whereas centers for fetal diagnosis and treatment start with vesicoamniotic shunt around midpregnancy in lower urinary tract obstruction combined with oligo- or anhydramnios (91 % 1-year survival with a mean 5.8-year survival and one third who need dialysis and transplantation).

Maintenance of urine evacuation and avoidance of urinary tract infection belong to the urgent measures. Because the substantial obstruction concerns the lower urinary tract in the majority of cases, this therapeutic option may be achieved by frequent clean intermittent catheterization and overnight catheter drainage, long-term urinary catheterization by the urachus, percutaneous suprapubic catheter drainage or cystostomy, and if the upper urinary tract obstruction is significant, by percutaneous nephro-, pyelo, or ureterostomy.

The meantime may be used for **surgical correction of the urethra** depending on the encountered anomaly and **orchidopexy**. Orchidopexy by Fowler-Stephens in one or two stages is best performed at this age and needs mobilization of the testis together with a strip of pelvic peritoneum.

Major reconstructive procedures of the upper urinary tract, bladder augmentation, or bladder replacement methods including urinary diversions need special skills and should be performed before renal transplantations. Permanent urinary diversions may be avoided by the former measures in a majority of cases.

Abdominal flaccidity may be improved by an (possibly laparoscopic-assisted) **abdominal wall reconstruction** that includes a bilateral and vertical fascial plication in two layers (Monfort procedure) and may be modified by a new umbilicus (created from an island flap based on the fascial plate at the iliac crest).

Prognosis concerning survival depends on the presence of lung hypoplasia, renal dysplasia, or secondary development of renal failure (up to one third), or development of urosepsis. Normal puberty and sex life is possible in >90 % with >50 % bilateral and >30 unilateral testis palpable in the scrotal pouch after Fowler-Stephens, but infertility must be expected in all.

27.1.3 Ureteroceles

Occurrence, Forms, Classification
In ureteroceles, the intravesical (or intraurethral) part of the ureter reveals a cystic dilatation that protrudes in the bladder or urethral lumen. Its orifice is either stenotic and hardly recognizable or wide with possible reflux. Ureteroceles occur at autopsy more frequently than diagnosed in life and concern probably mostly the adult type.

Three fourths of **ureteroceles are associated with complete ureteral duplication**, concern the upper moiety of the kidney, and are mainly observed in female children #. One fourth concerns **one or both single kidneys** and present as infantile or adult type.

In the first form, the ureterocele is often **ectopic** (the ureterocele is partly or completely situated in the bladder neck or urethra), whereas the **intravesical ureterocele** lies mostly completely within the bladder and belongs to a single ureter. Nevertheless, not all ureteroceles with duplex collecting system are ectopic and not all single system ureteroceles are exclusively intravesical.

The **external appearance** of the ureteroceles may be different on clinical examination,

radiological imaging, endoscopy, and surgery depending on the size, shape, and precise site of ureterocele; the size of its orifice, whether it is sessile or pedunculated; its submucous expansion in caudal direction; and the strength of the adjacent detrusor muscle. The same is true for their **effect on the ipsi- and/or contralateral ureter** (megaureter), **on the adjacent bladder wall** (formation of a diverticulum, invagination), and **on the bladder neck and urethra** (urinary retention or incontinence). Therefore, several categories of ureterocele with possible dynamic changes may be encountered of which some are depicted in Fig. 27.2.

Clinical Presentation
Ureteroceles of appropriate size may be recognized by prenatal ultrasound due to a filling defect of the bladder.

They manifest postnatally by *urinary tract infection and less frequently by disorders of micturition (complete or partial urinary retention, e.g., dribbling, interrupted micturition, or different degrees of incontinence), abdominal pain, or an interlabial mass (prolapsing ureterocele in the girl).*

The early manifestation of ureterocele concerns ureteroceles combined with duplex ureteral system and less frequently the infantile type of ureteroceles with single ureter. The adult type of ureterocele is either an *incidental finding* or becomes symptomatic due to *urolithiasis or urinary tract infection* beyond childhood.

Differential Diagnosis, Work-Ups
It includes disorders with urinary tract infection, of micturition, with recurrent abdominal pain, and rarely with an intralabial mass or urolithiasis of the upper urinary tract.

Ultrasound of the full bladder reveals a roundish, thick-walled cystic structure in relation to trigonum and bladder wall. It allows differentiation between duplex (lateralization of the kidney by an upper pole megaureter) and single ureter kidney and shows a possible alteration of the upper pole or lower kidney structure and more frequently dilatation of the ipsi- and occasionally of the contralateral ureter. Differentiation may be difficult in extreme megaureter.

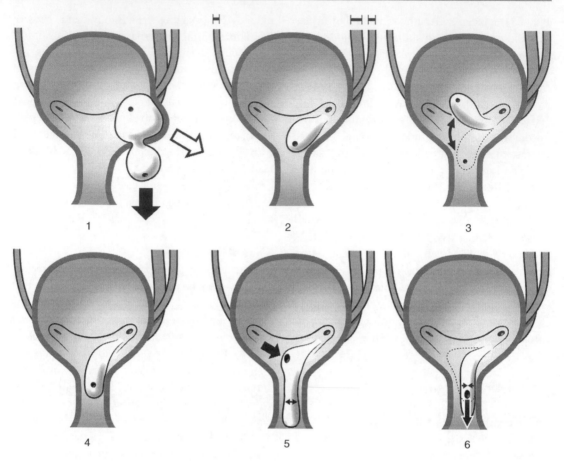

Fig. 27.2 Types of ureterocele. *1*: Orthotopic ureterocele with megaureter. Diverticulization of left bladder wall due to detrusor weakness $\Rightarrow$ or extravesicalization of ureterocele at endoscopy $\rightarrow$; *2*: sessile intravesical ureterocele in left complete duplication, megaureter of the cranial moiety of the kidney. *3*: Pedunculated ureterocele in left complete ureteral duplication, megaureter of the cranial moiety of the kidney. Different positions of the ureterocele of which one is prolapsed into the bladder neck. *4*: Ectopic ureterocele in complete ureteral duplication, constant bladder neck obstruction due to stenotic orifice. *5*: Cecoureterocele with wide orifice $\rightarrow$ obstruction of the bladder neck and urethral micturition due to reflux into the orifice (<–>). *6*: Ectopic ureterocele with wide orifice. Minimal obstruction of the bladder neck at micturition due to emptying of ureterocele (>–<) (Added to and redrawn according to Franc (1998))

VCUG shows reflux in the ipsi- and/or contralateral ureter or ureterocele, distal extension of ureterocele, voiding pattern of the bladder, and the dynamics of the ureterocele (emptying, filling, prolapse, or invagination at micturition).

IVU and urethrocystoscopy including inspection of the external genitals and colposcopy complete the work-ups (function of the involved renal moiety, examination of urethra, visualization of ureterocele #, ureteral orifices, and retrograde pyelography, and permits interventional surgery). **DMSA** scintigraphy is used for determination of the differential function of the upper and lower renal moiety or of the whole kidney. **MRI** is occasionally useful because it demonstrates an excellent overview of the whole system independent of function ##.

Treatment, Prognosis
The indications depend on the function of the involved upper pole or kidney and the site of ureterocele.

In general, intravesical ureterocele resection with reconstruction of bladder wall, ureteral modellage, and reimplantation en bloc should be avoided if possible. Best results of endoscopic ureterocele punction are achieved in orthotopic single ureter ureterocele.

1. Complete functional loss or differential function ≤10 %:

    Surgery is started with upper pole and subtotal ureter resection after deflation of the distal ureter and ligation close to the bladder. Further bladder intervention is only performed if necessary on follow-up. Alternative option: Endoscopic punction of the ureterocele. Further surgery is performed, if symptomatic reflux occurs or the patient remains symptomatic.

2. Sufficient residual function: Resection of the involved megaureter and interpyelic anastomosis. Further bladder intervention is performed only if necessary on follow-up. Alternative option: Endoscopic punction of the ureterocele. Further surgery, if symptomatic reflux occurs or the patients remains symptomatic.

The prognosis is excellent after complete resection of the upper pole or kidney and the corresponding ureter or after interpyelic anastomosis and resection of the involved ureter. The adult type of ureterocele needs regular long-term follow-ups.

27.2   Ureteral Duplications

Occurrence, Pathoanatomy

Ureteral duplication of one or less frequently of both kidney(s) occurs in 0.5–1.0 % of the population and preferred in females.

If two ureteral buds develop from the Wolffian duct, two separate ureters and collecting system of the ipsilateral kidney are formed. The ureter from the cranial renal moiety crosses first twice in front of the caudal ureter from medial to lateral and vice versa, then behind it from medial to lateral at the level of the bladder, and enters the bladder below the orifice of the caudal ureter (**complete ureteral duplication** (Fig. 27.3)).

The involved kidney is somewhat larger and the smaller upper moiety is delineated from the lower moiety only by a superficial furrow and

separate main branches of the renal artery and vein. Eccentric origin of the ureteral bud is usually combined with an ectopic ureteral orifice and a hypo- or dysplastic moiety.

If the ureteral bud forks outside of the Wolffian duct in two ureters, incomplete duplications develop with a common orifice and possibly with a distal common segment and a proximal duplex part. Depending on the site of duplication, a V- (with a common segment that includes only the transvesical ureter) or a Y-type of **incomplete duplication** is encountered (Fig. 27.4). Incomplete duplication occurs only in about 15 % of duplications. In about 50 %, the bifurcation concerns the middle part of the ureter.

Clinical Significance

- Up to 50 % of ureteral duplications are symptomless and may be recognized only as incidental finding at work-ups performed for other reasons.
- The complete ureteral duplication becomes more frequently symptomatic than the incomplete forms. Although recurrent urinary tract infection is the most common clinical presentation, ureteral duplication may be hidden behind a colorfully shimmering symptomatology.
- Dys- and hypoplastic renal moieties with a long-standing disorder usually need resection for permanent cure.

27.2.1 Complete Ureteral Duplication

Clinical Presentation

If both ureters enter the bladder, the following possibilities arise arranged in order of decreasing frequency: (1) The orifice of the caudal ureter may be lateralized (B, C, or D position in relation of the lateral cornu of the trigonum) leading to reflux in >90 % ##. About 30 % of duplex system has significant reflux; (2) the ostium of the cranial ureter is stenotic or exhibits a ureterocele leading to megaureter. Greater than 10 % of duplex system has a ureterocele; (3) both anomalies are combined.

Recurrent urinary tract infection is observed more frequently than disorders of micturition,

Fig. 27.3 Complete ureteral duplication in which two ureters enter the bladder, or one of them has an ectopic orifice outside the bladder. In the picture on the *left side*, the lower pole ureter enters the bladder in the cranial and the upper pole ureter in the caudal trigonum. In the drawing on the *right side*, the lower pole ureter enters bladder inside the trigonum, and the upper pole ureter enters the urinary tract distal from the trigonum in the bladder neck, urethra, seminal vesicle, vagina, or vulva. The orifice of the ectopic ureter may exhibit reflux and/or ureterocele

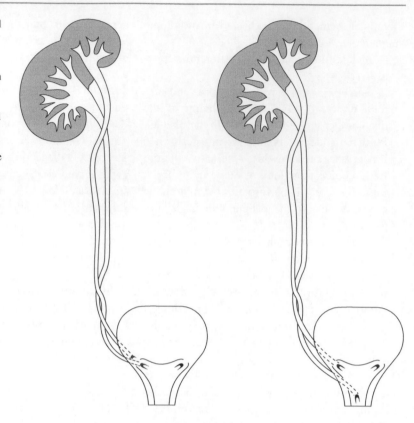

recurrent abdominal pain, and/or abdominal tumor.

If the cranial ureter (combined with ureterocele or not) enters the bladder neck, posterior urethra within the limits of the external sphincter, seminal vesicle, or ejaculatory duct in boys, and the urethra beyond the external sphincter or vagina in girls >30 % of duplex system, the following symptomatology may be encountered: *recurrent urinary tract infection and abdominal pain, abdominal tumor, urinary retention, and scrotal and testicular swelling (because of recurrent epididymitis and seminal vesiculitis)* in boys or *urinary incontinence or urine dribbling combined with normal micturition, enuresis, recurrent urinary tract infection (because of reflux), and intralabial masses* in girls.

Normal micturition combined with urine dribbling that cannot be influenced voluntarily is characteristic for girls with ectopic entrance of the cranial ureter in the distal urethra, vulva, and vagina. *It may be recognized by close inspection of the external genitals. The ectopic orifice may*

present as additional small opening, vulvar ectopic ureterocele, or may be hidden behind the normal urethral orifice.

Differential Diagnosis, Work-Ups

It includes all disorders with the already quoted leading symptoms and signs especially the infrequent ones such as disorders of micturition including urine dribbling, intralabial masses in girls, and urinary retention or scrotal and testicular swelling in boys.

In addition to ultrasound and VCUG, endoscopy has a major significance for work-up:

It is possible to visualize the site (lateralization or extravesical site) and shape of the ureteral orifice (gaping orifice #, ureterocele with stenosis, or large orifice). DMSA and other scintiscans are used for detection of the relative function of the involved renal moiety, the presence of pyelonephritic focuses or scars, and tracer out- and backflow. For precise topographical and pathoanatomical delineation of the anomalies, MRI with contrast is useful.

Fig. 27.4 Incomplete ureteral duplication in which there is a common distal ureter. If the common ureter is long as shown in the picture on the *left side*, the incomplete ureteral duplication may be called Y-type and in case of short common ureter as shown in the picture on the *right side*, V-type

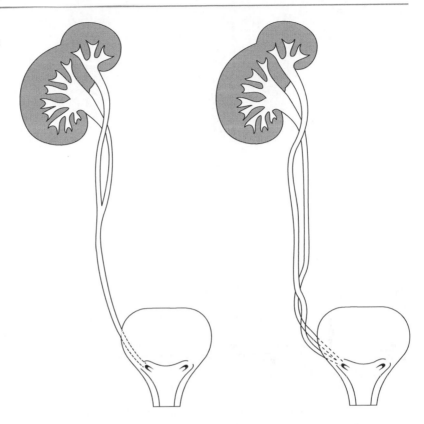

Treatment, Prognosis

The indication of reconstructive surgery or heminephrectomy depends on the morphology and function of the involved renal moiety, ureter, and possible presence of a lateralized or ectopic ureteral orifice, ureterocele, or ureteral stenosis:

1. Reflux of the caudal ureter # and/or ureterocele of the cranial ureter needs common sheet reimplantation (both intravesical ureters en bloc), in combination with ureterocele, aditional resection if the corresponding renal moiety has a sufficient function.
2. In megaureter due to severe reflux or ureterocele, type I or II ureteropyelostomy (interpyelic anastomosis) with resection of the involved ureter may be considered (Fig. 27.5);
3. If the relative renal function of the involved moiety is ≤10 %, heminephrectomy is performed # or nephrectomy, if both moieties are destroyed.

In extravesical ureter of the boy, the upper moiety of the kidney has usually lost its function due to obstruction and/or reflux and is mostly combined with megaureter. Both need resection by upper pole heminephrectomy and ureterectomy. Ureteroureterostomy (by inguinotomy) or interpyelic anastomosis may be performed in girls with ectopic ureter and in boys if the renal function is preserved. The residual or complete ureter respectively is resected.

Successful surgery leads to permanent cure in the majority of cases.

27.2.2 Incomplete Ureteral Duplication

Clinical Presentation

The Y- and the V-type of incomplete ureteral duplication may become symptomatic. The symptoms of the former are caused by a so-called **yo-yo reflux** within the proximal duplex segment or **obstruction** of the pelvicureteral junction or the ureter at the transition in the common segment, and of the latter due to severe **reflux** of the common ureteral orifice.

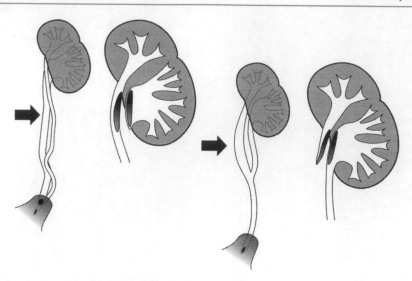

Fig. 27.5 Examples of surgical techniques in complete and incomplete ureteral duplication. The drawing on the *left side* shows dilatation of the ureter of the lower kidney because of severe vesicoureteral reflux. The problem of reflux and gross dilatation may be resolved by an interpyelic anastomosis (type I) combined with complete resection of the caudal ureter or by low ureteroureteros- tomy with resection of the caudal ureter stump. In the drawing on the *right side*, the incomplete duplication with high junction has led to a yo-yo reflux. The problem is resolved by an interpyelic anastomosis (type II) between the pelvis of the cranial moiety and caudal pelvis combined with resection of the dilated cranial ureter

The main clinical presentation is *recurrent urinary tract infection and abdominal pain due to the yo-yo phenomenon.*

Differential Diagnosis, Work-Ups

The recurrent abdominal pain needs specific con- sideration in the differential diagnosis, and the work-ups must be supplemented by IVU or scin- tiscan with video documentation of the contrast or tracer with search for yo-yo reflux #. The unco- ordinated peristalsis in both ureters leads to a back- and forward movement of the urine in both ureters and insufficient outflow in the common segment. In turn, urinary stasis triggers abdomi- nal pain and urinary tract infection

Treatment, Prognosis

Severe reflux of the V-type needs – after resec- tion of the common vesical part – reimplantation of both ureters en bloc without separation of the ureters from each other. Appropriate length of the common tunnel is necessary (≥3 times the diam- eter of both ureters).

If the complaints of the Y-type are confirmed by characteristic cineradiographic findings, interpyelic anastomosis type I or II is indicated #, ureteropyelic

anastomosis type I between cranial ureter and cau- dal pelvis is indicated if the caudal ureter must be resected because of dilatation, and ureteropelvic anastomosis type II between cranial ureter and cau- dal pelvis is indicated if the cranial ureter is dilated and must be resected (Fig. 27.5).

Correct indication and successfully performed surgery is followed by permanent cure in the majority of cases.

27.3   Fusion Anomalies of the Kidney

27.3.1 Horseshoe Kidney

Occurrence, Pathoanatomy

Horseshoe kidney is the most common fusion anomaly and has a similar incidence to renal ectopia. In >90 %, the lower poles are joined together (rarely the upper poles) by normal, dys- plastic, or fibrous renal tissue in front of the aorta (rarely behind the aorta). The isthmus is located either at the normal level of the lower poles or beneath the inferior mesenteric artery and in one fifth in the pelvis.

Horseshoe kidney may be combined with dysplasia, some ectopia, and variable rotation of each kidney. The single ureter has a high pelvic junction, runs in an anterior direction over the isthmus or lower pole, may be superimposed by crossing vessels, and lies altogether closer to the midline lateralized. The isthmus may be supplied by different sources, and even the main vascular supply to the kidneys may cross it.

Clinical Significance

- Depending on the pathoanatomical findings, horseshoe kidney may become symptomatic.
- The risk of Wilms' tumor in children # and of renal cell or collecting system carcinoma in adults is several times increased.
- Surgery in horseshoe kidney is a challenge for the pediatric surgeon and urologist/vascular surgeon (*e.g.*, tumor or aortic aneurism).

Clinical Presentation

The majority of horseshoe kidneys are asymptomatic and recognized incidentally, but up to one third may become symptomatic from child- to adulthood.

The symptomatology consists *either of urological symptoms and signs such as urinary tract infection, recurrent abdominal pain, hematuria, and abdominal tumor* (due to hydronephrosis with pelvicureteral or high ureteral obstruction, reflux, or urolithiasis) *or less frequently of ischemic abdominal pain* (because of intermittent obstruction of the inferior mesenteric artery). Several pathophysiological mechanisms may lead to a *suspected surgical abdomen* (renal calculus colic, upper urinary tract obstruction, intestinal ischemia).

Associated malformations are observed in more than three fourths of horseshoe kidneys and include mainly the CNS, gastrointestinal, skeletal, and cardiovascular system. Turner syndrome belongs to the disorders associated with renal anomalies such as horseshoe kidney.

Work-Ups, Differential Diagnosis

For rapid confirmation of horseshoe kidney and possible functional deficit of parts of it, DMSA scintiscan is very useful.

Ultrasound, VCUG (vesicoureteral reflux), and IVU (indirect signs of horseshoe kidney such as abnormal longitudinal axes, *e.g.*, V-shaped cranial divergence, and calices superimposed over the pelvis or medially of it with parasagittal orientation, anterior course of the proximal ureter over the isthmus or lower renal pole in lateral view) add further informations. 3D contrast CT, 3D spect (single-photon emission computed tomography), or MRI angio- and urography may be used preoperatively for precise anatomical and functional informations.

The differential diagnosis includes disorders of the quoted symptoms and signs.

Treatment, Prognosis

Surgery is indicated in case of upper urinary tract obstruction, symptomatic or severe reflux, intermittent ischemic attacks confirmed by precise history and radiological imaging, or tumor.

Except for ureteral reimplantation, the access depends on the planned intervention (type and laterality) and the position of horseshoe kidney and its parts. Instead of the usual extraperitoneal anterolateral approach, a transverse transperitoneal incision may facilitate reconstructive or resective surgery. It includes Anderson-Hynes pyeloplasty, ureterocalicostomy (Fig. 27.6), antireflux surgery, and rarely division or resection of the isthmus. The latter must consider the abnormal blood supply of the isthmus.

If the appropriate procedure is possible and skillfully performed, the outcome is excellent.

27.3.2 Crossed Renal Ectopia

The type of crossed renal ectopia with fusion with the contralateral kidney is the second most common fusion anomaly. It is often combined with other malformations of many organ systems including VACTRL syndrome.

27.4 Renal Ectopia

Occurrence, Types

Ectopia is observed in < to >1:1,000 individuals and in three locations: pelvic (below the aortic bifurcation), lumbar # (above the iliac crest), or intrathoracic and may occur as crossed ectopia.

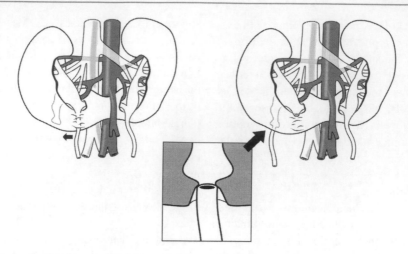

Fig. 27.6 Most frequent type of horseshoe kidney and treatment of the ureteropelvic junction obstruction on the *right side* by calicoureterostomy. Drawing on the *left side*: the ureteropelvic junction of the right side is embedded in the renal parenchyma and surrounded by the dense fibrous tissue. Mobilization of proximal ureter leaves a devitalized segment. Therefore, calicoureterostomy may be an alternative method as demonstrated in the drawing on the *right side* and more precisely in the *middle* at the *bottom*

Pelvic ectopia with the kidney either in front of the sacrum or the iliac bone is the most common location. Crossed ectopia appears mostly as anomaly in which the upper pole is fused with the lower pole of the contralateral kidney. Crossed ectopia without fusion as solitary kidney or bilateral ectopia occurs much less frequently.

Clinical Significance

- If renal ectopia becomes symptomatic, the abnormal pathoanatomy (abnormal shape, variable rotation, extrarenal calices, and deviation of blood supply and ureter from the normal anatomy and topography) needs precise evaluation by contrast CT or angio MRI before intervention.

Clinical Presentation

Renal ectopia is mostly an incidental finding. *Occasionally, the anomaly is detected because of urinary tract infection, recurrent abdominal pain, lower abdominal or intrathoracic tumor, urolithiasis* (upper urinary tract obstruction or reflux), *or signs of obstructive ileus, sometimes at work-up of associated genital or contralateral urological anomalies*, and rarely as part of Mayer-Rokitansky-Küster-Hauser syndrome. In case of a seemingly single kidney, ectopic kidney must be considered.

Work-Ups, Differential Diagnosis

DMSA scintiscan is very useful for detection of a supposed renal ectopia. In addition to ultrasound, VCUG, and IVU, contrast CT or MRI uro- and angiogram lead to more specific topographicoanatomical informations needed for surgery.

The differential diagnosis includes abdominal tumor specifically of the retroperitoneum or pelvis and in the intrathoracic type, lung sequestration, inflammatory and neoplastic lung tumor, or congenital diaphragmatic hernia. Ptotic kidney as differential diagnosis of lumbar ectopia plays a minor role in childhood.

Treatment, Prognosis

Both depend on the underlying cause (upper urinary tract obstruction, reflux, or acquired disorders (urolithiasis, tumor, or trauma)) and the skills of the pediatric surgeon because of the unusual location and topography of the renal ectopia.

27.5   Renal Aplasia, Hypoplasia, and Dysplasia

Occurrence

All three anomalies occur uni- or bilaterally, or combined. Unilateral renal aplasia has a prevalence of about 1:1,000 live births, whereas the bilateral form and the other anomalies are encountered less frequently as isolated disorders.

27.5.1   Renal Aplasia

Pathoanatomy
In renal aplasia, the kidney(s) and ureter(s) are missing, whereas in renal agenesis, a rudimentary proton is present. Renal aplasia may be a part of **adysplasia** in which a spectrum of aplasia, hypoplasia, and dysplasia is found in the same patient. Uni- and bilateral aplasia may be also a part of **VACTERL syndrome** and bilateral agenesia belongs together with a characteristic face and malformations of the lower extremities to the **Potter syndrome**.

Clinical Significance
From a pediatric surgical or urological point of view, the following observations are important:
- Although the contralateral kidney is mostly morphologically and functionally normal, dysplasia or malformations may occur (*e.g.*, adysplasia).
- In reality, a second ectopic kidney without or with dysplasia may exist.
- Unilateral renal aplasia influences the indication of surgery in the remaining kidney.
- In case of bilateral renal aplasia, the newborn dies due to lung hypoplasia. Bilateral aplasia must be excluded therefore before surgery, for example, reconstruction of esophageal atresia in VACTERL syndrome.

Work-Ups, Differential Diagnosis, Treatment, Prognosis
Unilateral aplasia needs evaluation of the single kidney, exclusion of an ectopic kidney, and regular ultrasound follow-ups. Sports with major risks of trauma to the flank, long-term application of nonsteroidal antirheumatics, and other nephrotoxic drugs should be avoided. Prognosis of children with unilateral aplasia is usually excellent. In newborns with or without foreseen surgery, bilateral renal aplasia should be excluded by clinical examination and if needed by ultrasound.

27.5.2   Renal Hypoplasia or Dysplasia

Pathoanatomy
In hypoplasia, the kidney is small and has fewer calices (<10). A small kidney with possible cysts is typical for dysplasia. It comprises disorganized, undifferentiated, metaplastic, and possibly ectopic tissue. Dysplasia concerns either the whole kidney(s) # or is an integrated part of another malformation of the kidney, for example, upper moiety of a renal duplex system or isthmus of horseshoe kidney. Both anomalies may concern parts of the kidney, one or both kidneys, or occur in combination.

Clinical Significance
- Hypoplasia has mainly a differential diagnostic significance.
- Complete or partially dysplastic kidney(s) are prone to urinary tract infection.
- It (they) may be a part of several urological malformations such as obstructive uropathies and may therefore influence the prognostic outlook.
- Bilateral renal dysplasia may lead to oligohydramnios, renal failure at birth, at 2–4 years of age, or later.
- In case of ignorance of history and pre- or postnatal clinical and radiological findings, a small kidney with irregular contour or similar localized signs compatible with dysplasia may lead to an incorrect interpretation as sequels of acquired disorders, for example, reflux nephropathy.
- Localized or diffuse renal dysplasia may be the cause of renal hypertension that may be cured by partial renal resection or nephrectomy.

Work-Ups, Differential Diagnosis, Treatment, Prognosis
In contrast to hypolasia, dysplasia displays a kidney with irregular contour or shape on radiological imaging. The same concerns the texture and differentiation on ultrasound in hypoplastic versus dysplastic kidney. The **differential diagnosis of a small kidney** depends on the age and history. In newborns, mainly dysplasia, hypoplasia, and **oligomeganephronia** (decreased

number of enlarged glomeruli) must be considered and in older children, in addition, **acquired disorders**, for example, former renal trauma. Differentiation is possible by history and radiological imaging to a certain degree and more reliable by DMSA scintigram or renal biopsy. Recurrent urinary tract infection or arterial hypertension because of localized or diffuse dysplasia may be cured by partial renal resection or nephrectomy. Localized dysplasia of one renal moiety needs resective surgery that includes the ureter.

27.6   Cystic Disorders of the Kidney

27.6.1 Multicystic Renal Dysplasia

Occurrence, Pathoanatomy
Multicystic renal dysplasia belongs to the most common differential diagnoses of prenatal hydronephrosis on ultrasound and of a palpable abdominal tumor in the newborn.

In 95 %, only one kidney is involved. It consists of multiple cysts of different size and dysplastic tissue. The cysts communicate neither with each other nor the collecting system. Calices, pelvis, and proximal ureter are absent #; usually, a distal ureter exists with a blind end. Segmental multicystic dysplastic kidney occurs mostly in the upper pole of a duplex kidney. Multicystic renal dysplasia and the segmental type may be associated with ureterocele.

According to the natural history, >20 % of the multicystic renal dysplasias disappear on ultrasound after 3–5 years, and 50 % remain unchanged on sonography.

Clinical Significance
- Multicystic renal dysplasia may present as a large, space-occupying mass in the newborn.
- Occurrence of reflux in the ureteral stump of the involved side and possible malformation of the contralateral kidney carry the risk of recurrent urinary tract infections.
- In spite of involution of the cystic part in about 50 % of the cases, the dysplastic residue is at minor risk of several complications.

Clinical Presentation
In addition to the possible prenatal diagnosis or suspicion that must be confirmed postnatally, *a visible and/or palpable abdominal tumor and/or recurrent urinary tract infections* are the main clinical presentation.

Associated malformations include reflux of the ipsilateral ureteral stump, absence, ectopia, or dysplasia, reflux, or obstructive uropathy of the contralateral kidney. Although multicystic renal dysplasia is not a transmitted anomaly of the collecting system, it may be encountered in kindreds.

Differential Diagnosis, Work-Ups
It includes mainly disorders of the prenatal ultrasound diagnosis "hydronephrosis" and after birth, of abdominal tumor and recurrent urinary tract infection, especially advanced cases of PUJ obstruction or obstructive ureter.

The work-ups are necessary because of the differential diagnosis and possible associated malformations and consist minimally of ultrasound and VCUG. DTPA and DMSA scintigraphy demonstrates absent function of the involved kidney.

Treatment, Prognosis
Surgery is indicated in symptomatic reflux of the ureteral stump # or if the contralateral and single kidney is involved. Because some of the ureteroceles combined with multicystic renal dysplasia do not collapse in spite of an expectant approach, early endoscopic punction is a valuable option.

The indication of resection of the multicystic renal dysplasia is controversial:
1. The expectant approach applies regular ultrasound follow-ups until the disappearance of the cystic part of the malformation and presents the following observations as an argument in favor of this option: significant chance of spontaneous resolution, avoidance of unnecessary operation, and infrequent occurrence of complications in childhood.
2. Surgery may be chosen for the following reasons:
   - Multicystic renal dysplasia may present as a large, space-occupying mass.

- Confusion with advanced PUJ obstruction is possible.
- Involution may take a long time, and if it occurs, dysplastic tissue is left behind.
- Elements of nephroblastomatosis occur in children and different malignant renal tumors or renal hypertension in adults.
- Infection and hemorrhage of the cyst can be avoided.
- A life with subjective uncertainty (parent's point of view), innumerable follow-ups (viewpoint of the insurance), and prolongation of an unresolved problem into adulthood must be considered.

Surgery is best performed in the neonatal period or early infancy, or if the size of the malformation remains unchanged. Although the mass may be very large, complete resection is possible by an extraperitoneal approach and if necessary, by punction of the larger cysts without the risk of postoperative ileus due to adhesions.

Prognosis is excellent after complete resection.

27.6.2 Autosomal Recessive Polycystic Kidney Disease (ARPKD)

Occurrence, Pathoanatomy
It occurs in 1:10,000–20,000 live births and is recognizable in the second half of pregnancy by ultrasound.

The kidneys are enlarged by diffuse, minute cysts and dilated collecting tubules. The kidneys have a spongy appearance with radial arrangement of fusiform cysts even visible by the naked eye.

Clinical Significance
- Prenatal ultrasound combined with a positive family history, advances in neonatal intensive care, and dialysis techniques have led to survival of some individuals.
- Surviving children need lifelong surveillance, intensive medical treatment, and possibly renal and hepatic transplantation.
- The expression of ARPKD may vary in the same family and generation. Therefore, less severe and/or delayed clinical courses are possible.

Clinical Presentation
Unborn patients with advanced disease suffer from oligohydramnios. Ultrasound shows large kidneys with hyperechogenicity, oligohydramnion, and empty bladder.

After birth, death is possible due to lung hypoplasia or renal failure. The majority who survive infancy reaches adolescence (except for death because of renal failure, portal hypertension, or cholangitis).

In the surviving children, *large kidneys are palpable*, *and early arterial hypertension* may be recorded. *Signs of congenital hepatic fibrosis develop in older children.*

Work-Up, Differential Diagnosis
The ultrasound shows large kidneys with increased echogenicity and loss of corticomedullary differentiation. Pooling of contrast in the collecting tubules leads to a dimmed appearance of the large kidneys (sunburst phenomenon) in the IVU. Occasionally, larger cysts (<2 cm) may be present. Liver ultrasound displays increased echogenicity and dilated intrahepatic ducts. Urinalysis and renal and hepatic serum markers are very important. If MRI does not confirm the diagnosis, percutaneous renal and/or hepatic biopsy may be indicated for differential diagnosis and staging.

The differential diagnosis includes ADPKD and other disorders with enlarged kidneys. The former differential diagnosis may be difficult by ultrasound.

Treatment, Prognosis
It includes treatment of renal failure and hypertension (hemodialysis, renal transplantation) and later of cholangitis, hepatic failure, and portal hypertension. DNA analysis and genetic counselling is important in cases with ARPKD not yet known in the family or spontaneous mutation.

27.6.3 Autosomal Dominant Polycystic Kidney Disease (ADPKD)

Occurrence, Pathoanatomy
It is less frequent than ARPKD (1:50,000 live births), and newborns are rarely and older children occasionally symptomatic.

Progressive development of countless cysts is observed in both kidneys that are of different sizes, compress, and replace the normal renal tissue within several decades. The disorder is caused by mutations of the PKD 1 or 2 gene (and other genes) that correspond to the clinical types 1 (85 %) and 2.

Clinical Significance
- Almost all patients reach end-stage renal failure during adulthood.
- Cysts are prone to hemorrhage or infection.
- >50 % of the patients develop arterial hypertension and/or >5–15 % intracranial aneurysms before end-stage renal failure.

Clinical Presentation
The disorder may be recognized by prenatal ultrasound and lead to oligohydramnios. The few symptomatic newborns display *respiratory failure and enlarged kidneys. Early clinical presentation is similar to that of adults.* Associated mitral valve prolapse, endocardial fibroelastosis, and intracranial aneurysms may also occur and occasionally **hypertrophic pyloric stenosis**.

End-stage renal failure occurs at a median age of 54 years in type 1 and 74 years in type 2. Although the time of end-stage renal failure may be variable within the same family or between families, it develops rapidly within a few years from an initially normal serum creatinine value.

The previous and oligosymptomatic period starts in the third or fourth decade with possible **arterial hypertension**, cyst hemorrhage, cyst infection, or pyelonephritis. Cyst hemorrhage and infection may lead to *flank and abdominal pain of variable degree up to acute severe attacks, possible microscopic or gross hematuria in the former, and fever and increased inflammatory markers in the latter.*

Cysts are observed in liver, pancreas, spleen, and arachnoidea. Cysts in the liver lead to progressive hepatomegaly as *a space-occupying abdominal mass.* In addition to *hypertension and spontaneous intracranial hemorrhage* due to intracranial aneurysms, valvular heart disease, dissection of coronary arteries, and dilatation of the aorta may become symptomatic.

Differential Diagnosis, Work-Ups
It includes disorders with bilateral renal enlargement, renal cyst(s), arterial hypertension, hepatomegaly, and end-stage renal insufficiency. ARPDK, simple cyst, megacalycosis, and multicystic renal dysplasia (in the rare unilateral ADPKD involvement) must be considered especially in children.

For diagnosis of ADPDK, positive family history, ultrasound, and DNA analysis are used. Ultrasound diagnosis is based on a minimal number of cysts in both or each kidney(s) and the age of the patient, for example, <40 years: at least three cysts in one or both kidney(s). The very large kidneys are lobular and display stretching and distortion of the calices by the cysts. Serial MRI may be used for prognostication by renal volumetry (the renal volume is determined by the volume of the cysts).

Treatment, Prognosis
It includes medical treatment of hypertension, symptomatic treatment of cyst hemorrhage and antibiotics for cyst infection or pyelonephritis (differentiation possible by PET/CT with 18F-FDG accumulation in cyst infection), and expectant or surgical treatment of the complications. Renal insufficiency needs hemodialysis and renal transplantation (peritoneal dialysis may be difficult due to hepatomegaly and the possibility of cyst infection). Inhibitors of cyst growth may become available in the future.

27.6.4 Localized Formation of Cysts

Simple or solitary renal cyst, **pyelogenic cyst**, and **hydrocalicosis** (megacalicosis) are examples of localized cysts. Whereas simple renal cyst is a cystic hamartoma without communication with the urine-collecting system, pyelogenic cyst and hydrocalycosis have a connection with it. Hydrocalycosis concerns either one calyx or a group of calices and is congenital or acquired. Because of the preferred site in the upper pole, especially the acquired forms are also called

upper calyx syndrome. Upper calyx syndrome may be observed after renal injury, after complicated nephrolithiasis, and after localized scarring due to reflux.

Occurrence

In contrast to the very rare congenital forms of localized cysts, acquired forms are observed somewhat more frequently.

Clinical Significance

- Each of the described cysts can gradually increase in size and behave like a space-occupying mass.
- The simple renal cyst # may mimic a Wilms' tumor.
- Hydrocalycosis with or without stricture of the calyceal neck may lead to recurrent urinary tract infection and stone formation.

Clinical Presentation

A simple renal cyst is mostly an incidental finding of ultrasound. The other cysts may lead to *recurrent urinary tract infection, hematuria, flank and abdominal pain*, and rarely to a palpable abdominal tumor or renal hypertension.

Differential Diagnosis, Work-Ups

It includes disorders with the quoted symptomatology and radiological imaging of Wilms' tumor, posttraumatic pseudocyst of the kidney, or ADPKD and ARPKD.

Ultrasound shows a solitary cystic mass with displacement of the pyelocalyceal system in simple cyst or distortion of one calyx or of a group of calices in upper calyx syndrome. Better description of all cysts and their differential diagnoses is possible by CT with i.v. contrast, retrograde pyelography, or IVU.

Treatment, Prognosis

Enucleation of a simple cyst or partial renal resection is necessary in case of continuously enlarging or already large simple cyst and for differential diagnosis or in symptomatic upper calyx syndrome #.

Prognosis is excellent, if the indication is correct.

27.7 Vesicoureteral Reflux (VUR, Reflux)

Occurrence

Reflux is a common disposing condition of urinary tract infection. Up to 30 % of hydronephrosis recognized by prenatal ultrasound are due to or associated with VUR, and vesicoureteral reflux is encountered in up to 50 % of children presenting with urinary tract infection.

Differentiation is useful between **fetal reflux** that is observed preferentially in boys and recognized at birth on work-up of prenatal hydronephrosis # and **classic reflux** that manifests clinically mainly in young girls.

Clinical Significance

- In children with urinary tract infection, reflux may increase the risk of pyelonephritis.
- One third to half of newborns with fetal reflux display a restricted function of one or both kidneys because of renal dysplasia, and renal hypertension and/or failure in the neonate or early in life are not excluded.
- Classic reflux, especially if bilateral and of high grade (grade IV and V) may lead to diffuse or localized renal scarring after upper urinary tract infection and possible hypertension and/or end-stage renal failure at puberty, in adolescence, or early adulthood.

Forms, Causes, and Grading of Reflux

The **primary reflux** results from congenital malformation, delayed maturation, or acquired causes such as cystitis.

1. Anomaly of the vesicoureteral junction (deficiency of the flap valve mechanism or short intravesical submucosal tunnel) is observed in the following disorders:
   - Uni- or bilateral gapping or golf hole orifice in single kidneys #
   - Gapping orifice of the caudal ureter in complete ureteral duplication (>90 %) or incomplete ureteral duplication with low junction (occasionally)
   - Deficiency of flap valve mechanism in ectopic ureter(s) without or with ureterocele

- Short intravesical submucosal tunnel or flap valve deficiency in bladder exstrophy and prune-belly syndrome
2. Delayed maturation of the flap valve mechanism
3. Caused by different stages or forms of cystitis

Secondary reflux is caused by disorders outside of the vesicoureteral junction and includes:

- Periureteral diverticulum (with gradual extravesicularization of the orifice #)
- Contralateral ureterocele
- Inferior obstructive uropathies such as posterior urethral valves
- **Functional voiding disorders**, neurogenic bladder (increased storage and voiding pressure)

According to an international consensus and relating to the radiological findings at voiding cystourethrography (VCU) at (slow and continuous) filling of the bladder and/or micturition, the degree of reflux is divided into five grades (Fig. 27.7):

Grade I and II correspond to a reflux in the ureter or ureter and pelvicalyceal system=**slight reflux**. Grade III (moderate reflux) and grades IV or V are combined with progressive dilatation of ureter, pelvis, and calices that become hardly recognizable as such in grades IV and V=**severe reflux**.

Clinical Presentation

Fetal reflux needs confirmation of reflux and grading by VCU because neither pre- nor postnatal ultrasound can almost certainly determine which newborn needs further evaluation for reflux. Severe fetal reflux may lead to *hypertension and/or end-stage renal failure in the neonate or early in life.*

No reflux-specific symptoms and signs exist. Urinary tract infection is the most common

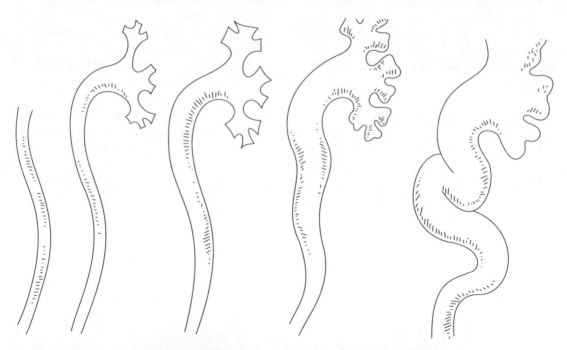

Fig. 27.7 Drawing of graduation of reflux (classification according to the degree of reflux) corresponding to an international consensus. The degree of vesicoureteral reflux increases from the *left* to the *right side* in the picture. Grade I and II on the *left side* in the drawing are slight types of reflux; during micturition, the ureter or, in addition, the pelvis is filled with contrast in the VCUG. In grade III (moderate reflux in the *middle* of the drawing), the ureter, pelvis, and calices are dilated but the fornixes have a sharp shape. In grade IV, also the fornixes are dilated and blunt, and in grade V (both on the *right side* in the picture), the deformations are grotesque and the ureter is tortuous. The two last-mentioned grades are severe types of reflux

clinical presentation either as recurrent simple or as acute complicated urinary tract infection. Enuresis or incontinence due to delayed learning of controlled micturition beyond the age of 5 years (in case of severe reflux, no sufficient bladder volume is attained that is necessary for bladder maturation), and rarely *hematurias* (about 3 %) are additional signs.

In **secondary reflux**, *the symptomatology of the underlying disorder may be in the foreground*, for example, symptomatology of the different functional voiding disorders.

Differential Diagnosis, Work-Ups

It includes disorders with urinary tract infection, enuresis, and urinary incontinence.

The primary work-ups are ultrasound and VCU with contrast. Ultrasound must include the morphology of the bladder and renal parenchyma (signs of cystitis, renal scarring, and size). Measurement of arterial pressure, urinalysis (sediment and cultures), and renal serum parameters are very important.

99 Technetium dimercaptosuccinic acid (DMSA) is useful for evaluation of complicated urinary tract infection and should be used at initial work-up and on follow-up for exclusion of preexisting or developing renal scarring. 99 Technetium mercaptoacetyltriglycine (MAG-3) may be applied combined with catheter drainage of the bladder and furosemide application for evaluation of the relative function of the involved kidney and for follow-up in case of decreased renal growth or signs of scarring.

At the beginning of treatment in the first decade of life, about 50 % of the children has already some renal scarring, 15 % localized thinning of parenchyma #, and 5 % small kidney #.

For evaluation of the form and cause of the reflux and the condition of the bladder, cystoscopy is indispensable (shape of the orifice, measurement of the length of submucosal tunnel, signs and type of cystitis). Functional voiding disorders and neurogenic bladder must be excluded if necessary by a precise history and urodynamic studies.

Treatment, Prognosis

The possible strategies of treatment are:

1. Nonoperative treatment in the majority of reflux cases
2. Elective surgery in a group of children with well-defined criteria of reflux
3. Operative treatment in the majority of reflux cases

Nonoperative treatment means avoidance of urinary tract infection by continuous prophylactic antibiotics until spontaneous disappearance of reflux or conversion to a low grade. It needs numerous follow-ups with urinalysis and radiological imaging, and long-term medication.

This approach is based on the international reflux study with a European and American branch performed in the 1990s of the last century. It demonstrated that spontaneous resolution of reflux is possible and that the percentage of new renal scarring and of preexisting scars that increase in size is identical in children with nonoperative and surgical treatment. The chance of spontaneous reflux resolution during a 5-year observation time is greater in unilateral or newly detected reflux cases than in refluxes that are bilateral or remain unchanged grade III or IV during 1 year. The study is based on IVU evaluation of renal scarring, and several questions have not been answered: The possibility of congenital anomalies of the ureteral orifices and the occurrence of renal scarring in the first 6 months has not been considered in both groups. Although the surgical cases had less pyelonephrites than the nonoperative group, the cases with postoperative scarring were not considered as possible explanation of earlier complicated urinary tract infection.

Surgery or subtrigonal injection is indicated in following conditions (with some restriction on injection therapy):

VUR of the caudal ureter in complete duplication
Paraostial diverticulum[a]
Selected cases of ureteral ectopy (without/with duplication, with/without ureterocele) and/or orthotopic ureterocele
Grade V (and grade IV and III) reflux with/without gapping or golf hole orifice

Breakthrough infection or insufficient adherence of the parents in the nonoperative group

Persistence of moderate and severe reflux until puberty

Reflux in bladder exstrophy, posterior urethral valves, and prune-belly syndrome (after alleviation of infravesical obstruction in the latter two)

[a]It is possible that the outcome of paraostial (paraureteral) diverticulum is similar to the common reflux. But the likelihood of spontaneous resolution in severe reflux is only one fifth in a median follow-up time of about 4 years. Therefore, surgery is indicated in severe, progressing, and persisting cases.

If surgery or subtrigonal injection is indicated or chosen, it should be performed as early as possible, for example, in infancy, because reflux in children is especially prone to pyelonephritis in the first 2 years of life.

In **fetal reflux**, the indication of surgery is restricted (except for a single functioning kidney) for the following reasons: The resolution rate or the rate of conversion to low grades may be greater than in the classical reflux, resolution of the postulated underlying infravesical obstruction may occur, and surgery needs special expertise.

In functional **voiding disorders and neurogenic bladder**, primary reflux surgery is contraindicated.

Subtrigonal injection by a bulging agent is an attractive method of nonoperative or operative treatment. 0.3–2.0 ml of stabilized nonanimal hyaluronic acid/dextranomer gel (Deflux®) is injected with the subureteral (STING and intraureteral) technique in general anesthesia and an outpatient setting. **STING technique**: After punction of the bladder mucosa at the site of ureteral orifice at 6 o'clock and 2–3 mm below the ostium, the needle is introduced in a depth of 4–5 mm along the ureter, and 0.1–0.2 ml Deflux® is slowly injected in the submucous space and thereafter an additional amount of 0.5–1.0–2.0 ml. The opening of the ureter should be elevated and closed by the bolus that is visible indirectly by marked eventration of the mucous membrane and a shape of the orifice like a sickle.

It may be repeated 2–3 times, and its application in grade IV reflux, refluxing ureteral duplication, and paraostial diverticulum is controversial. Good indications are grade I, II, and III refluxes of single kidneys.

The reported success rate depends on the characteristics of the treated population (reflux grades, types of primary reflux), the applied technique and experience, and the definition of "cure." So far, short-term cure (no reflux) is achieved in >60 % of the children (VCU 1.5–3 months postoperatively), and maximally 96 % of children remain free of dilatative reflux (grade III–V) in VCU 3–12 months postoperatively and 2–5 years later and display no febrile urinary tract infection in about the same percentage 7–12 years after subtrigonal injection with a postoperative rate of febrile UTI of only 3.4 %.

Postinterventional stenosis is observed in <1 % and resolves after temporary stent placement. Biodegradation and/or particle migration is obviously no major problem in contrast to older agents.

Ureteral reimplantation (ureterocystoneostomy according to **Politano-Leadbetter** or **Cohen Technique**) (for the still used extravesical Lich-Grégoir antireflux technique, the reader is referred to the literature):

After a transverse suprapubic incision in a skin crease, a longitudinal midline incision of the abdominal and anterior bladder wall is performed extraperitoneally, and the distal refluxing ureter(s) is (are) mobilized close to the entrance in the bladder wall. Care is taken not to injure the vas deferens in boys and the nerve supply to the bladder and blood supply of the ureter in both sexes.

After circumcision of the ureteral orifice including a rim of few millimeters of mucosa, the ureter intubated by a splint is mobilized completely from its connections to the bladder wall in a cranial direction, and the wall is incised well above the site of the former orifice. Afterward, the mobilized ureter is pulled through the new incision inside of the bladder. After closing the hole in the detrusor at the site of ureteral mobilization with single sutures and longitudinal incision of the caudal border of the new detrusor muscle incision for a few millimeters, a submucous tunnel is created between the former old orifice and the site of the new bladder incision with cutting movements of a special pair of scissors. After pull-through of the ureter underneath the tunnel, its end is (without or with additional resection of its end for some millimeters depending on its vitality) sutured to the cranial mucosa at the site of the former orifice in its cranial semicircle and anchored to the mucosa and trigonal muscles at its caudal semicircle.

The reimplanted ureter may be splinted, the bladder is completely drained by a suprapubic catheter, the prevesical space by a closed suction system, and bladder and access are closed stepwise with diverting the two or three catheters through and close to the incision. Some of the quoted details are aimed to avoid postoperative complications such a postoperative stenosis due to ureteral kinking or devitalization or reflux recurrence due to a primarily or secondarily too short tunnel. The tunnel length should amount to 3–5 times the ureteral diameter.

If the **Cohen technique** is applied, one or both ureters are mobilized in its (their) intravesical (and prevesical part). One or two subcutaneous tunnel(s) are created between the site(s) of the former ostium and above (and below) the contralateral orifice. After pull-through of one or both ureters, the site of mobilization is checked for a larger gap or ureteral kinking and corrected by either a muscle suture or small incision. The formation of the new orifice is analogous to the Leadbetter technique.

The disadvantage of Cohen techniques is the transposition of the orifice of the ipsilateral ureter to the contralateral side. If postoperative retrograde ureteral catheterization becomes ever necessary, a special technique must be applied with percutaneous punction of the bladder close to the involved orifice and percutaneous introduction of the catheter under endoscopic control.

Gross ureteral dilatation needs ureteral remodelling as quoted under the headline "obstructive megaureter."

Prognosis

Reflux can be cured in up to 98 % by surgery. Reflux recurrence and postoperative ureteral stenosis are observed in 2–3 % and may be higher in reflux surgery of infancy depending on the expertise of the surgeon. Postoperative diverticulum needs only surgery, if the child becomes symptomatic and residual contrast is observed in the VCU.

In contrast to boys in which lower urinary tract infections are observed mainly in infancy and otherwise in postoperative complications, recurrent lower urinary tract infections may be observed in the later postoperative clinical course in about one third of the girls, especially after start of sexual intercourse or during pregnancy. It can be explained by a decreased defense mechanism of the bladder mucosa against infection. Renal hypertension and/or renal end-stage failure occurs according to the natural history of not or insufficiently treated patients (and in some of the children with surgery) first at puberty and mainly in young adults. In teenagers <15 years of age with end-stage renal insufficiency, about one fourth are related to urinary tract malformations and one third of this subgroup to vesicoureteral reflux.

27.8 Bladder Diverticulum

Occurrence, Types

The different types of bladder diverticula are listed in order of frequencies:

- Pseudodiverticula as sequel of bladder hypertrophy due to lower obstructive uropathy, for example, severe forms of posterior urethral valves # or neurogenic bladder in meningomyelocele
- Diverticula after ureteral reimplantation (at the site of former ureteral entrance)
- Urachal diverticulum (at the dome of the bladder) #
- Isolated diverticulum of the bladder trigonum, for example, paraostial diverticulum #

Clinical Significance

- Stasis of urine in the diverticulum may lead to urinary tract infection depending on the type and width of the diverticular neck.
- Paraostial diverticulum leads to reflux, if the ureteric orifice is included in the wall of the gradually increasing diverticulum.

Clinical Presentation

Urinary tract infections, stone formation within the diverticulum, hematuria, and enuresis are the encountered clinical signs.

A second micturition on command and residual urine on bladder catheterization shortly after the first micturition may be an additional sign of a large diverticulum.

Some diverticula are incidental findings on radiological imaging or cystoscopy.

Differential Diagnosis, Work-Ups
The differential diagnoses are disorders with the quoted symptomatology and in case of significant residual urine, lower obstructive uropathies, reflux, and functional voiding disorders.

Ultrasound and VCU including lateral, retrovesical, and parallel views in relation to the bladder wall: Isolated diverticula lie close to the trigonum and may be single or multiple up to three. Contrast in the diverticulum after micturition corresponds to insufficient drainage. Rarely, CT or MRI with contrast is needed. Cystoscopy demonstrates the dynamic of the diverticulum during bladder emptying and filling, and the type of diverticulum, although it may difficult to recognize all diverticula.

Treatment, Prognosis
Pseudodiverticula need correction of the obstruction of the lower urinary tract that is followed by radiological disappearance after valve ablation in posterior urethral valves or CIC and overnight catheter drainage in neurogenic bladder.

Postoperative diverticula need only surgical resection with closure of the muscular defect if they are symptomatic, and contrast retention is observed in the VCU.

Isolated diverticula, especially the paraostial form needs resection, closure of the muscular defect, and possibly reimplantation of the ipsilateral ureter. See also indication of surgery in vesicoureteral reflux.

27.9   Cystitis

Cystitis is a frequent disorder in the daily clinical routine. Foul-smelling urine, pain in the suprapubic region (abdominal pain), burning and dysuria, pollakiuria, frequent urge, different forms of enuresis, and sometimes hematuria characterize the frequent disorder that occurs mainly in girls.

Nevertheless, the possibility exists that other dangerous disorders are overlooked because of the alarming clinical presentation of cystitis, for example, pelvic appendicitis or that common pediatric urological interventions are considered as failed due to simple urinary tract infection after ureteral reimplantation.

In addition, cystitis may be combined with reflux that disappears after cure of cystitis or persists due scarring and shrinkage.

27.9.1 Granular Cystitis

Occurrence, Pathoanatomy
Granular cystitis is a relatively frequent form of cystitis in which the bladder mucosa is covered with minute, semispherical, and glassy vesicles # and occasionally also with hemorrhagic vesicles (**hemorrhagic granular cystitis**). In contrast to the most common variety (**idiopathic granular cystitis**) with diffuse involvement of trigonum and bladder wall, the **symptomatic granular cystitis** concerns only a localized area, for example, in vicinity of a refluxing ureteral orifice and is also encountered in boys.

Clinical Significance
- Idiopathic granular cystitis is a chronic intermittent disorder that accompanies girls over several years and may persist into adulthood.
- Granular cystitis may be combined with reflux like any cystitis. Permanent reflux may develop because of a scarring process.

Clinical Presentation
Because about half of the cases are associated with simple urinary tract infection, the already quoted *symptoms and signs of cystitis* may be present, or *some of them*, even if the urine cultures are sterile.

The majority of girls from preschool age until puberty presents with *secondary enuresis and other forms of wetting*.

In case of persistent reflux, the chance of complicated urinary tract infection is increased with all the inherent complications of renal scarring.

Differential Diagnosis, Work-Ups

Other disorders with chronic intermittent urinary tract infection, other types of cystitis, for instance bullous cystitis, and mainly functional voiding disorders belong to the possible differential diagnoses.

Suspected granular cystitis is best confirmed by cystoscopy. Ultrasound and VCU (after alleviation of urinary tract infection) are performed for exclusion of reflux in general or other anomalies in symptomatic granular cystitis of the boy. Irregularities of the bladder wall in ultrasound and VCU are indications of chronic cystitis. Urinalysis is performed for exclusion of infection and evaluation of resistance against antibiotics. Repeated urinalyses and less frequent endoscopies should be performed for follow-up.

Treatment, Prognosis

Treatment is nonoperative except for secondary reflux. Therapeutic and prophylactic antibiotics are indicated in case of associated urinary tract infection and/or reflux. It is not excluded that granular cystitis is caused by reflux of bath water and toilet additives in the bladder. Therefore, all girls with granular cystitis should avoid baths and swimming pools and use only showers. Constant bladder voiding 6–8 times a day and frequent drinking of suitable liquids seem to be beneficial as well.

In about one third, complete recovery is observed within 1 year. The remainder of the girls suffer from persistent endoscopic findings combined with recurrent symptomatology until puberty. Recurrences have also been observed in adulthood.

27.10 Dysfunctional Voiding, Neurogenic Bladder, and Obstructive Uropathies of the Lower Urinary Tract

Urinary tract infection may be an important presenting sign in dysfunctional voiding, neurogenic bladder, and obstructive uropathies of the lower urinary tract. Because mainly, disorders of micturition, for example, daytime wetting, lead mostly to medical consultation except for phimosis, these pathologies are dealt with in the chapter "disorders of micturition."

27.10.1 Phimosis

Occurrence, Pathoanatomy

Phimosis is a very frequent disorder. Retraction of the prepuce is very difficult and leads to formation of a bloodless constricting ring # and lacerations with bleeding.

Retraction of the prepuce is impossible in >90 % of newborns for physiological reasons. On the other hand, obstruction to micturition corresponds likewise to phimosis in this age group.

Clinical Significance

- Phimosis is prone to complications such as balanoposthitis (inflammation of glans and penis) and obstruction of micturition with consequences for urethra, bladder, and, if long-lasting and severe, for the upper urinary tract.
- Phimosis may be associated with secondary sequels like meatal stenosis or ascending urinary tract infection and preposition to paraphimosis, zipper injury, HIV infection, and penis carcinoma. Some of these predispositions apply also more or less to an intact and not constricting prepuce.

Clinical Presentation

The urinary stream may be weak, and micturition occurs only as dribbling. Occasionally, the prepuce enlarges at micturition like a balloon.

The trial to retract the prepuce leads to a constricting ring, and severe pain is provoked depending on the applied force, and the prepuce may tear and bleed. The same maneuver applied during infancy is probably one of the causes of phimosis.

Balanoposthitis *leads to itch and pain of the prepuce if touched. Swelling, redness, and purulent or hemorrhagic discharge are additional signs #. If the whole penis is involved, disorders* of micturition such as acute urinary retention and dysuria are observed.

In **meatal stenosis**, the orifice presents – instead of a longitudinal-oval – as a minute opening like a point, and the urinary stream is thin and forceful.

In **paraphimosis**, manipulations have led to retraction of the prepuce that is swollen and painful #. Reduction is impossible for the patient due to the severe pain and swelling.

Differential Diagnosis, Work-Ups

It includes disorders of micturition (lower obstructive uropathy, functional voiding disorders), burning and dysuria (simple urinary tract infection, cystitis), and inflammation of scrotum and testis which spreads out to glans and penis.

Suspected meatal stenosis is confirmed by calibration after local application of an anesthetizing cream and starting with the thinnest Hegar's dilators.

Treatment, Prognosis

Balanoposthitis needs local anti-inflammatory treatment (if severe, combined with systemic antibiotics) with cataplasms or baths and the associated urinary retention enemas before catheterization or suprapubic cystostomy.

Paraphimosis is cured either by slow and concentric compression of the prepuce and expression of the edema or by dorsal longitudinal incision of the preputial leaves in general anesthesia.

Every **phimosis** with or without complications is an indication of elective total or partial circumcision in general anesthesia. Total circumcision is an absolute indication after balanoposthitis, in xerotic balanitis, paraphimosis, fetal reflux, and disorders that need frequent catheterization, for example, spina bifida.

In Europe, many parents prefer partial circumcision for aesthetical reasons. This view is supported by some men's liberation groups who complain about less sexual sensation after complete circumcision. On the other hand, the quoted

complications may also occur after partial circumcision.

The risk of complications is low in circumcision (0.19 %) of which posthemorrhage and infection are the most common; urinary tract or generalized infections occur much less frequently. Complications of ritual circumcision need special considerations.

Webcodes

The following webcodes can be used on www.psurg.net for further images and data.

2701 Obstructive megaureter	2716 Postoperative IVU, interpyelic anastomosis
2702 Snake head configuration	2717 Horseshoe kidney, Wilms' tumor
2703 IVU with fluoroscopy	2718 Lumbar ectopia and renal dysplasia
2704 IVU, nonobstructive megaureter	2719 Multicystic renal dysplasia
2705 Wrinkling abdominal skin, prune-belly syndrome	2720 Refluxing ureteral stump
2707 Post. urethral ureterocele, gaping orifice & intussusception	2722 Upper calyx syndrome after renal injury
2708 MRI, dysplastic left upper pole	2723 Bilateral fetal reflux, grade 4–5 and 3
2709 MRI, left megaureter, small ureterocele	2724 Gaping/golf hole orifice single kidney
2710 VCUG, gross reflux right lower renal moiety	2725 Paraureteral diverticulum, reflux
2711 Retrograde pyelography, right upper moiety	2726 Localized scarring left kidney
2712 Left duplex ureter, gaping orifice	2727 Generalized scarring right kidney
2713 IVU/VCUG pre-/postoperative refluxing caudal ureter	2728 VCUG, valve bladder, pseudodiverticula
2714 Dysplastic refluxing lower moiety	2729 Urachal diverticulum
2715 IVU, symptomatic incomplete ureteral duplication	2730 Paraureteral diverticulum
	2731 Granular cystitis
	2732 Phimosis, constricting ring
	2733 Balanoposthitis
	2734 Paraphimosis

Bibliography

General: Urinary Tract Infection, Pyelonephritis and Renovascular Hypertension, and Urinary Tract Anomalies

Armengol CE, Hendley JO, Schlager TA (2001) Should we abandon standard microscopy when screening for urinary tract infections in young children? Pediatr Infect Dis 20:1176–1177

Becker AM (2009) Postnatal evaluation of infants with an abnormal antenatal renal sonogram. Curr Opin Pediatr 21:207–213

Benador D, Benador N, Slosman D et al (1997) Are younger children at highest risk of renal sequelae after pyelonephritis? Lancet 349:17–19

Burnei G, Burnei A, Hodorogea D, Drăghici I, Georgescu I, Vlad C, Gavriliu S (2009) Diagnosis and complications of renovascular hypertension in children: literature data and clinical observations. J Med Life 2:18–28

Farnham SB, Adams MC, Brock JW 3rd, Pope JC 4th (2005) Pediatric urological causes of hypertension. J Urol 173:697–704

Gorelick MH, Shaw KN (2000) Clinical decision rule to identify febrile young girls at risk for urinary tract infection. Arch Pediatr Adolesc Med 154:368–390

Grapin C, Auber F, de Vries P, Audry G, Helardot P (2003) Postnatal management of urinary tract anomalies after antenatal diagnosis. J Gynecol Obstet Biol Reprod (Paris) 32:300–313

Hendren WH et al (1982) Surgically correctable hypertension of renal origin in childhood. Am J Surg 143:432

Hoberman A, Chao HP, Keller DM, Hickey R, Davis HW, Elllis D (1993) Prevalence of urinary tract infection in febrile infants. J Pediatr 123:17–23

Hoberman A, Charron M, Hickey RW et al (2003) Imaging studies after a first febrile urinary tract infection in young children. N Engl J Med 348:195–202

Kaplan RE, Springate JE, Feld EG (1997) Screening dip stick urinalysis: a time to change. Pediatrics 100:919–921

Landau D, Turner ME, Brennan J, Majd M (1994) The value of urinalysis in differentiating acute pyelonephritis from lower urinary tract infection in febrile infants. Pediatr Infect Dis J 13:777–781

Michael M, Hodson EM, Craig JC et al (2002) Short compared with standard duration of antibiotic treatment for urinary tract infection: a systematic review of randomised controlled trials. Arch Dis Child 87:118–123

Mingin GC, Hinds A, Nguyen HT, Baskin LS (2004) Children with a febrile urinary tract infection and a negative radiological work-up: factors predictive of recurrence. Urology 63:562–565, discussion 565

Newman TB, Bernzweig JA, Takayama JL et al (2002) Urine testing and urinary tract infections in febrile infants seen in office settings: the pediatric research in office Settings' febrile infant study. Arch Pediatr Adolesc Med 156:44–54

Sheih CP, Liu MB, Hung CS, Yank KH, Chen WY, Lin CY et al (1989) Renal abnormalities in schoolchildren. Pediatrics 84:1086–1090

Williams G, Lee A, Craig J (2001) Antibiotics for the prevention of urinary tract infection in children: a systematic review of randomized controlled trials. J Pediatr 138:868–874

Section 27.1

Bukowski TP, Smith CA (2000) Monfort abdominoplasty with neoumbilical modification. J Urol 164:1711–1713

Byun E, Merguerian PA (2006) A meta-analysis of surgical practice patterns in the endoscopic management of ureteroceles. J Urol 176:1871–1877, discussion 1877

Dénes FT, Arap MA, Giron AM, Silva FA, Arap S (2004) Comprehensive surgical treatment of prune belly syndrome: 17 years' experience with 32 patients. Urology 64:789–793, discussion 793–794

Franc JD et al (1998a) In: O'Neill JA Jr (ed) Pediatric surgery, vol II, 5th edn. Mosby, St. Louis

Hendren WH, Mitchell ME (1979) Surgical correction of ureteroceles. J Urol 121:590–597

Hendren WH, Carr MC, Adams MC (1998) Megaureter and Prune-Belly syndrome. In: O'Neill JA Jr et al (eds) Pediatric surgery, vol II, 5th edn. Mosby, St. Louis

Levine E, Taub PJ, Franco I (2007) Laparoscopic-assisted abdominal wall reconstruction in prune-belly syndrome. Ann Plast Surg 58:162–165

Patil KK, Duffy PG, Woodhouse CR, Ransley PG (2004) Long-term outcome of Fowler-Stephens orchidopexy in boys with prune-belly syndrome. J Urol 171:1666–1669

Pfister RC, Hendren WH (1978) Primary megaureter in children and adults. Clinical and pathophysiological features of 150 ureters. Urology 12:161–176

Prieto J, Ziada A, Baker L, Snodgrass W (2009) Ureteroureterostomy via inguinal incision for ectopic ureters and ureteroceles without ipsilateral lower pole reflux. J Urol 181:1844–1848, discussion 1848–1850

Stehr M, Metzger R, Schuster T, Porn U, Dietz HG (2002) Management of the primary obstructed megaureter (PMO) and indication for operative treatment. Eur J Pediatr Surg 12:32–37

Woods AG, Brandon DH (2007) Prune belly syndrome. A focused physical assessment. Adv Neonatal Care 7:132–143, quiz 144–145

Yoo E, Kim H, Chung S (2007) Bladder surgery as first-line treatment of complete duplex system complicated with ureterocele. J Pediatr Urol 3:291–294

Ziylan O, Oktar T, Korgali E, Nane I, Alp T, Ander H (2005) Lower urinary tract reconstruction in ectopic ureteroceles. Urol Int 74:123–126

Section 27.2

Afshar K, Papanikolaou F, Malek R, Bagli D, Pipppi-Salle JL, Khoury A (2005a) Vesicoureteral reflux and complete ureteral duplication. Conservative or surgical management? J Urol 173:1725–1727

Bettex M, Kummer-Vago M, Kuffer F (1970) Ureteroneocystostomy in refluxing ureteric duplications: indications, technique and results. J Pediatr Surg 5:622–627

Chacko JK, Koyle MA, Mingin GC, Furness PD 3rd (2007) Ipsilateral ureteroureterostomy in the surgical management of the severely dilated ureter in ureteral duplication. J Urol 178:1689–1692

Franc JD et al (1998b) Ureteral duplication and ureterocele. In: O'Neill JA Jr (ed) Pediatric surgery, vol II. Mosby, St. Louis

Ganz A, Roloff J, Walz PH (1996) Der "ectopic pathway" – Fakt oder Fiktion? Akt Urol 27:419–421

Grob C, Bettex M (1976) Die ektopische Uretermündung. Bericht über 18 Fälle (The ectopic ureteral orifice). Z Kinderchir 19:279–289

Leissner J, Filipas D, Buff S, Gottscholl M, Fisch M, Beetz R, Schumacher R, Hohenfellner R (1998) Operative Therapiekonzepte bei Doppelnieren. Akt Urol 29:135–138

Schaerli AF, Bettex M (1973) Die Behandlung der Doppelniere durch die interpyelische Anastomose. Akt Urol 4:245–253

Shah HN, Sodha H, Khandkar AA, Kharodawala S, Hedge SS, Bansal M (2008) Endoscopic management of adult orthotopic ureterocele and associated calculi with holmium laser: experience with 16 patients over 4 years and review of the literature. J Endourol 22:489–496

Steffens J, Oberschulte-Beckmann D, Siller V, Röttger P (1998) Ektoper, refluxiver, in eine Samenblasenzyste mündender Ureter mit ipsilateraler zystischer Nierendysplasie. Akt Urol 29:264–266

Storm DW, Modi A, Jayanthi VR (2010) Laparoscopic ipsilateral ureteroureterostomy in the management of ureteral ectopia in infants and children. J Pediatr Urol 7:529–533

Section 27.3

Bouckaert JI, Kuffer F, Bettex M (1970) Die Hufeisenniere. Z Kinderchir 8:268–281

Melchior SW, Fichtner JD, Nierhoff C, Hohenfellner R (1998) Therapie der symptommatischen Hufeisenniere. Akt Urol 29:267–271

Mouriquand P (1998) Renal fusion and ectopia. In: O'Neill JA Jr et al (eds) Pediatric surgery, vol II, 5th edn. Mosby, St. Louis

Section 27.4

Strand WR (2004) Initial management of complex pediatric disorders: prune-belly syndrome, posterior urethral valves. Urol Clin North Am 31:399–415, vii

Section 27.5

Kaplan BS (1998) Agenesis, dysplasia, and cystic disease. In: O'Neill JA Jr et al (eds) Pediatric surgery, vol II, 5th edn. Mosby, St. Louis

Section 27.6

Abdulhannan P, Stahlschmidt J, Subramaniam R (2011) Multicystic dysplastic kidney disease and hypertension: clinical and pathological correlation. J Pediatr Urol 7:566–568

Chiappinelli A, Savanelli A, Farina A, Settimi A (2011) Multicystic dysplastic kidney: our experience in nonsurgical management. Pediatr Surg Int 27:775–779

de Lichtenberg MH, Nielsen OS (1989) Infected renal cyst simulating acute abdomen. Acta Chir Scand 1055:135

Frishman E, Orron DE, Heiman Z, Kessler A, Kaver I, Graif M (1994) Infected renal cysts: sonographic diagnosis and management. J Ultrasound Med 13:7–10

Guay-Woodford LM, Desmond RA (2003) Autosomal recessive polycystic kidney disease: the clinical experience in North America. Pediatrics 111: 1072–1080

Hayes WN, Watson AR, Trent and Anglia MCDK Study Group (2012) Unilateral multicystic dysplastic kidney: does initial size matter? Pediatr Nephrol 27:1335–1340

Lin CC, Tsai JD, Sheu JC, Lu HJ, Chang BP (2010) Segmental multicystic dysplastic kidney in children: clinical presentation, imaging finding, management, and outcome. J Pediatr Surg 45:1856–1862

Padevit C, Jaeger P (2005) Infizierte solitäre Nierenzyste: eine seltene Ursache von Flankenschmerzen. Schweiz Med Forum 5:153–154

Pei Y, Obaji J, Dupuis A, Paterson AD, Magistroni R, Dicks E et al (2009) Unified criteria for ultrasonographic diagnosis of ADPKD. J Am Soc Nephrol 20(1):205–212

Shneider BL, Magid MS (2005) Liver disease in autosomal recessive polycystic kidney disease. Pediatr Transplant 9:634–639

Torres VE, Harris PC, Pirson Y (2007) Autosomal dominant polycystic kidney disease. Lancet 369(9569): 1287–1301

Wacksman J, Phipps L (1993) Report of the multicystic kidney registry: preliminary findings. J Urol 150: 1870–1872

Section 27.7

Elder JS (1992) Commentary: importance of antenatal diagnosis of vesicoureteral reflux. J Urol 148:1750–1754

Elder JS, Peters CA, Arant BS Jr, Ewalt DH, Hawtrey CE, Hurwitz RS et al (1997) Pediatric reflux guidelines panel summary report on the management of primary vesicoureteral reflux in children. J Urol 157:1846–1851

Jacobson SH, Hansson S, Jakobsson B (1999) Vesico-ureteric reflux: occurrence and long-term risks. Acta Paeditr Suppl 88:22–30

Jodal U, Koskimies O, Hanson E, Lohr G, Olbing H, Smellie J et al (1992) Infection patterns in children with vesicoureteral reflux randomly allocated to operation or long-term antibacterial prophylaxis. The International Reflux Study in Children. J Urol 148:1650–1652

Kirsch AJ, Hensle T, Scherz HC, Koyle M (2006) Injection therapy: advancing the treatment of vesicoureteral reflux. J Pediatr Urol 2:539–544

Läckgren G (2003) Endoscopic treatment of vesicoureteral reflux and urinary incontinence in children. AUA update series, vol XXII, Lesson 37:294–299

Olbing H, Claesson I, Ebel KD, Seppänen U, Smellie JM, Tamminen-Möbius T, and Wikstad on behalf of the International Reflux Study in Children (1992) Renal scars and parenchymal thinning in children with vesicoureteral reflux: a 5-year report of the International Reflux Study in children (European Branch). J Urol 148:1653–1656

Olbing H, Hirche K, Koskimies O et al (2000) Renal growth in children with severe vesicoureteral reflux: 10-year prospective study of medical versus surgical treatment: the International Reflux Study in Children (European branch). Radiology 216:731–737

Rizzoni G, Dello Strologo L (1989) Aetiologie terminaler Niereninsuffizienz bei Kindern: ein epidemiologischer Ueberblick. Ann Nestlé 47:139–146

Roussey-Kesler G, Gadjos V, Idres N, Horen B, Leclair LI, Raymond F, Grellier A, Hazart I, de Parscau L, Salomon R, Champion G, Leroy V, Guigonis V, Siret D, Palcoux JB, Taque S, Lemoigne A, Nguyen JM, Guyot C (2008) Antibiotic prophylaxis of recurrent urinary tract infection in children with Low grade vesicoureteral reflux: results from a prospective randomized study. J Urol 179:674–679

Smelli JM, Tamminen-Möbius T, Olbing H, Claesson I, Wikstad I, Jodal U, Seppänen U (1992) Five-year study of medical or surgical treatment in children with severe reflux: radiological renal findings. The International Reflux Study in Children. Pediatr Nephrol 6:223–230

Smellie JM, Jodal U, Lax H et al (2001a) Outcome at 10 years of severe vesicoureteral reflux managed medically: report of the International Reflux Study in Children. J Pediatr 139:656–663

Smellie JM, Barrat TM, Chantler C et al (2001b) Medical versus surgical treatment in children with severe bilateral vesicoureteral reflux and bilateral nephropathy: a randomised trial. Lancet 357:1329–1333

Stenberg A, Läckgren G (2007) Treatment of vesicoureteral reflux in children using stabilized non-animal hyaluronic acid/dextranomer gel (NASHA/DX): a long-term observational study. J Pediatr Urol 3:80–85

Tamminen-Möbius T, Brunier E, Ebel KD, Lebowitz R, Olbing H, Seppänen U, Sixt R, on behalf of the International Reflux Study in Children (1992) Cessation of vesicoureteral reflux for 5 years in infants and children allocated to medical treatment. J Urol 148:1662–1666

Tibballs JM, De Bruyn R (1996) Primary vesicoureteral reflux – how useful is postnatal diagnosis. Arch Dis Child 75:444–447

Weiss R, Duckett J, Spitzer A (1992) Results of a randomized clinical trial of medical versus surgical management of infants and children with grades II and IV primary vesicoureteral reflux (United States). The International Reflux Study in Children. J Urol 148:1667–1673

Wheeler D, Vimalachandra D, Hodson EM, Roy LP, Smith G, Craig JC (2003) Antibiotics and surgery for vesicoureteral reflux: a meta-analysis of randomised controlled trials. Arch Dis Child 88:688–694

Section 27.8

Afshar K, Malek R, Bakhshi M, Papanikolaou F, Farhat W, Bagli D, Khoury AE, Pippi-Salle JL (2005b) Should the presence of congenital para-ureteral diverticulum affect the management of vesico-ureteral reflux? J Urol 174:1590–1593

Section 27.9

Raez M (1977) Zur Aetiologie der Cystitis granularis. Nachweis eines Harnröhren-Blasen-Refluxes von Badewasser beim Baden und Waschen von kleinen Mädchen. Akt Urol 8:151–158

Section 27.10

Akporiaye LE, Jordan GH, Devine C Jr, American
    Urological Association, Inc (eds) (1997) Balanitis
    xerotica obliterans (BXO), vol XVI, AUA update
    series. Office of Education, Houston, Lesson 21

Craig JC, Knight JF, Sureshkumar P et al (1996) Effect of
    circumcision on the incidence of urinary tract infec-
    tion in preschool boys. J Pediatr 128:23–27

Das S, Tunuguntla HS (2000) Balanitis xerotica obliterans
    – a review. World J Urol 18:382–387

Ellis DG, Mann CM Jr (1998) Abnormalities of the
    urethra, penis, and scrotum. In: O'Neill JA Jr et al
    (eds) Pediatric surgery, vol II, 5th edn. Mosby, St.
    Louis

Horowitz M, Gershbein AB (2001) Gomco circumcision:
    when is it safe? J Pediatr Surg 36:1047–1049

Morris BJ (2007) Why circumcision is a biomedical
    imperative for the 21th century. Bioessays
    29:1147–1158

Pugliese JM, Morey AF, Peterson AC (2007) Lichen scle-
    rosus: review of the literature and current recommen-
    dations for management. J Urol 178:2268–2276.
    Comment in: J Urol (2009) 181:1502–1503

Wiswell TE, Geschke DW (1989) Risks from circumcision
    during the first month of life compared with those for
    uncircumcised boys. Pediatrics 83:1011–1015

Distorted micturition is a frequent presenting sign in childhood that draws attention of the parents especially in all kinds of wetting. In reality, the appearance of distorted micturition is many and diverse; it may be classified diagrammatically into five categories:

1. Acute or chronic urinary retention
2. Continuous leaking (as urine flow or dribbling) or intermittent uncontrolled micturition – incontinence or overflow incontinence
3. Abnormal course of micturition (see lower obstructive uropathies)
4. Abnormal direction of micturition: Deflection, doubling of, or fan-like urinary stream, ballooning of the urethra or prepuce, and exit of urine at abnormal sites
5. Symptomatology of dysfunctional voiding: Daytime wetting or urinary tract infection, and more specifically, delayed bladder maturation with pollakiuria due to a small bladder volume or absent control, frequent urge and hold maneuvers, prolonged micturitions in portions, etc.

Overlapping of these categories may occur in the single pathologies, and the symptomatology of dysfunctional voiding is also observed in pathoanatomically caused disorders.

Nevertheless, a **specific history**, **voiding diary**, and **precise clinical examination** (especially of the external genitals and micturition) permit the practitioner to classify micturition into one or several categories, often to list the differential diagnosis, or at least to differentiate between disorders with pathoanatomical or functional cause.

In the former case, **radiological imaging** (ultrasound and VCU) and **endoscopy** are in the foreground of work-ups, whereas in the latter case, **uroflowmetry** or **cystomanometry** combined with bladder ultrasound are useful tools.

It is important to know, that pathoanatomical disorders may be hidden by apparent dysfunctional voiding, that pathoanatomical pathologies may be combined with dysfunctional voiding (vicious circle), or that functional voiding disorders leave pathoanatomical sequels.

A frequently observed symptom is **pollakiuria**. It occurs in many disorders and means ≥ 5 (8) micturition in schoolchildren during the day. In addition to cystourethritis and pelvic appendicitis (as example of a disorder close to the bladder), the subsequently quoted lower obstructive uropathies and dysfunctional voiding must be considered; furthermore, postoperative and postradiation small bladder volumes may lead to possibly temporary pollakiuria, for instance after bladder reconstruction or undiversion of end or loop ureterostomies.

Enuresis is often quoted in relation to distorted micturition. In a restrictive linguistic use, enuresis means a delayed maturation of the controlled micturition. The following signs are characteristic for **primary enuresis**:

Table 28.1 Differential diagnosis of pediatric urological causes of distorted voiding

	Category 3[a]
Obstructive uropathies of the lower urinary tract	
o Bladder neck obstructions	Also cat 1
o Müllerian duct remnants, utricle cyst	Also cat 2
● Posterior urethral valves	Also cat 1, 2, 5
o Other rare urethral pathologies	Also cat 1, 2 and local findings
o Urethral stricture	Also cat 1, 2
● Meatal stenosis	Also cat 4, 2 and local findings
o Urethral diverticulum	Also cat 1, 2 and leading signs
● Phimosis	Also cat 4, 2 and local findings
● Labial synechia	Also cat 4, 2 and local findings
● Interlabial masses	Also cat 4, 2 and local findings, leading signs
Neurogenic bladder, functional voiding disorders	
o Neurogenic bladder	Cat **1** or **2**
● Dysfunctional voiding	Cat **5**, also 1, 2, 3
Acute and chronic urinary retention	
● Acute urinary retention	Cat **1**, also 2
o Chronic urinary retention	Cat **1** and **2**
Clefts of bladder and/or urethra, ureteral duplication	
● Bladder exstrophy	Cat **2**
● Epispadias	Cat **2**
● Complete ureteral duplication	Cat **2**, normal micturitions
o Other pathologies	Cat **2** – additional or important sign

[a]All pathoanatomical disorders except for clefts and duplications have category 3 and possibly other categories

- Familiality is often present. If one parent has been stricken by enuresis, about 40 %, and if both parents have been involved in enuresis, about 70 % of their children will have enuresis.
- Enuresis is a self-restricted disorder. About 10 % of the age group 5–6 years has enuresis, but only ≥1 % is still involved at age 18 years. Primary enuresis impairs self-esteem but never the urinary tract and kidneys.
- Voluntary control of micturition is usually attained by 4–6 years of age. Not realized,

mainly nocturnal micturitions with complete bladder voiding beyond the age of 6 years are regarded as primary enuresis.

In a further linguistic usage, the term "enuresis" is handled differently: **Secondary enuresis** means uncontrolled wetting after an interval of ≥6 months between attainment of controlled micturition and enuresis, **diurnal enuresis** means either daytime uncontrolled micturition equal to or combined with primary enuresis or voiding postponement, and **enuresis a diversity of wetting**. Accordingly, it is usually not defined, if single symptoms and signs of a disease are listed, which type of wetting is dealt with and the acting term "enuresis" is quoted.

In Table 28.1, the pediatric urological pathologies of distorted micturition are listed and the relevant or frequent disorders emphasized. In addition, the corresponding categories of distorted micturition are quoted for each disorder as differential diagnostic tool.

28.1 Obstructive Uropathies of the Lower Urinary Tract

An abnormal course of the micturition (category 3) is in the foreground of lower obstructive uropathies: a weak or thin, or a forceful urinary stream, dysuria, delayed start of micturition, abrupt interruption of micturition, or postmicturition dribbling. But other categories of micturition may be observed as well.

28.1.1 Bladder Neck Obstruction

Occurrence

Actual obstruction due to an autochthonous disorder of the bladder neck (by malformation, inflammation, trauma, or tumor) is rare. The obstruction is mostly caused by **intrinsic and extrinsic** obstruction.

Clinical Significance
- If bladder neck obstruction is suspected, it must be looked for an intrinsic or extrinsic disorder: Large intravesical # or ectopic ureterocele, polyp and other tumors, urethral stone,

former urethral injury, introduced foreign body, or a space-occupying pelvic mass close to the bladder neck.

Clinical Presentation

Acute or chronic urinary retention and hindered micturition (dribbling, interrupted, or micturition initiated by the abdominal press) are the possible clinical signs.

Differential Diagnosis, Work-Ups

It includes other disorders with obstruction of the lower urinary tract especially of the urethra posterior, for example, primary bladder neck dysfunction, and occasionally dysfunctional voiding and neurogenic bladder. Radiological imaging and endoscopy may simulate bladder neck obstruction because of dilatation of the posterior urethra leading to prominence of the bladder neck, for example, in urethral valves.

Primary bladder neck dysfunction (insufficient opening) may be missed, because it manifests with symptoms of the lower urinary tract and may be combined with dysfunctional voiding. Diagnosis is only possible with video-assisted urodynamic examinations, which display the site of obstruction on fluoroscopy. Treatment occurs with adrenergic antagonists.

VCU and urethrocystoscopy are the main diagnostic tools. It may be supplemented by urodynamics in suspected dysfunctional voiding and neurogenic bladder and by MRI in pelvic tumor with bladder neck involvement.

Treatment, Prognosis

It depends on the cause of bladder neck obstruction and is dealt with in the corresponding disorders.

28.1.2 Prostatic Utricle Cyst (Utricular Cyst), Remnants of the Müllerian Ducts

Occurrence, Pathoanatomy

The prostatic utricle (a pit in the seminal colliculus) and testicular appendages are relatively frequent remnants of the Müllerian ducts. If the production of anti-Müllerian hormone is insufficient in boys, parts or all of the female Müllerian ducts persist leading to a cyst of the utricule or even to a rudimental vagina, uterus, and fallopian tubes #. In clinically relevant Müllerian duct remnants, the ejaculatory ducts have a close anatomical relation to the utricular cyst or even enter it.

Clinical Significance

- Actually, rare persistent Müllerian duct remnants occur more frequently in severe forms of hypospadias, prune-belly syndrome, and disorders of sex differentiation.
- Utricular cysts may become symptomatic already in childhood by recurrent epididymitis and distortion of micturition, and in adults by infertility.

Clinical Presentation

Recurrent testicular and/or scrotal swelling (due to ascending epididymitis), impedement to micturition (signs of lower obstructive uropathy), and postmicturition wetting or dribbling are the clinical signs. In addition, the utricular cyst may become symptomatic after hypospadias repair (due to urethral stenosis at the side of anastomosis). It may lead to perineal pain, urinary tract infection, and palpable pelvic mass that may be felt as supraprostatic midline mass on rectal examination.

In adults, work-ups of infertility yield possibly a cyst of the utricule with azoo- or oligospermia. Rarely, a malignancy of the utricular cyst has been described.

Differential Diagnosis, Work-Ups

It includes disorders with (recurrent) testicular and scrotal swelling, simple urinary tract infection, distorted micturition, and wetting or pelvic tumor.

Endoscopy with contrast filling of the cyst # and VCU are diagnostic. Rectal ultrasound and MRI are additional options.

Treatment, Prognosis

Symptomatic or large cysts, the latter especially before hypospadias repair need resection. The posterior approach must avoid injury to the ejaculatory ducts #. Endoscopic incision of the cyst may be an alternative to open surgery.

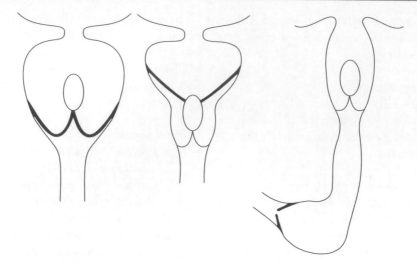

Fig. 28.1 Diagrammatic drawings of posterior and anterior urethral valves. The row shows on the *left side* the classic posterior urethral valves type I. The valves look like sails or nests of swallows, lead to nearly spherical dilatation of the posterior urethra, and feign bladder neck obstruction. In the *middle*, the rare type III posterior urethral valves are depicted that correspond to a diaphragm with a central hole. Anterior urethral valves of the membranaceous urethra are demonstrated on the *right side*; they have diaphragm-like structures with a central hole

Alleviation of symptoms and signs is successful in children but fertility remains open.

28.1.3 Posterior Urethral Valves

Occurrence, Pathoanatomy, Types

Posterior urethral valves are one of the most common obstructive disorders of the urethra in male newborns and infants.

They are sail-like structures that have developed instead of the normal folds originating from the inferior aspect of the seminal colliculus and display different degrees of obstruction depending on their thickness and extension in the anterior direction (with possible fusion with each other). This description corresponds to the most common **type I** according to Young #. The much less frequent **type III** is a diaphragm-like structure with a central hole in the region of the verumontanum or membranaceous urethra (Fig. 28.1).

Clinical Significance

- Posterior urethral valves are an important cause of oligohydramnion, lung hypoplasia, and fetal ascites that may be treated with vesicoamniotic shunt.

- Posterior urethral valves belong to the most common causes of lower obstructive uropathy in male newborns and infants.
- The large variability of pathoanatomical severity of the posterior urethral valves is responsible of the many and diverse clinical presentation and its time of manifestation from the newborn period to school age.
- In severe cases of posterior urethral valves, involvement of the kidneys up to end-stage renal failure and histological anomalies of the bladder with severe consequences for bladder function lead to a chronic disease in spite of surgical correction of the valves.

Clinical Presentation

Prenatal diagnosis is possible in severe cases by ultrasound and analysis of urine and amniotic fluid. Bilateral hydroureteronephrosis, a constantly filled, distended bladder, possible fetal ascites, and oligohydramnion are the main findings.

After birth, the **severe cases** develop *RDS, signs of renal insufficiency, chronic urinary retention with possible urine overflow or dribbling, and fatal outcome is possible due to renal failure or respiratory insufficiency #*.

If the distorted micturition of the children with **moderate degree** of valves is not recognized *(weak urinary stream, dribbling micturition),* upper urinary tract infections or urosepsis are the leading signs. **Slight forms** are often not recognized until school age because urinary tract infections become less common with time, and *the signs of distorted micturition may be minimal or atypical (delayed start of and prolonged micturition, use of abdominal pressure, weak stream, and wetting)* #.

Differential Diagnosis, Work-Ups

It depends on the age of the child at clinical presentation and/or the severity of the posterior urethral valves.

In **newborns with severe disease**, disorders with RDS, signs of renal insufficiency, urinary retention, and occasionally abdominal tumor due to urinary ascites must be considered. **Later in life**, disorders with distorted micturition (category 3) or urinary tract infection are in the fore.

The rare **anterior urethral valves** are either an isolated disorder or combined with the distal part of a urethral diverticulum, may concern the whole anterior urethra (bulbar, penoscrotal junction, or pendulous part), and may display a diaphragm-like configuration with a central hole. Their clinical presentation is variable depending on the severity of obstruction (e.g., similar to severe forms of posterior urethral valves).

Diagnosis of **slight forms** of posterior urethral valves is very tricky because other disorders such as dysfunctional voiding are mostly considered first.

The clinical suspicion of posterior urethral valves is confirmed by **VCU** and **ultrasound**: The posterior urethra is grotesquely dilated and elongated and combined with a prominent bladder neck that appears narrow and an abrupt transition from the wide urethra posterior to the narrow-appearing membranaceous urethra #. The valves are not depicted except for an occasional linear lucency at the site of the valves #. Often, reflux into the ejaculatory ducts may be seen. The bladder wall is thick with an irregular inner surface due to cystitis and hypertrophy and displays diverticula and possibly unilateral or bilateral reflux in 50 % of the patients. In anterior urethral valves, there is an abrupt change of the caliber at the side of the valve.

The ultrasound is useful for demonstration of megaureters (due to secondary obstruction or severe reflux), hydronephrosis and/or dysplasia (increased lucency and cysts), measurement of thickness of bladder wall and volume, and demonstration of diverticules. Perineal ultrasound displays the dilated posterior urethra.

Slight forms of valves may be missed by VCU. Therefore, all valves should be confirmed by **endoscopy** immediately before endoscopic valve ablation. The inner surface of the bladder is trabeculated and inflamed (cystitis and hypertrophy).

Other work-ups include determination of serum and urine **electrolytes and creatinine** before and after bladder drainage by permanent transurethral catheter or cystostomy, and **scintiscan** for evaluation of renal function after valve ablation, and on follow-up.

Treatment, Prognosis

After a bladder catheter with continuous derivation of urine has been performed with careful supervision and appropriate replacement of urine and electrolyte loss by peroral nutrition and an i.v. infusion, some stabilization occurs within 2–4 weeks with normalization of electrolytes and a possible trend toward normalization of renal parameters.

Transurethral ablation of the valves should be performed whenever possible in early infancy ##. In premature or small-for-date infants, preliminary **vesicostomy** may be an alternative to long-term transurethral bladder drainage. Percutaneous nephrostomies or loop enterostomies are rarely necessary.

If the infants thrive, have regular bladder evacuations, and their renal parameters display a continuous trend toward normalization or display no deterioration, the upper urinary tract should not be operated, because spontaneous recovery of reflux and megaureter is often observed.

Severe and moderate cases with involvement of bladder, upper urinary tract, and kidneys need **regular and long-term follow-ups** of function of these compartments. Persistent mega- or refluxing ureters may need ureteral reimplantation. Unilateral nephroureterectomy in case of lost function is controversial, if renal transplantation must be foreseen. Peritoneal dialysis and renal transplantation are further steps in case of end-stage renal failure. In addition, clinical, sonographic, and urodynamic follow-ups of bladder function are very important because up to one third or more of the children has functional bladder disorders already in infancy in spite of otherwise favorable outcome.

The term **"valve bladder syndrome"** is used for children and adolescents with persistent or progressive hydroureteronephrosis and increasing renal failure in whom successful urethral valve ablation without or with temporary urinary diversion has been performed. The term has been used for different ages and functional stages of the valve bladder, and its cause is discussed controversially: functional disorders of the bladder in the first years of life and thereafter that is observed in at least one third or even more of the valve patients (high voiding pressure, uninhibited contractions, small capacity, and myogenic failure of the bladder), or the bladder functions as end organ of polyuria, residual urine (urine from reflux or functional ureterovesical junction obstruction at bladder filling), and bladder insensitivity.

The results of different study groups about **clinical presentation and urodynamic findings** in patients after valve ablation differ in several aspects. Nevertheless, a correlation exists between clinical and urodynamic findings, the different urodynamic properties seem to be associated with different age groups (small, noncompliant, and instable bladders in pre- and large, hypotonic bladders with hypocontractility in postpubertal boys), and the urodynamic findings may change in the individual patient as the years go by (low capacity and hypertonicity below 3 years of age followed by normal capacity and normotonicity between 4 and 6 years with large capacity and hypotonicity afterward). *Polyuria, decreased bladder sensitivity to volume, inability to appreciate fullness, residual urine >20 % of capacity, and large bladder capacity* have been found in schoolchildren with valve bladder syndrome.

Depending on the assumed cause, different therapeutic approaches are proposed: (1) **Early** urodynamic work-ups in the infant is followed by CIC and/or anticholinergics in noncompliant bladders, or (2) timed and frequent voiding, double voiding or CIC after micturition, and nocturnal bladder emptying similar to the daytime regimen or use of an indwelling nocturnal catheter with continuous bladder drainage starts at first manifestation of valve bladder syndrome with **beginning school age**. The latter regimen has led to decreasing hydroureteronephrosis in all and decrease or stabilization of serum creatinine in three fourths.

The former **prognostic statement** that one third of the patients die of renal failure, one third survive with different degrees of restricted renal and/or bladder function, and one third are completely cured is probably too pessimistic. According to a multicentric study in which children have been compared with either a diagnosis in the newborn period or during infancy, 10 and 1 % died in the first year of life and 25 and 8 % displayed renal insufficiency after 5 years. Prognostic unfavorable factors were (1) a low birth weight, (2) values of creatinine of >200 μmol/l at diagnosis and ≥100 μmol/l after commencement of treatment, and (3) bilateral reflux grade IV to V and wetting beyond 5 years of age.

Whereas the macroscopic urethral and vesical changes demonstrated by radiological imaging normalize nearly completely (disappearance of abnormal bladder shape, wall irregularities, and diverticules, normal calibers of the urethra) within the first 3–6 months and 1–2 years, respectively, renal and bladder function may be a matter of concern.

Whereas renal function may be set in advance already at birth due to renal dysplasia, less or more recovery is possible after introduction of treatment, and/or deterioration toward end-stage renal failure may become manifest first during school age or specifically at puberty. One third of children with valve bladder syndrome are differently amenable to nonoperative treatment (e.g., CIC and overnight continuous bladder drainage), and some may need bladder augmentation.

28.1.4 Other Rare Urethral Pathologies

In addition to the anterior urethral valves that have been quoted already as differential diagnosis of posterior urethral valves, megalourethra, Cowper's gland anomalies, and male urethral duplications belong to this group.

Occurrence, Pathoanatomy
Megalourethra occurs in two varieties. The less severe scaphoid form has a defective corpus spongiosum and the fusiform-type deficient corpora cavernosa and corpus spongiosum. Depending on the form of megalourethra, the ventral wall of the urethra is ballooning during micturition, or the whole penis becomes distended with the presenting sign megalopenis.

Cowper's gland anomalies occur as simple, perforated, imperforated, or ruptured syringocele and have different appearances on endoscopy of the membranaceous urethra, for example, simple syringocele appears as a duct that enters the urethra.

Male urethral duplications have many and diverse forms, they occur at the ventral or dorsal part of the penis, and lie mostly in the sagittal plain. The abortive forms have a cutaneous opening, a duct with blind end, and no urine transportation. In complete duplications, two separate urethras are present, whereas incomplete forms mean a second urethra that originates from the proximal main urethra and opens somewhere on the penis or perineum. Some urine transportation is observed in both types.

Clinical Significance
- The quoted disorders must be considered if other causes of megalopenis, distorted micturition, urinary tract infection, hematuria, or perineal mass are excluded.

Clinical Presentation
The leading sign of the two types of **megalourethra** is *either an excentric ventral or a complete swelling of the penis during micturition (megalopenis). The corpus spongiosum is not palpable in the scaphoid type and corpus spongiosum and corpora cavernosa in the fusiform type, respectively.* The former type is further characterized by *glans tilting*

in a ventral direction with the impression of a penile curvature and redundant skin. Severe forms may lead to *lower and upper urinary tract obstruction.*

The symptomatology of the **bulbourethral gland anomalies** is variable and includes *hematuria or urinary tract infection, distorted micturition, and perineal mass.*

In **urethral duplications**, the characteristic signs are *abnormal penile or perineal openings # with or without wetting combined with normal micturition or double urinary stream and urinary tract infection.*

Differential Diagnosis, Work-Ups
It includes specifically urethral diverticulum or penis curvature with or without hypospadias in **megalourethra** (megalopenis), perineal testis (and anterior urethral valves at endoscopy) in **Cowper's gland anomalies**, perianal fistula in some **urethral duplications**, and in general, disorders with the quoted clinical signs.

Ultrasound is useful for confirmation of both megalourethra types and Cowper's gland anomalies and for exclusion of associated urological malformations in the former disorder or in urethral duplications. The types of Cowper's gland anomalies are best evaluated by endoscopy, and urethral duplications need examination with a tiny probe, VCU or antero- or retrograde fistulography, and MRI (MRI is expensive but permits delineation of the majority of male penile and urethral anomalies).

Treatment, Prognosis
Surgery of the scaphoid type of megalourethra includes degloving of the penile skin beyond the urethral dilatation, ventral resection of the enlarged urethra, and closure of urethra and skin. Cowper's gland syringocele needs endoscopic marsupialization into the urethra or resection. In urethral duplications, the abortive forms may be excised for aesthetic reasons. The symptomatic types need possibly staged resection or urethroplasty in complete duplications.

The outcome is permanent cure, if the aim of the different procedures is achieved, especially in Cowper's gland anomalies and urethral duplication.

28.1.5 Urethral Stenosis and Stricture

Occurrence, Causes

Urethral stenosis and stricture is either congenital or acquired and more common in boys (1 in >10,000 boys). Examples of the rare congenital stenosis up to atresia are those of prune-belly syndrome or those at the proximal to middle junction of the bulbar urethra. The majority of urethral strictures are acquired and may concern any part of the urethra. The causes are arranged in order of frequency:

- Inflammation, for example, permanent bladder catheter, balanitis xerotica obliterans, herpes simplex, and gonorrheal urethritis
- Iatrogenic, for example, traumatic catheterization or endoscopy, and urethral or paraurethral surgery (surgery of hypospadias or anorectal malformations)
- Urethral injury, for example, pelvic fracture, straddle injury, manipulation by the patient, and mountain cycling

Clinical Significance

- Treatment of urethral stenosis and stricture may be troublesome, and recurrences must be considered always.

Clinical Presentation

Symptoms and signs of acquired strictures develop often slowly and progressively after one of the incriminated causes except after urethral injury. If such a cause is not known, specific questions in the history and the clinical examination may reveal it.

Hindered micturition, a thin and weak urinary stream, postmicturition dribbling, and a feeling of incomplete emptying in older children are the symptomatology. Dribbling micturition or even acute and chronic urinary retention, hematuria, and urinary tract infection are observed in advanced stages. A correlation between the severity of complaints and the values of urinary flow rates does not necessarily exist.

Differential Diagnosis, Work-Ups

It includes disorders with distorted micturition (categories 3, 1, and 2) and specifically intraluminal disorders must be considered such as polyp, stone, or foreign body.

The work-ups depend on the suspected or probable cause and should evaluate the site, extension, and number of strictures. Retro- or anterograde urethrography (after bladder filling with contrast by IVU or percutaneous punction) or VCU display the stricture(s), their site, length, and severity with proximal urethral dilatation and distal attenuation of the urethra. Ultrasound is used to measure bladder thickness, residual urine, and possible consequences for the upper urinary tract but also for initial assessment and follow-up of the involved urethra.

Uroflowmetry measures objectively the grade of stricture and may be useful for differentiation of other causes of distorted micturition such as dysfunctional voiding. In stricture, the curve demonstrates a low peak flow rate and a flat flow pattern instead of the normal bell-shaped curve with a flow rate of 15 ml/s. Grading of the severity of stricture involves flow rates >10 ml, <10 ml, and <5 ml/s. The last grade is in accordance to a severe stricture with the risk of urinary retention.

Treatment, Prognosis

Both depend to a large extent on the cause, site, degree, and length of stenosis or stricture, the condition of the adjacent tissue, and the treatment options needed for it. Whereas congenital stenosis or atresia needs urethroplasty, acquired strictures require several therapeutic options with specific indications and stepwise application: (1) **dilatation or visual internal urethrotomy,** (2) **anastomotic urethroplasty** (excision of the stricture and end-to-end anastomosis), or (3) **substitution urethroplasty** (stricturotomy combined with a patch or circumferential repair with a flap with own blood supply or free graft in two or one stage[s]).

Dilatation or **internal urethrotomy** have equally a cure rate of about 50 % and are used mainly in short bulbar strictures. Children need general anesthesia. Complications are bleeding, infection including septicemia, and perforation. Recurrences occur within weeks to months up to 2 years at the latest. Repeated dilatation should only be performed in case of infrequent recurrences and as temporary measure.

Anastomotic urethroplasty is useful for short strictures (1–2 cm) of the bulbar or membranaceous urethra. It needs mobilization of the urethra. The indication for this type of surgery can be enlarged by performance of straightening maneuvers of the natural urethral curve. In the penile urethra, anastomotic urethroplasty may compromise the erectile function. Otherwise, the recurrence rate is lower than in the following procedures.

Stricturotomy combined with a patch is superior to a circumferential repair if the involved urethra must not be completely excised (e.g., after previous surgery for hypospadias). If the involved urethra must be completely resected, replacement of the urethral segment with a graft such as buccal mucosa or from other donor sites yields similar results as a flap except for a too long distance or intensive scarring of the adjacent tissue. In this case, a flap of local genital skin that is based on the dartos layer of the penis should be performed. Two-stage surgery may be superior to one- stage. Extensive scarring and multiple strictures may end up with a continent urinary diversion.

All strictures need clinical long-term follow-up combined with uroflowmetry and possibly radiological imaging.

28.1.6 Meatal Stenosis

Occurrence, Causes
Meatal stenoses are common in boys and unusual in girls.

The congenital form is frequent in more distal hypospadias and is a part of the rare so-called hypospadias of the girl. Otherwise, the majority of meatal stenoses are acquired: postcircumcisional in places with frequent intervention, after balanoposthitis in phimosis, as part of balanitis xerotica obliterans (lichen sclerosus), due to herpes simplex, after penile and urethral surgery, or manipulation by the patient.

Clinical Significance
- Meatal stenosis may escape notice by the parents even in advanced stages with repercussions upon bladder and upper urinary tract.

Clinical Presentation
Micturition occurs under pressure or is weak. The urinary stream is thin with possible deviation from the direction of the penis shaft or fan-like, and postmicturition dribbling may be observed. In advanced stages or severe forms, even chronic urinary retention and dribbling micturition are observed #.

Inspection of the foreskin, glans, and penis displays possibly an underlying cause but is not sufficient for evaluation of meatal size.

Differential Diagnosis, Work-Ups
It includes disorders with lower obstructive uropathy, especially of the anterior urethra to which some signs of bladder and posterior urethra disorders do not apply. Stones, foreign bodies, tumors (e.g., polyp), and diverticula must be considered specifically #.

Observation of the urinary stream, calibration starting with the smallest Hegar's dilators, and occasionally antero- or retrograde urethrography or VCU yield reliable data: The distally or in its whole length dilated urethra stops abruptly with transition in a minute contrast spot. In girls, the normal meatal diameter increases from 0 to 10 years of age from 5 to 7 mm with a mean deviation of 0.6–1.1 mm, and meatal stenosis is rare #. Although meatal anomalies exist in girls, they cannot be related to variations of the urethra as seen in routine VCU, and urethral calibrations are necessary for confirmation of stenosis.

Treatment, Prognosis
Treatment is surgical. After midline incision of the ventral glandular urethra for several millimeters (e.g., one third of whole length), the inner plane is sewn with the outer with small, resorbable, and unwoven threads in general anesthesia, or ventral midline is first clamped alternatively and then incised in local anesthesia with EMLA®. **Xerotic balanitis** recognizable by white patches of foreskin and glans, herpes simplex, and other local manifestations of dermatoses need first dermatological consultation and treatment before meatotomy.

In xerotic balanitis, total circumcision is indispensable, and if the meatus is involved as well, replacement urethroplasty with a pedicle graft of the foreskin is superior to meatotomy. Prognosis depends on the cause of meatal stenosis. Bougienage has often only a temporary effect, for example, during dermatological treatment. Long-term follow-ups are necessary.

28.1.7 Urethral Diverticulum

Occurrence, Pathoanatomy
Urethral diverticula are congenital or acquired and occur rarely in girls. The more common acquired forms develop in connection with postinfectious or posttraumatic urethral stricture and its treatment, after urethroplasties of hypospadias, or ligation of rectourethral fistulas in anorectal anomalies.

Especially the congenital forms have a narrow or wide communication between the urethra and diverticulum, have an oblong shape lying along the urethra with a proximal or distal extension of different length # or a sac-like shape, and originate from the ventral side of the urethra. A typical form is a sac-like diverticulum with a broad base that fills during micturition in its distal part and pushes the anterior edge of its opening to the urethra like a valve against the urethral lumen.

Clinical Significance
- The congenital diverticula are rare causes of distorted micturition and disfigurement of the penis in contrast to acquired forms that are observed more frequently in a hospital-based population.

Clinical Presentation
Concerning the obstructive symptomatology, *the clinical presentation is variable* depending on the size, shape, and drainage mechanism of the diverticulum: *from urinary retention in the newborn with repercussions upon bladder and upper urinary tract and overflow incontinence to weakness of the urinary stream and postmicturition wetting due to emptying of the diverticule. In addition, cystourethritis with dysuria, hematuria, and formation of concrements may be observed.*

Occasionally, *localized swelling may be seen and palpated at the ventral side of the penoscrotal transition zone or penis shaft or a more diffuse swelling along the urethra like the megalourethra types # or posturethroplasty forms*, caused by the dilated neourethra with meatal stenosis. *The described swellings are best observed at or shortly after micturition and may be reduced in size by finger pressure for evacuation of residual urine.*

Differential Diagnosis, Work-Ups
In the newborn with urinary retention, posterior urethral valves or other causes of urinary retention must be considered and in addition, with penis disfigurement, megalourethra. Later in life, other disorders with distorted micturition, for example, utricular cyst or with cystourethritis including hematuria, are in the fore of differential diagnosis.

VCU # or retrograde urethrography (with video display and demonstration of the lateral aspect of the urethra) and urethrocystoscopy are often diagnostic.

Treatment, Prognosis
Symptomatic diverticula need operative treatment with either endoscopic unroofing of the diverticulum or open resection (large and disfiguring or postoperative diverticula). Usually, the urethral symptomatology can be cured.

28.1.8 Labial Synechia (Fusion)

Occurrence, Cause
Fusion of the labia minora is a frequent disorder in female toddlers. It is caused by poor and inadequate hygienics and relative estrogen deficit.

It may concern the whole vestibule or only its anterior part. If the fusion extends close to the clitoris and in front of the urethral meatus, lower urinary tract obstruction develops or backward deviation of the urinary stream occurs with wetting of the thighs.

Clinical Significance
- Urethrovestibulovaginal urine reflux in severe cases leads to chronic vulvovaginitis, cystoure-

thritis, and postmicturition wetting from the vagina.

- Mothers are often afraid that their daughters have some type of gynatresia.

Clinical Presentation

It seems at first sight that the labia minora are joined together and that the shallow vulva has no urethral meatus, vestibule, and hymen. After bilateral, gentle traction of the labia maiora to both sides, a minute line of separation or a thin, transparent membrane with a tiny opening at its anterior end becomes visible that extends from the posterior commissure to the frenulum of the clitoris # or concerns only the anterior part.

Differential Diagnosis, Work-Ups

It includes some type of gynatresia or lichen sclerosus of the vulva (vulvitis xerotica obliterans). **Vulvitis xerotica obliterans** is an analogous disorder to balanitis xerotica obliterans. Vulvitis xerotica and gynatresias may be differentiated by their typical finding of the skin or labial fusion or short vagina in some of the latter.

No further work-ups are necessary except for bacterial examination and resistance of the recovered catheter urine and swabs and biopsy in suspected vulvitis xerotica.

Treatment, Prognosis

The labial fusion is divided by a probe that is introduced in the anterior small opening and guided along the line of separation up to the posterior commissure after application of EMLA® or in short general anesthesia #.

Follow-ups are necessary for control of the recommended appropriate hygienics due the possibility of recurrences. The application of anti-inflammatory cream is followed by estrogen cream.

28.1.9 Interlabial (Intralabial) Masses

They may lead to obstruction of the lower urethral end. Because interlabial masses of the girl and pubertal and postpubertal teenagers are usually visible from the outside, this presenting sign is dealt with in Chap. 29.

28.2 Neurogenic Bladder

Causes, Occurrence

The majority of meningomyelocele has a neurogenic bladder (>90 %). Less frequent causes are minimal spinal dysraphism, sacral agenesis, anorectal and cloacal malformations, acquired disorders such as spinal cord injury, and cerebral palsy and learning disability. The neurogenic bladder of the less frequent causes behaves often similar to that of meningomyelocele.

Clinical Significance

- Specific types of neurogenic bladder lead to upper urinary obstruction or reflux and progressive renal insufficiency.
- In other bladder types with poor storage capacity and compliance, the urinary incontinence prevents social acceptance and integration.

Types

Depending on hyperactivity or inactivity of the sphincter and detrusor muscle, different types and subtypes may be observed. From a practical point of view, three groups of abnormal bladder functions can be listed in order of their frequency in a population of spina bifida children:

1. Hyperactive sphincter and detrusor-sphincter dyssynergy lead to functional obstruction combined with hyperactive detrusor or less frequently with inactive detrusor (≤two thirds of all spina bifida children).
2. Inactive sphincter leads to incontinence with inactive and less frequently hyperactive detrusor (one third).
3. Normal bladder function (<10 %).

The bladder capacity is low in the subgroup with sphincter and detrusor hyperactivity and in the subgroup with sphincter incontinence and detrusor hyperactivity. The former subgroup is at considerable risk of upper urinary tract obstruction, reflux, progressive renal insufficiency, and bladder with irreversible poor storage capacity and compliance #.

Clinical Presentation

The distorted micturition manifests *either to chronic urinary retention with more or less frequent overflow incontinence and signs of secondary involvement of the ureters and kidneys or with different degrees of incontinence.*

Simple urinary tract infections are frequent but hardly recognizable clinically, and the type with chronic urinary retention is particularly at risk for complicated urinary tract infections.

Differential Diagnosis, Work-Ups

If the cause of distorted micturition is known by history and clinical examination, no other differential diagnosis must be considered except for a secondary disorder.

The work-ups include ultrasound, VCU, urodynamics with pelvic floor electromyography. If impaired renal function is suspected or reflux is present, renal scarring due to pyelonephritis must be excluded, or reflux must be followed by contrast or isotope cystography.

Urodynamics display the type of neurogenic bladder as baseline (in the newborn) and on follow-ups (the type of neurogenic bladder may change with time) and guide the appropriate treatment and prognostication (especially in the subtype with hyperactive sphincter and detrusor).

The combination with ultrasound and VCU (with video registration in the bladder filling and emptying phase) yields further information about morphological and functional sequels of neurogenic bladder: bladder wall thickness and other signs of hypertrophy, volume and residual urine, and dilatation and reflux of the upper urinary tract and involvement of the kidneys (hydronephrosis, thinning and alteration of the structure of parenchyma, renal growth).

Treatment, Prognosis

The type with detrusor-sphincter dyssynergy needs either vesicostomy or clean intermittent catheterization (CIC), antibiotics, and systemic or topical oxybutynin ##. The latter is not necessary if the detrusor is inactive.

The treatment of the type with sphincter inactivity is more demanding, especially in case of detrusor hyperactivity. CIC and antibiotics must

be supplemented by interventions to increase bladder neck competence that extends from injection of bulking agents, lengthening of bladder neck, and artificial sphincter to bladder neck closure combined with catheterizable continent reservoir. If the detrusor is hyperactive, bladder augmentation may be needed.

Untreated detrusor-sphincter dyssynergy has led in the past for the majority of the patients to end-stage renal failure and bladder shrinkage at puberty. It can be prevented by the quoted treatment if it is performed continuously and lifelong. If all available measures can be chosen according to the individual requirements, socially acceptable continence is achieved for the majority of patients with sphincter inactivity.

28.3 Dysfunctional Voiding (Functional Urinary Incontinence, Dysfunctional Elimination Syndromes)

Occurrence, Definition

Dysfunctional voiding is a frequent disorder that starts at the age of nursery school at the earliest, involves more frequently girls ($\geq$10 % of the schoolchildren), and may be caused by withholding behaviors acquired in the period of achievement of continence.

It consists of daytime urinary leaking and/or urinary tract infections, displays different types of clinical presentation with possible combination or order of occurrence in the same patient, and is not caused by a known neurological or pathoanatomical disorder.

Clinical Significance

- Daytime wetting is a considerable stress for schoolchildren and their parents.
- Dysfunctional voiding is often a major cause of urinary tract infection, megaureter, and reflux and may be combined with constipation or fecal soiling and vice versa.
- Dysfunctional voiding may escape the diagnosis because it is not considered, and complete clinical presentation develops only after a couple of time.

Clinical Presentation

The two main clinical presentations are either *daytime wetting and/or recurrent or chronic urinary tract infection*. The following patterns of dysfunctional elimination syndromes can be differentiated:

1. **Urge Syndrome (Instable Bladder)**

   It consists of *frequent* attacks *of the need to void the bladder (urge) possibly combined with suprapubic or perianal pain and motorial maneuvers to withhold micturition (doubling up the legs, squatting). Damping of the panties and underpants, pollakiuria, and possibly leaking at night complete this conspicuous clinical presentation.* Conscientious children and their parents know every restroom on the way home or where they live.

   The causally inhibited and involuntary contractions of the detrusor muscle lead to the described urge symptomatology and precocious and possibly incomplete bladder emptying (small functional bladder capacity). Inhibited detrusor contractions may be triggered also by stress leading to increased intra-abdominal pressure #. The described detrusor activity and the voluntary hold maneuvers lead repeatedly to high intravesical pressures and secondary reflux and incomplete bladder voiding because of incomplete pelvic floor relaxation to residual urine and urinary tract infection.

2. **Staccato** Voiding. It is also called "seized-up micturition" because *micturition is interrupted several times* by bursts of pelvic floor contractions #. Staccato voiding belongs together with following types to the group of dysfunctional voiding that has in common a detrusor-sphincter dyssynergy. The urine flow rate is decreased, and the urine flow time is increased. After each prolonged micturition, significant residual urine can be observed.

3. In **fractionated voiding** (interrupted voiding), *the child empties the bladder rarely and incompletely with several phases of micturition and small volumes. The need to void is diminished, and bladder emptying occurs only by a Valsalva maneuver* that increases the intra-abdominal pressure. Therefore, gross residual urine leads to urinary tract infection, and *urinary leaking occurs due to overflow incontinence.*

   Examples of severe end stages of fractionated voiding are the lazy bladder syndrome and Hinman syndrome. Detrusor contractions are completely absent, and some bladder emptying is only possible by straining in **lazy bladder syndrome**. A bladder with a very large volume and gross postmicturition residual urine is the sequel.

   The end stage is reached in **Hinman syndrome** over a stage with detrusor overactivity that is followed by a stage of bladder-sphincter dyssynergy and ends in a detrusor decompensation. The bladder wall is trabeculated, thickened, and combined with reflux.

4. **Voiding postponement (diurnal enuresis)** means that the *involved children withhold micturition because of their obsessiveness to play or a loathing for school toilets until the micturition cannot be held anymore and involuntary micturition occurs.*

Differential Diagnosis, Work-Ups

If the four categories of distorted micturition are considered, the main symptoms of dysfunctional voiding "daytime wetting and urinary tract infection" are in the fore and determine the possible differential diagnoses. It includes **giggle micturition** (sudden and involuntary complete bladder emptying related to laughing), **numerous disorders leading to urinary tract infection**, and **neurogenic bladder**. Because chronic urinary retention, intermittent and uncontrolled micturition, and abnormal course of micturition belong also to the repertoire of some types of dysfunctional elimination syndromes, several of the disorders quoted in Table 28.1 must be considered as well, for example, in prolonged micturition of staccato voiding, minor forms of posterior urethral valves. **Secondary radiological sequels of dysfunctional elimination syndromes** such as reflux, megaureter, bladder diverticula, bladder hypertrophy, and so-called wide bladder neck anomaly (spinning-top configuration of the posterior urethra) must be taken also into account in the differential diagnosis.

The principal work-up tools are a **precise history and clinical examination** (pattern of micturition; conspicuous findings of the external genitals; signs of minimal spinal dysraphism on the back; neurological signs of extremities, buttocks, anus, and perineum; signs of constipation or fecal soiling; and observation of micturition), a **voiding diary** of 24 h and several days (filled in by the parents and including number, time, and volume of single micturition, and time and number of wetting), urine sediment and cultures, and **ultrasound of kidneys, ureters, and bladder**.

Depending on the results, urodynamics are the next step after eradication of a possible urinary tract infection. They include **uroflowmetry** combined with electromyography (emg) of pelvic floor muscles # and **bladder manometry** combined with emg and recording of intra-abdominal pressure. The latter examination is indicated in the group with dysfunctional voiding and in case of urge syndrome not responding to anticholinergic drugs. It may be combined as video-urodynamic studies with radiological imaging by fluoroscopy.

Bladder ultrasound adds useful informations about bladder morphology (thickness and irregularities of bladder wall, severe reflux or megaureter, diverticula) and function (functional bladder volume, postmicturition residual urine).

Treatment, Prognosis

The following treatment options of dysfunctional elimination syndromes are applied depending on the type of distorted micturition and often in combination:

- Long-term antibiotic prophylaxis, especially in residual urine with regular urine culture and evaluation of resistance.
- Long-term anticholinergic medication, mainly in instable bladder; the muscarinic receptor antagonists are oxybutynin, tolterodine, and others. The adverse effects "dry mouth, constipation, headache, and blurred vision" may lead to discontinuation in about 10 % of the patients. The possibility of increased residual urine must be considered. Alternatively, repeated injections of botulinum neurotoxin type A at several sites of the detrusor muscle have been applied (grade B level of evidence for dysfunctional voiding and grade A for neurogenic bladder).

- Treatment of associated constipation and/or encopresis.
- Behavioral treatment that includes demonstration of the type of dysfunctional voiding to parents and child, implementation of a daily schedule of registration and activities concerning micturition, regular exercises for withholding, completeness of micturition, or modification of learned voiding patterns by a physiotherapist and possibly supplemented by biofeedback techniques (e.g., repeated visualization of the urodynamic characteristics) or psychological guidance are all very important in the detrusor-sphincter dyssynergy type.

Existing evidence is inconclusive for the urethral application of botulinum neurotoxin type A in detrusor-sphincter dyssynergy.

If hard data are missing on urodynamics relating to dysfunctional voiding or if the treatment is ineffective in spite of good adherence, a pathoanatomical cause should be considered, for example, slight forms of posterior urethral valves. On the other hand, primary reflux surgery is contraindicated in dysfunctional voiding, and dysfunctional voiding must be considered if reflux surgery has failed.

Except for voiding postponement, the treatment of dysfunctional voiding may be lengthy and lasts several months to years (in up to one fifth). Treatment is more rapidly successful in instable bladder than in detrusor-sphincter dyssynergy; ≥ 70 % of the former type is cured or ameliorated within 3 months in comparison to ≥ 50 % in the latter type. The treatment may influence recurrent urinary tract infections and reflux significantly.

28.4 Acute and Chronic Urinary Retention

Occurrence

Acute or chronic urinary retention is a frequent type of distorted micturition either for the general practitioner, pediatric urologist or surgeon, or at the emergency department, after general anesthesia, instrumental or operative intervention, and therefore an important presenting sign.

Clinical Significance

- Acute urinary retention requires rapid intervention due to the urgent symptomatology.
- The quoted remark applies less to the chronic form due to intermittent overflow. Nevertheless, urgent evaluation of the cause is in the foreground as well.

28.4.1 Acute Urinary Retention

Causes

Acute urinary retention is mostly observed in disorders that lead to dysuria and/or to inflammatory swelling and irritation of penis, scrotum, and perigenital or perianal region. Such disorders are:

- Cystourethritis, balanoposthitis.
- Local injuries by toilet seat, bicycle saddle or bar, manipulations with foreign bodies, or passage of renal stones.
- Causes of testicular or scrotal swelling.
- Mechanical or chemical irritations that are caused by too tight clothes, bath salts, drugs, urine, or diarrhea may lead to acute urinary retention as well.

In in- or outpatients, acute urinary retention is mainly observed after continual including self-controlled application of analgetics or after urethral surgery.

Clinical Presentation

Depending on the age, *acute urinary retention is communicated by crying or restlessness, or intermittent, increasing, and severe lower abdominal pain and strong desire to urinate.*

A roundish hard or firm mass is seen and palpated in the suprapubic midline region with dullness on percussion that may extend to the navel and can be palpated by rectal examination that is especially useful in infants in whom the bladder is covered partially by the pelvis.

History and local findings permit the diagnosis of acute urinary retention together with the knowledge of the accompanying circumstances and hints of the probable cause.

Differential Diagnosis, Work-Ups

It includes other causes of surgical abdomen or abdominal tumor; and in newborns, possibly **physiological anuria**, because the first micturition occurs in 90 % in the first 24 h and in the remaining, within 48 h at latest.

And independent of age, **hypovolemic anuria** after surgery or trauma with insufficient replacement of blood volume must be considered.

In case of doubt, ultrasound is useful. In acute urinary retention, the bladder is usually much larger than the age-dependent bladder capacity.

Treatment, Prognosis

Depending on the cause of acute urinary retention, considering the anxiety of small children or an acute postoperative state after urethral surgery, anti-inflammatory cataplasms or a sitz bath, an enema or catheterization, and a permanent bladder catheter or suprapubic percutaneous cystostomy may be appropriate.

Between the already quoted causes of acute urinary retention and those mentioned in the next section about chronic urinary retention exists a continuous transition.

28.4.2 Chronic Urinary Retention

Chronic urinary retention leads to *overflow incontinence with intermittent dribbling or incomplete micturitions that bring some relief from lower abdominal pain. Wetting and the risk of urinary tract infections are in the foreground.*

Posterior urethral valves and some less frequent lower obstructive uropathies in the newborn and **neurogenic bladder or dysfunctional voiding** are the main causes of chronic urinary retention.

28.5 Bladder Exstrophy, Epispadias, Cloacal Anomalies, and Duplex Kidney

In bladder exstrophy, epispadias grade 2–3, cloacal anomalies, and complete ureteral duplication with an ectopic ureteral orifice beyond the external sphincter muscle, a *constant or intermittent urine dribbling or flow is observed combined with regular micturition in the last-mentioned disorder.*

Involuntary loss of urine or dribbling may be an additional sign or one of the relevant signs in numerous disorders. They are quoted in the differential diagnosis of distorted micturition, for instance, continuous or intermittent dribbling in some complete ureteral duplications, urethral diverticula, ballooning phimosis, or labial fusion.

Webcodes

The following webcodes can be used on www.psurg.net for further images and data.

2801 Large intravesical ureterocele	2813 VCUG, meatal stenosis
2802 Rudimentary vagina, uterus, fallopian tubes	2814 Meatal stenosis in the girl
2803 Utricular cyst, contrast filling	2815 Polyp, membranaceous urethra
2804 Cyst of utricle, operative findings	2816 VCUG, oblong urethral diverticulum
2805 Type I posterior urethral valves, verumontanum	2817 Megalopenis, urethral diverticulum
2806 Posterior urethral valves, upper urinary system	2818 VCUG, distal urethral diverticulum
2807 Uroflowmetry, slight degree urethral valves	2819 Labial fusion
2808 VCUG, posterior urethral valves, bladder reflux	2820 Labial fusion, after division
2809 VCUG, lucency at the site of valves	2821 Neurogenic bladder, advanced detrusor-sphincter dyssynergy
2810 Posterior urethral valves, endoscopy	2822 IVU, dilatation upper urinary tract, neurogenic bladder and
2811 Posterior urethral valves, after valve ablation	2823 Normalization upper tract after CIC
2812 Incomplete urethral duplication, perianal opening	2824 Cystoelectromanometry, urge syndrome
	2825 Uroflowmetry, staccato voiding
	2826 Uroflowmetry, detrusor-sphincter dyssynergy

Bibliography

General: Penile Lesions, End-Stage Renal Disease, and Enuresis

Kirkham AP, Illing RO, Minhas S, Allen C (2008) MR imaging of nonmalignant penile lesions. Radiographics 28:837–853

Largo RH, Gianciaruso M, Prader A (1978) Die Entwicklung der Darm- und Blasenkontrolle von der Geburt bis zum 18. Lebensjahr. Longitudinale Studie. Schweiz Med Wschr 108:155–160

McDonald SP, for the Australian and New Zealand Paediatric Nephrology Association (2004) Long-term survival of children with end-stage renal disease. N Engl J Med 350:2654–2662

Robson WLM, Leung AKC, Van Howe R (2005) Primary and secondary nocturnal enuresis: similarities in presentation. Pediatrics 115:956–959

Ruano R (2011) Fetal surgery for severe lower urinary tract obstruction. Prenat Diagn 31:667–674

Wiersma R (2009) Urethro-ejaculatory duct reflux in children: an updated review. Eur J Pediatr Surg 19: 374–376

Section 28.1.1

Grafstein NH, Combs AJ, Glassberg KI (2005) Primary bladder neck dysfunction: an overlooked entity in children. Curr Urol Rep 6:133–139

Section 28.1.2

Gygi C, Plaschkes J, Carvajal MI, Kaiser G (1994) Prostatic utricle: an unusual case report. Eur J Pediatr Surg 4:211–213

Hendry WF, Pryor JP (1992) Müllerian duct (prostatic utricle) cyst: diagnosis and treatment in subfertile males. Br J Urol 69:79–82

Kaplan GW, Picconi JR, Schuhrke TD (1977) Posterior approach to Müllerian duct and seminal vesical cysts. Birth Defects Orig Artic Ser 13(5):241–245

Monfort G (1982) Transvesical approach to utricular cysts. J Pediatr Surg 17:406–409

Schuhrke TD, Kaplan GW (1978) Prostatic utricle cysts (Müllerian duct cyst). J Urol 119:765–767

Section 28.1.3

Bani Hani O, Prelog K, Smith GH (2006) A method to assess posterior urethral valve ablation. J Urol 176: 303–305

Berrocal T, Lopez-Pereira P, Arjonilla A, Gutierrez J (2002) Anomalies of the distal ureter, bladder, and urethra in children: embryologic, radiologic, and pathologic features. Radiographics 22:1139–1146

Biard JM, Johnson MP, Carr MC, Wilson RD, Hedrick HL, Pavlock C, Adzick NS (2005) Long-term outcomes in children treated by prenatal vesicoamniotic shunting for lower urinary tract obstruction. Obstet Gynecol 106:503–508

Carr MC, Snyder HM (2004) Urethral valves. Fate of the bladder and upper urinary tract. Urologe A 43: 408–413

Desai DY (2007) A review of urodynamic evaluation in children and its role in the management of boys with posterior urethral valves. Indian J Urol 23: 435–442

Duckett JW, Baskin LS (1998) Hypospadias. In: O'Neill JA Jr et al (eds) Pediatric surgery, vol II, 5th edn. Mosby, St. Louis

Ellis DG, Mann CM Jr (1998) Abnormalities of the urethra, penis, and scrotum. In: O'Neill JA Jr et al (eds) Pediatric surgery, vol II, 5th edn. Mosby, St. Louis

Glassberg KI (2001) The valve bladder syndrome: 20 years later. J Urol 166:1406–1414

Glassberg KI (2002) Editorial: the valve bladder syndrome. J Urol 167:298–299

Hodges SJ, Patel B, McLone G, Atala A (2009) Posterior urethral valves. Scientific World Journal 9: 1119–1126

Kajbafzadeh A (2005a) Congenital urethral anomalies in boys. Part I: posterior urethral valves. Urol J 2:59–78

Kajbafzadeh A (2005b) Congenital urethral anomalies in boys. Part II. Urol J 2:125–131

Karmarkar SJ (2001) Long-term results of surgery for posterior urethral valves: a review. Pediatr Surg Int 17: 8–10

Koff SA, Mutabagani KH, Jayanthi VR (2002) The valve bladder syndrome: pathophysiology and treatment with nocturnal bladder emptying. J Urol 167: 291–297

Lal R, Bhatnagar V, Agarwala S, Grover VP, Mitra DK (1999) Urodynamic evaluation in boys for posterior urethral valves. Pediatr Surg Int 15:358–362

Mildenberger H, Habenicht R, Zimmermann H (1989) Infants with posterior urethral valves: a retrospective study and consequences for therapy. Prog Pediatr Surg 23:104–112

Patil KK, Wilcox DT, Samuel M, Duffy PG, Ransley PG, Gonzalez R (2003) Management of urinary extravasation in 18 boys with posterior urethral valves. J Urol 169:1508–1511, discussion 1511

Puri A, Grover VP, Agarwala S, Mitra DK, Bhatnagar V (2002) Initial surgical treatment as a determinant of bladder dysfunction in posterior urethral valves. Pediatr Surg Int 18:438–443

Quintero RA, Johnson MP, Romero R, Smith C, Arias F, Guevara-Zuloaga F, Cotton DB, Evans MI (1995) In-utero percutaneous cystoscopy in the management of fetal lower obstructive uropathy. Lancet 346:537–540

Schober JM, Dulabon LM, Woodhouse CR (2004) Outcome of valve ablation in late-presenting posterior urethral valves. BJU Int 94:616–619

Section 28.1.4

Perovic S, Djakovic N, Hohenfellner M (2004) Penile and urethral anomalies. Urologe A 43:394–401

Weissmüller J (1985) Harnröhrenduplikation beim Mann. Urologe 24:274–279

Section 28.1.5

Meeks JJ, Erickson BA, Granieri MA, Gonzalez CM (2009) Stricture recurrence after urethroplasty: a systematic review. J Urol 182:1266–1270. Comment in: J Urol (2009) 182:1259–1260

Mundy AR (2006) Management of urethral strictures. Postgrad Med J 82:489–493

Section 28.1.6

Klingler J (1970) Der Durchmesser des Meatus externus urethrae bei Mädchen von 0–10 Jahren. Urol Int 25:551–562

Pompino HJ, Hoffmann D (1984) Anomalies of the external urethral orifice in girls. Prog Pediatr Surg 17:49–56

Section 28.1.7

Sheldon CA, Snyder HM III (1998) Structural Disorders of the Bladder, Augmentation. In: O'Neill JA Jr et al (eds) Pediatric surgery, vol II, 5th edn. Mosby, St. Louis

Sections 28.1.8 and 28.1.9

Centeno-Wolf N, Chardot C, Le Coultre CP, La Scala GC (2008) Infected urocolpos and generalized peritonitis secondary to labia minora adhesions. J Pediatr Surg 43:e35–e39

Section 28.2.1

Apostolidis A, Dasgupta P, Denys P, Elneil S, Fowler CJ, Giannantoni A, Karsenty G, Schulte-Baukloh H, Schurch B, Wyndaele JJ, European Consensus Panel (2009) Recommendations on the use of botulinum toxin in the treatment of lower urinary tract disorders and pelvic floor dysfunctions: a European consensus report. Eur Urol 55:100–119

Bauer SB (2008) Neurogenic bladder: etiology and assessment. Pediatr Nephrol 23(23):541–551

de Jong TPVM, Chrzan R, Klijn AJ, Dik P (2008) Treatment of the neurogenic bladder in spina bifida. Pediatr Nephrol 23:889–896

Gamé X, Mouracade P, Chartier-Kastker E et al (2009) Botulinum toxin-A (Botox) intradetrusor injections in children with neurogenic detrusor overactivity/neurogenic overactive bladder: a systematic literature review. J Pediatr Urol 5:156–164

Lazarus J (2009) Intravesical oxybutynin in the pediatric neurogenic bladder. Nat Rev Urol 6:671–674

Misseri R, Rosenbaum DH, Rink RC (2008) Reflux in cystoplasties. Arch Esp Urol 61:213–217

Section 28.2.2

Abrams P, Andersson KE (2007) Muscarinic receptor antagonists for overactive bladder. BJU Int 100: 987–1006

Bauer SB (2002) Special considerations of overactive bladder in children. Urology 60(5 Suppl 1):43–48, discussion 49

Chase J, Austin P, Hoebeke P, McKenna P, International Children's Continence Society (2010) The management of dysfunctional voiding in children: a report from the Standardisation Committee of the International Children's Continence Society. J Urol 183:1296–1302

Glassberg KI, Combs AJ (2009) Nonneurogenic voiding disorders: what's new? Curr Opin Urol 19:412–418

Hoebeke P, Van Laecke E, Raes A, Van Gool JD, Vande Walle J (1999) Anomalies of the external urethral meatus in girls with non-neurogenic bladder sphincter dysfunction. BJU Int 83:294–298

Houle AM, Gilmour RF, Churchill BM, Gaumaond M, Bissonnette B (1993) What volume Can a child normally store in the bladder at a safe pressure? J Urol 149:561–564

Kakizaki H, Moriya K, Ameda K, Shibata T, Tanaka H, Koyanagi T (2003) Diameter of the external urethral sphincter as a predictor of detrusor-sphincter incoordination in children: comparative study of voiding cystourethrography. J Urol 169:655–658

Nguyen MT, Pavlock CL, Zderic SA, Carr MC, Canning DA (2005) Overnight catheter drainage diuresis in children with poorly compliant bladders improves post-obstructive and urinary incontinence. J Urol 174:1633–1636, discussion 1636

Nijman RJ (2004) Role of antimuscarinics in the treatment of nonneurogenic daytime urinary incontinence in children. Urology 63(3 Suppl 1):45–50

Pompino HJ, Bodecker RH, Trammer UA (1995) Urethral valves during the first year of life – a retrospective, multicenter study. Eur J Pediatr Surg 5:3–8

Schulman SL, Duckett JW (1998) Disorders of bladder function. In: O'Neill JA Jr et al (eds) Pediatric surgery, vol II, 5th edn. Mosby, St. Louis

van Gool JD, Hjalmas K, Tamminen-Möbius T, Olbing H, on behalf of the International Reflux Study in Children (1992) Historical clues to the complex of dysfunctional voiding, urinary tract infection and vesicoureteral reflux. J Urol 148:1699–1702

Section 28.3

Asgari SA, Mansour Ghanaie M, Simforoosh N, Kajbafzadeh A, Zare' A (2005) Acute urinary retention in children. Urol J 2:23–27

Garcia-Nieto V, Navarro JF, Sanchez-Almeida E et al (1997) Standards for ultrasound guidance of suprapubic aspiration. Pediatr Nephrol 11:607–609

Kaefer M, Zurakowski D, Bauer SB et al (1997) Estimating normal bladder capacity in children. J Urol 158: 2261–2264

Munir V, Barnett P, South M (2002) Does the use of volumetric bladder ultrasound improve the success rate of suprapubic aspiration of urine? Pediatr Emerg Care 18:346–349

Peter JR, Steinhardt GF (1993) Acute urinary retention in children. Pediatr Emerg Care 9:205–207

Section 28.4

Brock JW III, O'Neill JA Jr (1998) Bladder exstrophy. In: O'Neill JA Jr et al (eds) Pediatric surgery, vol II, 5th edn. Mosby, St. Louis

Genital bleeding in the girl is an important differential diagnosis of hematuria, lower gastrointestinal hemorrhage, and bleeding from falls astride including impalement injuries. Genital bleedings can be differentiated between physiological and pathological hemorrhages.

29.1 Physiological Hemorrhages

They occur in the first week of the neonatal period as **withdrawal bleeding** after the discontinuation of the maternal estrogens: A vaginal discharge with occult blood is observed in one third of the newborns and a visible hemorrhage starting the second day after birth in about 3 %.

In addition, **menarche** at the beginning of the maturation period and later menstruation belong to the physiological bleedings. Menarche starts at about 12 years of life with a variation of 8(6)–16 years. Menarche before 8 years of age corresponds to a precocious puberty and if it starts after 16 years, to a delayed puberty and if it is absent, to a primary amenorrhea.

29.2 Pathological Hemorrhages and Vaginal Discharge

All other genital bleedings are pathological that occur also after the physiological endocrinologically quiescent period. Pathological genital bleedings manifest in the prepubertal girl rarely as abundant hemorrhage; mostly, only blood traces

at the external genitals # or spots are encountered in the nappies or panties that lead to medical consultation. Up to 20 % of the gynecological disorders in prepubertal girls concern genital bleeding.

The possible causes are partially age-dependent and encompass the disorders listed in Table 29.1. The cause of pathological genital

Table 29.1 Causes[a] of pathological genital bleedings in the girl

Neonatal period
o Birth injuries
o Congenital tumors
o Malformations
First month of life until menarche
• Vulvovaginitis
• Foreign bodies of the vagina
• Trauma (falling astride including impalement injuries, sexual abuse)
• Tumors (rhabdomyosarcoma, endodermal sinus tumor)
• Precocious puberty
Menarche and thereafter
• Trauma, multisystemic organ injury, sexual abuse, defloration bleeding
• Vulvovaginitis
• Foreign bodies of the vagina
• Dysfunctional bleedings (e.g., anovulation [estrogen-breakthrough bleeding])
o Tumors (cervical or endometrial polyps, submucosal leiomyomas, uterine and cervical carcinoma)
o Hypothyroidism, bleeding disorders

[a]The majority of the pathoanatomical groups occur at any age, but the prevalence of the form of injury or type of tumor changes with age

bleeding is best evaluated by history, physical examination (inspection and rectoabdominal examination), and vaginoscopy with hydrodistention (2–3 mm endoscope) especially in prepubertal girls. Up to 75–85 % of the causes can be recognized by these tools. Ultrasound cannot replace vaginoscopy although ultrasonography may be useful. Genital injuries, vulvovaginitis, and vaginal foreign bodies belong to the most common causes of genital bleedings in prepubertal girls.

29.2.1 Benign and Malignant Tumors

Occurrence

In general, malignant tumors arise mainly from the vagina and uterus, whereas benign tumors occur predominantly in the vulva. Benign and malignant tumors have a similar prevalence and occur in ≤5 to ≤20 % of prepubertal girls with genital bleeding.

Congenital tumors of the vulva are occasionally observed **in newborns** and are more frequently a cause of bleeding than malformations and birth injuries. Examples are the angioleiomyofibroma, perineal lipoma, and vascular malformations that protrude as polypoid masses from the external genitals. **After it**, hemangiomas, lymphangiomas, neurofibromas, and other benign tumors are observed and occasionally, papilloma of the vagina.

Rhabdomyosarcoma (often as botryoid variant) is the principal malignoma, although endodermal sinus tumors may be observed in a similar frequency. It occurs mainly **in infants and small children** and arises from vagina, cervix, and uterus or bladder. Malignancies are encountered in ≤5 to >5 % (if bleeding is related to the genital tract) of prepubertal girls and in more, if only a population of small children is evaluated. **In adolescence**, adenocarcinoma of the vagina and other benign and malignant tumors may be observed.

Clinical Significance

- Genital bleeding in prepubertal girls needs evaluation by colposcopy for exclusion of a malignant tumor.

Clinical Presentation

Tumor of the vulva presents as *mass, structure alteration, discoloration, and in the congenital form, as vascular malformations and hemangiomas with a blood-tinged discharge. The congenital tumor may give the impression of a malignancy because of its exophytic and bizarre appearance and neurofibroma of the clitoris of ambiguous external genitals due to a pseudopenis.*

Rhabdomyosarcoma and endodermal sinus tumor lead to a lower abdominal mass, vaginal discharge and bleeding, and prolapsing interlabial mass. In bladder involvement, lower abdominal tumor, chronic urinary retention, hematuria, and prolapsing interlabial mass # are the presenting signs.

The time comes only to a few weeks between first genital bleeding and appearance of a tumor protruding from the vagina. The tumor is lobulated with a grape-like surface.

Differential Diagnosis, Work-Ups

The differential diagnosis includes, depending on the age, congenital tumors #, lichen sclerosus, psoriasis and dermatitis, external genital warts, genital herpes, and other findings of possibly sexually transmitted diseases, gangrene of the external genitals (ecthyma gangrenosum in pseudomonas aeruginosa bacteremia), and candidiasis vulvovaginitis following menarche.

In addition to a precise history (including the possibility of sexual abuse or foreign body insertion) and clinical examination, genital examination and colposcopy # in general anesthesia must be performed combined with biopsy and/or swabs for bacteriology if indicated.

Treatment, Prognosis

Benign tumors should be excised completely combined with histological work-up. Treatment modifications are necessary in hemangioma and plexiform neurofibroma.

Rhabdomyosarcoma and endodermal sinus tumor need a sufficiently large biopsy for histology and biological typification and staging by ultrasound, MRI, and CT.

Treatment includes multiagent chemotherapy and limited radiation. In about one third of the genital cases, secondary hysterectomy, vaginectomy, and/or cystectomy are necessary due to residual organ involvement with tumor.

Genital location of rhabdomyosarcoma (vaginal, uterine, and paratesticular tumor) has a favorable prognosis with >90 % 4-year survival.

29.2.2 Vulvovaginitis

Occurrence, Types

Vulvovaginitis is the most frequent gynecological disorder in premenarchal girls and the most frequent cause of vaginal bleeding in this age group #. Vulvovaginitis is related to poor hygiene and/or oxyuriasis and is observed mainly in toddlers and preschool age, although upper respiratory tract infection in the previous month may also play an important role.

In the literature, unspecific and specific vulvovainitis is differentiated. The common nonspecific type is caused by mixed fecal flora, whereas in the specific type, single germs are responsible such as Hemophilus influenzae or β-hemolytic streptococci of group A, or sexually transmitted diseases (e.g., gonorrhea).

Clinical Significance

- Vulvovaginitis manifests with a vaginal discharge intermingled with blood and may be an important differential diagnosis of genital hemorrhage in this age group.

Clinical Presentation

Genital pain, vaginal discharge, and local itch are the preferred symptoms and signs in vulvovaginitis, but *bloody spots in the clothes may be observed in at least 20 %* of the children and become a matter of concern to the mother.

At clinical examination, *redness of the external genitals is present in >80 %, and a vaginal discharge is recognizable in one third of the involved girls*. Nevertheless, the local findings may be inconspicuous in a minority of patients.

Differential Diagnosis, Work-Ups

Although the majority of vulvovaginites in the preferred age group are caused by poor genital hygiene and/or oxyuriasis, the possibility of specific vulvovaginitis, foreign body, sexual abuse, or venereal diseases in teenagers and in all girls after sexual abuse must be considered. Stool incontinence, soiling, and encopresis or urinary tract infection may be associated with vulvovaginitis. Simple **vulvitis** is the most common differential diagnosis. In isolated inflammatory lesions of the external genitals such as ecthyma gangrenosum, pseudomonas septicemia must be considered.

Foreign bodies are excluded by history, local findings (foreign body leads usually to purulent and malodorous vaginal discharge), ultrasound of the vagina, and endoscopy. The suspicion of **sexual abuse** may arise by the history of caregivers and neighbors and induce thorough genital examination in general anesthesia.

Vulvovaginitis needs swabs for Gram stain, cultures, and resistance evaluation including the exclusion of venereal diseases and urine examination by bladder punction or catheterization.

Treatment, Prognosis

The common vulvovaginitis needs instruction for appropriate local cleaning, elimination of potential irritants, possibly topical antibiotics, and steroids or p.o. vermicide medication. The specific vulvovaginitis needs systemic antibiotics.

The prognosis depends on the cause and adherence of mother or caregiver.

29.2.3 Vaginal Foreign Body

Occurrence, Causes

Vaginal foreign bodies are observed in ≤5 % of prepubertal outpatients with gynecological disorders, in ≤10 % with vaginal discharge, and in up to 30 % with vaginal bleeding.

Involved are mostly toddlers and preschool children of whom >50 % recall that some objects have been inserted by themselves or playmates. A large variety of single or multiple objects # is used once or repeatedly. Later in life, tampons and other articles left behind in the vagina must be considered. In general, foreign bodies may be left there for a period of few days to years.

Clinical Significance

- Vaginal foreign body may be an indicator of sexual abuse.
- A persistent and purulent, malodorous vaginal discharge that is unresponsive to treatment may be caused by a vaginal foreign body.

Clinical Presentation

Vaginal bleeding or bloodstained, malodorous vaginal discharge is the main presentation. Often, a *positive history of foreign body insertion* can be ascertained, and occasionally, *the foreign body may be seen* especially in prone knee-chest position or *palpated by rectal examination*. Rarely, a foreign body is an incidental finding at vaginoscopy.

Differential Diagnosis, Work-Ups

The differential diagnoses are those of vaginal bleeding or discharge. The possibility of sexual abuse cannot be excluded from the beginning.

The work-ups include ultrasound and mainly vaginoscopy. The ultrasound displays echoes and acoustic shadows caused by the foreign body and as indirect sign, indentation of the posterior bladder wall #. Because tumors, foreign bodies, or signs of sexual abuse may be missed by radiological imaging, vaginoscopy should be performed in every case of vaginal bleeding or suspected foreign body. Depending on the history and clinical findings, not only swabs for Gram stain and cultures, but also evaluation of venereal diseases is necessary.

Treatment, Prognosis

The foreign body should be removed by endoscopy in general anesthesia because irrigation may be only successful, if the foreign body is visible. In case of suspected sexual abuse, careful examination of the vulva, hymen, and vagina, and photographic documentation (after seeking permission from the parents) are necessary. The interpretation of possible findings must rely on the large normal anatomic variations in pre- and postmenarchal girls. Immediate vaginal irrigation with a nonirritant antiseptic fluid is the only measure needed after foreign body removal (e.g., solution of povidone iodine).

29.2.4 Genital Injuries

Occurrence, Types

If all types are summarized, genital injuries occur quite frequently and unintentional genital injuries may account for up to 40 % of children hospitalized for lower genital problems (median age 7 years). They encompass straddle injuries because of playing or sports activities including impalement injuries #, genital injuries as part of a multisystemic organ injury, for example, due to motor vehicle accident, and sexual assaults. The latter need special consideration.

Clinical Significance

- Genital injuries are often underestimated after a quick glance at it.
- The possibility of associated urethral, perineal, and/or anorectal injury needs special consideration.

Clinical Presentation

Genital bleeding #, prominent swelling, and disfigurement of the external genitals # are the main presenting signs.

Specific injuries of the labia majora and minora, clitoris, vagina, cervix, and lower abdominal organs depend on whether blunt, pointed and cutting, or a combination of both forces have been effective. *On close and thorough examination, the injuries are often more severe than initially thought ##.*

Associated injuries of the urethra concern the external meatus or the bladder neck including vagina. In anorectal injuries, lesions of the external sphincter, levator muscle, and rectal wall must be considered.

Differential Diagnosis, Work-Ups

The quoted presenting signs of trauma to the external genitals and anorectal injuries up to rectal wall laceration may be caused by **sexual assault** especially by community and war violence.

Evaluation of genital injuries in children needs clinical examination in general anesthesia including vaginoscopy and possibly cysto- and anorectoscopy. Depending on the history and clinical findings, MRI and/or CT with contrast are necessary for the evaluation of pelvic and lower abdominal involvement.

Treatment, Prognosis
In severe cases, blood transfusions are necessary in addition to tetanus prophylaxis, antibiotics, and transurethral or suprapubic bladder catheter. The injuries need careful anatomical repair and possibly drainage and/or temporary colostomy. The encountered injury must be precisely documented with regard to possible later forensic demands.

Prognosis depends on the type and severity of the injury. Although injuries of the external genitals heal rapidly, follow-ups are necessary for possible sequels, for instance, secondary hymenal closure.

29.2.5 Sexual Abuse

Occurrence, Definitions, Terms
Sexual abuse is observed as domestic, community, or war violence. Penetrative sexual abuse occurs during childhood in 5–10 % of the girls and in up to 5 % of the boys in developed countries (possible underreportment of sexual abuse in boys), any type of sexual abuse is observed three times as much, and only a fraction of these occurrences are officially reported. Forty to seventy percent of the raped women concern girls below 18–15 years of age in some countries.

Several definitions of sexual abuse exist. It encompasses a wide range of sexual victimization from cyberspace violence (by which girls become victims or perpetrators of cyberbullying), photographing, viewing for sexual gratification, exposure of the child to pornographic material or to adult sexual activity and to genital fondling, and attempted or successful penetration of any of the child's orifices. Depending on the circumstances of sexual abuse, the terms assault and rape are used. The perpetrators are relatives, friends, and neighbors in domestic sexual abuse, and in community sexual violence, classmates, people with educational functions, and strangers. The involved youngsters are dependent and immature,

do not completely understand what is going on, and are unable for an informed consent.

Clinical Significance
- Sexual abuse leads to immediate physical and psychic injury and shock of the involved child or teenager.
- Sexual abuse may have several short- and long-term physical and psychic sequels.
- Former includes possibly fatal injuries of the genitals or anorectum, sexually transmitted diseases, involuntary pregnancy, and posttraumatic stress disorder.
- The latter concerns eating disorders, substance abuse including alcohol and smoking, self-mutilation, high-risk sexual behavior, adolescent pregnancy, and delinquency mainly in teenagers and at any age up to adulthood, diminished self-esteem, anxiety, revictimization, and depression.

Clinical Presentation
In **acute situations**, the genital or anorectal findings are similar to straddle or impalement injuries. Perianal (e.g., radial fissures extending from the anus), hymenal, or vaginal trauma suggests a penetrating mechanism either unintentional or from sexual assault. The latter is true especially in extensive and severe perianal, hymenal, or vaginal injury, enlarged introitus, hymenal attenuation or tears, if the general examination discloses concurrent nonurogenital injuries due to the fight against the aggressor, and if there is a lack of correlation between history and physical findings or the patient is younger than 9 months.

In **chronic situations**, sexually transmitted diseases, foreign bodies, and vaginal discharge or bleeding are or may be an indication of possible sexual abuse. Although many children and especially adolescents do not bring to light their experience of abuse for months and years, several aspects of sexual abuse are different in prepubertal girls and boys from those of teenagers.

In prepubertal children, parents or caregivers are more likely involved in disclosure of sexual abuse due to their close contact with the child or *medical and behavioral aberrations*. On the other hand, sexual abuse may be a familial secret that is withheld for several years. In the majority of cases, the practitioner or pediatrician is contacted in a **nonacute situation** in which up to 90 % of the children display no physical signs.

On visual examination, nonspecific erythema of the vulva or bruising of the trunk or legs may be found in up to half of the 10 % children with physical harm, and the other half may display less or more conspicuous signs such as the following: *severe erythema of the vulva, vaginal discharge, notched hymen, tears or tags of the anus, and/or signs of sexually transmitted diseases, for example, genital herpes simplex or perianal warts*. It is important to know that the acute signs such abrasion, swelling, or hematomas (including injuries of the posterior fourchettes) disappear rapidly within 1–2 weeks, but tears of the clitoris, narrow posterior rims at the point of injury, and irregular hymenal edges remain until adolescence.

In the acute stage of sexual abuse and in nonacute stages with a relevant history and noteworthy signs, **referral to a (pediatric) sexual assault center** is indicated:

A *history of genital bleeding, plausible disclosure especially with genital-genital contact or ejaculation, short time of last incident, visible injury of the genitals, vaginal discharge, and bleeding need immediate referral*, whereas elective referral is sufficient in the nonacute situation except for the few cases with noteworthy signs.

In **postpubertal teenagers**, community- and rape-related sexual abuse becomes more frequent and, although a detailed and consistent history can be reported more reliably than in prepubertal children, the teenagers do not speak to the parents or seek acute medical care, and forensic nurses may be the first clinicians who obtain the relevant informations. The demeanor and intelligence of some teenagers may influence their credibility as witness to the abuse.

In contrast to prepubertal girls, the numerous nonspecific genital findings of a normal population are not well known in postpubertal girls and possible findings of consensual intercourse, use of tampons, and sequels of self-inflicted injury may interfere with the interpretation of the encountered findings.

The majority of a group of postpubertal girls ($n=77$, median age 15 years) have reported with decreasing percentage intrafamilial abuse, repeated abuse, and onset prior to menarche. Three fourths had genital and one fifth anal penetration, and about 60 % had deep hymenal clefts and/or vestibular scars and >10 % unspecific anal findings.

Differential Diagnosis, Work-Ups

If only the genital findings are interpreted, several differential diagnoses may arise: In the **acute stage**, other causes of genital bleeding or nonintentional genital injury including self-inflicted injury may simulate sexual abuse. But tears and other injuries of the hymen are rare in accidental injury and are observed in <5 %.

Congenital minor abnormalities #, sequels of acquired disorders of the external genitals, for example, impalement injuries #, numerous unspecific genital findings, signs after consensual intercourse, tampon use, or self-inflicted injury play an important role in the differential diagnosis in the subacute and **chronic stage**. Vulvitis is an example of an unspecific genital finding that may be caused by poor hygiene, irritation by bubble or soap baths, or urinary tract infection.

The work-ups should be performed whenever possible in a **sexual assault referral center with pediatric affiliation**. Such centers cover the medical and the forensic needs of standardized **history**, **clinical examination**, **documentation and sampling**, and **treatment** including psychosocial crisis support and have trained people at their disposal. For instance, nurses trained in sexual offenses investigative techniques or female and male doctors trained in medical and forensic examinations are available.

Children and adolescents referred to such a center should neither drink or eat, nor urinate or smoke, and they should not bathe nor change their clothes. For informed consent that includes several options of investigations and measures, the caregiver or depending on the age the teenager itself is responsible (after assessment along a specific guide and opportunity for discussion with an appropriate adult).

In general, a medicolegal diagnosis of **an alleged nonacute** sexual abuse relies on a detailed history. The physical examination can identify genital findings compatible with sexual abuse. On the other hand, absence of typical genital findings does not rule out sexual abuse. In **acute situations**, the genital or anorectal findings are similar to straddle or impalement injuries and need no further interpretation, if the history is compatible with the findings.

The majority of **prepubertal girls** will not have a full-thickness transection of the posterior rim of the hymen without a history of genital trauma from sexual abuse. A posterior rim of minimally 1 mm should always be present # without sexual abuse, and the size of the hymenal opening is not useful.

In **pubertal and postpubertal girls** (without experience of consensual intercourse), repeated abusive genital perforation leaves deep posterior clefts and/or vestibular scars and a hymenal opening that allows examination with a 17–25-mm speculum.

Treatment, Prognosis
Acute medical care should always have priority over forensic considerations and collection of early evidence. Possible urgent treatment options are surgery of acute genital trauma, emergency contraception, commencement of treatment of sexually transmitted diseases especially HIV postexposure prophylaxis within 72 h and support in psychosocial crisis.

Although the prevalence of sexually transmitted diseases is low with <10 % in a population of sexually abused children, caution is indicated because half of the infected children are asymptomatic at the moment of consultation, the predictive value of many tests is low, and the treatment must possibly be postponed. To the sexually transmitted diseases belong syphilis, gonorrhea, chlamydia trachomatis, condylomata acuminata (human papilloma virus), genital herpes simplex, and human immunodeficiency virus. Syphilis presents mostly with condylomata lata and gonorrhea with early-onset purulent vulvovaginitis. Anogenital warts are often combined with anorectal and cervicovaginal location #

(notice perianal tag). The risk of acquisition depends on the type of sexual abuse and the prevalence of infection in the abusing population. Sexually transmitted diseases in children are mostly transmitted by sexual abuse and less frequently during delivery, by accidental contact with an infected caregiver, or by autoinfection from a nonanogenital site.

Long-term treatment may become a lifelong task because of the psychic and possibly physical sequels. For several reasons, long-term outcomes of different forms and degrees of sexual abuse and of different treatment strategies are not yet available.

The expectations of parents and referring physicians are high in contrast to the usual outcome of such sexual assault referral centers as a mean of definitively establishing evidence of sexual abuse. In nonacute, asymptomatic cases, physical examination rarely yields specific findings of possible sexual abuse. Only 8 % needs emergency evaluation and noteworthy findings are present in one fifth.

29.3   Interlabial (Intralabial) Masses

The interlabial mass is a leading sign and may lead to obstruction of the lower urinary tract in girls. The following disorders may be present as interlabial mass:

- **Urethral Prolapse #**. The hardly recognizable urethral meatus is surrounded by a bluish, red and possibly bleeding rim of mucous membrane. It presents with *hematuria or genital bleeding and is observed more frequently in black girls.*
- **Prolapsing Duplex or Single Kidney Ureterocele**. In ectopic ureterocele (mostly a unilateral duplex kidney ureterocele) of the girl, the ureter enters the vagina and much less frequently the distal urethra, cervix, or uterus, and the associated ureterocele may prolapse in the interlabial zone. It is larger than urethral prolapse, appears in the introitus of the vagina, and the urethral meatus is recognizable in front of the mass. *Urinary retention or continuous urine dribbling – urinary incontinence*

combined with normal micturitions – is the classic clinical presentation in girls. Work-ups are performed to recognize unilateral duplex kidney, simple kidney, or bilateral duplex kidney with ectopic ureterocele(s) and the condition of the involved ureter and kidney moiety(ies) or single kidney. They are followed by resections or preservation of ureter and kidney depending on the results.

- **Paraurethral Cyst #, Urethral Polyp, and Papilloma #.** The former disorder lies beside the meatus and introitus that may be displaced by the cysts. The urethral polyp protrudes through the meatus. *Both disorders may distort micturition, and polyp and papilloma may bleed.*
- **Vaginal # and Hymenal Cyst**. The former lies lateral from the vaginal wall and may displace the vagina to the contralateral site. They are palpable on rectal examination and recognizable by lower abdominal ultrasound. Hymenal cysts occur at the anterior boundaries of the hymen. Therefore, the vagina is accessible dorsally from them. *Distorted micturition is possible by hymenal cysts.*
- **Muco-(metro) colpos** is caused by hymenal atresia that is one type of the possible gynatresias. In newborns and infants, the closed, gray bluish hymen protrudes through the interlabial zone, and the urethral meatus is recognizable in front of it or may be hidden by it ##. A mass corresponding to the dilated vagina and possibly uterus is palpable by abdominal and rectal examination. *Bladder voiding and defecation may be hindered by the gross muco-(metro)colpos.*
- **Genital rhabdomyosarcoma** protrudes from the vagina through the vestibulum. The mass has a grapefruit-like structure and *leads to genital bleeding*.
- **Vaginal prolapse ##** occurs without or in pelvic floor paresis (e.g., spina bifida).

Differential Diagnosis, Work-Ups

The differential diagnosis arises in the individual case from the presenting and associated signs, and the characteristic local findings are unmistakable in some of them.

If a **prolapsing ectopic ureterocele** is suspected, radiological imaging with ultrasound and MRI yields the diagnostic duplex kidney combined with abnormal site and course of the upper pole ureter, and biopsy confirms a suspected **rhabdomyosarcoma**.

Treatment Prognosis

Both depend on the diagnosis and the possible therapeutic options. In urethral prolapse, treatment depends on the stage of prolapse: symptomatic treatment in minor forms and early stage with anti-inflammatory medicaments and sitz baths and resection and primary anastomosis in severe and advanced stages. **Prolapsing ectopic ureterocele** needs preliminary endoscopic punction that is followed by secondary upper pole resection and ureterectomy. **Paraurethral cysts** need marsupialization with the urethra, **urethral polyp** resection, and **muco-(metro) colpos** cruciform incision with resection of the edges. The outcome is uneventful in most disorders if the appropriate treatment is chosen.

Webcodes

The following webcodes can be used on www.psurg.net for further images and data.

2901 Blood traces, external genitals	2913 Congenital hymenal appendages
2902 Interlabial mass, rhabdomyosarcoma	2914 Secondary hymenal closure after injury
2903 Angioleiomyofibroma, newborn	2915 Normal posterior hymenal rim, prepubertal girl
2904 Rhabdomyosarcoma, endoscopy	2916 Perianal warts
2905 Chronic vulvovaginitis	2917 Urethral prolapse
2906 Vaginal foreign bodies	2918 Paraurethral cyst
2907 Ultrasound, vaginal foreign body	2919 Urethral papilloma
2908 Impalement injury, external genitals	2920 Paravaginal maldevelopmental cyst
2909 Straddle injury, genital bleeding	2921 Hymenal atresia, newborn

2910 Straddle injury, swelling	2922 Hymenal atresia, postpubertal girl
2911 Straddle injury at first sight	2923 Vaginal prolapse
2912 Straddle injury, close examination, avulsion labium minus	2924 Vaginal prolapse after reduction

Bibliography

General: Differential Diagnosis of Genital Bleeding, Endoscopy

Bevan JA, Maloney KW, Hillery CA et al (2001) Bleeding disorders: a common cause of menorrhagia in adolescents. J Pediatr 138:856–861

Navratil F (2001) Die gynäkologische Untersuchung bei kleinen Mädchen Wann ist sie sinnvoll? Pädiatrie 1:4–7

Parker JD, Hibbert ML, Dainty LD, Larsen FW, Dance VD (2000) Microhydrovaginoscopy in examining children. Obstet Gynecol 96:772–774

Ragni MV, Bontempo FA, Hassett AC (1999) von Willebrand's disease and bleeding in women. Hemophilia 5:313–317

Sections 29.1, 29.2.1–29.2.3

Castellino SM, Martinez-Borges AR, McLean TW (2009) Pediatric genitourinary tumors. Curr Opin Oncol 21:278–283

Cowan BD, Morrison JC (1991) Management of abnormal genital bleeding in girls and women. N Engl J Med 324:1710–1715

Cuadros J, Mazon A, Martinez R, Gonzalez P, Gil-Setas A, Flores U, Orden B, Gomez-Herruz P, Millan R, Spanish Study Group for Primary Care Infection (2004) The aetiology of paediatric inflammatory vulvovaginitis. Eur J Pediatr 163:105–107, Erratum in: Eur J Pediatr (2004) 163:283

Fischer GO (2002) Vulval disease in prepubertal girls. Australas J Dermatol 42:225–234; quiz 235–236

Giusti RM, Iwamoto K, Hatch EE (1995) Diethylstilbestrol revisited: a review of the long-term health effects. Ann Intern Med 122:778–788

Heinz M (2001) Genitalinfektionen in Kindheit und Adoleszenz Prävalenz, Diagnostik und Therapie. Pädiatrie 1:9–13

Heinz M, Schweizerische Arbeitsgruppe für Kinder- und Jugendgynäkologie (2004) Zyklusstörungen bei jungen Mädchen Amenorrhö, Regeltypus- und Regeltempostörungen. Pädiatrie 1:16–19

Imai A, Horibe S, Tamaya T (1995) Genital bleeding in premenarcheal children. Int J Gynaecol Obstet 49:41–45

Jones R (1996) Childhood vulvovaginitis and vaginal discharge in general practice. Fam Pract 13:369–372

Paradise JE, Willis ED (1985) Probability of vaginal foreign body in girls with genital complaints. Am J Dis Child 139:472–476

Pascual-Castroviejo I, Lopez-Pereira P, Savasta S, Lopez-Gutierrez JC, Lago CM, Cisternino M (2008) Neurofibromatosis type 1 with external genitalia involvement presentation of 4 patients. J Pediatr Surg 43:1998–2203

Renteria SC, Hirrle B, Schweizerische Arbeitsgruppe für Kinder- und Jugendgynäkologie (2005) Vulvaerkrankungen beim Mädchen im Kindesalter Orientierungshilfe für Differentialdiagnostik und Therapie in der Praxis. Pädiatrie 1:13–16

Smith YR, Berman DR, Quint EH (2002) Premenarchal vaginal discharge: findings of procedures to rule out foreign bodies. J Pediatr Adolesc Gynecol 15:227–230

Stricker T, Navratil F, Sennhauser FH (2004) Vaginal foreign bodies. J Paediatr Child Health 40:205–207

Striegel AM, Myers JB, Sorensen MD, Furness PD, Koyle MA (2006) Vaginal discharge and bleeding in girls younger than 6 years. J Urol 176:2632–2635

Vogel AM, Alesbury JM, Burrows PE, Fishman SJ (2006) Vascular anomalies of the female external genitalia. J Pediatr Surg 41:993–999

Sections 29.2.4–29.2.5

Berenson AB, Chacko MR, Wiemann CM et al (2002) Use of hymenal measurements in the diagnosis of previous penetration. Pediatrics 109:228–235

Berkoff MC, Zolotor AJ, Makoroff KL, Thackeray JD, Shapiro RA, Runyan DK (2008) Has this prepubertal girl been sexually abused? JAMA 300:2779–2792

Boos SC (1999) Experience and reason accidental hymenal injury mimicking sexual trauma. Pediatrics 103:1287–1290

Byard RW, Donald TG, Rutty GN (2008) Non-traumatic causes of perianal hemorrhage and excoriation in the young. Forensic Sci Med Pathol 4:159–163

Cremer M, Masch R (2010) Emergency contraception: past, present, and future. Minerva Ginecol 62:361–371

Dowd MD, Fitzmaurice L, Knapp JF, Mooney D (1994) The interpretation of urogenital findings in children with straddle injuries. J Pediatr Surg 29:7–10

Edgardh K, von Krogh G, Ormstad K (1999) Adolescent girls investigated for sexual abuse: history, physical findings and legal outcome. Forensic Sci Int 104:1–15

Elder DE (2007) Interpretations of anogenital findings in the living child: implications for the paediatric forensic autopsy. J Forensic Leg Med 14:482–488

Fegert JM (2007) Child sexual abuse. Bundesgesundheitsblatt Gesundheitsforschung Gesundheitsschutz 50:78–89

Garcia VE, Sheldon C (1998) Genitourinary tract trauma. In: O'Neill JA Jr et al (eds) Pediatric surgery, 5th edn, 1. Mosby, St. Louis

Gilbert R, Widom CS, Browne K, Fergusson D, Webb E, Janson S (2009) Burden and consequences of child maltreatment in high-income countries. Lancet 373: 68–81

Heger AH, Tiscont L, Guerra L, Lister J, Zaragoza T, McConnell G, Morahan M (2002) Appearance of the genitalia in girls selected for nonabuse: review of hymenal morphology and non-specific findings. J Pediatr Adolesc Gynecol 15:27–35

Lalor K, McElvaney R (2010) Child sexual abuse, links to later sexual exploitation/high-risk sexual behavior, and prevention/treatment programs. Trauma Violence Abuse 11:159–177

Lynch JM, Gardner MJ, Alabanese CT (1995) Blunt urogenital trauma in prepubescent female patients: more than meets the eye! Pediatr Emerg Care 11: 372–375

McCann J, Voris J, Simon M (1992) Genital injuries resulting from sexual abuse: a longitudinal study. Pediatrics 89:307–317

Saint-Martin P, Bouyssy M, Jacquet A, O'Byrne P (2007) Sexual assault: medicolegal findings and legal outcomes (analysis of 756 cases). J Gynecol Obstet Biol Reprod (Paris) 36:588–594

Shapiro RA, Makoroff KL (2006) Sexually transmitted diseases in sexually abused girls and adolescents. Curr Opin Obstet Gynecol 18:492–497

Smith WG, Metcalfe M, Cormode EJ, Holder N (2005) Approach to evaluation of sexual assault in children. Experience of a secondary-level regional pediatric sexual assault clinic. Can Fam Physician 51:1347–1351

Sommers MS (2007) Defining patterns of genital injuries from sexual assault: a review. Trauma Violence Abuse 8:270–280

Tolle MA, Schwarzwald HL (2010) Postexposure prophylaxis against human immunodeficiency virus. Am Fam Physician 82:161–166

Wiese M, Armitage C, Delaforce J, Welch J (2005) Emergency care for complaints of sexual assault. J R Soc Med 98:49–53

Section 29.3

Falandry L (1994) Prolapse of the urethra in black girls. Personal experience in 11 cases. Med Trop (Mars) 54:152–156

Fletcher SG, Lemack GE (2008) Benign masses of the female periurethral tissues and anterior vaginal wall. Curr Urol Rep 9:389–396

Grande Moreillo C, Rodo Salas J, Morales Fochs L (2000) Ectopic ureter as cause of urinary incontinence in Girls. Actas Urol Esp 24:314–318

The two terms are often mixed up with each other. They refer to disorders of the scrotal skin, scrotal content, or to both. Scrotal swelling is potentially a pediatric surgical emergency (**acute scrotum #**).

It is useful to look at the presence or absence of the skin creases, color, and thickness of the **scrotal skin,** as well as at the location of these changes (one or both scrotal halves, penis, groin, or perineum). The same applies to the **scrotal content**: Testis, epididymis, and spermatic cord must be examined for different features.

Testicular torsion leads initially to a slight swelling of the testicle and through it to an increase of the volume of the scrotal content. The scrotal skin is increasingly involved only in the further clinical course. Therefore, different clinical presentations can be observed in the same disorder **depending on the stage of testicular torsion**.

The percentage of the responsible disorders depends on the origin of the evaluated patients: medical practice, emergency department, or pediatric surgical inpatient population. Epididymitis, testicular torsion, and torsion of the testicular appendages belong to the most frequent causes of acute scrotum in a children's hospital emergency department. The differential diagnoses of testicular and/or scrotal swelling (pain) are listed in Table 30.1.

Although a part of the quoted pathologies display a **preferred age of presentation**, the majority actually occurs at any age of childhood. Examples are the age distribution of testicular torsion with two peaks in the neonatal period and

Table 30.1 Differential diagnoses of testicular and scrotal swelling (pain)

- Testicular torsion
- Epididymitis
- Torsion of the testicular and paratesticular appendages
- Scrotal injury, zipper entrapment
- Testicular hydrocele or hydrocele of the cord and complete inguinal hernia
- Acute idiopathic scrotal edema
- o Insect sting and bite
- o Scrotal swelling in Henoch-Schönlein purpura
- o Orchitis
- o Other (inflammatory) disorders of the scrotum
- o Peritoneal disorders with scrotal swelling
- o Varicocele
- Testicular tumor
- o Idiopathic infarction of testis and tunica vaginalis, spontaneous thrombosis of the plexus pampiniformis, torsion of a cyst of the tunica vaginalis

at puberty, the preferred age of torsion of testicular appendages with 10 years, of idiopathic scrotal edema below 7 years, and of orchitis beyond 11 years of age.

In addition to **history and carefully evaluated local clinical findings, ultrasound or scintiscan** belongs to the usual work-ups. But they do not replace the former tools because these are the basis of indication and interpretation of the latter.

By ultrasound, a so-called **microlithiasis** may be recognized by chance. It consists of multiple, dot-like hyperechogenic focuses distributed over the testicular parenchyma and is often associated

Fig. 30.1 Drawing of the two main types of torsion of the testis. (**a**) The spermatic cord is twisted above the tunica vaginalis. (**b**) The torsion lies within the testicular tunica vaginalis. The pathology in (**a**) is called supravaginal torsion that is observed perinatally. The findings in (**b**) correspond to an intravaginal torsion that occurs mostly at puberty. A rare type of torsion is twisting at the level of the connection between the testis and epididymis. I owe this drawing to Marcel Bettex who was my teacher in pediatric surgery

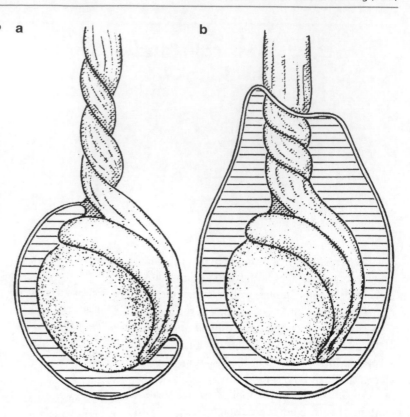

with a testicular tumor in adulthood. So far, this association does not apply to children.

30.1   Testicular Torsion (Torsion of the Spermatic Cord)

Occurrence, Pathoanatomy, Types

Testicular torsion may occur at any age of childhood, although its percentage is increased in the perinatal period and at puberty. The median age of testicular torsion is 14 years in a large cohort of children and adults.

Cryptorchidism is an important predisposing factor of testicular torsion as well as the bell clapper deformity of the testicle in which the tunica vaginalis has a high insertion and reflecting fold on the spermatic cord. Bilateral occurrence of this aberration explains the frequency of the asynchronous and rare synchronous bilateral testicular torsions.

The intravaginal type of testicular torsion is six times as much observed as the supravaginal

type in which torsion of the spermatic cord occurs outside and above the tunica vaginalis #. The supravaginal type is mainly observed in the perinatal period and may also present as isolated infarction of testis and tunica vaginalis (Fig. 30.1). Torsion of the mesorchium is a rare form of testicular torsion. Torsion of the testis occurs either in a clockwise or in a counterclockwise direction. Twisting of the testis is ≥360° in severe cases. In one third of the cases, recurrent testicular torsion may be observed with spontaneous recovery.

Clinical Significance

- Delayed diagnosis and surgery of testicular torsion lead to irreversible testicular loss and if bilateral to complete infertility.
- The recurrent type of testicular torsion may be one of the many causes of pain in the groin.

Clinical Presentation

Immediate or gradually increasing severe testicular pain that occurs spontaneously or after sports activities *is the leading symptom of testicular torsion (96 %). It may be combined with unspecific signs such as vomiting and pain radiating in the groin and lower abdomen.*

In the **early stage**, *a swollen testis is visible within the scrotum # which has a high and twisted or horizontal position #* (the horizontal position is significantly associated with bell clapper deformity) *and is extremely painful on palpation. The cremasteric reflex is absent.* Provocation of the cremasteric reflex is usually possible in all boys older than 2 1/2 years of age, and its absence is therefore a reliable sign of testicular torsion in preschool and older boys. *Occasionally, a localized and small retraction of the ipsilateral scrotal skin is recognizable as additional sign #.*

In **advanced stages**, *inflammation of the scrotal skin with edema and redness superimposes the changes of the testis # which becomes a large and tough mass.* In general, typical signs of testicular torsion are present in at least three fourths.

Most children with **recurrent testicular torsion** have a bell clapper malformation that is also present in the majority of cases on the contralateral side. It occurs at all ages and is characterized *by rapid onset of severe testicular pain and spontaneous resolution.* The reported rate of such episodes ranges from 1 to 30 before surgery. Recurrent testicular torsion holds the danger of final unresolved torsion with potential loss of the testicle. Elective bilateral testicular fixation is recommended after confirmation of an episode by ultrasound (due to the challenging clinical condition a spectrum of different sonographic features may be present). Because final unresolvable torsion may occur already after two episodes, the indication of surgery should not be expectant, particularly since the results of elective surgery are excellent with resolution of the episodes.

Perinatal (intrauterine) testicular torsion corresponds to supravaginal torsion, occurs before birth to 30 days after it, and is mostly unilateral. The bilateral form (<10 %) is observed in two thirds synchronously and in one third asynchronously. The newborns are usually born at term after a difficult delivery in some. The clinical presentation includes *dark red scrotal skin # and enlarged, tender, and firm or hard testis in high position.* Idiopathic infarction of testis and tunica vaginalis is a possible differential diagnosis. Amelioration of the surgical results is possible by (a) early detection by conscious search of the typical clinical findings in every newborn, (b) immediate surgery with detorsion and prophylactic fixation of the contralateral side, and (c) preservation of not completely necrotic testes (maintenance of endocrine function). Up to one fourth of the testes may be preserved (mean time of surgery 45 h) with good results. In bilateral form, the results are probably worse with <10 % good results.

Differential Diagnosis, Work-Ups

It includes disorders with testicular and/or scrotal swelling and pain, and occasionally, a surgical abdomen. A rare differential diagnosis is torsion of a cyst within the tunica vaginalis. The early stage of testicular torsion should be recognized by clinical examination. In advanced stages, testicular tumor or an inflammatory process may be considered. Testicular tumor is usually a painless mass without sign of scrotal inflammation. The **typical testicular torsion is recognizable by history and clinical examination provided the physician knows the symptomatology**.

Possible work-ups are gray scale or **color Doppler sonography** (pulsed Doppler with mechanical sectorial scanning) and scintiscan. Ultrasound is especially indicated in equivocal findings or if another disorder than testicular torsion is possible. Ultrasound must specifically consider the intraparenchymal arteries. False-negative results occur in >1 %, the findings depict a momentary stage, recurrent testicular torsions may be missed, and subacute stages may be interpreted as testicular tumor.

Sonography should include testis, epididymis, and spermatic cord. Whirlpool sign is the most specific and sensitive sign of complete and incomplete testicular torsion. Absent central arterial perfusion with/without abnormal parenchymal echogenicity or absent venous blood flow and reduced central arterial perfusion are other characteristic signs. Heterogeneous echogenicity (focal hyper/hypoechogenicity) is an indication of irreversible testicular damage.

Treatment, Prognosis

Immediate surgery is indicated in case of typical testicular torsion, in cases confirmed by ultrasound, and if testicular torsion cannot be excluded due to clinical suspicion in spite of an apparently normal ultrasound. **Ultrasound should not prevent or postpone prompt surgical exploration in case of severe symptomatology**.

The access is either transscrotal or inguinal and includes careful inspection of the degree of torsion # and recovery of the testis after retorsion # with possible biopsy in doubtful cases.

After retorsion, the testicle of both sides are fixed with nonabsorbable sutures between testis and tunica dartos to avoid retorsion of the ipsilateral and torsion of the contralateral side. Testicular ablation is only indicated in irreversible interruption of the blood supply #. Torsion does not necessarily cause the circulation to cease. Preserving surgery can be attempted in some cases, although <15 % retain normal trophicity and <10 % need secondary resection because of purulent testicular necrosis ##.

In large cohorts, the number of patients who need ablation is <20 %. After a testicular torsion of >24 h duration and ≥360° torsion, loss or atrophy of the testis must be expected in >50 % of the patients, and the same may occur already after ≥4 h and ≥360°. If only the length of torsion is considered, a small percentage needs ablation after <24 h and after >24 h 80 %. Up to 50 % of the seemingly normal testes suffer from >20 % loss of their volume or even atrophy in comparison to the contralateral side, and about 40 % of the patients display later in life oligozoospermatism possibly because of a primary malformation. In adults, autoimmunological reactions with subsequent male infertility have been observed and decreased testosterone secretion in one third without influence on virilization, libido, and sexual potency in adolescents and young adults.

All testicular fixation techniques are not entirely reliable in preventing recurrence. It occurs rarely and may be observed a few days up to >25 years after initial orchidopexy. Albeit rare, atrophy, gangrene, and seriously damaged testes are reported in recurrences that need orchiectomy. A four-point orchidopexy is quoted instead of fixation in a line as superior method against recurrence.

30.2   Epididymitis

Occurrence, Pathoanatomy, Causes

Epididymitis # is observed at any age in childhood. It occurs more frequently than thought in earlier times, and its prevalence is similar to that of torsion of the spermatic cord or testicular appendages.

Epididymitis is related to orchitis because a focus in the epididymis may spread to the testis (epididymo-orchitis) and involvement of one organ may lead to an associated swelling of the other. Epididymitis is usually a unilateral disorder, although bilateral forms are observed occasionally. In acute epididymitis, the symptomatology lasts <6 weeks and in chronic epididymitis, >3 months.

In childhood, the preferred **causes** of epididymitis are different from those of adults, and the age groups play an important role in this respect (young and prepubertal boys vs. adolescent boys). In infancy, epididymitis may be observed as **part of a systemic infection** and in prepubertal boys, as **first manifestation of pediatric urological malformations**, especially obstruction of the lower urinary tract. In school-children, **dysfunctional voiding** is an important cause of epididymitis and at puberty, sexually transmitted diseases such as those generated by **Chlamydia trachomatis** and **Neisseria gonorrhoeae**. The following groups of etiopathogenesis can be differentiated:

- Infectious epididymitis (retrograde propagation through the vas deferens or by the bloodstream), enterobacteria, Gram negative germs, sexually transmitted diseases, viruses, tuberculosis (the epididymis is the most common site of genitourinary tuberculosis), or bilharziosis (usually combined with urinary tract bilharziosis)
- Traumatic epididymitis (caused by genitourinary injuries)
- Chemical epididymitis (caused by urethrovasal reflux and combined with infection), lower

urinary tract malformation, dysfunctional voiding, idiopathic urethroseminal reflux
- Epididymitis as part of a systemic disease (granulomatous, allergic, immunodeficiency disorders)
- Idiopathic epididymitis

Urological malformations are responsible in 10–15 % of the children with epididymitis. If the patients with dysfunctional voiding and with miscellaneous causes are included, much more children will have a concrete cause of epididymitis. In this context, vesicoureteral reflux; complete ureteral duplication; infravesical obstruction such as posterior urethral valves, meatal stenosis, and neurogenic bladder; permanent bladder catheter, CIC, or vesicourethral instrumentation and endourethral procedures; anorectal malformations, hypospadias, or persistent Müllerian duct structures; detrusor-sphincter dyssynergy or lazy bladder syndrome must be considered.

In general, the scrotum should always be inspected and palpated in urinary tract infection, and absent symptomatology and/or findings of urinary tract infection do not exclude epididymitis.

Clinical Significance
- Epididymitis is a frequent cause of acute scrotum and is often not recognized.
- Epididymitis has often a hidden cause that must be looked for, and if these causes are not recognized and treated, epididymitis will recur.

Clinical Presentation
It may be similar to a more advanced stage of testicular torsion. *The most frequent symptoms and signs are scrotal pain, swelling (100 %), tenderness of the epididymis (<100 %), and redness of the scrotum (65–75 %) #. Reactive testicular hydrocele, nausea, vomiting, and sign of urinary tract infection are much less frequently observed.* Sexually transmitted epididymitis is possibly combined with signs of urethritis. Comparing patients with testicular torsion and epididymitis, tenderness of the testis and absent cremasteric reflex occur also in epididymitis albeit less frequently and tenderness of the epididymis also in testicular torsion.

For differentiation of epididymitis from testicular torsion, the following signs may be looked for: *Resting of the scrotum in a raised position lessens discomfort and pain,* and *an enlarged and painful mass may be felt that can be delineated from the testis* in older children.

Differential Diagnosis, Work-Ups
The differential diagnosis includes all disorders leading to an acute scrotum, especially more advanced stage of testicular torsion and idiopathic scrotal edema.

The work-ups encompass the inflammatory blood parameters, urine sediment, and cultures. Depending on the suspected cause and age of the patient, blood, stool, and CSF cultures, Gram stain and cultures from urethral swab (Chlamydia trachomatis, gonorrhea), histology and cultures from epididymis biopsy, specific blood examinations, and radiological imaging including ultrasound # for differential diagnosis of acute scrotum become necessary. Ultrasound and scintiscan shows a straight spermatic cord, absent focal testicular lesions, enlargement of the epididymis and/or testis # with increased blood flow # or tracer accumulation and possible formation of abscess (≤ 5 %).

The initially quoted examinations should be performed, if epididymitis is probable. Nevertheless, fever, leukocytosis, and/or pyuria are observed at most in 20–40 % of children with epididymitis.

Treatment, Prognosis
Treatment is usually **nonoperative** with bed rest, raised position of the scrotum, local cold, and antiphlogistics. Antibiotics are only indicated in proven or suspected bacterial infection, for example, p.o. ceftriaxone for gonococci and macrolides or second-generation quinolones for gonococci and Chlamydia trachomatis and cotrimoxazole or second-generation quinolones for enterobacteria (in severe cases, parenteral aminoglycoside combined with cephalosporin).

Surgical revision is indicated in case of epididymitis with abscess, if testicular torsion cannot be excluded, in equivocal cases, or for biopsy, for example, urogenital tuberculosis or bilharziosis.

The **prognosis** is good without infertility and/or atrophy of the epididymis except for bilaterality of large abscess with organ destruction.

Further work-ups after treatment are necessary, if no definite cause has been recognized such as epididymitis in the context of a systemic Haemophilus influenzae infection in infancy or a sexually transmitted disease in adolescence:

(a) In urinary tract symptomatology or infection particularly with enterobacteria, recurrent epididymitis, and/or in small children, ultrasound of kidneys and bladder is indicated possibly completed by IVU, VCU, and cystourethroscopy for exclusion of urinary tract malformations. In idiopathic urethrovasal reflux, suprapubic VCU is recommended.

(b) Depending on the results of a precise history of bladder voiding, in absence of the conditions quoted in (a), presence of sterile urine, and/or in schoolchildren, urodynamics are necessary combined with ultrasound and VCU for exclusion of dysfunctional voiding. The measures to be taken depend on the result of the work-ups quoted above.

30.3   Torsion of the Testicular and Paratesticular Appendages

Pathoanatomy, Occurrence

Appendages of testis, epididymis, and cord are residuals of embryonal development that may be the subjects of spontaneous torsion or edema and ischemia related to hormonally induced enlargement.

Torsion of the testicular and paratesticular appendages and possibly spontaneous ischemia belong to the most common causes of acute scrotum even if not to the most frequent cause, may occur rarely asynchronously or synchronously on both sides, and concern testicular appendages at surgery in about 90 % #. Although all ages may be involved, a peak exists around 10 years of age.

Clinical Significance

• Torsion of the testicular appendages belongs together with epididymitis to the most frequent differential diagnosis of acute scrotum.

Clinical Presentation

The leading sign is acute pain within the scrotum. Pathognomonic findings are a visible blue spot # and/or palpable tender nodule or painful point at the anterior surface or upper pole of the testis. The nodule may be mobile. These findings are observed only in up to 20 %. Reactive testicular hydrocele may overlap these findings.

The severity of inflammation at histological examination of the removed appendices correlates with the length of symptomatology and presence of classic findings.

Differential Diagnosis, Work-Ups

It includes disorders with acute scrotum and mainly testicular torsion.

Gray scale and color Doppler **sonography** display several features suggesting testicular appendage and its torsion: Extratesticular upper pole nodule that may be pedunculated, has a central hypoechogenic area, an increased blood flow, and is larger than 5.6 mm. Possible secondary inflammatory changes in up to 50 % of the cases including testicular hydrocele, enlarged epididymis, swollen scrotal wall, and testis may lead to an erroneous diagnosis of epididymitis, idiopathic scrotal edema, orchitis, or testicular torsion.

Treatment, Prognosis

Although nonoperative treatment with anti-inflammatory agents is recommended by some because of the possibility to depict the twisted appendage in some cases or to display features compatible with it by ultrasound (95 % CI of 45–85 % for sensitivity and of 75–100 % for specificity), surgery with ablation of the twisted appendage relieves immediately the pain and excludes with certainty other causes of acute scrotum especially testicular torsion.

The prognosis after surgery is excellent except for rare asynchronous contralateral torsion of testicular or paratesticular appendages.

30.4   Scrotal Injury, Zipper Entrapment

Occurrence, Type, and Sites of Injury

Most scrotal injuries occur between the ages 10 and 30 years and are blunt traumas because of falls astride (e.g., on a bicycle frame), athletic activities, or motor vehicle accidents. Open injuries to which belong the degloving trauma with scrotal avulsion #, penetrating injuries (stab wounds, self-mutilation, and gunshots), and animal attacks, thermal, or surgical injuries are less common.

The injuries may lead to **hematoma** (intratesticular or extratesticular [scrotal wall, epididymis, or cord] hematomas), **hydrocele**, **hematocele**, **testicular fracture or rupture**, and rarely to intratesticular pseudoaneurysm.

Clinical Significance
- Scrotal injury is an important differential diagnosis of acute scrotum.
- It may be overlooked in multisystemic organ injury.
- Delayed or inaccurate diagnosis, especially of severe intratesticular hematoma or rupture may lead to testicular loss or atrophy.
- Scrotal injury may lead to testicular torsion, epididymitis, or epididymo-orchitis

Clinical Presentation
Except for missed or concealed informations, scrotal trauma is usually recognized *by a corresponding history with scrotal pain and local genital findings of scrotum and possibly penis.*

At clinical examination, *abrasions, bruises #, scrotal swelling, possible wounds, and signs of involvement of the scrotal content may be found. The testis may be tender and enlarged, retracted in the groin, or cannot be palpated due to hydrocele or hematocele.* In **zipper injury**, the prepuce is usually entrapped.

Differential Diagnosis, Work-Ups
The differential diagnosis includes disorders of acute scrotum, especially advanced stages of testicular torsion, scrotal swelling in Henoch-Schönlein purpura, or coagulation disorders.

First-line work-up tool is gray scale and color Doppler ultrasound, especially for evaluation of scrotal content. **Hematoma** leads to focal hyperechogenicity without internal flow and on follow-up, to hypoechogenicity and heterogenicity in complex hematomas and thickening of the scrotal wall. In **hydrocele**, the fluid collection is anechogenic, and **hematocele** is uniformly echogenic with a similar follow-up like hematoma. Complex layering of the hematoma is possible. **Testicular fracture** displays a linear echoic band across the testicular parenchyma, but fractures are not identifiable in large hematomas. Internal flow and intact tunica albuginea must be checked for. In **testicular rupture**, the margins of the tunica albuginea are poorly defined or lost, and extrusion of testicular content is visible. Unfortunately, the accuracy of ultrasound-based diagnosis of rupture is between >50 and >90 % sensivity and specifity, and the loss of tunica contour is combined with heterogeneous echotexture of the parenchyma. MRI is an alternative diagnostic tool in equivocal cases.

Treatment, Prognosis
Emergency surgery is indicated, if rupture or nonperfusion of testis (large intratesticular hematoma without/with testicular fracture) is proven by ultrasound or clinically suspected in spite of equivocal sonographic findings. The same applies to scrotal lacerations and degloving and open injuries that need emergency skin repair or revision.

Surgery in testicular rupture and nonperfusion includes control of active bleeding, evacuation of hematoma, debridement, possible drainage, and closure of the tunica albuginea. In degloving injuries, closure of the skin is often possible due to the elasticity and abundance of scrotal skin. Nevertheless, skin grafting may become necessary, for example, expanded mesh grafts. Most surgical cases need antibiotics.

The other injuries are treated conservatively with bed rest, raised positioning of the scrotum, and analgesics.

In **zipper injury**, division of the zipper bar by small and strong pliers frees the caught prepuce. Elective circumcision is indicated thereafter.

Prognosis depends on the type of injury and the promptness of surgery. In testicular rupture and nonperfusion, the testis may be retained in 80–90 % by correct indication and rapid surgery. In open injury, the prognosis depends on the type and degree of destruction.

Fig. 30.2 Testicular hydrocele. The drawing shows on the *left side* a testicular hydrocele that is locally the only disorder because the processus peritonealis vaginalis is atretic. In the *middle of the row*: the testicular hydrocele is combined with a minute sinus tract to the peritoneal cavity. If it is not considered at surgery, recurrence of hydrocele may occur. On the *right side*: the testicular hydrocele is combined with a sack of a possible inguinal hernia, and it must be considered at surgery to avoid manifestation of inguinal hernia. In case of gross testicular hydrocele, simultaneous small inguinal hernia with protrusion of some abdominal content may be overlooked

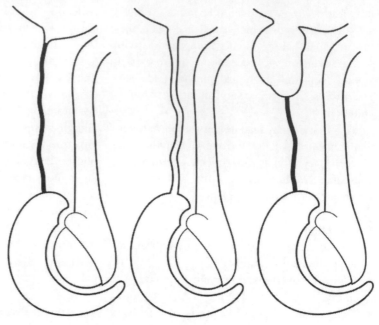

30.5 Testicular Hydrocele or Hydrocele of the Cord and Complete Inguinal Hernia

Occurrence

All three disorders are frequent differential diagnoses of scrotal and testicular swelling.

Clinical Significance

- **Acute or recurrent communicating hydrocele** (narrow peritoneovaginal process communicating with the hydrocele) or **symptomatic hydrocele** (reactive to an intrascrotal process) and **incarcerated complete inguinal hernia** (inguinoscrotal hernia) are subgroups of the disorders quoted in the title that need specific attention in the differential diagnosis of acute scrotum.

Clinical Presentation

The acute or recurrent hydrocele manifests *as intrascrotal swelling that is cystic and possibly hard to firm or fluctuant on palpation and translucent on diaphanoscopy. The overlying scrotum may be reddened* without or with infection of the hydrocele #.

Clinical differentiation from other causes may be difficult in acute incarcerated complete inguinal hernia. *The extremely painful and tender mass is firm, elastic, and continues from the groin to the external inguinal ring and scrotum. The overlying skin is dark red #. It is possibly combined with clinical and radiological signs of obstructive ileus.*

Treatment

Whereas incarcerated complete inguinal hernia needs immediate surgery by inguinal access, the acute or symptomatic hydrocele has more likely a differential diagnostic significance and needs possibly further work-ups and elective surgery (Fig. 30.2).

30.6 Acute Idiopathic Scrotal Edema (Scrotal Wall Edema)

Occurrence

Acute idiopathic scrotal edema occurs mainly in boys in the second half of the first decade (mean age 6 years) although it may be observed occasionally in younger and older children or even in adults. It amounts to <10 % of children with acute scrotum and has mostly an unrecognizable cause except for some adults, for example, **dengue fever** (characterized by fever, chills, bone pain, skin rash, gum bleeding, thrombocytopenia, and hemoconcentration).

Clinical Significance

- Idiopathic scrotal edema is a possible differential diagnosis of acute scrotum that needs no surgery.

Clinical Presentation

It consists of *unilateral and less frequently bilateral scrotal edema (effacement of the skin creases) combined with a more or less distinct redness # and nonfocal tenderness. It may characteristically extend from the whole scrotum to the ipsilateral groin, perineum, buttock, or penis #.* The child is otherwise unimpaired.

Differential Diagnosis, Work-Ups

It includes all other causes of acute scrotum including insect stings and bites, diaper dermatitis, and rarely scrotal cystic lymphangioma.

The blood inflammatory signs are usually normal except for moderate leukocytosis and occasional eosinophilia. For differentiation from testicular torsion or epididymitis, color Doppler ultrasound may be useful. It displays edematous scrotal wall thickening (thickness of >10 mm) with increased blood flow (fountain sign) that is compressible and enlargement of the ipsilateral inguinal lymph node. Testis and epididymis are mostly normal. Depending on the equipment and experience of examiner, false-negative results may be possible in case of testicular torsion.

Treatment, Prognosis

Bed rest and analgesics are sufficient because edema disappears spontaneously within a few days. Nevertheless, several relapses may occur in at least 20 % of the children within several years.

30.7 Insect Stings and Bites

After insect stings or bites, the practitioner is often consulted with delay, when an inflammation or allergic reaction spreads from the site of sting or bite.

If the scrotum is involved, these secondary reactions to stings or bites may present as acute scrotum and resemble an acute idiopathic scrotal edema. *In the center of the lesion, the original sting or bite may be recognizable* which aids in the correct differential diagnosis.

Treatment consists of local and systemic antihistaminics. The possibility of allergy to insect stings must always be considered. In case of **xodiasis (infestation with ticks)**, a possible endemic area must be considered. Ticks occur worldwide especially in dense deciduous wood, 1,500 m below sea level, and during warm weather. Ticks cling on the skin, suck blood, and may transmit Lyme borreliosis and meningoencephalitis depending on the endemic areas and in a relation of 30:1. Ticks should be carefully removed as soon as possible, and incomplete removal needs medical consultation. The site of infestation should be observed for 3 weeks regarding possible infection or redness. Whereas Lyme borreliosis is amenable to antibiotics, tick-borne encephalitis (early summer meningoencephalitis) can only be prevented by active vaccination.

30.8 Henoch-Schönlein Purpura with Scrotal Involvement

Occurrence

Henoch-Schönlein purpura is the most common systemic vasculitis in children. Rash of the extensor site of the lower trunk and extremities, arthralgia, and abdominal pain are the main symptoms. Scrotal involvement is observed in >20 % of boys. It concerns the scrotal skin and possibly also the scrotal content and is the most common site of nonrenal genitourinary disorders. In acute abdominal and flank pain, **obstructive ureteritis** must be considered.

Clinical Significance

- Scrotal involvement may be in the fore of Henoch-Schönlein purpura or even occur before the appearance of the classic signs.
- Rarely, scrotal involvement may be associated with testicular torsion.

Clinical Presentation

Scrotal swelling (>80 %), tenderness, and pain (<70 %) are the main symptoms and signs. Scrotal swelling may be grotesque # and accompanied with diffuse hemorrhage and redness #.

Patients with scrotal involvement display more frequently headache and localized edemas than those without it. No correlation exists between scrotal and possible renal involvement.

In contrast to acute idiopathic scrotal edema, the scrotal content is often not palpable in scrotal edema of Henoch-Schönlein purpura.

Differential Diagnosis, Work-Ups

In the differential diagnosis, mainly idiopathic scrotal edema, blunt scrotal injury, testicular torsion of advanced stage, and coagulopathies including thrombocytopenia must be considered, especially if the Henoch-Schönlein purpura is not obvious.

Work-ups are performed for exclusion of differential diagnostic relevant disorders, because Henoch-Schönlein purpura is a clinical diagnosis. They include inflammatory blood tests of which serum C3 may be increased, urinalysis, and possibly coagulation studies including thrombocyte count.

Sonography shows involvement of the scrotal skin and possibly swelling and hemorrhage of epididymis and testis and may exclude testicular torsion. Demonstration of the characteristics of testicular torsion may be difficult due to the grotesque scrotal edema.

Treatment, Prognosis

It includes, after exclusion of testicular torsion, bed rest, raised position of the scrotum, and symptomatic medication of the purpura. Usually, spontaneous recovery of the grotesque genital findings without sequels can be observed.

30.9   Orchitis

Occurrence

Orchitis is a relatively rare cause of testicular enlargement and is observed either because of a viral infection or an epididymitis with propagation to the testis. On the other hand, a testicular swelling in response to an insult is more frequently observed, for example, due to testicular torsion or blunt injury of the scrotal content, or as part of a generalized disorder, for example, in Henoch-Schönlein purpura.

Epidemic parotitis leads to the classic mumps orchitis in about 30 % of the pubertal or postpubertal teenagers. In countries with introduction of mumps vaccination, the time of appearance of epidemic parotitis is postponed to the early adulthood.

Clinical Significance

- One third of the patients with epidemic parotitis and complicated orchitis display later in life infertility.

Clinical Presentation

Unilateral or bilateral orchitis (10 %) occurs mostly 4–5 days after beginning of mumps and is recognizable by a visible and/or palpable scrotal swelling and fever that last for a mean time of 4–5 days. It may be accompanied by mumps meningitis or subclinical pancreatitis in about 30 %.

Because parotitis epidemica with orchitis occurs in the second decade of life, the swollen testis is easily palpable in contrast to small children. Reactive hydrocele may efface these findings.

Differential Diagnosis, Work-Ups

The diagnosis of mumps orchitis is evident, if endemic parotitis is proven clinically and serologically. In other cases, inflammatory blood signs and ultrasound permit the diagnosis of orchitis, for example, in case of mumps orchitis before occurrence of parotitis.

Treatment, Prognosis

It is symptomatic and includes interferon alpha in case of general impairment.

Long-term follow-up of pubertal and postpubertal patients with determination of the testicular size by comparing the size with an orchidometer enables some prognostication concerning fertility. Decreased testosterone and inhibin B levels may be encountered in one third already in the acute period and seminal abnormalities frequently in the first year after epidemic parotitis.

30.10 Other Inflammatory Disorders of the Scrotum

Occurrence, Causes

Other inflammatory disorders of the scrotum than the already quoted are rare. They include fat necrosis, cellulitis of the scrotum, and adjacent inflammatory disorders of penis, perineum, buttock, and lower abdomen.

Clinical Presentation

(Idiopathic) subcutaneous fat necrosis may arise spontaneously or after a soft tissue injury and is localized or diffuse and unilateral or bilateral. It leads to *an inflammatory swelling of the scrotum or to an intradermal mass.*

Cellulitis of the scrotum # that is possibly combined with gangrene and necrosis # is observed mainly in newborns and infants. This severe type of scrotal infection is usually based on a recognizable cause including septicemia, for instance, napkin dermatitis, circumcision, urethral stone impaction, or ecthyma gangrenosum.

A continuous transition exists between cellulitis of the scrotum and **inflammatory disorders of the adjacent regions**, for instance, in advanced balanoposthitis.

Proceeding and Treatment

In case of inflammatory findings of the scrotum, these differential diagnoses must be considered and confirmed by history, specific clinical findings, and inflammatory blood markers. Suspected fat necrosis can be confirmed by ultrasound. Primary treatment is usually medical and includes appropriate antibiotics.

30.11 Peritoneal Disorders

Occurrence, Pathoanatomy

Pre- and postnatally, especially in newborns and infants, but also in older children, the processus vaginalis is open or remains so.

Intrauterine or postpartal peritonitis and less frequently intra-abdominal tumors or other disorders propagate through the processus to the tunica vaginalis, and the peritoneal disorder becomes manifest by scrotal swelling.

Clinical Presentation

The characteristics of scrotal swelling depend on the specific peritoneal disorder. The scrotal swelling comes to be a mirror of the specific peritoneal disorder that is now visible from the outside and amenable to diagnostic work-up.

Examples are residuals of meconium peritonitis such as a dark brown discolored and enlarged scrotal compartment, hydrocele with palpable hard masses, or multiple calcifications within the scrotum; hydrocele due to chylous and other types of ascites; acute appendicitis or secondary peritonitis with infected testicular hydrocele; or abdominal non-Hodgkin's lymphoma with hydrocele because of tumorous ascites.

Proceedings and Treatment

History, specific general and local clinical findings, and appropriate work-ups confirm the clinical diagnosis. To the latter belong radiological imaging of the scrotum, puncture, and revision by inguinal access that enables simultaneous resection and closure of the open processus.

30.12 Varicocele

Occurrence, Pathoanatomy, and Pathophysiology

Varicocele occurs already in small and school-children. A distinct increase is observed during puberty up to values in adult men (e.g., 19 % at the age of 19 years or <10 to >25 % in different populations).

Eighty to ninety percent occurs on the left side, and the rest are bilateral or right-sided. Spermatic phlebography displays on the left side absence of valves in up to three fourths and reflux of blood through venous branches from the left kidney in the remaining. The altered flow characteristic leads to dilatation of the plexus pampiniformis and possibly to damage of the developing testis.

Clinical Significance

- The growth of the ipsilateral testicle remains behind by >20 % in about one fourth of adolescents with varicocele, and about 9 % of the young men have a small testis.
- In addition to the impaired testicular growth, the teenagers may have an abnormal sperm

count, and the histological findings of the testis are analogous to those of infertile men.

Clinical Presentation

Painless scrotal swelling and dragging sensations are the possible complaints.

The upper part of the left hemiscrotum is filled up with dilated venous vessels, the testis takes a horizontal position, and is possibly smaller than the contralateral testicle or its size is inappropriate to the age. Grade III varicocele looks similar to a sac of worms # in standing position, the soft mass is compressible and depends on the body position. Grade I and II varicocele is only palpable with and without a Valsalva maneuver.

Varicocele in small children and those on the right side are rarely related to a retroperitoneal mass (hydronephrosis, Wilms' tumor, or another retroperitoneal tumor).

Differential Diagnosis, Work-Ups

It includes all painless and soft masses of the scrotum. Grade III varicocele has a characteristic appearance.

Ultrasound is used for grading of the varicoceles and measurement of the testicular size. If the size of the testis is determined by comparison with an orchidometer or another method (measurement of testicular length or comparison with a stencil), the difference of testicular size is recognized in only ≥ 50 %. Radiological evaluation of the kidney for tumor is not necessary in the common left-sided varicocele.

Treatment, Prognosis

Surgery is based on the observation that testicular catch-up growth takes place in adolescents afterward (by 55 ± 39 % after the modified and by 67 ± 20 % after the classic Palomo method [$p = 0.58$]) and improvement of seminal quality in comparison with noncorrected patients. The indications of surgery are:
- Varicocele of small and schoolchildren and bilateral varicocele independent of age
- Varicocele of adolescents with an ipsilateral testicular size <20 % and/or abnormal semen

- Varicocele grade III with complaints

Surgery is best performed according to the modified or classic method of Palomo. The results of open or laparoscopic surgery are comparable. The latter procedure permits repair of bilateral forms by the same access.

Prognostic statements concern only testicular growth and semen analysis. It is not yet known if varicocele of the adolescence impairs fertility later in life and if this can be prevented by early surgery. Recurrences are observed in 3–4 %; postoperative hydrocele occurs less frequently after the modified technique with 3.2 % versus 7.7 %.

Recurrences or persistent varicocele needs pre- or intraoperative spermatic phlebography, and the results must be considered by the reoperation.

Adolescents with normal testicular size need annual follow-up for testicular size and possibly semen analysis.

30.13   Testicular Tumor

Occurrence, Pathoanatomy

Although testicular tumors occur at any age of childhood, more than 50 % are observed in the first 2 years. Only 1 % of childhood malignancies are testicular tumors, and 1 in 2–3 cases of neoplasms of the testis is benign. Testicular tumors are observed in Asia less frequently.

About 70 % are **germ cell tumors** of whom the malignant *yolk sac tumor* # and the often benign *teratomas* # and dermoid/epidermoid are the most frequent. Mixed germ cell tumors and seminomas are rare in childhood. The next most frequent group is the **stromal testicular tumors** (*Leydig cell*, Sertoli cell, and juvenile granulosa cell tumor). The third group includes special types of tumor: involvement of the testicle(s) by *leukemia or malignant lymphoma* # (histological involvement occurs in about 20 % of lymphoblastic leukemias, and testicular tumor may be a primary manifestation of Burkitt's lymphoma), paratesticular tumors like *rhabdomyosarcoma*, melanotic neuroectodermal tumor of infancy, and gonadoblastoma in mixed gonadal dysgenesis (25 % risk of unilateral or bilateral involvement of streak gonads with possible malignant degeneration). Benign tumors are lipoma, lipoblastoma, leiomyoma, and hemangioma of the cord or scrotal soft tissue.

Clinical Significance

- Testicular tumor must be suspected in every painless, gradually developing scrotal or testicular mass.

Clinical Presentation

A painless and nontender mass in the scrotum that is related to the testis or cord, or an unexplained testicular growth is the main sign of testicular tumor. Therefore, several months may pass by until a physician is consulted #.

The enlarged testis has an irregular shape except for secondary involvement by leukemia or lymphoma. Smaller tumor nodules may be palpated by a *specific technique* in which the thumb and index finger grasps the anterior and posterior testis including epididymis and cord and palpates the testicular surface by sliding movements.

In case *of precocious puberty,* a Leydig cell tumor must be considered and in case of *gynecomastia,* Leydig cell or Sertoli cell tumor due to an autochthonous production of testosterone or other hormones.

Differential Diagnosis, Work-Ups

The differential diagnosis includes disorders with a painless scrotal mass, especially advanced stages of testicular torsion or scrotal injury; furthermore, developmental disorders such as ectopic spleen #, polyorchidism, and spermatocele #; or tumors like scrotal lipoma #, lipoblastoma, or dermoid cyst of the scrotal raphe.

Spermatocele is a retention cyst of the epididymis and occurs mostly in adults. The painless cystic mass lies separate from the testis posteriorly close to the head of the epididymis, is freely movable and transilluminates. Ultrasound displays the falling snow sign. Complete resection is possible without harm to the epididymis.

Work-ups include gray scale and color Doppler ultrasound, and trunk CT and serum tumor markers like α-fetoprotein (AFP) and β-human chorionic gonadotropin (β-HCG), if a malignant tumor is suspected. A mass mixed with solid and cystic areas point to teratoma. AFP and β-HCG are increased in yolk sac tumor and embryonal carcinoma and mixed teratomas, respectively. Their normalization or persistently or renewed abnormal levels on follow-ups can be used for confirmation of complete or incomplete resection or relapse of the tumor. Trunk CT is performed for retroperitoneal lymph node and liver and/or lung metastatic disease. MRI of the testis may be useful for small testicular tumors (e.g., Leydig cell tumor) and precise delineation of the tumor # if an organ-sparing surgery can be considered.

Treatment, Prognosis

Malignant and possibly malignant tumors need bloodless high inguinal orchiectomy #, especially if frozen sections are necessary. **Dermoid cysts, benign teratomas, and other (initially) nonmalignant tumors** are or may be operated by enucleation # or partial resection.

Yolk sac tumors and other malignant germ cell tumors need special consideration:

Preoperative staging by radiological imaging and possibly by ipsilateral sampling of retroperitoneal lymph nodes at primary surgery by laparoscopy (lymph node metastasis occurs in <10 %) is necessary. Staging is as follows: Stage I=tumor limited to the testis and appropriate tumor resection has been performed; stage II=tumor resection by transscrotal orchiectomy with microscopic involvement of scrotum or cord; retroperitoneal lymph node involvement; increased or persistently abnormal tumor markers; stages III and IV=retroperitoneal lymph node involvement and distant metastatic disease, respectively.

Retroperitoneal lymph node sampling is indicated in the following conditions: (1) in case of lymph node involvement at initial CT or persistently abnormal tumor markers after orchiectomy, (2) in patients with recurrent disease or persistently abnormal tumor markers, and (3) in patients with stage III or IV. In **mixed and feminizing gonadal dysgenesis**, prophylactic resection of the streak gonads is indicated due to the risk of gonadoblastoma and malignant degeneration.

Prognosis depends on the type of tumor and its stage. Permanent cure is possible for all benign tumors including teratomas.

Webcodes

The following webcodes can be used on www.psurg.net for further images and data.

3001 Acute scrotum, testicular torsion	3021 Scrotal injury, visible hematoma
3002 Supra- and infratesticular torsion	3022 Acute testicular hydrocele left side
3003 Early stage, high testicular position	3023 Strangulated complete inguinal hernia rightside
3004 Early to intermediate stage, twisted testis	3024 Acute idiopathic scrotal edema of both sides
3005 Skin retraction, testicular torsion	3025 Acute idiopathic scrotal edema, including penis
3006 Late stage, scrotal involvement	3026 Henoch-Schönlein purpura, genital edema
3007 Unilateral perinatal testicular torsion	3027 Henoch-Schönlein purpura, diffusehemorrhage
3008 Testicular torsion, before retorsion and	3028 Scrotal cellulitis, inguinal lymphangitis
3009 After retorsion, clapper bell deformity	3029 Necrotizing scrotal cellulitis
3010 Far advanced testicular torsion	3030 Grade 3 varicocele, teenager
3011 Bilateral perinatal testicular torsion beforeand	3031 Malignant germ cell (yolk sac) tumor
3012 After retorsion	3032 Benign teratoma
3013 Epididymitis	3033 Gross involvement left testis, leukemia
3014 Left epididymitis	3034 Painless scrotal swelling, testicular malignancy
3015 Ultrasound, normal side and	3035 Ectopic spleen
3016 Ultrasound, epididymitis abnormal side	3036 spermatocele
3017 Ultrasound with Doppler, increased blood flow	3037 Scrotal lipoma
3018 Torsion testicular appendage, upper pole of testis	3038 MRI, paratesticular mass
3019 Blue spot sign, torsion testicular appendage	3039 High inguinal orchiectomy, testicular malignancy
3020 Scrotal avulsion, right hemiscrotum	3040 Residual testis after tumor enucleation, teratoma

Bibliography

General: Differential Diagnosis, Radiological Imaging, and Management Scrotal Swelling and Pain, and Microlithiasis

Dagash H, Mackinnon EA (2007) Testicular microlithiasis: what does it mean clinically? BJU Int 99:157–160

Dell'Acqua A, Toma P, Oddone M, Ciccone MA, Marsili E, Derchi LE (1999) Testicular microlithiasis: US finding in six pediatric cases and literature review. Eur Radiol 9:940–944

Ellis DG, Mann CM Jr (1998) Abnormalities of the urethra, penis, and scrotum. In: O'Neill JA Jr et al (eds) Pediatric surgery, vol II, 5th edn. Mosby, St Louis

Ganem JP, Workman KR, Shaban SF (1999) Testicular microlithiasis is associated with testicular pathology. Urology 53:209–213

Gatti JM, Patrick Murphy J (2007) Current management of the acute scrotum. Semin Pediatr Surg 16:58–63

Kass E, Stone KT, Cacciarelli AA, Mitchel B (1993) Do all children with an acute scrotum require exploration? J Urol 150:667–669

Kogan SJ (1987) Acute and chronic scrotal swelling. In: Gillenwater JY et al (eds) Adult and pediatric urology, vol II. Year Book Medical Publishers, Chicago

Lewis AG, Bukowski TP, Jarvis PD, Wachsman J, Sheldon CA (1995) Evaluation of acute scrotum in the emergency department. J Pediatr Surg 30:277–281; discussion 281–282

Melekos MD, Asbach HW, Markou SA (1988) Etiology of acute scrotum in 100 boys with regard to age distribution. J Urol 139:1023–1025

Van Glabeke E, Khairouni A, Larroquet M, Audry G, Gruner M (1999) Acute scrotal pain in children: results of 543 surgical explorations. Pediatr Surg Int 15:353–357

Vijayaraghavan SB (2006) Sonographic differential diagnosis of acute scrotum: real-time whirlpool sign, a key sign of torsion. J Ultrasound Med 25:563–574

Yazbeck S, Patriquin HB (1994) Accuracy of Doppler sonography in the evaluation of acute conditions of the scrotum in children. J Pediatr Surg 19:1270–1272

Section 30.1

Al-Hunayan AA, Hanafy AM, Kehinde EO, Al-Awadi KA, Ali YM, Al-Twheed AR, Abdulhalim H (2004) Testicular torsion: a perspective from the Middle East. Med Princ Pract 13:255–259

Al-Salem AH (2007) Intrauterine testicular torsion: a surgical emergency. J Pediatr Surg 42:1887–1891

Anderson JB, Williamson RC (1986) The fate of the human testes following unilateral torsion of the spermatic cord. Br J Urol 58:698–704

Antao B, MacKinnon AE (2006) Axial fixation of testes for prevention of recurrent testicular torsion. Surgeon 4:20–21

Baglaj M, Carachi R (2007) Neonatal bilateral testicular torsion: a plea for emergency exploration. J Urol 177: 2296–2299

Baker LA, Sigman D, Mathews RI, Benson J, Domico SG (2000) An analysis of clinical outcomes using color Doppler testicular ultrasound for testicular torsion. Pediatrics 105:604–607

Caesar RE, Kaplan GW (1994) The incidence of the cremasteric reflex in normal boys. J Urol 152:779–780

Callewaert PR, Van Kerrebroeck P (2010) New insights into perinatal testicular torsion. Eur J Pediatr 169:705–712

Chmelnik M, Schenk JP, Hinz U, Holland-Cunz S, Günther P (2010) Testicular torsion: sonomorphological appearance as a predictor for testicular viability and outcome in neonates and children. Pediatr Surg Int 26:281–286

Eaton SH, Cendron MA, Estrada CR, Bauer SB, Borer JG, Cilento BG, Diamond DA, Retik AB, Peters CA (2005) Intermittent testicular torsion: diagnostic features and management outcomes. J Urol 174:1532–1535; discussion 1535

Gesino A, Bachmann De Santos ME (2001) Spermatic cord torsion after testicular fixation. A different surgical approach and a revision of current techniques. Eur J Pediatr Surg 11:404–410

Hayn MH, Herz DB, Bellinger MF, Schneck FX (2008) Intermittent torsion of the spermatic cord portends an increased risk of acute testicular infarction. J Urol 180(4 Suppl):1729–1732

Hutson JM (1998) Undescended testis, torsion, and varicocele. In: O'Neill JA Jr et al (eds) Pediatric surgery, vol II, 5th edn. Mosby, St Louis

Matteson JR, Stock JA, Hanna MK et al (2001) Medicolegal aspects of testicular torsion. J Urol 57:783–787

Papatsoris AG, Mpadra FA, Karamouzis MV (2003) Posttraumatic testicular torsion. Ulus Travma Acil Cerrahi Derg 9:70–71

Pepe P, Panella P, Pennisi M, Aragona F (2006) Does color Doppler sonography improve the clinical assessment of patients with acute scrotum? Eur J Radiol 60:120–124

Rybkiewicz M (2001) Long-term and late results of treatment in patients with a history of testicular torsion. Ann Acad Med Stetin 47:61–75

Tryfonas G, Vlolaki A, Tsikopoulos G, Avtzoglou P, Zioutis L, Limas C, Gregoriadis G, Badouraki M (1994) Late postoperative results in male treated for testicular torsion during childhood. J Pediatr Surg 29:553–556

Van Glabeke E, Khairouni A, Larroquet M, Audry G, Gruner M (1998) Spermatic cord torsion in children. Prog Urol 8:244–248

Bennett RT, Gill B, Kogan SJ (1998) Epididymitis in children: the circumcisional factor? J Urol 160:1842–1844

Bukowski TP, Lewis AG, Reeves D, Wacksman J, Sheldon CA (1995) Epididymitis in older boys: dysfunctional voiding as an etiology. J Urol 154:762–765

Fall I, N'Doye M, Wandaogo A, Sankale AA, Diop A (1992) A case report of epididymo-testicular bilharziasis in a child. Ann Urol (Paris) 26:360–361

Gislason T, Noronha RF, Gregory JG (1980) Acute epididymitis in boys: a 5-year retrospective study. J Urol 124:533–534

Haecker FM, Hauri-Hohl A, von Schweinitz D (2005) Acute epididymitis in children: a 4-year retrospective study. Eur J Pediatr Surg 15:180–186

Hermansen MC, Chusid MJ, Sty JR (1980) Bacterial epididymo-orchitis in children and adolescents. Clin Pediatr (Phila) 19:812–815

Kadish HA, Bolte RG (1998) A retrospective review of pediatric patients with epididymitis, testicular torsion, and torsion of the testicular appendages. Pediatrics 102:73–76

Likitnukul S, McCracken GH Jr, Nelson JD, Votteler TP (1987) Epididymitis in children and adolescents. Am J Dis Child 141:41–44

Megalli M et al (1972) Reflux of urine into ejaculatory ducts as a cause of recurring epididymitis in children. J Urol 108:978

Thirumavalavan VS, Ransley PG (1992) Epididymitis in children and adolescents on clean intermittent catheterization. Eur Urol 22:53–56

Section 30.3

Baldisserotto M, de Souza JC, Pertence AP, Dora MD (2005) Color Doppler sonography of normal and torsed appendages in children. AJR Am J Roentgenol 184:1287–1292

Karmazyn B, Steinberg R, Livne P, Kornreich L, Grozovski S, Schwarz M, Ziv N, Freud E (2006) Duplex sonographic findings in children with torsion of the testicular appendages: overlap with epididymitis and epididymoorchitis. J Pediatr Surg 41:500–504

Monga M, Scarpero HM, Ortenberg J (1999) Metachronous bilateral torsion of the testicular appendices. Int J Urol 6:589–591

Rakha E, Puls F, Saidul I, Furness P (2006) Torsion of the testicular appendix: importance of associated acute inflammation. J Clin Pathol 59:831–834

Section 30.4

Bhatt S, Dogra VS (2008) Role of US in testicular and scrotal trauma. Radiographics 28:1617–1629

Leibovitch I, Mor Y (2005) The vicious cycling: bicycling related urogenital disorders. Eur Urol 47:277–286; discussion 286–287

Section 30.2

Baipai M, Nambhirajan L, Dave S, Gupta AK (2006) Surgery in tuberculosis. Indian J Pediatr 67(2 Suppl):S53–S57

Santucci RA, Bartley JM (2010) Urologic trauma guidelines: a 21st century update. Nat Rev Urol 7:510–519

Srinivasa RN, Akbar SA, Jafri SZ, Howells GA (2009) Genitourinary trauma: a pictorial essay. Emerg Radiol 16:21–33

van der Horst C, Naumann CM, Martinez-Portillo FJ, Jünemann KP (2005) External genital injuries. Diagnostics and treatment. Urologe A 44:898–903

Wessells H, Long L (2006) Penile and genital injuries. Urol Clin North Am 33:117–126, vii

Section 30.5

Lloyd DA, Rintala RJ (1998) Inguinal hernia and hydrocele. In: O'Neill JA Jr et al (eds) Pediatric surgery, vol II, 5th edn. Mosby, St Louis

Section 30.6

Geiger J, Epelman M, Darge K (2010) The fountain sign: a novel color Doppler sonographic finding for the diagnosis of acute idiopathic scrotal edema. J Ultrasound Med 29:1233–1237

Halb C, Eschard C, Lefebvre F, Brunel D, Abély M, Bernard P (2010) Acute idiopathic scrotal oedema in young boys: a report of ten cases and review of the literature. Ann Dermatol Venereol 137:775–781

Lee A, Park SJ, Lee HK, Hong HS, Lee BH, Kim DH (2009) Acute idiopathic scrotal edema: ultrasonographic findings at an emergency unit. Eur Radiol 19:2075–2080

Section 30.7

Golden DBK, Kagey-Sobotka A, Norman PS et al (2004) Outcomes of allergy to insect stings in children, with and without venom immunotherapy. N Eng J Med 351:668–674

Section 30.8

Ha TS, Lee JS (2007) Scrotal involvement in childhood Henoch-Schönlein purpura. Acta Paediatr 96:552–555

Kaiser G, Kuffer F, Gugler E (1970) Hodenschwellung bei anaphylaktoider Purpura Schönlein-Henoch-Glanzmann. Mschr Kinderheilk 118:119–122

Soreide K (2005) Surgical management of nonrenal genitourinary manifestations in children with Henoch-Schönlein purpura. J Pediatr Surg 40:1243–1247

Wiersma R (2009) Urethro-ejaculatory duct reflux in children: an updated review. Eur J Pediatr Surg 19: 374–376

Section 30.9

Ternavasio-de la Vega HG, Boronat M, Ojeda A, Garcia-Delgado Y, Angel-Moreno A, Carranza-Rodriquez C, Bellini R, Frances A, Novoa FJ, Perez-Arellano JL (2010) Mumps orchitis in the post-vaccine era (1967–2009): a single-center series of 67 patients and review of clinical outcome and trends. Medicine (Baltimore) 89:96–116

Section 30.10

Cabrera H, Skoczdopole L, Marini M, Della Giovanna P, Saponaro A, Echeverria C (2002) Necrotizing gangrene of the genitalia and perineum. Int J Dermatol 41:847–851

Kaiser G (1974) Spontane Komplikationen der Urolithiasis im Kindesalter. Helv Chir Acta 41:323–326

Rabinowitz R, Lewin EB (1980) Gangrene of the genitalia in children with pseudomonas sepsis. J Urol 124:431–432

Section 30.11

Friedman SC, Sheynkin YR (1995) Acute scrotal symptoms due to perforated appendix in children: case report and review of the literature. Pediatr Emerg Care 11:181–182

Roberts JP, Malone PS, Moore I (1995) Diagnosis of meconium peritonitis by orchidopexy. Eur J Pediatr Surg 5:50–51

Section 30.12

Atassi O, Kass EJ, Steinert BW (1995) Testicular growth after successful varicocele correction in adolescents: comparison of artery sparing techniques with the Palomo procedure. J Urol 153:482–483

Barroso U Jr, Andrade DM, Novaes H, Netto JM, Andrade J (2009) Surgical treatment of varicocele in children with open and laparoscopic Palomo technique: a systematic review of the literature. J Urol 181:2724–2728

Campagnola S, Flessati P, Fasoli L, Sulpasso M, Pea M (1999) A rare case of acute scrotum. Thrombophlebitis from ectasia of the left pampiniforme plexus. Minerva Urol Nefrol 51:163–165

Cromie WJ (1987) Varicocele and other abnormalities of the testis. In: Gillenwater JY et al (eds) Adult and pediatric urology, vol II. Year Book Medical Publishers, Chicago

Diamond DA, Xuewu J, Cilento BG Jr et al (2009) Varicocele surgery: a decade's experience at a children's hospital. BJU Int 104:246–249

El-saeity NS, Sidhu PS (2006) "Scrotal varicocele, exclude a renal tumor". Is this evidence based? Clin Radiol 61:593–599

Glassberg KI, Badalato GM, Poon SA, Mercado MA, Raimondi PM, Gasalberti A (2011) Evaluation and management of the persistent/recurrent varicocele. Urology 77:1194–1198

Kass EJ, Belman B (1987) Reversal of testicular growth failure by varicocele ligation. J Urol 137:475–476

Salzhauer EW, Sokol A, Glassberg KI (2004) Paternity after adolescent varicocele repair. Pediatrics 114:1631–1633

Wagner L, Tostain J, Comité Andrologie de l'Association Française d'Urologie (2007) Varicocele and male infertility: AFU 2006 guidelines. Prog Urol 17:12–17

Walker AR, Kogan BA (2010) Cost-benefit analysis of scrotal ultrasound in the treatment of adolescents with varicocele. J Urol 183:2008–2011

Wyllie GG (1985) Varicocele and puberty – the critical factor? Br J Urol 57:194–196

Section 30.13

Agarwal PK, Palmer JS (2006) Testicular and paratesticular neoplasms in prepubertal males. J Urol 176:875–881

Ahmed HU, Arya M, Muneer A, Mushtag I, Sebire NJ (2010) Testicular and paratesticular tumours in the prepubertal population. Lancet Oncol 11:476–483

Andrassy RJ, Corpron C, Ritchey M (1998) Testicular tumor. In: O'Neill JA Jr et al (eds) Pediatric surgery, vol I, 5th edn. Mosby, St Louis

Arda SI, Senocak ME, Gögüs S, Büyükpamukcu N (1993) A case of benign intrascrotal lipoblastoma clinically mimicking testicular torsion and review of the literature. J Pediatr Surg 28:259–261

Del Sordo R, Cavaliere A, Sidoni A, Colella R, Bellezza G (2007) Intrascrotal lipoblastoma: a case report and review of the literature. J Pediatr Surg 42:E9–E11

Häcker A, Hatzinger M, Grobholz R, Alken P, Hoang-Böhm J (2006) Scrotal lymphangioma – a rare cause of acute scrotal pain in childhood. Aktuelle Urol 37:445–448; quiz 421–422

Kramer AS, Kelalis PP (1987) Pediatric urologic oncology. In: Gillenwater JY et al (eds) Adult and pediatric urology, vol II. Year Book Medical Publishers, Chicago

Oottamasathien S, Thomas JC, Adams MC, DeMarco RT, Brock JW 3rd, Pope JC 4th (2007) Testicular tumours in children: a single-institutional experience. BJU Int 99:1123–1126

Sastri J, Dedhia R, Laskar S, Shet T, Kurkure P, Muckaden M (2006) Extra-renal Wilms' tumour – is it different? Pediatr Nephrol 21:591–596

Sung T, Riedlinger WF, Diamond DA, Chow JS (2006) Solid extratesticular masses in children: radiographic and pathologic correlation. AJR Am J Roentgenol 186:483–490

Teixeira RL, Rossini A, Paim NP (2009) Testicular tumors in childhood. Rev Col Bras Cir 36:85–89

Occurrence, Clinical Significance

Cryptorchidism is a frequent disorder: 2–5 % of the neonates born at term and about 20 % of those with a birth weight <2,500 g have cryptorchidism (i.e., bilateral altogether in 45 %), and still 1 % at the age of 1 year and somewhat less after the end of growth. Recently, the prevalence of cryptorchidism is increasing in some developed countries. Its clinical significance is many and diverse:

- Possible impairment of fertility (reduced germ cell number at birth or general depletion of germ and to a lesser degree of Leydig cells after birth and specifically loss from 6 months to 4 years of age [due to maternal lifestyle or exposition to diethylstilbestrol and factors related to failing descent]).
- Increased risk of testicular malignancy (2.75–8 times increased risk of neoplasm for the undescended testis).
- Pathologies which become visible and palpable in descended testes, for example, testicular torsion # or tumor, may be hidden.
- Psychological effect on the developed young man is possible.

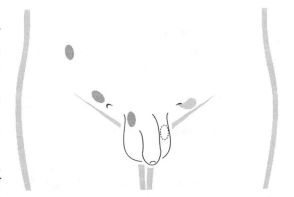

Fig. 31.1 Diagrammatic drawing of the topographically possible sites in the two main types of cryptorchidism; on the *right side* of the patient: in retention of the testis and on the *left side*: in testicular ectopy. C – external inguinal *ring*. On the *right side*: the testis does not or only minimally descend – intra-abdominal (abdominal) testicular retention; it descends along the normal route and remains in the inguinal channel – canalicular testicular retention, or at the entrance of the scrotum – high scrotal retention. On the *left side*, the testis diverges from the normal route of descent and lies in front of the external inguinal *ring* diverging in a lateral direction underneath the Scarpa's fascia – prefascial ectopy of the testis (sliding testis) – or it lies somewhere outside the external inguinal *ring*. Precise assignment to the different types and forms may be possible sometimes only during surgery

31.1 Testicular Retention and Ectopy

Empty scrotum # is observed in two types of cryptorchidism (Fig. 31.1):

- Testes that retain a position on the normal route of testicular descent (testicular retention): abdominal (<10 %), canalicular, or high scrotal position (testis at the entrance of scrotal compartment)
- Testes that deviate from the normal route of decent and remain there (testicular ectopy): prefascial, perineal #, pubopenile, femoral, and transverse forms (both testes migrate toward the same scrotal compartment)

G.L. Kaiser, *Symptoms and Signs in Pediatric Surgery*,
DOI 10.1007/978-3-642-31161-1_31, © Springer-Verlag Berlin Heidelberg 2012

31.1.1 Abdominal Testis

The intra-abdominal testis is either peeping (partially lying in the inguinal channel) or lies close to the internal inguinal ring # or in a variable distance of ≤ or ≥2.5 cm from it in direction of the kidney, is uni- or bilateral, of normal size, small or dysplastic, and displays rarely a tumor.

31.1.2 Prefascial Ectopy or Sliding Testis

The sliding testis is a form of cryptorchidism in which the testicle lies underneath the subcutaneous fascia and is reflected laterally to the external inguinal ring #. It is the most common form of cryptorchidism, and its precise definition is only possible at surgery.

31.1.3 The Transverse Ectopy

Transverse ectopy presents either as unilateral impalpable testis with two testes on the contralateral side or as unilateral inguinal hernia (that hides the testes) combined with contralateral impalpable testis. The latter presentation may be an indication of a persistent Müllerian duct syndrome.

31.2 Secondary Cryptorchidism

Secondary cryptorchidism may be observed spontaneously in a small part of boys with an undescended testis at birth and at the age of 3 months but intrascrotal position with 1 year (**late ascending testis**) or after inguinal hernia repair especially in premature infants.

In operative **acquired undescended testis**, the often normal-sized testis lies in 85 % in a superficial inguinal pouch and has usually a normal attachment of the gubernaculums, and an open processus vaginalis is encountered in >50 %. Prompt orchidopexy is indicated with excellent results, if it is performed by an experienced surgeon.

Indications of possible **late ascending testis** are:

- A history as quoted above (definite descent occurs in the majority of term infants in the first 3–6 months of life).
- Testes of children with cerebral palsy and other associated disorders (in two thirds of the patients).
- One fourth of retractile testis develops sometimes into a late ascending testis.

The late ascending testis accounts for ≤5 % of cryptorchidism, is more frequent on the left side, and displays the same possible histological abnormalities as undescended testes (decreased testicular volume, mean tubular diameter, and testicular fertility index).

31.3 Clinical Presentation and Skills in Cryptorchidism

An empty scrotum with or without a palpable testis is probably more frequently observed by medical check-up than by observation of mother or father.

The **examination** should be performed in a quiet and lying child without any haste and with warm hands. **Inspection** shows if one or both testicles do not lie in the corresponding scrotal compartment and if they lie somewhere else. In unilateral forms, the ipsilateral scrotal compartment is underdeveloped and in bilateral forms the whole scrotum. Two hands are necessary for **palpation** of the testis and its site: The left hand lies flat over the ventral iliac spine and expresses smoothly the inguinal channel, whereas the right hand tries to grasp the testis starting from the scrotum #.

The Scorer index corresponds to the distance measured between the upper pubic border and the middle of the testis in cm; values ≤7 cm are abnormal. If the testis is not palpable, examination is repeated in the so-called tailor's sitting position (Fig. 31.2). In spite of indisputable value of the clinical examination, the precise type and site of the testis can only be recognized by surgery.

At clinical examination, **size and consistency** of the involved and contralateral testis and **stage of sexual development** including penis length

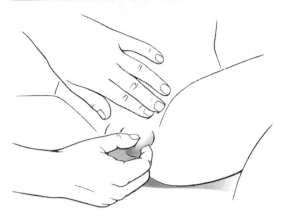

Fig. 31.2 Drawing of the clinical examination of a boy with suspected *left-sided* cryptorchidism. In the cross-legged position (so-called tailor's seat), the patient sits with abducted and angled legs. During palpation of the left scrotum and of the soft tissue above it by the *right hand*, the *left hand* strips off the inguinal channel smoothly in a distal direction: (a) In high scrotal retention, the testis is palpable at the entrance of the scrotum; (b) in prefascial ectopy (sliding testis), the testis can be palpated and seemingly moved into the scrotum, but the testis slides again in its original position on release of the traction; (c) in low canalicular retention, the testis is palpable, but moving it in the direction of the scrotum is impossible; (d) in abdominal and high canalicular retention, a testis is not palpable at all in spite of a correct technique of clinical examination. In case of obesity and/or testicular hypoplasia, this statement also concerns the types mentioned in (a) to (c)

should be determined, and the **sites of possible testicular ectopy** evaluated including the contralateral scrotal compartment. Measurement of testicular size is possible by comparison with Prader's orchidometer, a set of elliptic areas, stencils according to Takiharo, by determination of testicular length, or by ultrasound. If the latter tool is applied, the prepubertal size of undescended testes does not differ significantly from that of normal reference values of descended testes in relation to age and location in the prepubertal period.

Cryptorchidism is a frequent associated disorder of hereditary syndromes and other syndromic anomalies, abdominal wall defects, urological malformations (e.g., obstructive uropathies of the lower urinary tract, severe hypospadias, etc.), and myelomeningocele. Hypothalamic pituitary dysfunction may be associated with cryptorchidism as well.

31.4 Differential Diagnosis and Work-Ups in Cryptorchidism

It includes in case of nonpalpable testis **uni- or bilateral anorchism** # (primary malformation or secondary testicular loss by peri- or postnatal torsion, incarcerated inguinal hernia, or other disorders), **retractile testis**, and **polyorchidism**. In case of palpable testis, inguinal lymphadenopathy and inguinal hernia must be considered.

The mother reports on occasional scrotal position of the testis, development of the corresponding scrotum, the testicle can be placed in the scrotum without great traction #, remains there for a while, or retracts immediately, spontaneously, or after touching of the inner side of the thigh are typical signs of **retractile testis**. It occurs on one side or bilaterally. Three fourth of the cases recover spontaneously by the age of 14 years, but one fourth need later surgery due to evolution of a late ascending testis and/or decreasing testicular size. **Polyorchidism** means >2 histologically proven testes (usually 3, <5 % 4). Two thirds are left-sided, drained by a vas deferens, and the supernumerary testis is smaller and lies mostly higher. Polyorchidism is mostly found at surgery for inguinal hernia, cryptorchidism, testicular torsion or pain, and less frequently as accessory scrotal mass. US or MRI is indicated in complications or equivocal findings. Surgery must consider the underlying complications and patho-anatomical findings and consists of preservation or resection in case of cryptorchic supernumerary testis (>5 % malignancies).

In case of **nonpalpable testis**, ultrasound of the groin # and clinical examination in general anesthesia are useful tools, if an intervention is planned anyway.

Uni- or bilateral impalpable testis needs **diagnostic laparoscopy** # that is superior to determination of testosterone and anti-Müllerian hormone without and with human chorionic gonadotropin stimulation, abdominal ultrasound, or MRI for exclusion of any testicular tissue in the latter condition (visualization of dys- or neoplastic testis, precise localization of abdominal testis (es), nonpalpable canalicular, or lower localized testis in contrast to insufficient specificity and sensitivity of radiological imaging).

On the other hand, the mentioned **hormonal status and chromosomal sex** should be applied for sex differentiation in case of nonpalpable testis and if other signs of hypovirilization (hypospadias, micropenis) are present.

Diagnostic laparoscopy is not superior to inguinal revision in one third but has in two thirds of the patients several advantages #: Laparotomy may be avoided by it in nearly 15 %; it yields an abdominal testis in roughly 2/5, a canalicular testis 1/5, and anorchism in 2/5.

31.5 Treatment and Prognosis of Cryptorchidism

The majority of testes with cryptorchidism at birth descend spontaneously within the first year of life only in 6.9 % and mainly in the first 6 months of life, and rarely after 6 months **in contrast to the common opinion** that this is true for the majority of cases. **Watchful waiting** ends up at the age of 6 months of life, and consultation of a pediatric surgeon is indicated.

Human chorionic gonadotropin (hCG) or **luteinizing hormone-releasing hormone** (LH-RH), for instance, as nasal spray, has a real chance of success in retractile testis, late ascending testis, or bilateral testis with high scrotal position. The combination of these drugs yields not better results, and human menopausal gonadotropin is ineffective. Because late ascending testis has the same histological abnormalities as undescended testes, surgery should not be postponed too long.

There is sufficiently strong evidence that gonadotropin-releasing hormone application in the first month increases by activation of transformation of gonocytes into dark adult spermatogonia together with early orchidopexy the fertility.

In cryptorchidism, **orchidopexy** is indicated in the second half of infancy. Because the frequency of recurrence and severe complications (testicular atrophy) increases significantly if the median age of surgery is lowered, the technically demanding orchidopexy of infants and small children should be performed only in specialized centers. If cryptorchidism is recognized beyond the age of 3 years, surgery should be performed before school age.

Cryptorchidism combined with testicular torsion, inguinal hernia, hydrocele of the cord, and varicocele is an absolute indication for orchidopexy. The same applies to late ascending and retractile testis that persists or develops decreased testicular volume.

Of the available techniques, the Schoemaker procedure has gained a wide acceptance. The transscrotal approach avoids an additional groin incision and achieves similar results in palpable testes. Nevertheless, a second incision becomes necessary in 4.4 % in large cohorts, and transverse orchidopexy is not suitable for all recurrences.

Schoemaker procedure: After an inguinotomy through a transverse skin crease above the inguinal ligament and division of the external aponeurosis, the testis is mobilized from the surrounding adhesion and its gubernaculums is divided as distal as possible. Precise inspection of the testis and its adnexes yields in order of frequency:

Open processus vaginalis; **long-loop vas deferens** #; and much less frequently, **segmental atresia of the vas** # or **failure of fusion of testis and epididymis** # (complete separation is a rare condition). The former anomaly should be operated like the not infrequently encountered testicular appendages; the latter malformations should be protocolled.

Funicolysis is the most crucial part of orchidopexy because the testis should be positioned in the scrotum without any tension. It includes division of some or all cremasteric fibers with electrocautery, separation of an open processus vaginalis, possibly retroperitoneal mobilization of testicular vessels and vas deferens, and pull-through of the testis and its adnexes behind the epigastric vessels ##.

After introduction of a finger in the corresponding scrotum #, the scrotal skin is incised in longitudinal direction and a sufficiently large pouch is created between skin and tunica dartos. After incision of the latter, the testis is pushed through the incision and positioned in the pouch #. Sutures of the dartos incision without obstruction of testicular blood supply reduce its size and avoid retraction of the testis.

After closure of the incisions, the correct site of the testis within the scrotum is checked.

In **uni- and bilateral abdominal cryptorchidism**, the Fowler-Stephens procedure is considered the treatment of choice especially in high testicular position. In the first stage, the testicular vessels are clipped or cauterized, and in the second stage, orchidopexy is performed. Both stages can be performed by laparoscopy and the second stage by inguinotomy, if the testis becomes palpable or descends spontaneously after the first stage. The gubernaculums should be preserved. After the first stage, at least 50 % of the testes remain in the same position, and the remainder descend somewhat or ascend less often. Between first and second stage, an interval of 6 months is proposed, and the second stage should be finished at the age of 1 year. Laparoscopic orchidopexy may be complicated by bladder injury during creation of a transperitoneal tunnel for the cryptorchid testis (up to 3 %). Permanent catheter drainage, careful perivesical dissection, and refilling of the bladder after surgery are useful tools to avoid bladder injury.

Recently, the indication of Fowler-Stephens procedure for abdominal testicular retention has been questioned because better results are attained without clipping of the testicular vessels. Accordingly, laparoscopic or open surgery with mobilization of the testicular vessels should be performed whenever possible instead.

Redo orchidopexy for recurrent undescended testis is a challenging operation that needs an experienced surgeon who applies the same principle as for primary orchidopexy including cord transposition behind the epigastric vessels or laparoscopic mobilization of the testicular vessels. It is successful in 95 %.

The **prognosis** includes the outcome of medical or surgical treatment and those concerning the risks of cryptorchidism especially infertility and testicular malignancy.

The **early success** is defined as a complete descent of the testis with the same volume (and texture) as preoperatively. It is observed after **hCG** for palpable testis in >25–35 % and depends on the initial site of the testis. LH-RH yields similar results. After **orchidopexy** for palpable testis, the success rate is about 98 % with maintenance of the results after 6 months. Early complications are hematoma, infection, secondary atrophy, obstruction of the vas deferens, and initially insufficient position. They are avoidable and observed in <2 %. Recurrences should not exceed 2 %. Surgery at 9 months has a beneficial effect on the growth of previous undescended testis. The results in **nonpalpable testes** depend on the applied technique and amount to >85–90 %. After two-stage Fowler-Stephens with clipping of the testicular vessels, the incidence of atrophy is higher (about 10 %) than in procedures without clipping, and the viable testis remains smaller than the contralateral descended testis after 10 years.

Fertility is tested by fertility indices, semen analysis, and paternity. **Paternity** after successful orchidopexy of palpable testes in school age has been observed in unilateral cryptorchidism in 80 % and in 60 % in bilateral forms, whereas bilateral nonpalpable testes have been associated with zero paternity. More recently, it has been demonstrated that paternity does not appear to be compromised after unilateral cryptorchidism compared with a control group (89.7 % success of attempted paternity with a mean time to conception of 7.1 ± 0.7 months. Except for a lower inhibin level and considerable variation of the sperm parameters, hormonal and sperm parameters did not differ significantly). In azoospermic men with former uni- or bilateral cryptorchidism, surgical sperm extraction (TESE) is possible in 65 and in 75 % if the testicular volume is >10 cm^3 and/or the FSH is normal. After TESE, in vitro fertilization, and intracytoplasmic sperm injection (ICSI), the figures of fertilization, pregnancy, and live birth have been reported as >40, 30, and 20 %, and physical health at 5.5 years of age of term-born singletons after ICSI is comparable to that of spontaneously conceived children except for an increased risk of cryptorchidism (5.4 %).

The relative **risk of testicular malignancy** in a cryptorchidism case is 2.75–8 %. 0.6 % of adults with cryptorchidism have testicular malignancy at surgery, and cryptorchidism has been present in about 10 % of patient with a germ cell tumor. The risk to become ill with a testicular tumor between 20 and 40 years increases with bilaterality, abdominal site, dysplasia, and time before surgery of the undescended testis. Patients who undergo orchidopexy after 12 years or have no orchidopexy at all, the probability of testicular cancer is two to six times higher than in those with prepubertal orchidopexy. Older patients without former orchidopexy and involved in tumor will suffer in three fourths from seminoma, whereas those with corrected cryptorchidism are more likely affected by another malignancy. In unilateral undescended testis, the contralateral descended testis carries no increased risk of tumor formation, and the risk of cancer is low in scrotal testicular remnants.

Webcodes

The following webcodes can be used on www.psurg.net for further images and data.

3101 Cryptorchidism, testicular torsion	3110 Canalicular testis, laparoscopy
3102 Empty scrotum, cryptorchidism	3111 Possible findings, laparoscopy
3103 Perineal testicular ectopy	3112 Long-loop vas deferens
3104 Abdominal testis	3113 Anomaly vas deferens
3105 Sliding testis, prefascial ectopy	3114 Incomplete fusion anomaly, epididymis/testis
3106 Examination with two hands	3115 Mobilized funiculus at surgery and
3107 Unilateral anorchism	3116 Tension-free transposition
3108 Retractile testis	3117 Introduction of finger and
3109 Ultrasound, nonpalpable testis	3118 Transposition of testis

Bibliography

General: Occurrence, Clinical Skills, Differential Diagnosis

Boisen KA, Kaleva M, Main KM et al (2004) Difference in prevalence of congenital cryptorchidism in infants between two Nordic countries. Lancet 363:1264–1269

Chipkevitch E, Nishimura RT, Tu DG, Galea-Rojas M (1996) Clinical measurement of testicular volume in adolescents: comparison of the reliability of 5 methods. J Urol 156:2050–2053

Hutson JM (1998) Undescended testis, torsion, and varicocele. In: O'Neill JA Jr et al (eds) Pediatric surgery, vol II, 5th edn. Mosby, St Louis

Hutson JM, Balic A, Nation T, Southwell B (2010) Cryptorchidism. Semin Pediatr Surg 19:215–224

Section 31.1

Berkowitz GS, Lapinski RH, Dolgin SE, Gazella JG, Bodian CA, Holzman IR (1993) Prevalence and natural history of cryptorchidism. Pediatrics 92:44–49

Hussain Taqvi SR, Akhtar J, Batool T, Tabassum R, Mirza F (2006) Correlation of the size of undescended testis with its location in various age groups. J Coll Physicians Surg Pak 16:594–597

La Scala GC, Ein SH (2004) Retractile testes: an outcome analysis on 150 patients. J Pediatr Surg 39:1014–1017

Wenzler DL, Bloom DA, Park JM (2004) What is the rate of spontaneous testicular descent in infants with cryptorchidism? J Urol 171:849–851

Section 31.2

Merjer RW, Hack WW, van der Voort-Doedens LM, Haasnoot K, Bos SD (2004) Surgical findings in acquired undescended testis. J Pediatr Surg 39:1242–1244

Yoshida T, Ohno K, Morotomi Y, Nakamura T, Azuma T, Yamada H, Hayashi H, Suehiro S (2009) Clinical and pathological features of ascending testis. Osaka City Med J 55:81–87

Zenaty D, Dijoud F, Morel Y, Cabrol S, Mouriquand P, Nicolino M, Bouvatier C, Pinto G, Lecointre C, Pienkowski C, Soskin S, Bost M, Bertrand AM, El-Ghoneimi A, Nihoul-Fekete C, Léeger J (2006) Bilateral anorchia in infancy: occurrence of micropenis and the effect of testosterone treatment. J Pediatr 149:687–691

Sections 31.3–31.4

Abbasoglu L, Salman FT, Gün F, Asicioglu C (2004) Polyorchidism presenting with undescended testis. Eur J Pediatr Surg 14:355–357

Koff WJ, Scaletscky R (1990) Malformations of the epididymis in undescended testis. J Urol 143:340–433

Savas M, Yeni E, Ciftci H, Cece H, Topal U, Utangac MM (2010) Polyorchidism: a three-case report and review of the literature. Andrologia 42:57–61

Wakeman D, Warner BW (2010) Urogenital nonunion – a rare anomaly associated with the undescended testis. Am J Surg 199:e59–e60

Section 31.5

Biers SM, Malone PS (2010) A critical appraisal of the evidence for improved fertility indices in undescended testes after gonadotropin-releasing hormone therapy and orchidopexy. J Pediatr Urol 6:239–246

Bukowski TP, Wacksman J, Billmire DA et al (1995) Testicular autotransplantation: a 17-year review of an effective approach to the management of the intra-abdominal testis. J Urol 154:558–561

Daher P, Nabbout P, Feghali J, Riachi E (2009) Is the Fowler-Stephens procedure still indicated for the treatment of nonpalpable intraabdominal testis? J Pediatr Surg 44:1999–2003

De Schepper J, Belva F, Schiettecatte J, Anckaert E, Tournaye H, Bonduelle M (2009) Testicular growth and tubular function in prepubertal boys conceived by intracytoplasmic sperm injection. Horm Res 71:359–363

Gapany C, Frey P, Cachat F, Gudinchet F, Jichlinski P, Meyrat BJ, Ramseyer P, Theintz P, Burnand B (2008) Management of cryptorchidism in children: guidelines. Swiss Med Wkly 138:492–498

Esposito C, De Lucia A, Palmieri A, Centonze A, Damiano R, Savanelli A, Valerio G, Settimi A (2003) Comparison of five different hormonal treatment protocols for children with cryptorchidism. Scand J Urol Nephrol 37:246–249

Gordon M, Cervellioni RM, Morabito A, Bianchi A (2010) 20 years of transscrotal orchidopexy for undescended testis: results and outcomes. J Pediatr Urol 6:506–512

Kjaer S, Mikines KJ (2006) HCG in the treatment of cryptorchidism. The effect of age and position of the testis. Ugeskr Laeger 168:1448–1451

Kollin C, Hesser U, Ritzen EM, Karpe B (2006) Testicular growth from birth to two years of age, and effect of orchidopexy at age nine months: a randomized, controlled study. Acta Paediatr 95:318–324

Ludwig AK, Katalinic A, Thyen U, Sutcliffe AG, Dietrich K, Ludwig M (2009) Physical health at 5.5 years of age of term-born singletons after intracytoplasmic sperm injection: results of prospective, controlled, single-blinded study. Fertil Steril 91:115–124

Marcelli F, Robin G, Lefebvre-Khalil V, Marchetti C, Lemaitre L, Mitchell V, Rigot JM (2008) Results of surgical testicular sperm extractions [TESE] in a population of azoospermic patients with a history of cryptorchidism based on a 10-year experience of 142 patients. Prog Urol 18:657–662

McAlleer IM et al (1995) Fertility index analysis in cryptorchidism. J Urol 153:1255

Miller KD, Coughlin MT, Lee PA (2001) Fertility after unilateral cryptorchidism. Paternity, time to conception, pretreatment testicular location and size, hormone and sperm parameters. Horm Res 55:249–253

Moller H, Cortes D, Engholm G, Thorup J (1998) Risk of testicular cancer with cryptorchidism and with testicular biopsy: cohort study. BMJ 317(7160):729

Nouira F, Ben Ahmed Y, Jlidi S, Sarrai N, Chariag A, Ghorbel S, Khemakhem R, Chaouachi B (2011) Management of perineal ectopic testes. Tunis Med 89: 47–49

Puri P, O'Donnell B (1988) Semen analysis of patients who had orchidopexy at or after seven years of age. Lancet II:1051–1052

Schindler AM, Diaz P, Cuendet A, Sizonenko PC (1987) Cryptorchidism: a morphological study of 670 biopsies. Helv Paediatr Acta 42:145–158

Stec AA, Tanaka ST, Adams MC, Pope JC 4th, Thomas JC, Brock HW 3rd (2009) Orchidopexy for intra-abdominal testes: factors predicting success. J Urol 182: 1917–1920

Thorup J, Jensen CL, Langballe O, Petersen BL, Cortes D (2011) The challenge of early surgery for cryptorchidism. Scand J Urol Nephrol 45:184–189

Vinardi S, Magro P, Manenti M, Lala R, Costantinos S, Cortese MG, Canavese F (2001) Testicular function in men treated in childhood for undescended testes. J Pediatr Surg 36:385–388

Wood HM, Elder JS (2009) Cryptorchidism and testicular cancer: separating fact from fiction. J Urol 181: 452–461

Zerella JT, McGill LC (1993) Survival of nonpalpable testicles after orchidopexy. J Pediatr Surg 28:51–253

Conspicuous External Genitals in the Boy

Many and diverse pathologies manifest as conspicuous external genitals. The visible genitals may be assigned to a boy or a girl, or assignment occurs first to a wrong sex or is not possible at all (ambiguous external genitals). Therefore, classification in one of the three groups (male or female conspicuous external genitals, and external genitals in disorders of sex development) may be impossible at the first look because effacement of the clinical presentation does not render a correct delineation. In Table 32.1, most relevant pathologies that lead to conspicuous external genitals in the boy are listed and differentiated according to their clinical significance.

32.1 Epispadias

Occurrence, Clinical Significance

Epispadias is either an integrated part of bladder exstrophy or occurs without bladder involvement. It may be interpreted as a variation of the bladder exstrophy complex. In contrast to hypospadias, isolated epispadias occurs 50 times less fre-

Table 32.1 Differential diagnosis of conspicuous and abnormal external genitals in the boy

- Epispadias (bladder exstrophy complex)
- Hypospadias
- Micropenis, pseudomicropenis
- o Penis torsion and lateral deviation
- o Rare malformations of the penis
- Priapism

quently and is encountered in the daily work of a primary care provider only exceptionally. The clinical significance of a dorsally cleft penis concerns the following topics:

- It may be a cause of urinary incontinence.
- The esthetical appearance is impaired.
- It may be a hindrance of normal sexual intercourse and fathering.
- Minor forms of the less frequent female epispadias may be a diagnostic challenge.

Clinical Presentation, Clinical Skills

Depending on the grade of epispadias, only *the glans is divided on its dorsal aspect, the urethral orifice lies in the penoglandular furrow, and the foreskin is formed nearly exclusively on the ventral side –* **grade I epispadias** with usually maintained urinary continence. In **grade II # and III epispadias**, *the penis is foreshortened and deviated in a dorsal direction due to a chordee. Only after traction on the epispadic prepuce in a ventral direction, the full extent of the anomaly becomes visible: The urethral plate has failed to tubularize and continues to the bladder neck as a broad groove where a skin fold crosses the penis like a bridge. The ejaculatori ducts and testes including their adnexes are formed normally.*

Differential Diagnosis, Work-Ups

If careful examination is performed, a correct diagnosis and grading are possible, and no other disorder must be considered.

The spatial arrangement and pathoanatomical findings of pelvis, hip, and symphysis are similar to bladder exstrophy as the anus with its ventral transposition. Kidneys and the upper urinary tract are usually normal; nevertheless, ultrasound of kidneys, upper urinary tract, and hips, as well as plain pelvis x-ray, should be performed as initial examination.

Surgery is performed in two stages: Reconstruction of the penis in the first year of life with transfer of the urethral plate and urethral reconstruction on the ventral site of the penis with possible lengthening and continuation in the bladder neck, release of the chordee which retracts the penis in a dorsal direction, transposition of mobilized corpora cavernosa on the dorsal side of the penis and connection in the penile midline, and glanduloplasty. At the age of 4 years, bladder neck reconstruction is performed according to Young-Dees-Leadbetter.

32.2 Hypospadias

Occurrence, Clinical Significance
A urethral plate of variable distance at the ventral side of the penis # instead of a urethra which is covered by normal skin occurs frequently (1 in 300 or less live births), and familiality is observed in a small proportion. The frequency of hypospadias has increased in the last two to three decades in some developed countries; so-called hypospadias of the girl are very rare.

The clinical significance is many and diverse:
• Esthetical appearance of the penis is impaired.
• Micturition may be distorted.
• In case of concomitant penis curvature or relatively small penis, sexual intercourse may be hindered.
• External genitals of the boy may be mixed up with those of a girl or a child with ambiguous external genitals in very proximal forms.
• Disorders of fertility can be observed due to proximal site of the meatus and associated utricular cyst.

Forms, Components, Associated Malformations
Depending on the site of the urethral orifice along the penis, different forms can be differentiated. The native condition may conceal the final

findings; the meatus is situated more proximal after correction of a curvature or excision of the most distal part of the urethra with absent corpus spongiosum #. The individual classification of hypospadias should take into consideration the final status.

In case of **anterior hypospadias**, the meatus lies at the ventral surface of the glans (glanular), close to the balanopenile furrow (coronal #), and in the distal third of penis shaft (anterior penile subtype). They belong to the minor or slight forms of hypospadias and occur in ≥50 %.

In case of **middle hypospadias**, the meatus lies in the middle third of the shaft # (≥20 %).

In case of **posterior hypospadias**, the meatus lies in the proximal third of the shaft (posterior penile), at the base of the shaft (penoscrotal), between the scrotal halves (scrotal ##), or behind the scrotum (perineal subtype #). It concerns ≥30 % and belongs to the severe or major forms.

In contrast to the quoted classification, the Barcat classification counts the anterior and the posterior penile subtype among the middle hypospadias.

In addition to the abnormal site of the urethral orifice and absent ventral prepuce and urethra, several abnormalities of glans and penis including its skin may be observed: **Meatal stenosis** and **tilting of the glans** # (mainly in anterior forms), **chordee** leading to a curvature ## of glans and penis, **bifid scrotum #**, **torsion of the penis**, and **penoscrotal transposition** (the latter four abnormalities occur mainly in posterior hypospadias and in 25 % of all hypospadias). **Chordee** may also exist **without hypospadias ##**.

Cryptorchidism and inguinal hernia belong to the classic associated malformations, less in distal and more in proximal forms of hypospadias (</>5 %). Utricular cyst is encountered frequently in proximal hypospadias. Other urological malformations of kidneys and upper urinary tract are observed only in about 5 % except for an increased risk, if one or several extragenital anomalies are present with or without the quoted classical malformations. In such cases and proximal forms, further urological work-ups are necessary (reflux, renal agenesis, and UPJ junction obstruction belong to the most common).

Clinical Presentation, Clinical Skills

The uniform and characteristic signs of all forms of hypospadias are an incomplete formation of the ventral combined with an excess of the dorsal prepuce like a hood and a wide glans #. The latter sign is used for prenatal diagnosis of hypospadias by ultrasound.

The site of the meatus and the described components permit a preliminary determination of the form of hypospadias (Fig. 32.1). *For a precise inspection, the penis can be unfolded by upward traction on the dorsal prepuce. A lateral view of the penis without or with spontaneous erection demonstrates a possible curvature* and its dimension.

The urinary stream is increasingly deviated to the bottom, the more the urethral orifice lies in the proximal direction of the shaft. Therefore, children with a scrotal or perineal subtype of posterior hypospadias urinate in a sitting position because they would wet otherwise the clothes. In *meatal stenosis, the slightly deviated urinary stream is thin, and micturition occurs under pressure.*

In the scrotal and perineal subtype, *the scrotum is divided in two halves. The hardly visible penis and/or empty scrotal compartments (associated cryptorchidism) that cover the penis give the impression of female or ambiguous external genitals* (vaginal hypospadias #).

Differential Diagnosis, Work-Ups

A precise clinical examination permits mostly a correct diagnosis except for a vulviform hypospadias with or without cryptorchidism.

Posterior forms need VCU or retrograde urethrography and possibly urethrocystoscopy for recognition and characterization of a utricular cyst. If hypospadias is combined with one or more extraurological malformations or belongs to the severe form, radiological imaging starting with ultrasound should be performed for exclusion of possible urogenital anomalies.

Additional examinations are unnecessary if both testes are descended and the scrotum is developed. However, severe forms of hypospadias especially the vulviform subtypes need further work-ups for differential diagnostic delineation of the abnormal external genitals:

- Specific family and pregnancy history, precise evaluation of the local findings, and record of possibly associated malformations.
- Sex chromatin bodies, chromosomal analysis, and ultrasound of kidneys, whole urinary tract, gonads, and possible Müllerian structures. If a utriculus is present, additional Müllerian structures are outlined by retrograde contrast application at cystourethroscopy or MRI.
- Luteinizing hormone, follicle-stimulating hormone, testosterone, adrenal steroids, and others belong to the specific hormonal evaluation of such cases.

Treatment, Prognosis

In anterior forms, the indication of surgery is mainly based on esthetical reasons except for the anterior penile subtype and meatal stenosis. Meatal stenosis is confirmed by observation of the micturition and calibration of the orifice with small Hegar's dilators and corrected already in the newborn.

In moderate and severe forms, surgery is also indicated for functional reasons, for example, the ability to stand to urinate.

The optimal time for surgery is the second half of infancy or even earlier (avoidance of an adverse reaction of the child to the hospitalization in toddlers). Surgery in small children beyond infancy has the advantage that the penile structures are larger, and some parents have reservations about surgery in infancy.

In **anterior forms**, remodeling of the glans and formation of the most distal urethra or transfer of the orifice toward the tip of the glans by local tissue are combined with removal, correction, or reconstruction of the prepuce. Examples of applied techniques are MAGPI (meatal advancement glanduloplasty) procedure, Mathieu-Rhigini procedure, or tubularized incised hypospadias repair.

In spite of all therapeutic enthusiasm to transfer the meatus to the tip of the glans, it must be considered that the urethral orifice is situated at the tip of the glans only in 55 % of normal men and that it opens between the tip and the penoscrotal furrow in an additional third without any hindrance to micturition or sexual intercourse (Fig. 32.2).

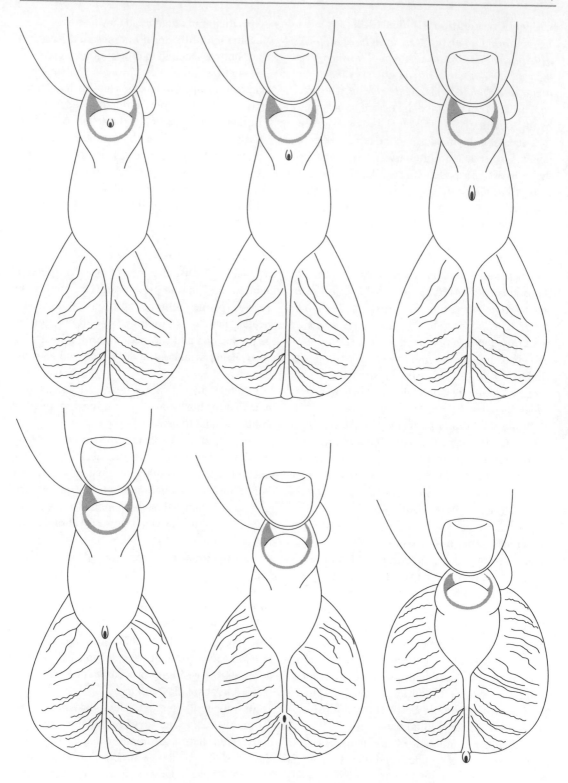

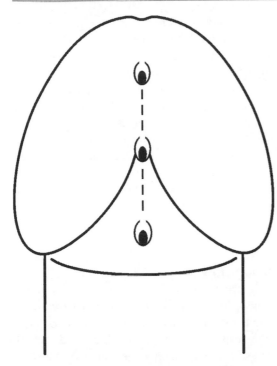

Fig. 32.2 Variations of the site of the external urethral meatus. In a large cohort of normal and asymptomatic men, the site of the external urethral meatus lies in the anterior, middle, or posterior third of the distance between the tip of the glans and the coronary sulcus. Therefore, only the last mentioned site corresponds to anterior type of hypospadias (Fichtner et al. (1995, p. 833))

If the meatus lies proximal to the penoglandular furrow, formation of a new urethra of variable length and the possible need of correction of ventral curvature is in the fore.

It can be performed with the **transverse preputial island flap technique** (Duckett) in which a flap of the inner layer of prepuce is tubularized and anastomosed with the residual urethra ##. The intervention must be combined with correction of a possible chordee (ventral penile curvature that is checked at surgery by artificial erection [after injection of saline] before and after resection of

the chordee), a possible torsion of the penis, and a possible bifid scrotum. Surgery is finished by glanduloplasty and covering of the penis with the degloved skin.

An alternative method is the **tubularized incised plate (TIP) hypospadias repair** (Snodgrass) in which the urethral plate alone is used for reconstruction of the urethra after a relaxing midline incision of sufficient depth that allows widening of the plate by minimum ≥10–12 mm. The flat or grooved urethral plate is initially separated from the glans wings by deep parallel longitudinal incisions (that should avoid glans or skin tissue on the side of the plate). They taper off in a circumferential incision of the ventral penile skin and dorsal inner layer of the prepuce that includes the orifice and leaves a subcoronal collar. After creation of a button-holed dartos pedicle that is used to cover the reconstructed urethra as second layer, glansplasty is performed, all skin edges are closed, and a smooth bladder stent is left in place for continuous drainage of urine for 5–7 days. A similar technique can also used for proximal hypospadias of all types in which complete degloving of the penis is always combined with artificial erection. Most of the penile curvatures can be handled by dorsal midline plication(s) of the tunica albuginea. An alternative method for hypospadias repair must be chosen if the urethral plate cannot be sufficiently widened or is thin and fragile, or if it contributes significantly to the ventral curvature and division of the plate is necessary. Staged repair or the quoted preputial island flap technique is a possible alternative procedure.

Prognosis

In tubularized incised plate hypospadias repair, the figures of fistulas, meatal stenosis, and partial or complete wound dehiscence are 4, 3, and 1 %

Fig. 32.1 Drawing of the different types of hypospadias in which the urethra is not formed as a tube and displays only a urethral plate on the ventral side of the penis for different distances. With increasing severity, the orifice shifts from the glans to the perineum that is shown in the drawing from the *top* on the *left side* to the *bottom* on the *right side*. The common sign of hypospadias is a prepuce

that is deformed on the dorsal side like a cape and divided on the ventral side. On the *top* of the *left side*, a normal situation is visible for comparison. In the *middle* of the *top row*, an anterior type of hypospadias, and on the *right side*, an intermediate or *middle* type is shown. The *bottom row* shows from *left* to *right* a penoscrotal, scrotal, and perineal type of hypospadias in experienced hands and more in the other quoted methods.

Psychosocial and social development is not impaired in patients with hypospadias, and no correlation exists between severity of hypospadias and psychosocial function. The involved adolescents avoid undressing in public because of the opinion that their genitals have not a satisfactory appearance. Sexual maturation is normal, but patients with operated hypospadias display greater difficulty in making contact with women and delayed initiation of full sexual activity.

Patients with former distal hypospadias have in the majority of cases no lasting effects in adulthood except for the appearance of the penis, but some degree of voiding problems have been observed in up to 40 % of adult men after surgery of severe hypospadias and sexual problems that concern erection, ejaculation, and sexual sensitivity in more than 20 %. Although sexuality is satisfactory overall, problems of erection (e.g., sensitive scar or soft appearing glans) and ejaculation (such as dribbling ejaculation) are often reported.

32.3   Micropenis

Occurrence, Clinical Significance

Micropenis means a length of the penis that is more than 2.5 standard deviations below the normal values # (the distance of the extended penis from its base over the symphysis to the tip of the glans is 3.5 ± 0.7 cm in normal newborns).

The clinical significance of micropenis is as follows:

- Fear that the penis of their child is too small is a relatively frequent cause of consultation.
- A true micropenis is mostly not present in such situation but another cause that simulates micropenis.
- True micropenis is a major concern of pubertal boys.

Forms

In addition to **micropenis** of normal shape and proportions because of **endocrinological disorders or as part of a specific syndrome**, a decreased length of the penis of different degrees

is observed **in the bladder exstrophy complex and subtypes of proximal hypospadias**. Such forms of micropenis differ from the former by their history and appearance (by sequels of surgery and possibly by their proportions).

In **isolated micropenis**, the androgen stimulation is either missing (hypothalamic insufficiency – secondary hypogonadotropic hypogonadism; 5-α-reductase deficiency, the rudimentary testes cannot produce androgens – primary hypogonadotropic hypogonadism) or less frequently, the penis cannot react to the available androgens due to a missing responsiveness.

Clinical Presentation, Clinical Skills

The penis should be visualized in its whole length, and its proportions must be evaluated. The penis length is determined on its dorsal side from the base to the tip and measured without and with extension (erection), and the results are compared with normal values.

Body length and weight, testicular location and size, and possible signs of sexual development belong also to the clinical examinations. Useful informations concern also pubertal development of the father.

Differential Diagnosis

The differential diagnosis of the causes of a seemingly micropenis (pseudomicropenis) is very important and often possible by clinical examination and knowledge of these causes:

- **Buried penis**: The actual length of the penis is hidden by prepubertal obesity in general and specifically by a suprapubic paunch. Compression and shift of the latter yields the actual size of the penis #.
- The overlaying skin is not sufficiently adherent to the penis (insufficient fixation by the suspensory ligament) – **concealed penis**. If the skin is pulled away from the penis, a penis of normal size becomes visible.
- **Webbed penis** ("palmure" of the penis) is similar to webbed fingers. A vertical scrotal fold leads to the underside of the penis # (triangular scrotal web that gives the impression of micropenis and may later hinder erection

and sexual intercourse). An acquired form may result after excess removal of foreskin at circumcision.

- **Trapped penis** means a penis that is raised by the suspensory ligament.

The differential diagnosis of micropenis must not only consider causes of pseudomicropenis but also the less frequent causes of ambiguous external genitals.

Work-Ups

Depending on the cause of micropenis, the testes are small and undescended or present only as testicular remnants. Such suspicious findings can be confirmed by ultrasound.

Medication of gonadotropin-releasing hormone leads mostly to production of luteinizing and follicle-stimulating hormone, whereupon the testes produce mostly androgens, or the penis reacts to androgen applied locally as androgen cream or systemically. This situation concerns the majority of patients with missing androgen stimulation.

In nonsyndromic micropenis or primary hypogonadism, sex chromatin, chromosomal analysis, and work-up of androgen-receptor deficiency are indicated; the latter disorder is also excluded by effective local androgen application #.

Treatment

Whereas watchful waiting is indicated in buried penis, the other disorders need surgery. In buried penis, a visible effect may be attained for psychological reasons by temporary local application of androgen cream. In webbed penis, correction can be attained by Z-plasty(ies) that should be performed before a possibly indicated circumcision.

32.4   Penis Torsion, Lateral Deviation of the Penis

Occurrence, Clinical Significance

In **penis torsion**, shaft and glans are turned in the longitudinal axis by 90° or more either in a counterclock- # or clockwise direction. Therefore, the slit-like meatus and frenulum are not lined up in a ventral but a lateral direction.

Lateral deviation is caused by asymmetrical development of the corpora cavernosa and becomes visible if the penis gets stiff at erection.

Penis torsion is a part of hypospadias or chordee without hypospadias, or less frequently an isolated malformation that may be a familial disorder. Penis torsion may also be an acquired disorder after circumcision or other types of penis surgery.

The clinical significance of torsion and lateral deviation is as follows:

- Both disorders interfere with a normal esthetical appearance and possibly with the function of the penis (deviation of urinary stream and disturbance of sexual intercourse).

Clinical Presentation

If looked from the front of the glans, meatus and frenulum are either directed in a left or right lateral direction #, or dorsal direction in relation to the longitudinal penis axis. The raphe of the penis runs spiral-shaped around the penis shaft.

Objective confirmation of lateral deviation of the penis needs observation of a spontaneous or artificial erection.

Treatment, Prognosis

Correction of **penis torsion** is indicated, if the torsion exceeds 90° and/or if the torsion is symptomatic (e.g., inappropriate wetting of the surroundings due to insufficient correction of the urinary stream by the patient).

Surgery consists of degloving the skin of the penis after a circumferential coronal incision, repositioning according to the type of torsion, and readaptation of the skin. In severe forms of penile torsion, possible abnormal relation of shaft and glans must be considered and specifically treated (relocation of the involved Buck's fascia).

Hypospadias repair, circumcisions, and other types of penis surgery should consider a possible associated torsion and/or avoid a postoperative torsion.

Lateral deviation should be operated at or after puberty if it interferes with micturition or sexual intercourse.

Both disorders can be corrected by appropriate surgery.

32.5 Other Rare Malformations of the Penis

Disorders, Pathoanatomy
Penoscrotal transposition, penis duplication, penis agenesis, and venous lakes of the glans are examples of such rare penile malformations.

In **penoscrotal transposition**, the spatial relation of the penis and the separate or fused scrotal compartments is wrong in the frontal plane (dorsal instead of ventral position). It is either incomplete or complete #, occurs in hypospadias, and ambiguous external genitals.

In **penile duplication**, the diphallus is either complete (glans and shaft) or incomplete (involving only the glans). It may be associated with urogenital or lower intestinal malformations.

In **penile agenesis**, the penis is lacking, the urethra is foreshortened (with a postsphincteric perianal meatus, presphincteric urethrorectal fistula, or atresia).

Clinical Significance
- Impaired esthetical appearance in all four anomalies.
- Penis duplication may be associated with more severe urogenital or lower intestinal malformations; penis agenesis has serious implications for assignment to an appropriate sex and possible disorders of micturition; and venous lakes may lead to penis bleeding, ulceration, and infection.
- Penis agenesis may have a differential diagnostic significance (e.g., micropenis, concealed penis, ambiguous external genitals, epispadias, and intrauterine amputation).

Clinical Presentation
Penoscrotal transposition is recognizable by the described inverse relation of penis and scrotum. In **penis duplication**, close inspection permits assignment to one of the two types. In **penis agenesis**, scrotum and testes are usually normal and combined with a foreshortened urethra with a perineal meatus, urine dribbling by the anus, or urinary retention. In **venous lakes,** the glans exhibits several bluish patches of the glans that correspond to vascular malformations.

Treatment, Prognosis
The scrotal compartments are relocated by rotational advancement flaps in penoscrotal transposition before or at hypospadias repair.

In penis duplication, preoperative genitourinary work-up is indicated and either the surplus glans or the less developed penis is removed. Penis agenesis: Sexual transformation is recommended during infancy with removal of both testes, formation of female external genitals including transposition of the urethral orifice between the reconstructed labia and early or delayed vaginal reconstruction.

Venous lakes: Permanent cure is possible by intralesional laser application.

32.6 Priapism

Occurrence, Clinical Significance
Priapism is less frequently observed in children except for specific disorders or groups of drugs. It presents an involuntary, prolonged, and possibly repeated (stuttering) erection that is unrelated to or persists beyond sexual stimulation. It includes exclusively the corpora cavernosa. All ages of childhood may be involved including newborns. The clinical significance is as follows:
- Priapism is a urological emergency that needs treatment for cessation of erection and possibly for pain relief.
- Fibrosis of the corpora cavernosa, erectile dysfunction, and impotence may result if the priapism is left untreated.

Clinical Presentation
Priapism presents either as low- (ischemic or venous) or high-flow (nonischemic or arterial) type. The clinical presentation of erection as defined above permits a clinical diagnosis. Erection is very painful (possibly resistent to analgetics) in low-flow erection and not painful in high-flow priapism that is combined with a

semirigid penis. In general, only the shaft is hard and not the glans.

A history of former erections and/or a possible underlying cause may confirm the suspected diagnosis. The most common causes in childhood are **sickle cell disease** (SS and AS sickle cell phenotypes, priapism occurs either as isolated complication or as part of general manifestation, low-flow type) or priapism after **perineal or penile injury** (high-flow type):

- Hematological and neoplastic disorders: sickle cell disease, leukemia, or other tumors
- Specific groups of drugs: antipsychotics, antidepressants, anticonvulsants, medicaments for treatment of attention deficit ADHD, TPN, or incidental ingestion of sildenafil citrate
- Infectious and other disorders: epidemic parotitis, Henoch-Schönlein purpura, Fabry disease
- Traumatic injuries: falls astride, overuse of cycling (perineal, penile, or penetrating trauma)
- Idiopathic priapism

Except for traumatic and the minority of idiopathic priapism, all other groups display a low-flow priapism (with vascular blockage or endothelial inflammatory activation) with a peak incidence of 5–10 years of age. In traumatic and a few idiopathic cases, a high-flow priapism is observed due to an arteriocavernous fistula. Low-flow priapism is associated with ischemia of the cavernous smooth muscle (paralysis, necrosis [by 48 h], and fibrosis).

Priapism may be accompanied by disorders of micturition or localized infections (e.g., cavernositis) or be a sign of a specific disorder such as appendicitis.

Differential Diagnosis, Work-Ups

In infants and small children, personal hygiene or surgery of the external genitals may lead to prolonged and repeated erections, or posttraumatic or inflammatory swelling of the penis may feign priapism.

The work-ups include perineal and penile color Doppler US (demonstration of turbulent flow in high-flow priapism), diagnostic puncture of corpora cavernosa (ph, PO_2, CO_2, and color of the blood [dark vs. bright red]), and superselec-tive arteriography of the internal pudendal artery or contrast-enhanced MR angiography.

In addition, work-ups are necessary of the underlying disorder (e.g., Hb electrophoresis in suspected sickle cell disease, SS > AS).

Treatment, Prognosis

Treatment is different for low-flow and high-flow priapism.

In the latter, superselective angiography (with a maximum of two sessions) is used for demonstration of the suspected penile arteriocavernous fistula and selective embolization with autologous blood clot or gel foam. On the other hand, conservative approach has been reported with spontaneous recovery within 2–5 weeks without long-term effect on the erectile tissue.

Low-flow priapism needs immediate treatment of the underlying cause and erected penis within 24 h by aspiration of the corpora cavernosa and lavage with sympathomimetics (norepinephrine) in general anesthesia. Although often a return to a flaccid penis occurs by these measures, a venous drainage of the corpora cavernosa must be performed in case of failure of lavage (shunt between corpora cavernosa and glans or corpus spongiosum, or as modification of the Winter's shunt (drawbacks by persistent venous leaks) multiple punctures using large bore needles which function as temporary cavernoglandular fistulas). In delayed cases, frozen sections of the cavernosus muscle are indicated because shunting is useless if necrosis has already occurred. Then, implantation of an erection prosthesis is necessary instead of a shunt to avoid complete fibrosis and shrinkage.

Treatment of the underlying disorder is specifically important in sickle cell disease. It includes rapid hydration (two to three times the maintenance fluid), hypertransfusion (with packed red blood cells) up to an Hb >10–12, and strong analgetics; or in case of leukemia, hyperhydration, hydroxyurea, and chemotherapy.

Prophylaxis and treatment of stuttering priapism include low-dose aspirin, ice packs, and if necessary the already quoted measures.

Prognosis depends on the duration of erection and the age of the patient (inverse relation). In low-flow priapism and priapism in sickle cell disease, the critical time is 24–48 h and 3 days, respectively. Impotence occurs in up to 50 % of the patients and is established after 1 year at latest.

Webcodes

The following webcodes can be used on www.psurg.net for further images and data.

3201 Epispadias of the boy, grade II	3214 After artificial erection
3202 Posterior hypospadias	3215 Wide glans in hypospadias
3203 (Short) absence of corpus spongiosum	3216 Vulviform hypospadias
3204 Subcoronal hypospadias	3217 Transverse preputial island flap for
3205 Middle hypospadias	3218 Hypospadias repair including glans channel
3206 Scrotal hypospadias before and	3219 Micropenis, hypospadias
3207 After elevation of the penis	3220 Buried penis, suprapubic paunch
3208 Perineal hypospadias	3221 Webbed penis and glans tilt
3209 Tilting of the glans	3222 Buried penis, response to local androgens
3210 Chordee before and after	3223 Penis torsion, counterclockwise direction
3211 Artificial erection, middle hypospadias	3224 Penis torsion, clockwise direction
3212 Bifid scrotum	3225 Penoscrotal transposition
3213 Chordee without hypospadias before and	

Bibliography

General: Differential Diagnosis

Colodny A (1987) Urethral lesions in infants and children. In: Gillenwater JY et al (eds) Adult and pediatric urology, vol II. Yearbook Medical Publishers, Chicago

Ellis DG, Mann CM Jr (1998) Abnormalities of the urethra, penis, and scrotum. In: O'Neill JA Jr et al (eds) Pediatric surgery, vol II, 5th edn. Mosby, St Louis

Hensle TW (1987) Genital anomalies. In: Gillenwater JY et al (eds) Adult and pediatric urology, vol II. Yearbook Medical Publishers, Chicago

Johnston JH (1982) Acquired lesions of the penis, the scrotum, and the testes. In: Williams DI, Johston JH (eds) Pediatric urology, 2nd edn. Butterworth Scientific, London

Klauber GT, Saut GR (1985) Disorders of the male external genitalia. In: Kelalis PP et al (eds) Clinical pediatric urology, vol I, 2nd edn. Saunders, Philadelphia

Section 32.1

Frimberger D (2011) Diagnosis and management of epispadias. Semin Pediatr Surg 20:85–90

Section 32.2

Aigrain Y, Cheikhelard A, Lottmann H, Lortat-Jabob S (2010) Hypospadias: surgery and complications. Horm Res Paediatr 74:218–222

Albers N, Ulrichs C, Glüer S, Hiort O, Sinnecker GH, Mildenberger H, Brodehl J (1997) Etiological classification of severe hypospadias: implications for prognosis and management. J Pediatr 131:386–392

Baskin LS, Ebbers MB (2006) Hypospadias: anatomy, etiology, and technique. J Pediatr Surg 41:463–472

Brock JW III, O'Neill JA Jr (1998) Bladder exstrophy. In: O'Neill JA Jr et al (eds) Pediatric surgery, vol II, 5th edn. Mosby, St Louis

Castagnetti M, El-Ghoneimi A (2010) Surgical management of primary severe hypospadias in children: systematic 20-year review. J Urol 184:1469–1474

Duckett JW, Baskin LS (1998) Hypospadias. In: O'Neill JA Jr et al (eds) Pediatric surgery, vol II, 5th edn. Mosby, St Louis

Fichtner J, Filipas D, Mottrie AM et al (1995) Analysis of meatal location in 500 men. Wide variation questions need for meatal advancement in all pediatric anterior hypospadias cases. J Urol 154:833–834

Fisch M (2004) Concepts for correction of penile hypospadias. Urologe A 43:202–207

Ishii T, Hayashi M, Suwanai A, Amano N, Hasegawa T (2010) The effect of intramuscular testosterone enanthate treatment on stretched penile length in prepubertal boys with hypospadias. Urology 76:97–100

Kelly JH (1998) Exstrophy and epispadias: Kelly's method of repair. In: O'Neill JA Jr et al (eds) Pediatric surgery, vol II, 5th edn. Mosby, St Louis

Lam PN, Greenfield SP, Williot P (2005) 2-Stage repair in infancy for severe hypospadias with chordee: long-term results after puberty. J Urol 174:1567–1572; discussion 1572

Manzoni G, Bracka A, Palminteri E, Marrocco G (2004) Hypospadias surgery: when, what and by whom? BJU Int 94:1188–1195

Markiewicz MR, Lukose MA, Margarone JE 3rd, Barbagli G, Miller KS, Chuang SK (2007) The oral mucosa graft: a systematic review. J Urol 178:387–394

Mieusset R, Soulié M (2005) Hypospadias: psychological, sexual, and reproductive consequences in adult life. J Androl 26:163–168

Milla SS, Chow JS, Lebowitz RL (2008) Imaging of hypospadias: pre- and postoperative appearances. Pediatr Radiol 38:202–208

Muruganandham K, Ansari MS, Dubey D, Mandhani A, Srivastava A, Kapoor R, Kumar A (2010) Urethrocutaneous fistula after hypospadias repair: outcome of three types of closure techniques. Pediatr Surg Int 26:305–308

Paulozzi LJ, Erickson JD, Jackson RJ (1997) Hypospadias trends in two US surveillance systems. Pediatrics 100: 831–834

Snodgrass WT (2002) Tubularized incised plate (TIP) hypospadias repair. Urol Clin North Am 29:285–290

Snodgrass WT (2008) Management of penile curvature in children. Curr Opin Urol 18:431–435

Thorup J, McLachlan Cortes D, Nation TR, Balic A, Southwell BR, Hutson JM (2010) What is new in cryptorchidism and hypospadias – a critical review on the testicular dysgenesis hypothesis. J Pediatr Surg 45: 2074–2086

Toppari J, Virtanen HE, Main KM, Skakkebaek NE (2010) Cryptorchidism and hypospadias as a sign of testicular dysgenesis syndrome (TDS): environmental connection. Birth Defects Res A Clin Mol Teratol 88: 910–919

Wilcox D, Snodgrass W (2006) Long-term outcome following hypospadias repair. World J Urol 24: 240–243

Section 32.3

Adan L, Couto-Silva AC, Trivin C, Metz C, Brauner R (2004) Congenital gonadotropin deficiency in boys: management during childhood. J Pediatr Endocrinol Metab 17:149–155

Bergeson PS, Hopkin RJ, Bailey RB Jr, NcGill LC, Piatt JP (1993) The inconspicuous penis. Pediatrics 92:794–799

Bhangoo A, Paris F, Philibert P, Audran F, Ten S, Sultan C (2010) Isolated micropenis reveals partial androgen insensitivity syndrome confirmed by molecular analysis. Asian J Androl 12:561–566

Cheng PK, Chanoine JP (2001) Should the definition of micropenis vary according to ethnicity? Horm Res 55:278–281

Feldman KW, Smith DW (1975) Fetal phallic growth and penile standards for the newborn male infants. J Pediatr 86:395

Grumbach MM (2005) A window of opportunity: the diagnosis of gonadotropin deficiency in the male infant. J Clin Endocrinol Metab 90:3122–3127

Lee PA, Houk CP (2004) Outcome studies among men with micropenis. J Pediatr Endocrinol Metab 17:1043–1053

Lumen N, Monstrey S, Selvaggi G, Ceulemans P, De Cuypere G, Van Laecke E, Hoebeke P (2008) Phalloplasty: a valuable treatment for males with penile insufficiency. Urology 71:272–276; discussion 276–277

Menon PS, Khatwa UA (2000) The child with micropenis. Indian J Pediatr 67:455–460

Paris F, De Ferran K, Bhangoo A, Ten S, Lahlou N, Audran F, Servant N, Poulat F, Philibert P, Sultan C (2011) Isolated 'idiopathic' micropenis: hidden genetic defects? Int J Androl 34:e518–e525

Summerton DJ, McNally J, Denny AJ, Malone PS (2000) Congenital megaprepuce: an emerging condition – how to recognize and treat it. BJU Int 86:519–522

Wisniewski AB, Migeon CJ (2002) Long-term perspectives for 46, XY patients affected by complete androgen insensitivity syndrome or congenital micropenis. Semin Reprod Med 20:279–304

Wisniewski AB, Migeon CJ, Gearhart JP, Rock JA, Berkovitz GD, Plotnick LP, Meyer-Bahlburg HF, Money J (2001) Congenital micropenis: long-term medical, surgical and psychosexual follow-up of individuals raised male or female. Horm Res 56:3–11

Section 32.4

Bar-Yosef Y, Binyamini J, Matzkin H, Ben-Chaim J (2007) Degloving and realignment – simple repair of isolated penile torsion. Urology 69:369–371

Fisher C, Park M (2004) Penile torsion repair using dorsal dartos flap rotation. J Urol 171:1903–1904

Paxson CL Jr, Corriere JN Jr, Morriss FH Jr, Adcock EW III (1977) Congenital torsion of the penis in father-son pairs. J Urol 118:881

Pomerantz P, Hanna M, Levitt S, Kogan S (1978) Isolated torsion of the penis. Urology 11:37–39

Sarkis PE, Sadasivam M (2007) Incidence and predictive factors of isolated neonatal penile glanular torsion. J Pediatr Urol 3:495–499

Shaeer O (2008) Torsion of the penis in adults: prevalence and surgical correction. J Sex Med 5:735–739

Section 32.5

Caldamone AA, Chen SC, Elder JS, Ritchey ML, Diamond DA, Koyle MA (1999) Congenital anterior urethrocutaneous fistula. J Urol 162:1430–1432

Rattan KN, Kajal P, Pathak M, Kadian YS, Gupta R (2010) Aphallia: experience with 3 cases. J Pediatr Surg 4:E13–E16

Section 32.6

Adetayo FO (2009) Outcome of management of acute prolonged priapism in patients with homozygous sickle cell disease. West Afr J Med 28:234–239

Cantasdemir M, Gulsen F, Solak S, Numan F (2011) Posttraumatic high-flow priapism in children treated with autologous blood clot embolization: long-term results and review of the literature. Pediatr Radiol 41:627–632

Corbetta JP, Duran V, Burek C, Sager C, Weller S, Paz E, Lopez JC (2011) High flow priapism: diagnosis and treatment in pediatric population. Pediatr Surg Int 27: 1217–1221

Fall B, Fall PA, Diao B, Sow Y, Dieng E, Sarr A, Ndoye AK, Sylla C, Ba M, Diagne BA (2010) Acute priapism associated with sickle cell disease in Senegal: clinical, therapeutic features and risk factors for erectile dysfunction. Med Trop (Mars) 70:475–478

Hekal IA, Meuleman EJH (2008) Idiopathic low-flow priapism in prepuberty: a case report of literature. Adv Urol 2008:549861

Maples BL, Hagemann TM (2004) Treatment of priapism in pediatric patients with sickle cell disease. Am J Health Syst Pharm 61:355–363

Raveenthiran V (2008) A modification of Winter's shunt in the treatment of pediatric low-flow priapism. J Pediatr Surg 43:2082–2086

Sandler G, Soundappan SS, Cass D (2008) Appendicitis and low-flow priapism in children. J Pediatr Surg 43: 2091–2095

Sood R, Wadhwa SN, Jain V (2006) Neonatal priapism associated with spontaneous bilateral pyocavernositis. Ann Acad Med Singapore 35:425–427

Towbin R, Hurh P, Baskin K, Cahill AM, Carr M, Canning D, Snyder H, Kaye R (2007) Priapism in children: treatment with embolotherapy. Pediatr Radiol 37: 483–487

Volmer BG, Nesslauer T, Kraemer SC, Goerich J, Basche S, Gottfried HW (2001) Prepubertal high flow priapism: incidence, diagnosis and treatment. J Urol 166: 1018–1023

Winter CC, McDowell G (1988) Experience with 105 patients with priapism: update review of all aspects. J Urol 140:980–983

Conspicuous External Genitals in a Girl

33

True malformations as causes of conspicuous external genitals occur less frequently in girls than in boys and often as varieties of normality and acquired pathologies (Table 33.1). The latter are important for differential diagnostic reasons because parents and the involved girl can be reassured and/or adequate treatment be carried out. On the other hand, early recognition of true anomalies is superior to diagnosis at puberty for psychological and therapeutical reasons.

33.1 Epispadias in a Girl

Occurrence, Clinical Significance

In contrast to the epispadias of a boy in whom the penis is intact as a whole, the clitoris is divided in female epispadias. Female epispadias is commonly considered as a disorder associated with urinary incontinence because grade III in which the anterior aspect of the urethra is completely divided as far as the bladder neck is the most obvious, whereas the seemingly less frequent grades II and I and especially the minor form are ignored completely (1:160,000 live births in girls and 1:70,000 in boys).

Clinical Significance

- Although grade III and II epispadias of the girl is combined with urinary incontinence, disorders of micturition may exist in grade I and the minor form as well.

Table 33.1 Differential diagnosis of the conspicuous external genitals in a girl

Malformations
• Bladder exstrophy, epispadias
o Hypospadias
• Interlabial masses[a]
• Imperforate hymen
o Other vaginal obstructions (vaginal atresia), vaginal agenesis
o Duplications of vagina and uterus
Variations of normality, acquired disorders
o Pseudohypertrophy of clitoris and/or labia, synechia of clitoris frenulum
o Pseudoimperforate hymen
• Labial synechia
• Injuries, female genital mutilation
o Tumors of the external genitals

[a]Interlabial masses are congenital malformations or less frequently acquired tumors

Clinical Presentation

In grade III epispadias, *the corresponding halves of the clitoris and its prepuce lie on the right and left side of the urethral plate with its funnel-shaped access to the bladder. The mons pubis is flat, and continuous dribbling can be observed* #. In grade II, the bladder neck is intact, and in grade I, *only the clitoris is divided.*

The minor form is characterized by a *drug-resistant wetting, diastasis of the symphysis palpable as a gap, oblong, and possibly patulous external urethral meatus, and possibly a bifid clitoris.* The bladder leaks if minimal pressure is applied to the lower abdomen.

Differential Diagnosis, Work-Ups

Grade I and the minor form may be missed and explained as nocturnal or daytime enuresis.

The work-ups include plain abdominal x-ray including the symphysis that shows diastasis and cystoelectromanometry in grade I and in the minor form (low leak pressure).

Treatment, Prognosis

Starting in infancy, the bladder neck is reconstructed according to Young-Dees-Leadbetter followed by urethroplasty and reconstruction of the external genitals. Acceptable continence is achieved in two thirds of the girls who need additional appropriate physiotherapy for bladder rehabilitation.

33.2 Hypospadias and Interlabial Masses

In so-called female hypospadias, the urethral meatus is placed above its normal site on the anterior vaginal wall and is combined with a significant stenosis. The hidden meatus is not recognized at first sight, and repeated dilatations or meatomy is necessary. The term female hypospadias has also been used for very short urethra in urogenital sinus.

For interlabial masses, see Chap. 29.

33.3 Congenital Obstructions of the Genital Tract (Gynatresias)

Duplications (anomalies of fusion) of uterus and vagina have been recognized in the past often only at puberty or thereafter. On the other hand, gynatresias may present already at birth.

33.3.1 Imperforate Hymen

Occurrence, Clinical Significance

Imperforate hymen is the most common congenital vaginal obstruction. Its clinical significance is as follows:

- If imperforate hymen is not recognized at birth or in the prepubertal girl by inspection of the external genitals, its manifestation as lower abdominal tumor is possible in the neonate, during childhood (due to mucometrocolpos), or at puberty and adolescence (due to hematometrocolpos).
- Cyclic abdominal pain and lower abdominal mass can be interpreted at puberty as surgical abdomen or abdominal tumor in spite of associated primary amenorrhea.
- Development of peritonitis (hemoperitoneum, ascending infection) or endometriosis is not excluded if imperforate hymen is not recognized before menarche.
- Menarche does not exclude completely congenital vaginal obstruction (unilateral obstruction of duplex vagina and uterus didelphys).

Clinical Presentation

In imperforate hymen, *the hymen is completely closed* # (Fig. 33.1 upper row).

Because imperforate hymen is not recognized at first sight, it is important that newborns are checked for it or another more proximal vaginal obstruction. *Usually a track of mucus is visible at the posterior commissure. If it is not present and the hymen is open, the vagina should be tested for obstruction by a probe. A length of less than the normal 4 cm is suspicious of another gynatresia than imperforate hymen. Acute urinary retention may be the first presenting sign of imperforate hymen.*

In some of the cases, **mucometrocolpos** has developed. *The whitish or gray bluish hymen protrudes between the labia (interlabial mass) and a cystic mass is palpable in the lower abdomen on rectoabdominal bimanual, and on rectal examination as an enlargement of the vagina in front of the rectum. The bluish transilluminating mass is combined with primary amenorrhea, cyclic abdominal pain, and tumor # if imperforate hymen is recognized only at puberty.*

Mucometrocolpos and hematometrocolpos may also lead to disorders of micturition (*urinary retention*) and stool evacuation (*constipation*) and obstruction of the upper urinary tract (*abdominal and flank pain and urinary tract infection*).

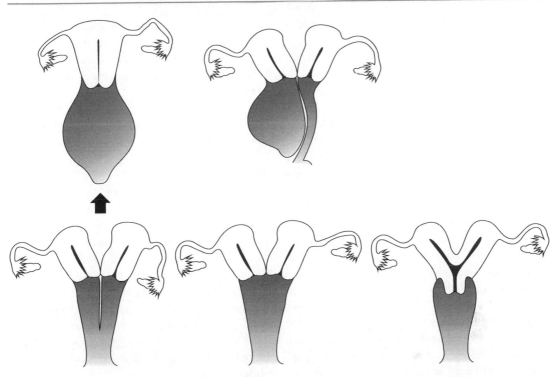

Fig. 33.1 Imperforate hymen and unilateral obstruction of duplex vagina in uterus didelphys and types of fusion anomalies of uterus and vagina. On the *left side* of the *top row*, a diagrammatic drawing of imperforate hymen is visible that is the most common congenital vaginal obstruction. The hymen protrudes between the labia and is *gray* or *bluish* depending on the age and development of the girl. Unilateral obstruction of duplex vagina and uterus didelphys that is recognizable in the drawing on the *right side* may mimic imperforate hymen at clinical examination. On the other hand, the possibility of this rare anom-aly is often not considered because menarche does occur by the contralateral vagina. The different types of fusion anomaly of uterus and vagina are depicted in the row at the *bottom* and are from the *left* to the *right side*: **Uterus didelphys** with two uteri, cervices, and vaginas, **uterus duplex bicollis** with a common vagina and two cervices and uteri, and **uterus duplex unicollis** (bicornuate uterus) with a common vagina and cervix and two uteri. These duplications can only be suspected from the outside if the dividing vaginal septum reaches the introitus

Differential Diagnosis, Work-Ups

It includes other causes of an interlabial mass, abdominal tumor, surgical abdomen, cyclic or chronic abdominal pain, urinary retention and constipation, and of another more proximal gynatresia.

Ultrasound shows a cystic pelvic and/or abdominal mass with some scattered echos.

CT or MRI permits characterization of the muco- or hematometrocolpos and its relation to the adjacent organs. VCU and contrast enema display additional information of the effects on the adjacent organs.

Treatment, Prognosis

It consists of crosswise incision of the hymen with resection of the edges #. The possible complications such as ascending adnexitis and peritonitis, abdominal adhesions, and endometriosis can impair a favorable outcome.

33.3.2 Other Transverse Congenital Vaginal Obstructions, Vaginal Agenesis

Occurrence, Pathoanatomy

The other transverse vaginal obstructions (vaginal atresias) occur less frequently than imperforate hymen and are encountered close and proximal to the hymen, at the transition from the middle to the proximal third of the vagina, and close to the cervix. The membranous occlusion is

complete or incomplete with a central opening #
and may be associated with partial anterior vaginal agenesis or persistent common urogenital
sinus.

In **vaginal agenesis**, the vagina or a major part
of it is absent, the external genitals and ovaries
are normal, and the uterus is either rudimentary
or normal. The disorder is also called Mayer-
Rokitansky-Küster-Hauser syndrome or MURCS
association (**M**üllerian duct and **r**enal aplasia and
cervicothoracic **s**omite association). It occurs in
1:5,000 female live births and may be associated
with urological (unilateral renal agenesis, uni- or
bilateral renal ectopy, or fusion anomalies in one
third) or skeletal malformations (of the spine,
extremities, ribs including Klippel-Feil syndrome) in >10 %.

Clinical Significance

- Because the external genitals are normal, both
  disorders are not recognized at birth except for
  cases with a strong suspicion because of prenatal ultrasound findings, routine examination
  of the vagina in the newborn, or a combination
  of associated malformations.
- Obstruction of the vagina leads in both disorders to the same complications as the quoted
  imperforate hymen.

Clinical Presentation

It may be similar to imperforate hymen except
for the external genitals that are normal in both
disorders. In MURCS association, urological and
skeletal anomalies may point to it. If the uterus of
MURCS association is rudimentary, *missing vaginal discharge before puberty and primary amenorrhea thereafter* are the only signs. If transverse
vaginal obstruction and MURCS association with
a normal uterus do not lead to mucometrocolpos,
work-ups of *primary amenorrhea, cyclic abdominal pain, and cystic abdominal tumor* lead to the
diagnosis.

Differential Diagnosis, Work-Ups

The important differential diagnoses are the same
as in imperforate hymen. The possible partial vaginal agenesis or urogenital sinus and associated

urological and skeletal anomalies may lead to
confusion about the correct diagnosis.

In addition to radiological imaging with ultrasound and MRI that permit characterization of
the different disorders, colposcopy and laparoscopy yield further informations. Ultrasound and
VUC are used for exclusion of urological
malformations.

Treatment, Prognosis

Transverse membranes of the vagina are best
crosswise incised with resection of the edges ###.

MURCS association with **complete or partial vaginal agenesis** needs vaginal replacement.
The time of intestinal replacement of the vagina
depends on the retained uterus function (functioning uterus needs surgery before commencement of menarche and rudimentary uterus before
initiation of sexual activity) and the interest of
the patient in sexual activity and motivation to
use the reconstructed vagina on a regular basis
postoperatively.

Surgery: After a transverse lower abdominal
incision, a segment of 8–10-cm length is chosen
from the distal sigmoid that is based on the left
colic artery. After closure of its proximal end, the
distal end is anastomosed with the perineal skin
or a vaginal remnant. In functioning uterus, the
proximal end of the sigmoid segment is anastomosed with it.

33.3.3 Duplications of Vagina and Uterus (Fusion Anomalies)

Occurrence, Types

Anomalies of fusion are caused by complete or
incomplete failure of union of the Müllerian ducts
and occur quite frequently.

In **uterus didelphys**, two uteri, two cervices,
and two vaginas are present. The two vaginas are
separated by a longitudinal septum that involves
the whole double vagina or only the proximal part
of it. If the common vagina has two separate uteri
and cervixes, a so-called **uterus duplex bicollis** is
present. If two separate uteri share a common cervix and vagina, the terms **uterus duplex unicollis**

or bicornuate uterus are applied. Occasionally, a duplex vagina may be obstructed in one of the two vaginas leading to unilateral muco- or hemato-/metrocolpos (**unilateral obstruction of duplex vagina**) (Fig. 33.1 upper row right side and lower row).

Clinical Significance
- Duplex vagina may lead to disorders of cohabitation later in life and, if combined with unilateral obstruction, to symptoms and signs of congenital vaginal obstruction.
- Duplications of the uterus may be associated with obstetrical and/or gynecological disorders later in life.

Clinical Presentation
Complete duplex vagina may be recognizable by *inspection of the external genitals #*, whereas duplications of the uterus may be clinically suspected in case of duplex vagina, unilateral obstruction of a duplex vagina, and associated specific urological malformations. In unilateral obstruction of duplex vagina, *the cyclic abdominal pain and a cystic abdominal mass do not subside in spite of menarche and menses.*

Differential Diagnosis, Work-Ups
It includes all types of congenital vaginal obstruction in case of unilateral obstruction of duplex vagina.

Reliable work-ups are colposcopy and laparoscopy that are diagnostic in uterus didelphys, uterus duplex bicollis, and uterus bicornuate, respectively. MRI is also diagnostic for all types of duplicity of uterus and vagina including unilateral obstruction of duplex vagina and for recognition of associated urological anomalies. In the latter anomaly, ultrasound and endoscopy display a normal vagina that is pushed to the ipsilateral side by a contralateral cystic mass and takes a tortuous course in the pelvis.

Treatment, Prognosis
The longitudinal membrane in duplex vagina needs complete division and, in case of unilateral

obstruction of duplex vagina, resection of the obstructive membrane or communication in case of a foreshortened ipsilateral vagina with the normal contralateral vagina as preliminary measure.

Sexual intercourse, conception, pregnancy, and birth may be possible in spite of uterus duplication.

33.3.4 Urogenital Sinus, Cloacal Anomalies

Pathoanatomy, Types, Occurrence
Urogenital sinus is a common tract into which urethra and vagina enter after a variable distance from the bladder and uterus, respectively. In cloacal anomalies, the anus is missing, and the terminal rectal fistula enters vagina or urogenital sinus at different levels.

In urogenital sinus, three types are observed depending on where the urethra and vagina enter the common channel: Close to bladder and uterus or to the perineum #, and in between these two types (Fig. 33.2 upper row). If the same criterium is applied in cloacal anomaly, four types arise depending on whether urethra, vagina, and rectal fistula enter the common channel close to their organ of origin or to the perineum, and/or whether the urethra or the rectum fistula enters proximally or distally: forms with either high or low connection of urethra and rectal fistula to the urogenital sinus, and forms with either high connection of the urethra and low connection of the rectal fistula to the urogenital sinus and vice versa (Fig. 33.2 lower row).

Common urogenital sinus occurs as a part of congenital adrenal hyperplasia or other disorders of sex development, as isolated disorder, or combined with anteriorly displaced anus cloacal anomaly.

Clinical Presentation
Urogenital sinus is characterized by the following findings of the external genitals: *Instead of a clitoris, often a penis-like hooded structure is visible that resembles a penis; only one orifice*

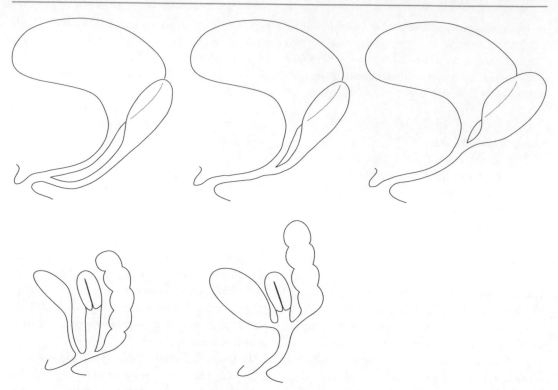

Fig. 33.2 The *top row* shows a genitogram in urogenital sinus and the row at the *bottom* a diagrammatic drawing of two forms of cloacal anomaly. *Top row* from the *left* to the *right side*: separation of the vagina from the urethra has occurred close to the external genitals, in the middle of the urogenital tract, and near to bladder and vagina. The row at the *bottom* demonstrates two of the many forms of cloacal anomaly in which urethra, vagina, and rectovaginal fistula merge with each other low and away from or high and close to the organs of origin. The common sign of the various forms of cloacal anomaly is one perineal opening with evacuation of urine, wind, and meconium

except of the anus is recognizable with spontaneous or dribbling micturition that is flanked by labioscrotal folds ##. **Cloacal anomalies** *have a similar appearance. The only opening evacuates in addition to urine also air and possibly meconium. The anus is missing, and the buttocks are flat* (Fig. 33.3). The perineal opening may be stenotic leading to dilatation of urogenital sinus and vagina by urine or meconium retention.

Possible bladder outlet insufficiency, lower urinary tract obstruction, and/or emptying of urine in the genital tract, urinary incontinence with constant dribbling or urinary retention (full bladder and possible upper urinary tract obstruction) are additional signs. Obstruction of the rectogenital fistula in cloacal anomalies leads to signs of lower abdominal obstructive ileus with distended belly and vomiting.

Differential Diagnosis, Work-Ups

It includes disorders with ambiguous external genitals, anorectal malformation, *disorders of bladder voiding, and obstructive ileus* of the newborn, and other disorders with urogenital sinus.

Work-ups include ultrasound that shows the different parts of the whole anomaly and possible dilatation of the involved hollow organs (bladder, upper urinary tract, vagina and uterus, and rectum). A precise description of the whole malformation is only possible by an integrated assessment of MRI, endoscopy #, and genitogram

Fig. 33.3 Types of female genital mutilation or female circumcision. *Top left*: survey of the three main types. *Bottom left*: Sunna circumcision means excision of the prepuce including a part or the whole of the clitoris. *Bottom middle*: excision circumcision includes removal of the clitoris and partial or total amputation of the labia minora. *Bottom right*: in pharaonic circumcision, a part or the whole of the external genitals is removed, and the vaginal introitus is sewed up except for a small opening close to the anus ⇑. *Top right*: presentation after pharaonic circumcision

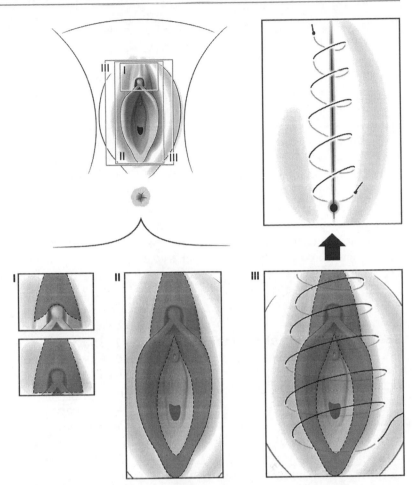

with contrast #. In addition, determination of chromosomal and gonadal sex is necessary.

Treatment, Prognosis

Surgery of urogenital sinus and/or cloacal anomaly requires precise work-up of the pathoanatomy that displays a wide individual range and concerns the low or high and intermediate site of connection of the different tracts and possible associated malformations such as lateralization of the ureteral orifices or longitudinal vaginal septum. Surgery is performed whenever possible in one session shortly after birth or during infancy with perineal, abdominoperineal, or posterior sagittal approach without or with laparotomy. The

approach depends on the site of connection of the different tracts and on the necessity to perform additional interventions for the associated anomalies, to reconstruct the urethra, pull-through, bring down, and reconstruct vagina and rectum.

Preliminary measures are dilatation or small posterior incision of the stenotic sinus and totally diverting colostomy (cloacal anomaly).

A bladder neck or very short urethra that empties in the urogenital sinus and high vagina is an example that needs abdominoperineal or posterior sagittal access (cloacal anomaly). The bladder neck or short urethra is disconnected from the vagina and its distal part reconstructed using the anterior wall of the vagina; the foreseen vagina is brought down and lengthened in its distal part by perineal skin flaps or a pedunculated segment of sigmoid. In case of cloaca, the rectum is pulled through posteriorly in a correct relation to the levator and external sphincter. Posterior sagittal approach is not performed if the length of the reconstructed urethra amounts to >3 cm.

In low connection, perineal anoplasty and flap vaginoplasty can be performed.

In general, acceptable functional and aesthetic results are achieved with urinary and fecal continence for the majority of cases except for cases with deficiencies of the sphincters or neurogenic bladder or anorectum. The latter children need bladder and anorectal rehabilitation such as CIC and enemas or some type of continent uro- and colostoma.

33.4   Variations of Normality, Acquired Disorders

Pseudohypertrophy of the clitoris, of the labia minora, synechia of the clitoris frenulum, and pseudohymenal atresia belong to variations of normality of the female external genitals. They may look like a severe disorder.

The normal size of the clitoris is 4 mm (up to 7), 5 mm (up to 11), and 7 mm (>14 years of age). In case of **pseudohypertrophy of the clitoris**, *excess prepuce lies over the clitoris # and may cover the entrance to the vagina.* The clitoris itself has a normal size. It is a good example that the external genitals of a girl must be carefully unfolded and washed before recovering urine.

In **pseudohypertrophy of the labia minora**, *a possibly transitory difference of the size of the labia minora in relation to the labia minora exists that are lying over the labia majora and look like an apron.* They may mimic abnormal external genitals and cause complaints depending on the clothes and activities. Spontaneous normalization may occur in the course of growth.

Synechia of the clitoris frenulum is *an adhesion of the foreskin* as a result of retention of smegma and may lead to pain and local infection.

Pseudohymenal atresia is an important **differential diagnosis** of the congenital gynatresias

and acquired labial synechia. In contrast to them, the labia minora or the hymen is not completely closed, but *the edges of the hymen lie close to the external urethral meatus, and/or the hymen has several holes like a sieve #.*

Clinical Presentation, Clinical Skills

The local findings correspond to those given above. **Pseudohypertrophy of the clitoris yields** *possibly false-positive results of urine examination.* **Pseudohypertrophy of the labia minora** may *mimic an anomaly of the external genitals and lead to pain and irritation, and the child may find it repulsive.* **Synechia of the clitoris frenulum** is combined with *pain and irritations* because of local infection.

Pseudohymenal atresia is recognizable *by the described local findings and whitish secretions that are evacuated in floods during crying or straining. Later in childhood, malodorous fluor leads to consultation because urine flows back in the vagina at micturition in a sitting position and is retained there or leads to wetting. Menstruation and cohabitation may be hindered in adolescence.*

The following clinical skills are useful to differentiate pseudohymenal atresia from imperforate hymen:

- If the intra-abdominal pressure is increased by coughing or straining, the edges of the hymen are retracted from the vagina and the introitus gets visible.
- The edges of the hymen can be unfolded if the finger that is introduced in the rectum for rectoabdominal examination pulls the anus in a posterior direction and downward.
- Vaginal fluor can be expressed by rectal examination.

Like pseudohymenal atresia, the other three disorders can be recognized by clinical examination, and other disorders can be excluded by the same way.

Treatment

Pseudohypertrophy of the clitoris and labia minora needs rarely surgical treatment except for advice about personal hygiene. Synechia of the clitoris can be treated by preputiolysis after a bath. In **pseudohymenal atresia**, resection of the edges to obtain an oblong introitus is indicated in general anesthesia.

33.5   Injuries of the External Genitals and Female Genital Mutilation

33.5.1 Injuries of the External Genitals

For injuries of the external genitals see Chap. 29.

33.5.2 Female Genital Mutilation (Female Genital Cutting, Female Circumcision)

Occurrence, Types of Mutilation

The term "female genital mutilation" (FGM) means partial or complete removal of each of the female external genitals or other injuries to it for cultural or other not therapeutic reasons. FGM is prevalent in 28 states of the sub-Saharan Africa and some regions of Asia (Middle East). Worldwide, >140 million girls and women live who had been circumcised, and each year, two million new cases are added.

The World Health Organization (WHO) classification differentiates the following four types (Fig. 33.3):
- Type I (Sunna) involves excision of the prepuce including a part or the whole of the clitoris.
- Type II (excision) means removal of the clitoris with partial or total amputation of the labia minora.
- Type III (infibulation or pharaonic incision) includes removal of a part or the whole of the external genitals combined with sewing up the vaginal introitus leaving only a small opening.
- Type IV includes many and diverse unclassifiable techniques such as punction, piercing, incision, and tearing of the clitoris. Extension or lengthening of clitoris and/or labia minora.
Burning out of clitoris and/or adjacent tissue
Tearing of the adjacent tissue (angurya incisions)

Application of corrosive substances or herbs that constrict the vagina, scraping of the vagina, pricking and piercing of clitoris or vulva

The interventions are usually performed without anesthesia and sterile instruments (knives, scissors, razors, pieces of broken glasses, scalpels) and in 70 % during childhood shortly after birth, at puberty, or before wedding. Recently, a trend has been observed to perform circumcision more and more often in younger children in some groups of immigrants to avoid unpleasant questions from the school authorities.

Clinical Significance
- FGM may lead to severe and life-threatening acute and chronic complications and restrictions of sexual function, obstetrical disorders of mother and child, and psychic disorders of the involved girls or women.
- The same applies to girls or women who immigrate. In addition, the confrontation with the opinions and requests of the western countries leads the involved girls and women and their families into uncertainty and severe stress.

Clinical Presentation
If not seen in the acute stage of mutilation, only type III is recognizable at the first glance. Infibulation has a small opening at the base of the vulva.

If the health-care services are consulted, findings of **acute or chronic complications** may be visible. They include in the **acute stage**: bleeding and/or wound infection with possible shock and/or septicemia including gangrene and tetanus. FGM may be associated with increased prevalence of HIV. Disorders of micturition (e.g., urinary retention) may also be present. Fractures and psychic trauma result from forceful peri- and postinterventional immobilization (e.g., tied legs), and performance of circumcision without anesthesia.

The **chronic stage** shows possibly keloids, chronic abscesses, neurinoma, or dermoid cyst of the external genitals, lower and upper urinary tract obstruction and/or infection, vaginal stenosis, vulvovaginitis, endometritis and adnexitis, hematocolpos and disorders of menstruation, dyspareunia, infertility, depression and other psychic disorders. In addition, birth may lead to severe disorders of mother (e.g., perineal tear and infection, postpartal hemorrhage) and child (e.g., insufficient monitoring of birth and child). In general, FGM is associated with some health consequences, but no statistically significant associations have been documented for a number of health conditions.

Discussion with the involved child or woman and their family about FGM is difficult because a big difference exists between the sociocultural and family expectations and the individual life experience of the involved patient and the ideas of the consulted medical staff, and the neutral term "female circumcision" should be used instead of female mutilation. The parents do not think that the complaints of their daughter are related to the former circumcision.

Differential Diagnosis, Work-Ups

Acute FGM includes accidental injury or sexual assault or rape. Because characteristic findings may be missing or hidden especially in the chronic stage, a precise history is very important.

The work-ups include careful clinical examination in general anesthesia including the use of small endoscopes, swabs, and photo documentation, ultrasound of urinary tract and kidneys, and vagina, uterus, and adnexe.

Treatment, Prognosis

FGM needs a multidisciplinary approach that meets all possible disorders and necessary treatments. Defibulation by anterior episiotomy is necessary at birth of a woman with infibulation. Depending on the local findings and the request of the patient, reconstruction of the external genitals must be performed electively.

Other medical or surgical treatment concerns urinary tract and other infections, psychiatric disorder, and repair of urogenital complications.

Usually former FGM is a long-term problem and needs long-term follow-up and/or treatment. Medicalization of female circumcision for reduction of harm is a questionable and dangerous practice (medicalization – FGM or pricking/nicking re-infundibulation carried out by doctors, nurses, or midwives).

Webcodes

The following webcodes can be used on www.psurg.net for further images and data.

3301 Epispadias in the girl, grade II	3309 Complete vaginal duplication
3302 Imperforate hymen, prepubertal girl	3310 Urogenital sinus, low union vagina and urethra
3303 Imperforate hymen, at puberty	3311 Urogenital sinus in associated ACH type 2
3304 Fresh hematocolpos after incision	3312 Urogenital sinus in associated ACH type 3
3305 Incomplete transverse membranous vaginal obstruction	3313 Endoscopy, urogenital sinus, high union vagina and urethra
3306 Complete membranous vaginal obstruction	3314 Genitogram, vagina, uterus, and fallopian tube
3307 Before final in- and excision	3315 True versus pseudohypertrophy of clitoris
3308 Old hemato-/metrocolpos after incision	3316 Incompletely open hymen

Bibliography

General: Clinical Skills, Differential Diagnosis

Hensle TW, Kennedy WA II (1998) Abnormalities of the female genital tract. In: O'Neill JA Jr et al (eds) Pediatric surgery, vol II, 5th edn. Mosby, St Louis, Hensle TW (1987) Genital anomalies

Terruhn V (1987) Fehlbildungen des weiblichen Genitale im Kindes- und Jugendalter und ihre Behandlung. In: Stolecke H, Terruhn V (eds) Pädiatrische Gynäkologie. Springer, Berlin

Sections 33.1–33.2

Allen L, Rodjani A, Kelly J et al (2004) Female epispadias: are we missing the diagnosis? BJU Int 94: 613–615

Sections 33.3.1–33.3.2

Barda G, Bernstein D, Arbel-Alon S, Zakut H, Menczer J (1997) Gynecologic problems of the lower genital tract in children and young adolescents. Harefuah 133(3–4):84–86, 168

Chang JW, Yang LY, Wang HH, Wang JK, Tiu CM (2007) Acute urinary retention as the presentation of imperforate hymen. J Chin Med Assoc 70:559–561

Ekenze SO, Mbadiwe OM, Ezegwui HU (2009) Lower genital tract lesions requiring surgical intervention in girls: perspective from a developing country. J Paediatr Child Health 45:610–613

Letts M, Haasbeek J (1990) Hematocolpos as a cause of back pain in premenarchal adolescents. J Pediatr Orthop 10:731–732

Lima M, Ruggeri G, Randi B, Domini M, Gargano T, La Pergola E, Gregori G (2010) Vaginal replacement in the pediatric age group: a 34-year experience of intestinal vaginoplasty in children and young girls. J Pediatr Surg 45:2087–2091

Loscalzo IL, Catapano M, Loscalzo J, Sama A (1995) Imperforate hymen with bilateral hydronephrosis: an unusual emergency department diagnosis. J Emerg Med 13:337–339

Posner JC, Spandorfer PR (2005) Early detection of imperforate hymen prevents morbidity from delays in diagnosis. Pediatrics 115:1008–1012

Stelling JR, Gray MR, Davis AJ, Cowan JM, Reindollar RH (2000) Dominant transmission of imperforate hymen. Fertil Steril 74:1241–1244

Thomas JC, Brock JW III (2007) Vaginal substitution: attempts to create the ideal replacement. J Urol 178:1855–1859

Tran ATB, Arensman RM, Falterman KW (1987) Diagnosis and management of hydrohematometrocolpos syndromes. Am J Dis Child 141:632–634

Yanza M-C, Sépou A, Nguembi E, Ngbale R, Gaunefet C, Nali MN (2003) Hymen imperforé: diagnostic négligé a la naissance, urgence chirurgicale à l'adolescence. Schweiz Med Forum 44:1063–1065

Yu TJ, Mc Lin (1993) Acute urinary retention in two patients with imperforate hymen. Scand J Urol Nephrol 27:543–544

Sections 33.3.3–33.3.4

Acien P, Acien M, Sanchez-Ferrer M (2004) Complex malformations of the female genital tract. New types and revision of classification. Hum Reprod 19:2377–2384

Acien P, Acien M, Fernadez F, Jose Mayol M, Aranda I (2010) The cavitated accessory uterine mass: a Müllerian anomaly in women with an otherwise normal uterus. Obstet Gynecol 116:1101–1109

Capito C, Echaieb A, Lortat-Jacob S, Thibaud E, Sarnacki S, Nihoul-Fékété C (2008) Pitfalls in the diagnosis and management of obstructive uterovaginal duplication: a series of 32 cases. Pediatrics 122:e891–e897

Cooney MJ, Benson CB, Doubilet PM (1998) Outcome of pregnancies in women with uterine duplication anomalies. J Clin Ultrasound 26:3–6

Hendren WH (1977) Surgical management of urogenital sinus abnormalities. J Pediatr Surg 12:339–357

Hendren WH (1982) Further experience in reconstructive surgery for cloacal anomalies. J Pediatr Surg 17:695–715; discussion 715–717

Hendren WH, Donahoe PK (1980) Correction of congenital abnormalities of the vagina and perineum. J Pediatr Surg 15:751–762; discussion 762–763

Levitt MA, Pena A (2010) Cloacal malformations: lessons learned from 490 cases. Semin Pediatr Surg 19:128–138

Lewis AD, Levine D (2010) Pregnancy complications in women with uterine duplication abnormalities. Ultrasound Q 26:193–200

Montevecchi L, Valle RF (2004) Resectoscopic treatment of complete longitudinal vagina septum. Int J Gynaecol Obstet 84:65–70

Nigam A, Puri M, Trivedi SS, Chattopadhyay B (2010) Septate uterus with hypoplastic left adnexa with cervical duplication and longitudinal vaginal septum: rare Mullerian anomaly. J Hum Reprod Sci 3:105–107

Orazi C, Lucchetti MC, Schingo PM, Marchetti P, Ferro F (2007) Herlyn-Werner-Wunderlich syndrome: uterus didelphys, blind hemivagina and ipsilateral renal agenesis. Sonographic and MR findings in 11 cases. Pediatr Radiol 37:657–665

Pena A, Bischoff A, Breech L, Louden E, Levitt MA (2010) Posterior cloaca – further experience and guidelines for the treatment of an unusual anorectal malformation. J Pediatr Surg 45:1234–1240

Philbois O, Guye E, Richard O, Tardieu D, Seffert P, Chavrier Y, Varlet F (2004) Role of laparoscopy in vaginal malformation. Surg Endosc 18:87–91

Ribeiro SC, Yamakami LY, Tormena RA, Pinheiro Wda S, Almeida JA, Baracat EC (2010) Septate uterus with cervical duplication and longitudinal vaginal septum. Rev Assoc Med Bras 56:254–256

Zhapa E, Rigamonti W, Castagnetti M (2010) Hydrosalpinx in a patient with complex genitourinary malformation. J Pediatr Surg 45:2265–2268

Section 33.5

Abdulcadir J, Margairaz C, Boulvain M, Irion O (2011) Care of women with female genital mutilation/cutting. Swiss Med Wkly 140:w13137. doi:10.4414/smw.2010.13137

Garcia VF, Sheldon C (1998) Genitourinary tract trauma. In: O'Neill JA Jr et al (eds) Pediatric surgery, vol I, 5th edn. Mosby, St Louis

Jäger F, Hohlfeld P (2009) Mädchenbeschneidung – konkrete Prävention in der Schweiz Ein Artikel für alle, die gefährdete Kinder oder Betroffene betreuen. Schweiz Med Forum 9:473–478

Magoha GA, Magoha OB (2000) Current global status of female genital mutilation: a review. East Afr Med J 77:268–772

Merritt DF (2008a) Genital trauma in children and adolescents. Clin Obstet Gynecol 51:237–284

Merritt DF (2008b) Genital trauma in children and adolescents. Clin Obstet Gynecol 51:237–258

Monjok E, Essien EJ, Holmes L Jr (2007) Female genital mutilation: potential for HIV transmission in sub-Saharan Africa and prospect for epidemiologic investigation and intervention. Afr J Reprod Health 11:33–42

Nour NM (2004) Female genital cutting: clinical and cultural guidelines. Obstet Gynecol Surv 59:272–279

Obermeyer CM (2005) The consequences of female circumcision for health and sexuality: an update on the evidence. Cult Health Sex 7:443–461

Renteria SC (2008) Female genital mutilation – need for answers at the age of adolescence. Rev Med Suisse 4:1445–1446, 1448–1450

Utz-Billing I, Kentenich H (2008) Female genital mutilation: an injury, physical and mental harm. J Psychosom Obstet Gynaecol 29:225–229

Ambiguous External Genitals, Disorders of Sex Development (DSD)

34

Ambiguous external genitals mean that their atypical appearance does not allow assignment to a male or female gender (Table 34.1).

Table 34.1 Differential diagnosis of ambiguous external genitals

Newborns
46, XX disorders of sex differentiation
● Congenital adrenal hyperplasia (CAH), complicated CAH
o Ovotesticular DSD (true hermaphroditism)
o Testicular DSD (XX-male)
46, XY disorders of sex differentiation
● Complete and incomplete androgen insensitivity syndrome (cAIC, pAIC)
● Defects of testosterone synthesis and dihydrotestosterone transformation
o Disorders with abnormal differentiation of the testis
o Oviduct persistence (persistent Müllerian duct syndrome)
Chromosomal disorders of sex differentiation
● Asymmetrical mixed gonadal dysgenesis
Infants and older children
46, XX disorders of sex differentiation
● Congenital adrenal hyperplasia (CAH), late-onset CAH, CAH in boys
46, XY disorders of sex differentiation
● Complete androgen insensitivity syndrome, testicular feminization
● Pure gonadal dysgenesis
o Oviduct persistence (persistent Müllerian duct syndrome)
Chromosomal disorders of sex differentiation
● Turner syndrome
● Klinefelter's syndrome

Occurrence, Clinical Significance

The prevalence of DSD is 1:4,500 (0.18–0.2:1,000) live births of which Turner syndrome and congenital adrenal hyperplasia are the most frequent. In Africa, the incidence of DSD seems to increase possibly because of environment pollution (e.g., pesticides against mosquito larvae). The clinical significance is as follows:

- Ambiguous external genitals and disorders of sex development impose strong psychological pressure on parents, physicians, and lifelong on the patients.
- Psychological pressure starts with their clinical recognition, in developed countries earlier (neonatal period) than in nondeveloped (throughout childhood or adulthood).
- Psychological pressure may lead to rejection, stigmatization, social exclusion, and suicide of the involved people.
- Decision about gender assignment, treatment options, and their schedule may be difficult but also controversial and crucial.
- Patients need mostly lifelong medical, psychological, and psychosexual treatment and guidance.
- Patients with hypovirilizing DSD and gonadal dysgenesis are at risk of germ cell tumors.

In the newborn and less frequently in infancy, urgency arises from it. It has mainly a psychological but also a differential diagnostic and therapeutic significance (expert medical guidance of the parents, detection of life-threatening conditions), and referral to a tertiary care center gets necessary. The medical care provider should avoid

G.L. Kaiser, *Symptoms and Signs in Pediatric Surgery*,
DOI 10.1007/978-3-642-31161-1_34, © Springer-Verlag Berlin Heidelberg 2012

comments such as "it is not clear if the newborn is a boy or a girl" or "it is an intersex" if confronted with such a child. Instead, the term "disorder of sex development" should be used. Comprehensive informations, prognostic statements, and the name of the specific diagnosis should only be provided by a pediatric endocrinologist and genetician and/or after appropriate work-up.

Clinical Presentation

Forms of clinical manifestations of ambiguous external genitals are the following:

- **Micropenis** and its relationship to the scrotum. Normal mean penile length and diameter of the newborn at term are 3.5±0.4 and 1 cm, respectively. Values of abnormal small penis are <1.5 and 0.7 cm.
- **Clitoris hypertrophy** #. Normal lengths are 4 (1 month–7 years), 5 (until 11 years), and 7 mm (after 14 years). A clitoris length of >10 mm corresponds to clitoris hypertrophy.
- **Posterior hypospadias** with/without bifid scrotum or penoscrotal transposition.
- **Posterior labial fusion, labioscrotal folds** #. Labia versus scrotum #.
- **Indicators of urogenital sinus**. Single funneled sinus in the depth of which the urethral and vaginal entrance is visible; single, narrow, and funneled sinus #; and small sinus opening at the base of the penis (type 5 intersexual external genitals with an orifice of the urogenital sinus at the tip of the penis analogous with male conditions does at first not remember the presence of a urogenital sinus).
- **Symmetrical or asymmetrical site of the gonads, their size, shape, and consistency, inguinal or labial mass** (palpable gonads in the scrotum, labioscrotal folds, or in front of the external inguinal ring are usually testicles and the presence of a Y is almost certain; ovaries do not descend).
- Cryptorchidism especially in nonpalpable testes.
- History of a disorder of sex development in the family (e.g., CAIS), discordance between (external) genitals and karyotype.

However, intersexual external genitals are not the single presentation of **disorders of sex development** (**intersex disorders**). They may be defined as congenital conditions in which chromosomal, gonadal, or anatomical sex is atypical.

In spite of normal external genitals, a disorder of sex development may be present, and the manifestations presented in the previous chapters "conspicuous external genitals in the boy and in the girl" cannot only exclude an intersex in case of classic appearance but also be an indication of a disorder of sex development. This is mainly true for hypoplastic genitals, micropenis, hypospadiases, and cryptorchidism. These abnormal findings are often or occasionally observed in syndromes, and they are even diagnostically relevant for the assignment to a specific syndrome or as an indicator of ambiguous genitals.

Work-Ups

They include in general:
- Electrolytes.
- Basal and stimulated hormone measurements (serum, urine), for example, increased plasma 17-OH-progesterone, for CAH (deficiency of 21-hydrolase) or hCG for testicular stimulation, if positive, for functional testicular tissue.
- Abdominopelvic imaging (ultrasound, MRI).
- Chromosomal analysis, karyotypizising, molecular genetic testing, for example, PCR analysis of SRY gene demonstrates presence of Y chromosome and is available in 1 day.
- Endoscopy, genitogram, laparoscopy including gonadal biopsy.
- Medical photographies need permission of the parents and in teenagers, of the patient.

Genetic testing is very important because some mutations are related to developmental abnormalities of the gonads (WT1 and SF1) and possibly of the ovaries (WNT4, DAX1, FOXL2, RSPO1) or to CAH (CYP21A2). Gonadal biopsies can be avoided if the diagnosis can be established biochemically or by gene studies. They are necessary if ovotestis or dysgenetic gonads are suspected.

Disorders of sex development with hypovirilization and gonadal dysgenesis are at **risk of germ cell tumors of the gonads**. They need clinical and radiological follow-up, morphological and histological evaluation of gonadal tissue, evaluation of tumor markers OCT3/4, TSPY double immunohistochemistry, and possibly gonadectomy.

An increasing number of intersex individuals is recognized today by prenatal ultrasound and chromosomal examination (early noninvasive fetal sexing) or postnatal screening. Nevertheless, it is important for the general practitioner or pediatric surgeon to consider the possibility of a disorder of sex development in the newborn and thereafter in spite of these tools.

Intersex disorders have been divided pragmatically in the past into four groups:

- Female pseudohermaphroditism: abnormal genital development in spite of normal XX-karyotype and ovaries because of a strong androgenic effect
- Male pseudohermaphroditism: abnormal genital development in spite of normal XY-karyotype and testicles because of an insufficient androgenic effect
- Disorders of development and differentiation of the gonads (that may be missing, incomplete, or asymmetrical): frequently in aberrations of the sex chromosomes
- Nonclassifiable forms

In 2005, a new classification system for intersex disorders has been recommended (Chicago Consensus) which encompasses children with congenitally abnormal gonadal, chromosomal, or anatomic gender. It has been followed by consensus statements on management of intersex disorders (societies LWPE and ESPE).

Intersex disorders are called **disorders of sex development (DSD),** and terms such as intersex, (pseudo)hermaphroditism, and sexual reversal should be avoided. Disorders of sex development are grouped into **three categories according to the karyotype: 46, XX DSD, 46, XY DSD, and sex chromosomal DSD**. Each category has several etiological subgroups, for example, 46, XX DSD encompasses disorders of gonadal (ovarian) development, disorders related to androgen excess, and other rare disorders.

The new taxonomy was accepted by many medical and lay experts. Nevertheless, several objections have been raised by others; for example,

the discarded histology of the gonads remains fundamental to the understanding of development of normal or aberrant sex by the medical students and residents in training and is a major determinant of clinical outcome. The new classification has led to a change in the distribution of etiological diagnoses. Although congenital adrenal hyperplasia and androgen insensitivity syndrome are still the most frequent DSD, Turner and vanishing testes syndrome belong now to the most common diagnoses as well. About 50 % belong to the 46, XY DSD and 25 % each to the 46, XX and sex chromosome DSD.

Treatment

General principles of work-up, parent's information, indication, treatment, and follow-up include routine use of **multidisciplinary diagnostic and expert surgical teams** (pediatric endocrinology, pediatric surgery and urology, genetics, psychology, and psychiatry), early gender assignment, full disclosure of final diagnosis and alternatives relating to surgery type and timing, and continuing psychosocial and psychosexual care.

In the past, three fourths of the patients have been reared as girls and one fourth as boys.

Hormonal therapy is used for:

- Survival such as cortisol and aldosterone in CAH
- Replacement of sex hormones, especially for stimulation of sexual development (such as penis growth in combination with hypospadias repair), pubertal changes, psychosexual development, and adult sexual behavior including bone mineral density
- Treatment of the unborn child with dexamethasone in maternal 21-hydroxylase deficiency

Surgery: The rationale for early reconstructive surgery includes several fields; avoidance of complications from the malformations and confusion about gender identity in case of atypical genital appearance are examples.

The feminizing genital surgery includes the following:

- Early separation of vagina and urethra combined with vaginal exteriorization and reconstruction of the external genitals

- Reduction of the clitoris (with preservation of sensation [glans and neurovascular bundle])
- Vaginoplasty in case of missing or short vagina for menstruation and/or sexual intercourse (in teenagers, because of potential scarring in early surgery)

The masculinizing genital surgery needs more surgical interventions that are challenging and complex. They include the following:

- Surgery of severe hypospadias including chordee resection and urethral reconstruction
- Orchidopexy
- Phalloplasty
- The implantation of testis prosthesis in the empty scrotum at the end of puberty

34.1 Newborns

In newborns, some of the known disorders of sex development can be diagnosed or suspected with the help of abnormal genital findings (ambiguous external genitals), and confirmed or rejected after appropriate work-ups and consultation with a pediatric endocrinologist.

34.1.1 46, XX Disorders of Sex Development (Female Pseudohermaphroditism)

34.1.1.1 Congenital Adrenal Hyperplasia (CAH)

Causes, Occurrence, Clinical Significance

CAH is caused by a genetically determined enzyme deficit (in >90 % by the P450-C21-enzyme [21-hydroxylase], less frequently by other enzymes) and rarely by placental androgen effect (virilizing tumor or androgen exposition of the mother) or postnatal androgen effect on the child. The defect of cortisol synthesis with accumulation of androgens leads to masculinization of the external genitals of different degrees.

CAH belongs with 50 % of all disorders of sex development (and in girls in an even higher percentage) to the most common abnormalities. In Switzerland, 1:8,000 live births are recorded every year since the introduction of newborn screening in 1992 of which 50 % are girls. The clinical significance is as follows:

- If the girls and boys with CAH are not recognized early in the neonatal period, those with a complicated CAH will escape the necessary early treatment.
- Boys with CAH will not be detected, and girls with AGS may suffer from delayed and complicated work-ups till final diagnosis.

Clinical Presentation

The combination of nonpalpable gonads with virilized external genitals is suspicious of female CAH and especially if ultrasound displays normal Müllerian structures.

The external genitals of the girls have different degrees of virilization and correspond to the types 1–5 of Prader. Stage 1 (isolated clitoris hypertrophy) and 5 (local findings analogous with male external genitals) are mostly overlooked. Increased pigmentation of the external genitals, nonvisible or nonpalpable gonads, and findings of urogenital sinus that are visible from the outside are compatible with stages 2–4 #. In boys, hyperpigmentation of the scrotum and a possibly large penis should alert the physician.

Complicated CAH is characterized by additional deficit of mineralocorticosteroids that leads to salt wasting (hyperkalemia and hyponatremia) with vomiting, diarrhea, and exsiccosis. The association of CAH with salt loss is independent of the severity of masculinization.

Differential Diagnosis, Work-Ups

It includes disorders with clitoris hypertrophy, with insufficient virilization (male pseudohermaphroditism), with external signs of urogenital sinus (anomalies of vagina and uterus or cloacal anomalies), with severe hypospadias, and in case of complicated CAH disorders, with vomiting of the newborn and young infant. In small-for-date newborns and pseudohypertrophy (excess prepuce), the clitoris may appear somewhat prominent. Transplacental virilization must be considered if the steroids are not increased; mixed gonadal dysgenesis, true hermaphroditism, or lack of anti-Müllerian hormone if gonads are not or only palpable on one side and no or abnormal Müllerian structures are present; or a female with nongonadal source of androgens if no gonads are palpable and the external genitals are ambiguous.

The work-ups include (1) determination of electrolytes and base excess, 17-α-hydroxyprogesteron, ACTH, cortisol, renin, 11-deoxycortisol, dehydroepiandrosterone and DHEA-S, androstenedione, and testosterone (before and after stimulation with human chorionic gonadotropin=hCG); (2) radiological imaging with abdominopelvic ultrasound, genitogram #, and MRI; (3) possibly laparoscopy and gonadal biopsy; (4) chromosomal analysis including karyotype and specific genes (lymph node cultures).

Treatment, Prognosis
The 46, XX masculinized patients are usually assigned to and reared as girls. Early surgery in infancy includes separation of vagina and urethra combined with vaginal exteriorization, reconstruction of the external genitals, and possibly clitoral reduction.

In modest genital ambiguity and clitoris enlargement, late vaginoplasty and genitoplasty may be an option. Possible exceptions are severely masculinized patients with diagnostic delay and community male preference who may be assigned to the male gender #.

Prenatal diagnosis and treatment is possible by HLA-typizising of parents and unborn patient and DNA analysis of CYP21-gene.

34.1.1.2 Ovotesticular Disorder of Sex development (True Hermaphroditism)
Occurrence, Clinical Significance
Individuals with true ovotesticular DSD have functioning ovarian and testicular tissue (50 % of the patients have an ovotestis on one and ovary or testis on the other side, and 25% have either bilateral ovotestis or testis on one and ovary on the other side). It is a rare disorder. The karyotypes are 46, XX and less frequently 46, XY or XX/XY mosaicism.

Its clinical significance is as follows:
- Early recognition and assignment to the suitable and desired gender may be very difficult for several reasons.

Clinical Presentation
The external genitals appear more frequently to be of male gender, although less virilized or rather female varieties do occur. The gonads are different relating to their site and size, consistency, and shape. The external genitals display clitoris hypertrophy, labioscrotal folds, or severe forms of hypospadias with bifid scrotum and penoscrotal transposition. Urogenital sinus is present in every case. The internal genitals contain Müllerian as well as Wolff's duct structures.

Differential Diagnosis, Work-Ups
It is similar to mixed gonadal dysgenesis. The typical asymmetry of the gonads is analogous to mixed GD.

Work-ups include radiological imaging; endoscopy; laparoscopy and biopsy; determination of testosterone, anti-Müllerian, and other hormones; and chromosomal analysis.

Treatment, Prognosis
Gender assignment may be very difficult. In case of true hermaphroditism, mixed gonadal dysgenesis, and less frequently in male hermaphroditism, fallopian tubes, uterus, and vagina must be removed after male gender assignment with preservation of the vasa deferentia.

34.1.1.3 Testicular DSD (XX Males)
In testicular DSD (XX males), the external genitals are mostly male and rarely ambiguous. The testes remain small and have a similar histology as in Klinefelter's syndrome #.

34.1.2 46, XY Disorder of Sex Development (Male Hermaphroditism #)

For normal virilization, early pituitary and testicular function, testosterone synthesis, transformation of testosterone to dihydrotestosterone, and androgen receptor of target tissues are necessary. Undervirilization or absent virilization occurs in the following conditions:

- In some disorders of Sect. 34.1.2.3
- Defect of testosterone synthesis
- Defect of 5-α-reductase (impairment by gene mutation, inhibitors)
- Defect of androgen receptor (impairment by gene mutation, antiandrogens)

In all defects, gene mutations and in the last two, environmental (e.g., industrial and agricultural chemicals) may act as endocrine disruptors and may mimic 5-α-reductase defect or partial androgen insensitivity syndrome. Undervirilization may lead to cryptorchidism, micropenis, hypospadias, and disorders of sex development (ambiguous external genitals). The effect on the external genitals is different depending on the cause and completeness of the quoted defects ###.

34.1.2.1   Complete and Incomplete Androgen Insensitivity Syndrome

Causes, Occurrence
Complete androgen insensitivity syndrome (CAIS) is the most common 46, XY disorder of sex development. **Testicular feminization** is the most common type of CAIS. The testes with histological findings of a cryptorchic testis produce testosterone and anti-Müllerian hormone. The external genitals are females, and the vagina is short #. The recessively inherited disorder is transmitted by the mother and occurs in 1:200 female newborns. It is not recognizable from the outside and therefore mostly not recognized or suspected in the newborn except for prenatal work-up because of familiality or due to precise examination of the external genitals including measurement of vaginal length for exclusion of congenital hymenal obstruction. *No Wolffian structures are present, urethra and vagina are completely separated with own orifice, and the external genitals are female combined with a blind vaginal pouch.*

Incomplete androgen insensitivity syndrome may be caused by environmental chemicals as well and leads to *undermasculinization with undescended testes, small prostate, clito-ris hypertrophy, possible low urogenital sinus, partial fusion of the labioscrotal folds, and blind vaginal pouch. At puberty, some virilization is possible.* For work-ups, differential diagnosis, and treatment, the reader is referred to Sect. 34.1.2.2 and 43.1.2.4.

34.1.2.2   Defect of Testosterone Synthesis and Dihydrotestosterone Transformation

Causes, Occurrence
At least five congenital enzyme defects lead to testosterone synthesis defects (**17,20-desmolase-**, 17-reductase-, **3-β-ol-dehydrogenase-**, 20,22-desmolase-, and 17-hydroxylase-defect). Of the last three disorders, the first two are combined also with a defect of cortisol and aldosterone synthesis (salt wasting) and 17-hydroxylase-defect only partially with cortisol synthesis. The inherited defect of transformation of testosterone to dihydrotestosterone is caused by **5-α-reductase-defect**. These rare disorders have an autosomal recessive or X-chromosomal inheritance, and some lead to undervirilization and ambiguous external genitals, male or female phenotype, and missing, complete, or incomplete male puberty with or without gynecomastia. There is no oviduct persistence due to the activity of anti-Müllerian hormone.

Clinical Significance
- Early recognition is very important for adequate and desired gender assignment and appropriate treatment and/or cortisol and aldosterone substitution in some.

Clinical Presentation
These types of XY DSD must be considered in an individual with familiality concerning a disorder of sex development or exposition to endocrine disruptors and male karyotype if symmetrical gonads are palpable and any degree of ambiguity from hypospadias to female appearance is present.

Some of the newborns cannot be differentiated from girls and show different degrees of incomplete virilization especially 17, 20-desmolase, 3-β-ol-dehydrogenase, and 5-α-reductase: micropenis, severe forms of hypospadias with bifid scrotum, and penoscrotal transposition or with micropenis, hypospadias, partially descended testes, residual vagina (e.g., 5-α-reductase-defect). *Testicles are always present, may be of normal size or small, descended or not descended, and are symmetrical.*

Differential Diagnosis, Work-Ups

It includes female pseudohermaphroditism, isolated severe hypospadias, micropenis, or cryptorchidism if only the most frequent disorders are quoted.

Work-up may be very complicated in some males with insufficient or absent masculinization. It includes the initially quoted examinations and specifically chromosomal sex, aberration of sex chromosomes, abdominal ultrasound, determination of the precursors of testosterone depending on the suspected site of enzyme block, for example, increase of plasma dehydroepiandrosterone in 3β-hydrosteroid dehydrogenase deficiency or lack of dihydrotestosterone in deficient transformation of testosterone, and molecular genetic examination.

Treatment

The patient should be assigned to and reared in the gender that carries the best prognosis for sex and reproductive function and for which the genitals and physiological appearance can be made to look most normal. If these guidelines are applied, most individuals must be assigned to the female and some to the male gender.

34.1.2.3 Disorders with Abnormal Differentiation of the Testis

Pathology, Clinical Features

The following rare disorders belong to this group: congenital pituitary hypofunction and disorders of hormonal timing, Leydig cell hypoplasia or aplasia, embryonic testicular regression syndrome, testicular dysgenesis, and congenital anorchia. Because of early anti-Müllerian hormone activity, no Müllerian structures are observed except for testicular dysgenesis.

In the disorders of pituitary gland and hormonal timing, *no gonads are palpable in contrast to the normal appearing phallus.*

In Leydig cell hypoplasia and aplasia, *the testes are partially descended, and no masculinization does occur. The patients have a female appearance.*

The testicular regression syndrome is characterized by early intrauterine degeneration, and normal testicular tissue is replaced by connective tissue. The external genitals are either ambiguous or female.

In testicular dysgenesis, *the testicles are very small and the external genitals either ambiguous or female.*

In congenital anorchia, degeneration of the testicles has occurred late in pregnancy. *The testicles are missing, and the external and internal genitals are male.*

The differential diagnosis of **absent gonads in spite of a normal appearing penis** includes congenital gonadotropin deficiency, hormonal timing problem, complete virilized CAH, anorchia, Klinefelter's syndrome, and the most frequent cryptorchidism.

34.1.2.4 Oviduct Persistence

Causes, Occurrence

In isolated oviduct persistence, the production of anti-Müllerian hormone by the testes is missing. This rare disorder is usually not recognized at birth except for discordant prenatal ultrasound in boys with gross Müllerian duct remnants. The patients display male external genitals and often incompletely descended testes with distorted development and possible azoospermia.

Clinical Presentation

Male pseudohermaphroditism must be considered *if demonstrable, symmetrical gonads (possibly recognizable as testes) are combined with micropenis and/or severe hypospadias #.*

In case of complete feminization, *symmetrical gonads may be detected in the groin* of which testicular feminization is an example.

Differential Diagnosis, Work-Ups

It includes disorders of female pseudohermaphroditism, isolated severe hypospadias, micropenis, or cryptorchidism, and other malformations of the external genitals, for example, penis agenesis. The palpation of gonads in the labioscrotal folds or inguinal region speaks against a 46, XX disorders of sex development.

Work-ups consist of abdominopelvic ultrasound, MRI, and if possible endoscopy and genitogram #. Usually, neither uterus and fallopian tubes nor vagina is present except for oviduct persistence. If normal testosterone excretion is observed after hCG, androgen resistance must be assumed, and testicular dysgenesis or distortion of biosynthesis if no testosterone excretion takes place.

Treatment, Prognosis

It encompasses the treatment of the disorders in sections 34.1.2.1 to 34.1.2.4. 46, XY undermasculinized patients are assigned to and reared as boys if testes and external genitals are sufficiently developed. Exceptions are individuals with dysgenetic gonads resulting in completely female external genitals and with complete androgen insensitivity syndrome (testicular biosynthesis defect) that are assigned to and reared as girls. Removal of the rudimentary and nonfunctioning testes is indicated in CAIS.

In case of sufficient masculinization and/or response to testosterone, reconstruction of the male external genitals is performed, and the oviduct resected #. Otherwise, assignment to female gender is indicated with reconstruction of vagina and adaption of the external genitals.

34.1.3 Chromosomal Disorders of Sex Development

34.1.3.1 Asymmetrical Mixed Gonadal Dysgenesis

Occurrence

Mixed gonadal dysgenesis belongs to the most common anomalies of sex chromosomes (45, X/46, XY and less frequently 46, XX/46, XY and other mosaicisms) and is likely to be recognized at birth.

Clinical Significance

- Necessity of early gender assignment
- The risk of malignant degeneration of the gonads (gonadoblastoma) is similar to pure

gonadal dysgenesis including some virilization

Clinical Presentation

It is dependent on the basic chromosomal aberration and development/differentiation of the gonads. *The external genitals are ambiguous but with only a weak masculinization for instance clitoris hypertrophy, indications of urogenital sinus, and signs similar to pure gonadal dysgenesis. Most frequently asymmetrically developed and localized gonads are observed: a dysgenetic or normal testis on one side # and a not visible and palpable streak gonad with a rudimentary fallopian tube # on the other side.*

Differential Diagnosis, Work-Ups

It includes female pseudohermaphroditism, pure gonadal dysgenesis, ovotesticular DSD, and other malformations with urogenital sinus. Pure gonadal dysgenesis has bilateral streak gonads with minimal hormone production and distinct female external genitals.

Chromosomal analysis, determination of androgen, and anti-Müllerian hormone levels, radiological imaging of the internal organs, localization and definition of the gonads by laparoscopy and biopsy, and endoscopy for evaluation of the urogenital sinus and its union are the most important work-up tools.

Treatment, Prognosis

Gender assignment and rearing is often female, the streak gonad and testis must be removed because of the risk of gonadoblastoma and virilization.

34.2   Infants and Older Children

The primary care provider encounters again and again children beyond the neonatal period in whom the suspicion of a disorder of sex development arises **due to other symptoms and signs than ambiguous external genitals,** for example, *short stature, severe hypospadias, inguinal hernia in a girl with missing fallopian tube or in a boy with Müllerian duct remnants, delayed or incomplete puberty, primary amenorrhea, breast* *development in a boy and virilization in a girl, gross hematuria in a boy,* and only occasionally ambiguous external genitals. In children of developing countries or with migration background, much more patients with ambiguous external genitals are encountered at any age of childhood than in developed countries in which newborns with ambiguous external genitals come early to the attention of the physicians.

34.2.1 46, XX DSD (Female Pseudohermaphroditism)

34.2.1.1 Congenital Adrenal Hyperplasia

In the context of adrenal cortical hypertrophy, **involved boys** must be considered in whom hyperpigmentation and possibly large penis has been overlooked. Those with a complicated form *start in the second to third week of life vomiting and refusing to drink;* they are considered to suffer from hypertrophic pyloric stenosis. Strong scrotal hyperpigmentation and a possibly large penis, hyperkalemia and hyponatremia speak in favor of CAH. In addition, **late-onset CAH** must be considered *if an accelerated growth of body length and premature pubarche is observed that has started early in childhood.* Whereas boys display infantile testicular sizes, girls develop hypertrophy of the clitoris but neither thelarche nor pubarche (precocious pseudopuberty).

34.2.2 46, XY DSD (Male Pseudohermaphroditism)

34.2.2.1 Testicular Feminization

This diagnosis is often missed in the newborn. These female patients *develop recurrent inguinal hernia and are therefore referred to the pediatric surgeon.* In contrast to normal girls with inguinal hernia, *these patients display preoperatively often gonads that are somewhat large and oblong on palpation, emerge repeatedly from the abdomen without incarceration, and are easy to reduce.*

At surgery, fallopian tubes are absent, and the gonads correspond neither macroscopically nor histologically to ovaries.

Testicular feminization occurs in 1:200 live born girls. Therefore, whenever female inguinal hernias are operated, this disorder should be excluded by inspection of ovaries and fallopian tubes. It belongs to the 46, XY # disorders of sex differentiation. The patients have no uterus, only a short vagina of 1–2-cm length, and sex-chromatin negative bodies. If not recognized before puberty, *primary amenorrhea, missing axillary and pubic hair, absent breast development, and occasionally ovarian tumor (originating from the gonad) are additional signs.* The patients are usually reared as girls, and some type of vaginal plasty should be performed before initiation of sexual activity.

34.2.2.2 Persistent Müllerian Duct Syndrome (Oviduct Persistence)

Isolated persistence of Müllerian duct structures (persistent Müllerian duct syndrome, oviduct persistence) belongs also to the 46, XY disorders of sex differentiation and is caused by a deficit of anti-Müllerian hormone ##. If oviduct persistence is associated with ambiguous external genitals, the diagnosis belongs to another subgroup of disorders of sex differentiation. Rudimentary forms of fallopian tubes, uterus, and vagina # are found at work-up, or only a utricular cyst may be encountered at the time of herniotomy, orchidopexy, and hypospadias or infertility work-ups.

Resection of the Müllerian duct structures and large utricular cysts are indicated to avoid inherent complications. At surgery, the dense interconnection of the vasa deferentia with the utricular cyst should be considered.

34.2.2.3 Pure Gonadal Dysgenesis

It is characterized by 46, XY chromosomes and bilateral streak gonads and has a recessive X-chromosomal inheritance.

Clinical Significance
- Streak gonads are at risk for gonadoblastoma.
- The disorder is often detected at expected puberty because of primary amenorrhea and other signs of absent female puberty.

Clinical Presentation

At birth, the individuals appear as girls and are reared accordingly. Some clitoris hypertrophy as well as some virilization is possible during growth. At the time of puberty, the corresponding female signs fail to develop.

Differential Diagnosis, Work-Ups

Especially testicular feminization must be considered. Work-ups include radiological work-up, laparoscopic gonadal biopsy, and chromosomal analysis.

Treatment

In pure gonadal dysgenesis, the gonads must be removed because of risk of malignant degeneration. Finally, vaginal plasty is necessary in case of missing or insufficiently developed vagina for intercourse.

34.2.3 Chromosomal Disorders of Sex Development

34.2.3.1 Turner Syndrome

Occurrence, Cause

Turner syndrome is usually not recognized at birth. It is one of the most common types of aneuploidy and occurs in 1:2,000 newborns with female appearance.

Fifty to sixty percent of the individuals have sex chromosome monosomy 45, X. The remainder has mosaicism with another (other) cell line(s) with complete, abnormal X or Y chromosome. Because of undetected mosaicism (e.g., in low frequency cell lines), these figures may change in the future (all Turner syndrome fetuses with spontaneous abortion have 45, X). In about two fifth of those with mosaicism and 5–10 % of the whole population, Y chromosome-derived material can be found.

Clinical Significance

- Turner syndrome belongs to the most common disorders of sex development according to the new classification.
- The clinical presentation is variable, and multisystemic involvement is characteristic.

- Patients with Y chromosome cell line are at risk for germ cell tumors
- Because of their multisystemic involvement, high morbidity, and increased mortality, a lifelong follow-up by a multidisciplinary team with a responsible coordinator for personal contact is necessary

Clinical Presentation

Turner syndrome is recognized because the children remain small and no or only late development of the breast is observed and no menarche in the teenagers.

The clinical examination displays variably dysmorphic signs of the face, webbed neck, low-set posterior hairline, hypoplasia of metacarpal and metatarsal bones of the fourth and fifth fingers and toes, and lymphedemas of hands and feet. Except for *edema of the hands and feet and a combination of the quoted findings*, rather *short stature, shield-shaped chest, primary amenorrhea and distorted puberty with slowly growing breasts and widely separated nipples*, or associated anomalies as *coarctation and horseshoe kidneys, ureteral duplications, or unilateral renal agenesia* will point to Turner syndrome. Accordingly, it is diagnosed at a variable age.

The external genitals are female, and the internal ones consist of small uterus and fallopian tubes, vagina, and streak gonads containing only ovarian stroma. Some virilization may occur at any time. In addition, arterial hypertension, hypothyroidism, celiac disease, and diabetes mellitus may be encountered.

In cases with Y chromosome-specific sequences, a high incidence of gonadoblastoma (>30 %) that are precursors of malignant germ cell tumors (e.g., dysgerminoma in 60 %) and nontumoral androgen-producing lesions are encountered.

Work-Ups, Differential Diagnosis

It includes cytogenetic analysis (e.g., evaluation of 30 metaphases of lymphocyte cultures from a peripheral lymph node), molecular DNA analysis (FISH, PCR) for mosaicism, SRY, and possibly other genes. In addition, work-ups for exclusion of the quoted associated disorders.

Treatment, Prognosis

In children, the delay of growth may be ameliorated by growth hormone. Application of estrogens becomes necessary from the age of 12 years and throughout the whole life to prevent osteoporosis. Girls with Y chromosome cell lines need strong supervision of their gonads by ultrasound and possibly bilateral gonadectomy. Regular and lifelong follow-up by a multidisciplinary team should be performed.

Patients with Turner syndrome are reared as girls. Normal sexual life is possible. Pregnancies and births have been possible after oocyte donation, but the patients need specialized management before and during pregnancy and birth.

34.2.3.2 Klinefelter's Syndrome

A patient who appears to be outwardly a boy may have a Klinefelder's syndrome before puberty *if gigantism (in which lower length is relatively large in relation to upper length, and arm span is larger than body length), eunuchoid proportions, and school or educational problems are present* and later, if in spite of delayed and incomplete puberty, *penis and testes are small (≤6 ml), secondary sex characteristics and muscles remain underdeveloped, and female pubarche and gynecomastia are present.*

The diagnosis is confirmed by positive sex-chromatin bodies, characteristic karyotype: X/XY and others, low testosterone and high FSH levels, and azoospermia.

The differential diagnosis encompasses patients with pre- or postnatally acquired bilateral anorchia or a secondary bilateral testicular loss, who has no androgen substitution and testicular prostheses.

Treatment includes testosterone supplementation for further male sex development and prophylaxis of osteoporosis and possible implantation of testicular prosthesis. Paternity may become possible by testicular sperm extraction.

34.2 Webcodes

The following webcodes can be used on www.psurg.net for further images and data.

3401 Clitoris hypertrophy, ACH	3411 Undervirilization, 46, XY DSD, with
3402 Labioscrotal folds, ACH	3412 Micropenis and feminized urethra and
3403 Right labial, left scrotal skin, mixed gonadal dysgenesis	3413 Vagina, genitography
3404 Urogenital sinus, ACH	3414 Testicular feminization
3405 Ambiguous external genitals, ACH	3415 Severe hypospadias with
3406 Genitography, urogenital sinus, ACH	3416 Oviduct persistence, genitography
3407 ACH, 46, XX, stage V	3417 Resected Müllerian structures
3408 Testicular DSD (XX-male), scrotum	3418 Mixed asymmetrical gonadal dysgenesis, left testis
3409 Testicular disorder of sex differentiation (DSD), micropenis	3419 Mixed asymmetrical gonadal dysgenesis, right streak gonad
3410 Undervirilization, 46, XY DSD	3420 Testicular feminization, 46, XY DSD

Bibliography

General: Classification, Radiological Imaging, Tumors, Ethical and Psychosocial Aspect, Treatment, Outcome

Aaronson IA, Aaronson AJ (2010) How should we classify intersex disorders? J Pediatr Urol 6:443–446

Ahmed SF, Morrison S, Hughes IA (2004) Intersex and gender assignment; the third way? Arch Dis Child 89:847–850

Bosinski HA (2006) Psychosocial aspect of intersex syndromes. Urologe A 45:981–991

Chang TS, Hwang WY (1984) Forearm flap in one-stage reconstruction of the penis. Plast Reconstr Surg 74:251

Chavhan GB, Parra DA, Oudjhane K, Miller SF, Babyn PS, Pippi Salle FL (2008) Imaging of ambiguous genitalia: classification and diagnostic approach. Radiographics 28:1891–1904

Creighton S (2001) Surgery for intersex. J R Soc Med 94:218–220

Crouch NS, Creighton SM (2004) Minimal surgical intervention in the management of intersex conditions. J Pediatr Endocrinol Metab 17:1591–1596

Donahoe PK, Schnitzer JJ (1998) Ambiguous genitalia in the newborn. In: O'Neill JA Jr et al (eds) Pediatric surgery, vol II, 5th edn. Mosby, St Louis

Duckett JW, Baskin LS (1993) Genitoplasty for intersex anomalies. Eur J Pediatr 152(Suppl 2):S80–S84

Erdogan S, Kara C, Ucaktürk A, Aydin M (2011) Etiological classification and clinical assessment of children and adolescents with disorders of sex development. J Clin Res Pediatr Endocrinol 3:77–83

Gnassingbe K, da Silva-Anoma S, Akakpo-Numado GK, Tekou AH, Kouame B, Aguehounde C, Coupris L, Galifer RB, Aubert D, Revillon Y (2009) Transfer of surgical competences in the treatment of intersex disorders in Togo. Afr J Paediatr Surg 6:82–84

Houk CP, Hughes IA, Ahmed SF, Lee PA, Writing Committee for the International Intersex Consensus Conference Participants (2006) Summary of consensus statement on intersex disorders and their management. International Intersex Consensus Conference. Pediatrics 118:753–757

Hughes IA, Houk C, Ahmed SF, Lee PA, Lawson Wilkins Pediatric Endocrine Society/European Society for Paediatric Endocrinology Consensus Group (2006a) Consensus statement on management of intersex disorders. J Pediatr Urol 2:148–162

Hughes IA, Houk C, Ahmed SF, Lee PA, LWPES Consensus Group; ESPE Consensus Group (2006b) Consensus statement on management of intersex disorders. Arch Dis Child 91:554–563

Josso N (1981) Physiology of sex differentiation. A guide to the understanding and management of the intersex child. Pediatr Adolesc Endocrinol 8:1–13, Karger, Basel

Lambert SM, Vilain EJ, Kolon TF (2010) A practical approach to ambiguous genitalia in the newborn period. Urol Clin North Am 37:195–205

Lee PA, Houk CP, Ahmed SF, Hughes IA (2006) Consensus statement on management of intersex disorders. Pediatrics 118:e488–e500

Petrykowski WV (1981) Embryology of genital malformations. Guidelines in diagnosis and treatment of intersex. In: Malformations of the external genitalia. Karger, Basel, Monogr Paediatr 12:1–30; discussion 31–32

Pleskacova J, Hersmus R, Oosterhuis JW, Setyawati BA, Faradz SM, Cools M, Wolffenbuttel KP, Lebl J, Drop SL, Looijenga LH (2010) Tumor risk in disorders of sex development. Sex Dev 4:259–269

Verwoerd-Dikkeboom CM, Koning AH, Groenenberg IA, Smith BJ, Benzinka C, Van Der Spek PJ, EA Steegers (2008) Using virtual reality for evaluation of fetal ambiguous genitalia. Ultrasound Obstet Gynecol 32:510–514

Vidal I, Gorduza DB, Haraux E, Gay CL, Chatelain P, Nicolino M, Mure PY, Mouriqunad P (2010) Surgical options in disorders of sex development (DSD) with ambiguous genitalia. Best Pract Res Clin Endocrinol Metab 24:311–324

Warne GL (2008) Long-term outcome of disorders of sex development. Sex Dev 2:268–277

Warne GL, Grover S, Zajac JD (2005a) Hormonal therapies for individuals with intersex conditions: protocol for use. Treat Endocrinol 4:19–29

Warne G, Grover S, Hutson J, Sinclair A, Metcalfe S, Northam E, Freeman J, Murdoch Childrens Research Institute Sex Study Group (2005b) A long-term outcome study of intersex conditions. J Pediatr Endocrinol Metab 18:555–567

Wiesemann C (2010) Ethical guidelines for the clinical management of intersex. Sex Dev 4:300–303

Specific Topics

Al-Maghribi H (2007) Congenital adrenal hyperplasia: problems with developmental anomalies of the external genitalia and sex assignment. Saudi J Kidney Dis Transpl 18:405–413

Brant WO, Rajimwale A, Lovell MA, Travers SH, Furness PD III, Sorensen M, Oottamasathien S, Koyle MA (2006) Gonadoblastoma and Turner syndrome. J Urol 175:1858–1860

Cabanes L, Chalas C, Christin-Maitre S, Donadille B, Felten ML, Gaxotte V, Jondeau G, Lansac E, Lansac J, Letur H, N'Diaye T, Ohl J, Pariente-Khayat A, Roulot D, Thepot F, Zénaty D (2010) Turner syndrome and pregnancy: clinical practice. Recommendations for the management of patients with Turner syndrome before and during pregnancy. Eur J Obstet Gynecol Reprod Biol 152:18–24

Carvajal Busslinger MI, Kulmann B, Kaiser G, Inaebnit D, Zuppinger K (1993) Persistent Müllerina duct syndrome: a case report. Eur J Pediatr 152(Suppl 2):S79

Chemes H, Muzulin PM, Venara MC, Muhlmann Mdel C, Martinez M, Gamboni M (2003) Early manifestations of testicular dysgenesis in children: pathological phenol-types, karyotype correlations and precursor stages of tumour development. APMIS 111:12–23; discussion 23–24

Federman DD, Donahoe PK (1995) Ambiguous genitalia – etiology, diagnosis, and therapy. Adv Endocrinol Metab 6:91–116

Husmann DA (2004) The androgen insensitivity micropenis: long-term follow-up into adulthood. J Pediatr Endocrinol Metab 17:1037–1041

Kousta E, Papathanasiou A, Skordis N (2010) Sex determination and disorders of sex development according to the revised nomenclature and classification in 46;XX individuals. Hormones (Athens) 9:218–231

L'Allemand D, Schweizerische Arbeitsgruppe für Kinder- und Jugendgynäkologie (2005) Mädchen mit Ulrich-Turner-Syndrom. Geschlechtsreifung und Behandlung bei Kinderwunsch im Ueberblick. Pädiatrie 3:20–23

Lean WL, Deshpande A, Hutson J, Grover SR (2005) Cosmetic and anatomic outcomes after feminizing surgery for ambiguous genitalia. J Pediatr Surg 40:1856–1860

Lipay MV, Bianco B, Verreschi IT (2005) Gonadal dysgenesis and tumors: genetic and clinical features. Arq Bras Endocrinol Metabol 49:60–70

Mahoudeau J, Reznik Y, Nivot S (1991) Clinical aspects of gonadal dysgenesis. Bull Assoc Anat (Nancy) 75:39–42

Mazur T (2005) Gender dysphoria and gender change in androgen insensitivity or micropenis. Arch Sex Behav 34:411–421

Mendonca BB, Costa EM, Belgorosky A, Rivarola MA, Domenice S (2010) 46, XY DSD due to impaired androgen production. Best Pract Res Clin Endocrinol Metab 24:243–262

Nihoul-Fékété C, Thibaud E, Lortat-Jacob S, Josso N (2006) Long-term surgical results and patient satisfaction with male pseudohermaphroditism or true hermaphroditism: a cohort of 63 patients. J Urol 175:1878–1884

Oliveira RM, Verreschi IT, Lipay MV, Eca LP, Guedes AD, Bianco B (2009) Y chromosome in Turner syndrome: review of the literature. Sao Paulo Med J 127:373–378

Parker KL, Wyatt DT, Blethen SL et al (2003) Screening girls with Turner syndrome: the National Cooperative Growth Study experience. J Pediatr 143:133–135

Schnitzer JJ, Donahoe PK (2001) Surgical treatment of congenital adrenal hyperplasia. Endocrinol Metab Clin North Am 30:137–154

Schober JM (2004) Feminizing genitoplasty. A synopsis of issues relating to genital surgery in intersex individuals. J Pediatr Endocrinol Metab 17:697–703

Sharma S, Gupta DK (2008a) Male genitoplasty for intersex disorders. Adv Urol 2008:685897

Sharma S, Gupta DK (2008b) Gender assignment and hormonal treatment for disorders of sexual differentiation. Pediatr Surg Int 24:1131–1135

Sultan C, Paris F, Terouanne B, Balaguer P, Georget V, Poujol N, Jeandel C, Lumbroso S, Nicolas JC (2001) Disorders linked to insufficient androgen action in male children. Hum Reprod Update 7:314–322

Völkl TM, Langer T, Aigner T, Greess H, Beck JD, Rauch AM, Dörr HG (2006) Klinefelter syndrome and mediastinal germ cell tumors. Am J Med Genet A 140:471–481

Part VI
Back

This chapter deals with congenital disorders of the back that are visible and/or palpable at birth but sometimes are not paid attention to. The most important disorders are listed in Table 35.1.

35.1 Myelomeningocele, Meningocele, Lipomyelomeningocele

Occurrence, Clinical Significance

Myelomeningocele (MMC) is the most frequent type of neural tube defect. It occurs in a ratio of 5 myeloceles to 3 anencephalies to 1 encephalocele. It is observed in 1 to>2:1,000 live births. The decreased incidence of myelomeningocele in some developed countries (0.35 in 1,000 live births) is caused by prenatal diagnosis and termination of pregnancy and to a lesser degree by prophylactic periconceptional folic acid administration. Its clinical significance is as follows:

- Newborns with MMC have different degrees of paraparesis and sensibility disorder of legs, trunk, and pelvic floor, functional disorders of bladder and anorectum, and often hydrocephalus that lead to a lifelong invalidity.
- Periconceptional prophylaxis with folic acid can diminish significantly the number of cases in women at risk but not completely eliminate them.

Forms and Types (Fig. 35.1)

The most frequent lumbosacral **MMC** is characterized by a macro- and microscopically malformation

Table 35.1 Differential diagnosis of masses, fistulas, and skin anomalies of the back

- Myelomeningocele, meningocele, and lipomyelomeningocele
- Minimal spinal dysraphism (occult spinal dysraphism, spina bifida occulta)
- o Sacrococcygeal teratoma
- Dermal sinus of the coccyx

of a lumbosacral segment of the spinal cord #. The medullary plate is not tubularized in an early stage of development, and the usually overlying meninges, spine (spinal arches and processes), truncal muscles, and skin are missing and/or underdeveloped and displaced. Less frequently involved sites are the sacral, thoracolumbar #, and thoracic region. The exposition of the spinal cord and its roots and tension on it during growth lead to the functional deficits.

In case of the ten times less frequent **meningocele**, the visible prominence consists only of epithelialized # and less frequently nonepithelialized meninges. The spinal cord is not involved.

Lipomyelomeningocele means either a lipoma that extends from the back to a normal or less frequently malformed spinal cord which is a part of it #.

Dysraphic lesions of the cervical spinal cord are uncommon. Open MMC and occult spinal dysraphism are associated more frequently with other spinal and CNS malformations, for example, Arnold-Chiari II malformation and hydrocephalus in open and Klippel-Feil syndrome type I in occult forms. The open MMC presents either as meningocele with possible split cord malformation or as

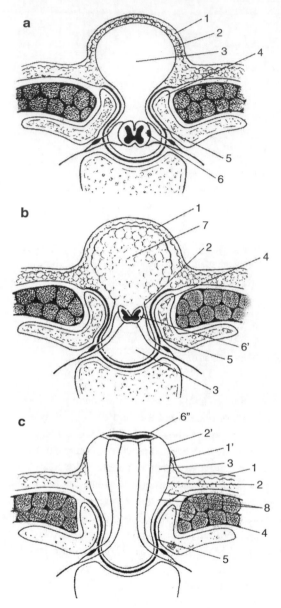

Fig. 35.1 Diagrammatic drawings of the dysraphic malformations of the spinal cord which are recognizable from the outside according to M. Bettex: (**a**) spinal cord is normal (*6*) and lies in the spinal canal. Sack-like continuation of the arachnoid underneath the skin, the dura tapers off at the level of spina bifida (*5*) = meningocele. (**b**) Spinal cord (*6*) is malformed and lies abnormally in the spinal canal (*3*). Over the spinal cord and in connection with it, a lipoma (*7*) is spreading out underneath the skin (*1*) = myelomeningocele with lipoma or lipomyelomeningocele. (**c**) The spinal cord (*6*) is malformed, lies outside the spinal canal, and is not covered by skin at its *top*. The arachnoid inserts at the borders of the exposed medullary plate (*2*) = myelomeningocele. (*4*) means in all drawins the open spinal arch

myelocystocele herniating posteriorly into a meningocele. Tethering of the cervical spinal cord occurs in both forms with late neurological deterioration. Therefore, at primary surgery, untethering of the spinal cord is an important part of surgery. The possible neurological dysfunction is not recognizable in the newborn.

Clinical Presentation, Clinical Skills

It includes the local findings, the neuromuscular findings of legs, trunk, and pelvic floor with resulting deformities (e.g., of the joints), indications of bladder and anorectal dysfunction, findings of the frequently associated hydrocephalus and obligatory Arnold-Chiari malformation II, and findings of associated malformations of the spine and other organs.

Local Findings

The bare medullary plate lies as an oblong and reddish or anchovy-like structure within a skin defect of different size in the midline of the dorsal lumbosacral region either at the level of the lateralized residuals of the vertebral arches # or at the top of a cystic mass #. Leaking of CSF may be observed at the cranial end of the medullary plate from the caudal end of the central channel or from rupture of the cele.

Neuromuscular Findings

In contrast to a clear transection of the spinal cord at the level of injury with a corresponding neurological level in trauma to the spinal cord, a mosaic-like deficit that extends over several segments may be observed. The motor deficit may be combined with some complicating reflex activity and some residual voluntary activity and sensation. It is mainly due to a lesion of the upper motor neuron.

Appearance and location of the quoted local findings permit only partly a statement about the extent of the neuromuscular deficits. Rather, the **knowledge of segmental innervation of the muscles and the possible patterns of involvement** according to **Stark types I and II a–c** are useful with regard to a precise documentation of neurological deficit. Type I pattern is observed in >25 % of the cases and means a flaccid paraparesis below a level of a segment with final innervation. Type II patterns are observed in about two thirds and are divided in the three subgroups a–c with decreasing incidence. Below the neurological level, a distinctly recognizable (type IIa) or a narrow, even imperceptible segment (type II b) with loss of motor, sensory, and reflex activity is present with spasticity and reflex activity below this segment #. In type IIc, an incomplete transection is present with partly preserved voluntary muscular activity and sensation, and reflex activity and spasticity.

Due to paresis of antagonists, imbalance of agonists and antagonists, or **reflex activity**, secondary luxations of the joints, deformities, and restrictions of the movements in hip, knee, and foot occur (e.g., neurogenic clubfoot #). Scoliosis and lordosis develop later on in addition to a possibly preexisting gibbus and other spine anomalies.

Complete **motor examination** includes separate examination of each side and muscle group according to the segmental innervation of the lower limb [Sharrard], observation of spontaneous movements or movements after stimulation with a pin (starting cranial of the suspected level) and grading of their strength (good, fair, poor, and none), and observation of possible reflex activity below the motor level or possible deformities of the lower extremities (hip, knee, and feet) which are secondary and may point to the motorial level [Stark].

The **sensory level** may be higher, lower, or asymmetrical. Its determination is performed with a pinprick starting from the sacral sensory dermatomes and observation of the reactions of the newborn (facial expression or crying) which occur delayed after several seconds.

Differentiation of **high and low types of MMC** is pragmatically very useful. A neurological level (corresponding to the last segment with voluntary innervation of the muscles) L2 and higher corresponds to a high and a neurological level of L3 and lower to a low type of MMC. The low types of MMC display the following findings #:

- Ability to walk independently can be attained much better because of the stabilization of the knee by the quadriceps muscle.

- Hydrocephalus occurs less frequently.
- Severe malformations of the spine such as kyphosis do not occur.

Signs of bladder and anorectal dysfunction (pelvic floor paresis #): Indications are frequent dribbling (spontaneously, at crying, or picking up), urinary retention, or residual urine that is hidden by overflow incontinence. Permanent evacuation of small stool portions or constipation is the indication of anorectal dysfunction, and a preserved bulbocavernosal reflex (pinching of the glans or clitoris is followed by contraction of the external sphincter muscle) speaks in favor of an intact reflex bow. Similar to the neuromuscular deficits, only 10 % of patients do not have a neurogenic bladder.

Hydrocephalus, Arnold-Chiari Malformation II, and Other Associated Anomalies

Hydrocephalus is present at birth in >80 % and becomes clinically apparent from birth until early infancy in the majority of cases. In the newborn, the head circumference does not necessarily correlate with the degree of hydrocephalus. It is caused by aqueductal stenosis and Arnold-Chiari malformation II in which parts of hindbrain are herniated in the upper cervical channel.

Arnold-Chiari malformation II leads permanently or intermittently during childhood to *deficits of the cranial nerves with stridor, dysphagia, and other symptoms and signs in about one third of the patients. Sometimes, already newborns may suffer from life-threatening attacks of cyanosis and apnea.*

Several associated anomalies of the spine and other organs occur such as gibbus and kyphosis of the spine and urological malformations. Other anomalies are quoted in the relevant chapters.

Differential Diagnosis, Work-Ups

No other disorders must be considered in the characteristic posterior MMC except for split notochord syndrome. In case of spontaneous survival combined with complete epithelization or in the rare anterior MMC, lipomyelomeningocele, and meningocele, coccygeal teratoma, neurogenic tumor (ganglioneuroma or neuroblastoma), or other presacral or lumbar neoplasm or developmental masses must be considered. High thoracic and cervical masses are mostly meningoceles with a good prognosis, whereas occipital, parietal, or frontal cystic masses are mostly cranial meningo- or encephalomeningoceles with equivocal prognosis except for frontal lesions with good outcome.

The work-ups include initially ultrasound and CT/MRI of skull and upper cervical spine (for hydrocephalus, Arnold-Chiari malformation II, hydromyelia) and thoracoabdominal plain x-ray (for spinal deformities, widened interpeduncular distances #, anomalies of the vertebrae).

Treatment

Prophylaxis of MMC is possible by supplementation of folic acid 3 months before conception and in the first trimester in a significant number of high-risk women. The remaining small risk is caused by an error of folic metabolism among other things. Fetal myelomeningocele repair is performed in specialized centers in the 19–25th week of gestation by hysterotomy. The outlook is favorable so far.

In **low types of MMC**, so-called total care is indicated. It includes (1) closure of the MMC combined with/without simultaneous shunt of the hydrocephalus within a few days after birth. The aim of surgery is to preserve the residual neuromuscular function and to prevent additional damage. Shunt surgery combined with MMC closure is controversial because of potential CSF infection from the MMC site; (2) delayed shunt surgery with timing dependent on the presence of an overt hydrocephalus at birth or the development of signs of increased intracranial pressure in early infancy; (3) rehabilitation of bladder and anorectal dysfunction, and neuromuscular deficits: clean intermittent catheterization (CIC) and systemic oxybutynin, physiotherapy according to Bobath or Vojta, and parenteral instruction belong to the cornerstones of early rehabilitation.

In **high types of MMC**, total care should only be initiated after several discussions and informed consent. Especially in thoracolumbar forms with severe hydrocephalus, kyphosis and gibbus, and associated severe anomalies or perinatal disorders, selection of nontreatment may be made. Nevertheless, these patients need also parenteral instruction for daily care, should be raised like other MMC patients, and if possible at home. In case of survival and demands of the parents, secondary total care is appropriate.

Surgery is performed in general anesthesia, prone position, and after measure has been taken to avoid temperature loss and to have an appropriate venous line and blood at the anesthesiologist's proposal.

Using magnification, an incision is made at the junction of normal skin and meninges of the MMC. After entering the cele, the neural plaque is isolated from the adjacent possibly epithelialized meninges, and all adhesions of the arachnoidea to the spinal cord and nerve roots are divided. Now the margins of the deficient paraspinal fascia become visible, and the neural plaque can be positioned in the residual spinal canal.

After circumferential incision of the central meningeal residuals, the borders can be closed with the dura at its inner surface in a watertight fashion and leaving sufficient space for CSF over the neural plaque.

After closure of the paraspinal fascia (without or with laterally developed flaps), the skin is subcutaneously mobilized and closed in the midline without tension (without or with Z-plasties).

Urological Work-Ups and Bladder Rehabilitation

In the newborn, **clean intermittent catheterization** (CIC), **antimuscarinic therapy** against detrusor hyperactivity (oxybutynin orally, intravesically, or transdermally), and **infection prophylaxis** (trimethoprim) are started in all patients after surgery for MMC combined with CIC instruction of the patients. Some of the work-ups are already performed such as **renal and bladder ultrasound** and **serum creatinine** beyond the first week of life.

Because the change from a paralyzed sphincter to a sphincter dyssyngergy is possible in the first 2–3 months of life, **measurement of residual urine** after voiding or leaking by catheterization, **urodynamics** with measurements of detrusor pressure and activity, and electromyography of external urethral sphincter, and **VCUG** in case of sphincter dyssynergy are performed thereafter.

After it, the type of **sphincter** activity (**intact-dyssynergic** with/without detrusor overactivity

#; partial or complete **denervation**; or **intact-synergic**) and **detrusor** activity (**overactivity**; normal; or diminished activity) can be determined. Elevated detrusor filling pressure, bladder sphincter dyssynergy, high voiding or leaking pressure (>40 cm H_2O), and reflux ≥grade 3 are absolute indications for CIC due to the inherent danger of urinary tract deterioration in up to two thirds of the population ##.

Sphincter dyssynergy (SDS) occurs in about 50 % of a spina bifida population and needs lifelong CIC, antimuscarinic therapy, and infection prophylaxis. With it, renal scarring and failure, and auto- or clamcystoplasty becomes necessary only in <5 %. Till school age, CIC is performed by the parents and thereafter by the patient itself. After the age of 1 year, infection prophylaxis may be stopped and followed by regular urine analyses (higher rate of bacteriuria vs. lower symptomatic urinary tract infection). Detrusor overactivity can be overcome by oxybutynin and alternatively by intravesical botulinum toxin injection that must be repeated because the effect lasts only 6–9 months and autoaugmentation.

In infants with **paralytic pelvic floor**, CIC is continued until surgery for incontinence and possible bladder augmentation. Afterward, CIC becomes indispensable.

Surgical procedures can be performed at any age depending on the urological findings and/or parent's and patient's (schoolchildren) requests.

Autoaugmentation (partial detrusorectomy) or clamcystoplasty (ileo- or colocystoplasty) is indicated in intractable SDS (serious detrusor overactivity in combination with poor bladder compliance and low capacity, e.g., voiding or leaking pressure >40 cm H_2O) or combined with surgery for incontinence. In **autoaugmentation**, the increased end-filling pressure is normalized, the gain in capacity is not very large, and muscarinic dependency for treatment of detrusor overactivity may be resolved in some of the patients. Its outcome is improved by intraoperative preservation of the bladder adventitia and closure after partial detrusorectomy and by postoperative intermittent expansion of the bladder. **Ileocystoplasty or colocystoplasty** increases the capacity and decreases the increased end-filling pressure significantly. It is constructed by a U-shaped cap of vascularized intestine that is anastomosed with the bladder incision extending from anterior bladder neck to the posterior trigonum. Afterward, the augmented bladder is extraperitonealized. The risk of spontaneous perforation is <2.5 %. Other risks are mucus production, recurrent urinary tract infections, electrolyte imbalance, stone formation, and late-occurring cancer.

Surgery for incontinence encompasses sling suspension, bladder neck surgery (e.g., Young-Dees-Leadbetter technique), injection of bulking agents in the bladder neck, or artificial sphincter implantation.

Abdominoperineal puboprostatic sling procedure in boys is faced with the technical difficulty to develop a plane between rectum and bladder neck that can be achieved best by an abdominoperineal approach. The main risks are false route (<10 %) or urethral perforation (<2 %). In girls, the bladder neck is visualized by an incision of the vagina at the same level (**transvaginal sling procedure**). There is a small risk of sling erosion. The success rate of sling procedures is about 80 %.

Catheterizable urostomas without or with bladder neck closure may be indicated for several reasons: need for transfer from the wheelchair to do CIC (burden to the parents and patient), preservation of child's privacy, intractable incontinence, false urethral routes because of CIC, and so forth.

It consists of a **continent appendicovesicostomy** or a **Monti procedure** (use of an ileal tube). At surgery, the conduit needs creation of an intravesical tunnel of sufficient length (depending on the diameter of the conduit and ≥2 cm length) and must be arranged according to its peristalsis in direction of the bladder. The conduit must pass the rectus muscle and may end in a lateral or median urostoma of the lower abdomen. Temporary complications are observed in up to 50 % and include stenosis of the stoma or at the bladder entrance site and leaking. Whereas stenosis of the urostoma may be prevented by an appropriate button, the latter two complications need frequently revision of the implantation site.

Cutaneous vesicostomy and **endoscopic external sphincterotomy** are possible but temporary measures to lower the intravesical pressure at the expense of continence.

Before 3 years of age, neurogenic stool incontinence is treated by dietetic measures and laxatives. After this age, patients who become symptomatic present with constant soiling and accidents (involuntary passage of stool), constant staining (fecal smearing present on the underwear or diapers), occasional staining, or stool impaction and encopresis. A patulous anus with no external sphincter contraction on stimuli and normal relaxation of the internal sphincter in contrast to a negative contraction of the external sphincter are the findings on anorectal manometry.

Daily evacuation regime by retrograde colonic catheter enemas after initial washouts for evacuation of all impacted stool is now the treatment that should be started as early as possible. With it, half of patients who are symptomatic because of neurological incontinence become completely clean, and the remaining have some staining because the internal sphincter prevents soiling if its relaxation is not triggered by a full ampulla.

Rarely antegrade colonic enema stoma (ACE) must be performed using either the appendix or a transverse tube created from the ileum that needs an appropriate submucosal colonic tunnel to prevent leakage and is supplemented by an appropriate stoma button.

Total care is a lifelong task that encompasses adaptation of the rehabilitation measures and orthopedic devices, medical and surgical treatment of the associated anomalies and secondary disorders arising during growth.

Prognosis

Seventy-five to eighty percent of the children will have normal intelligence though with partial deficits on neuropsychological testing. Ten to fifteen percent of surviving children in an unselected population are likely not to be socially competitive. About 80 % will be community ambulators by school age, and bladder and bowel control can be achieved in about 80–90 %. These results depend largely on the quality of follow-up by a multidisciplinary spina bifida team and the

adherence and motivation of parents and patients. The quoted results especially those of ambulation and bladder control are dynamic and may take a turn for the worse with adoption of the responsibility by the patient itself or because of worsening health conditions.

Many MMC patients are not adequately prepared for adulthood and to become independent. Realistic and active programs can improve the **autonomy**. In addition, arrangements for young dependent adults are necessary. Nevertheless, participation in the full range of adolescent activities is uncommon.

In nondeveloped countries, early **death** in childhood occurs frequently (e.g., 50 % of infant deaths are due to congenital anomalies especially MMC). Only 60 % or some more survives into adulthood in developed countries. Renal failure and cardiorespiratory disorders account for the majority of death although renal scarring and failure can be lowered to <5 % with appropriate bladder rehabilitation.

With age, spinal deformities become more pronounced (if spinal surgery is not performed), damage to the insensate joints occurs, the patient spends less time with dynamic physical activity, obesity takes place, and respiratory reserve worsens. Especially those with a high neurological level have an up to 50 % risk to lose their ability to walk beyond the first decade.

In adult MMC patients, **anesthesia and surgery** become much more risky than in healthy people of the same age for several reasons, for example, decrease of respiratory reserve and frequent latex allergy or limitation of possible position and danger of pressure scores.

Allergy to latex: A history of allergic reaction to latex products is observed in about one third of a spina bifida population, and at least 25 % have latex-specific immunoglobulin (Ig) E. It may be difficult to ascertain this complication because parents and patients are often not aware of possible latex allergy or the clinical manifestation may be subtle (e.g., local skin reaction to latex products). The involved patients have often other atopies and had significantly more operations in the past than not involved MMC patients. Life-threatening events with hypotension, bronchospasm, and other generalized allergic reactions occur mostly during general anesthesia but may also be observed during minor interventions and may be heralded by episodes of coughing or sneezing. Treatment includes identification of patients at risk by specific enquiry, skin testing and measurement of latex-specific (Ig) E, and provision of a latex-free environment for surgery and all performances in the hospital, at home, and the protected environment.

About one third of the MMC patients achieve a gainful **employment** and many of the other two thirds are able to work in a protected environment.

Development of normal **sexuality** is often impeded: in patients with severe disability, due to dependence on others and lack of privacy, and in less disabled, because of uncertainty of bladder and bowel control. In addition, preparations for adult sexual activities including ordinary facts of reproductive life and personal hygiene have not been met before.

In general, sexual activities of adolescent boys and girls are less than those of their peers. The majority of female MMC patients with a sensorial level below L2 will have sexual sensations and orgasms, whereas this is correct for only about one fifth of those with higher levels and urinary incontinence. Male MMC patients with intact sacral reflexes will have erections and ejaculations and be potent if combined with urinary continence. Absent penis sensibility in lesions below L1 can be resolved by bypass for sensorial innervation of the penis (connection of the ilioinguinal nerve with dorsal penis nerve). In case of absent sacral reflexes, potency may be present in two thirds of those with levels below D10 and <15 % with levels above D10.

Although sexual potency may be achieved with intracorporeal injection or sildenafil in reduced doses, it may be associated with azoospermia.

Pregnancy and labor are possible in female MMC patients, although the outcome is impaired by several risks: neural tube defect and prematurity (about one third) of the offsprings, urinary tract infection, increased bladder dysfunction, and immobility, and C-section due to disproportion (>1/3) of the mother.

35.2   Minimal Spinal Dysraphism (Occult Spinal Dysraphism, Spina Bifida Occulta)

Pathology, Occurrence

Minimal spinal dysraphism encompasses only minor alterations in closure of skin #, muscles, spine, meninges, and spinal cord, and Arnold-Chiari II malformation and hydrocephalus are usually not associated with it in contrast to myelomeningocele.

Spina bifida occulta is observed in >25 % of the MMC incidence without prenatal diagnosis. In developed countries, the incidence equals that of MMC (0.35:1,000 live births).

Clinical Significance

- Minimal spinal dysraphism is usually not recognized by prenatal ultrasound.
- Minimal spinal dysraphism is often a progressive disorder that leads to many and diverse symptoms and signs, for example, foot deformity, disorders of gait, and urinary incontinence.
- The single symptoms and signs are treated separately by different specialists and without lasting success in ignorance about minimal spinal dysraphism.

Forms

Many of the used terms are special forms of minimal spinal dysraphism, for example, subcutaneous lumbosacral lipoma, or describe a possible pathogenetic mechanism, for example, tethered spinal cord. Therefore, conceptional confusion may arise.

- Lipomeningomyelocele: A subcutaneous lipoma of the lumbosacral region tapers in a stalk ## that enters the subdural space through a hole in the dorsal fascia and dura and enlarges again to become a lipoma connected with the medullary cone or the cauda equina. In addition, a pouch of the arachnoid may lead through the stalk to the subcutaneous lipoma. Intraspinal lipoma belongs to the same disorder.
- The filum terminale is enlarged and tight, and the end of the conus lies very distal.

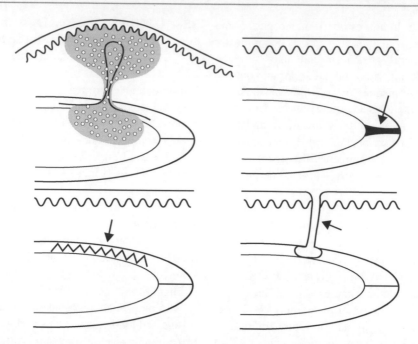

Fig. 35.2 Drawings of the pathoanatomical types of minimal spinal dysraphism. *Top left*: subcutaneous lipoma which continues like a sandglass through an opening in the fascia and dura to the conus and cauda equina. Both isolated intradural and subcutaneous lipoma occur as well. A protrusion of the arachnoid may proceed into the subcu-taneous lipoma. *Top right*: the terminal filum is tight and leads to tethering of the conus during growth. *Bottom left*: tight adhesions between conus and dura may also be present and lead to tethering. *Bottom right*: a fistula communicates between the skin surface and the intradural space with or without associated dermoid cyst

- Tight adhesions exist between dura and conus and may continue as a stalk to the subcutaneous tissue.
- A dermal sinus enters the intradural space or conus and may be associated with a dermoid cyst (Fig. 35.2).

In the individual case, any combination of these anomalies occurs in the four forms of minimal spinal dysraphism. They may be combined as well with diastematomyelia with or without an osseous spur, anterior MMC, and multiple malformations of the spine such as osseous spina bifida occulta, vertebral or sacral anomalies, and defects. The primary malformation of the spinal cord and of the overlying structures, and especially compression and traction of the conus (tethered spinal cord), leads to progressive neurological deficits and acute deteriorations during childhood and thereafter. The end of the conus lies usually at birth at the upper border of the third lumbar vertebral body (L1 and 2) and at the end of pubertal growth at the lower end of the first lumbar vertebral body (with variations of D10/L1 to the middle of L2). In spinal dysraphism, this cranial ascent is hindered and leads to tethered spinal cord. The underlying mechanism is related to impairment of oxidative metabolism. Traction and compression with secondary tethering is observed in 30 % of the spina bifida cases.

Clinical Presentation

The symptoms and signs of minimal spinal dysraphism consist of *two groups, those that are static and present from the beginning and act as markers of minimal spinal dysraphism (1) and those that are dynamic (2)*, often not recognizable in infancy. They appear slowly with advancing age with rapid progression during periods of rapid growth (pubertal growth spurt at latest) or after a trauma (although osseous spina bifida is not at increased risk for injury). Damage to spinal cord occurs at any age and is often progressive, and the observed symptoms are either single or combined:

- Congenital skin disorders of the lumbosacral region and malformations recognizable on plain x-rays or CT of the spine (1)

- Neurological and orthopedic disorders of the lower extremities and lower trunk (2)
- Neurological disorders of bladder and anorectal function (3)

Congenital Skin Disorders (>2/3 of the Cases)
They include: Lipomas (smooth asymmetrical masses that are bulging the skin and movable to the side), vascular malformations and hemangiomas (if two or more are present #, minimal spinal dysraphism will be present in 60 %), pigmented nevi, hairy patches #, skin scar like parchment, skin pit # and dermal sinus, cutaneous tails # or tail-like cutaneous appendages (usually midline lumbosacral region), and asymmetrical gluteal cleft. About 50 % are associated with meningocele or spina bifida occulta.

Neurological and Orthopedic Disorders
They concern often one leg or asymmetrically legs or buttocks: sensorial and motor deficits (muscular atrophy and diminished strength, absent tendon reflex or signs of spasticity, minimal sensorial deficit of the sacral dermatomes), deformities of the joints (e.g., neurogenic clubfoot #), lumbago, or scoliosis.

Neurogenic   Bladder   and   Anorectal Dysfunction may lead to urinary incontinence or constipation #. The individual type of bladder dysfunction may be different and can only be classified by urodynamics. They may lead to obstruction and reflux of the upper urinary tract, urinary tract infection, and renal insufficiency.

Urodynamics are usually normal in infancy and display rarely partial denervation of urethral sphincter or absent sphincter relaxation during detrusor contractions. In older children, extensive denervation of the sphincter and/or acontractile detrusor is mostly observed although detrusor sphincter dyssynergy may occur as well.

Differential Diagnosis, Work-Ups
It includes sequels of **poliomyelitis, cerebral palsy, spinal cord injury or tumor, late tethering after surgery of myelomeningocele**, and **spinal neurenteric cyst**. In contrast to the two first disorders, only spinal cord tumor, tethering after surgery of MMC, and neurenteric cyst are

progredient. The dermal sinus of the coccyx has usually no connection to the intradural space and is not a marker of minimal spinal dysraphism. The differential diagnosis of radiological imaging encompasses **sacral agenesis** and **split cord syndrome**.

The concept of the so-called **occult tethered cord syndrome** (=normally located conus tethered by a terminal filum) is controversial. It presents with neurogenic urinary incontinence that may be ameliorated by early surgery. Ultrasound up to 3 months of life is necessary to its recognition.

Spinal cord injury occurs less frequently than myelomeningocele and more frequently than spinal tumor. It is mainly caused by motor vehicle accident, falls (not necessarily from the height), diving or sports, penetrating injury, and by birth injury. The spinal cord damage is more frequently complete than partial and leads to flaccid para- or quadriplegia with hypotonia, areflexia, and sensorial loss or to focal deficits. Spinal cord injury **at birth** occurs in difficult deliveries due to abnormal cephalic (face) or breech presentation. The injury occurs mostly above C4 and less frequently below T4. Absent spontaneous breathing and flaccid quadriplegia or paraplegia after a difficult birth is typical for spinal cord injury and is confirmed by ultrasound and MRI.

The younger the child, the more the **cervical spine** is involved and the more spinal cord injuries without radiological abnormality of the skeleton (**SCIWORA**) may be observed with possible occurrence of delayed deficits (with or without initial transient neck pain or stiffness and neurological signs). The neurological deficit may be overlooked in cerebral contusion or multisystemic organ injury or in small children with reflectory withdrawal on pinching the legs. Neurogenic shock with hypotension, bradycardia, and warm extremities, Horner's syndrome, or other signs may point to (cervical) spinal cord injury.

The flaccid paraplegia is often replaced within several weeks by hyperreflexia and spasticity, and the initially acontractile bladder with a nonreactive sphincter by an overactive detrusor and sphincter dyssynergy or less frequently neither detrusor nor sphincter function is present.

The **work-ups** include plain x-ray of the spine and/or CT for evaluation of the skeleton and MRI for the depiction of the spinal cord. **Treatment** is mainly conservative except for penetrating injuries, reduction and stabilization of instable fractures, or irreducible luxations and includes initial resuscitation similar to head injury, insertion of gastric tube, and permanent bladder catheter.

During rehabilitation, the following **complications** must be considered: spontaneous fractures, contractures of the lower limbs, scoliosis, funnel chest, nephrolithiasis, and urinary tract infection. If the spinal cord injury is not associated with severe brain injury or preexisting cerebral disorder, the outlook for independence in daily life, schooling, apprenticeship, and partnership is good for the majority of patients. Recovery of paraplegia does not occur in complete lesions, whereas some recovery with lowering of the sensory level has been observed in patients with partial injury. Birth injury of spinal cord: Absence of respiration within 24 h and recovery of quadriplegia within 3 months mean respirator dependence and permanent quadriplegia.

Benign and malignant **spinal (intramedullary) tumors** lead after a shorter or a longer time (months to years) to localized nocturnal spinal pain, torticollis or scoliosis, myelopathic or radicular signs (gait alterations, paresthesia, focal paresis), and rarely to disorders of micturition or defecation.

MRI as primary work-up examination displays in the most common astrocytoma decreased density on T1-weighted images and associated cystic dilatation of the spinal cord above or below the mass, and distict enhancement of and cysts within the less frequent ependymomas. Both tumors need complete resection that is easier in the latter tumor.

Sacral agenesis means partial or complete absence of the sacral vertebral bodies (and several lumbar bones). It may be a part of minimal spinal dysraphism, isolated (e.g., in diabetic mother), or associated with **Currarino syndrome** (presacral mass, sacral agenesis, and anorectal malformation). Absence of the upper end of the gluteal cleft and flattened buttocks in the newborn and difficulty in toilet training later in life should alert the physician to sacral agenesis that is confirmed

by ultrasound, plain lateral x-ray of the lower spine, or MRI. Neurogenic bladder is observed in 90 % of children with either acontractile detrusor and complete sphincter denervation (incontinence) or overactive detrusor combined with sphincter dyssynergy (urinary tract infections and reflux). Treatment should consider the type of neurogenic bladder.

Split cord syndrome (diastematomyelia, diplomyelia) is divided into two types: Type I malformation consists of two dural sacs and a bony or fibrocartilaginous spur and type II of a single dural sac and intradural fibrous bands. Some diastematomyelias are recognizable by an osseous spur and bifid vertebral body on plain x-ray. The intervening mesenchymal elements contribute to symptomatic spinal dysraphism and need early untethering of the spinal cord.

Eighty-three to hundred percent of MMC patients have **after spina bifida repair** an asymptomatic in spite of low lying conus, and 13 % will develop tethered cord syndrome (prevalence of tethered cord syndrome after lipomeningocele is 23 %). Sensory loss or change of bladder or bowel function is claimed as indication of tethering, but the symptoms and signs of tethering are indistinguishable in myelomeningocele from other possible causes which must also be considered before revision. Such disorders are shunt insufficiency, intraspinal findings as in minimal spinal dysraphism, neurenteric or arachnoid cyst, and spinal cord hypoplasia or hydromyelia and syrinx.

Work-Ups

If the quoted neurological or orthopedic disorders are combined with malformations of the lumbosacral spine, minimal spinal dysraphism may be expected in about 90 %.

Such radiological anomalies (visible on plain x-rays or CT) are osseous spina bifida (occurs in <20 to >30 %), interpeduncular distances above the normal values visible by the naked eye or comparison with normal values, diastematomyelia, and vertebral or sacral defects. An increase of the lumbosacral angle (horizontal sacrum) may be a sign of tethering in open and minimal spinal dysraphism.

For confirmation of suspected minimal spinal dysraphism, **ultrasound** in the newborn and early infancy and **MRI** # in older children are the main diagnostic tools. In some of the patients, not only a tight filum but elongated conus may be visible as well. In addition, urodynamics, ultrasound of bladder and upper urinary tract, and anorectal pressure measurement are necessary that can be used for follow-up similar to precise neurological examination.

Treatment Prognosis

All children need lifelong multidisciplinary follow-up for recognition of development of back pain, neurological deficits (distal motor weakness and trophic and sensory disturbances in the legs), bladder and/or bowel dysfunction, and scoliosis or foot deformities or deterioration of pre-existing deficit especially in childhood and at puberty.

Surgery is **indicated** in spinal congenital dermal sinus and in minimal spinal dysraphism with appearance of upper motor signs and/or progression of lower motor signs and/or appearance of bladder and/or bowel dysfunction.

Indication of surgery is **controversial** because of the possible side effects (local and neurological complications and re-tethering) in asymptomatic children, in children with signs of spinal cord tethering but normal radiological finding or with stable deficits.

The observation that some asymptomatic children especially infants remain asymptomatic after prophylactic surgery, additional intraspinal anomalies are present (for instance, dermoid cyst, complex lipoma containing tissue of the three germinal layers, diastematomyelia), and that surgery is less laborious in small children are arguments in favor of prophylactic surgery especially in children with congenital lumbosacral lipomas or low conus (at L3 vertebral body level or lower) and short and thick filum.

Most children with minimal spinal dysraphism become symptomatic during childhood, at puberty, or thereafter, >35 % will have neurogenic bladder and at least 30 % of not symptomatic children develops during childhood and as late as at puberty signs of spinal cord tethering.

For surgery, magnification and neurological monitoring by evoked potentials is necessary. In case of **lipomyelomeningocele and congenital lumbosacral lipoma**, the subcutaneous part, the stalk, and as far as possible the intradural lipoma are removed (##), associated anomalies are corrected, and additional untethering and dural plasty are performed (the conus or cauda equina should be completely surrounded by CSF to avoid re-tethering).

The medullary conus jumps upward after operative division of **a thickened tight terminal filum**.

Neurogenic bladder needs similar measures as in MMC depending on the type of disorder.

Prognosis depends on the age and local findings at surgery, and whether the child is asymptomatic or has already deficits. Existing deficits have been maintained in two thirds on short-term follow-up and ameliorated or made worse each in one sixth, and no deficits have been observed on short-term follow-up so far in asymptomatic and early in infancy operated cases in an older study. The neurological symptoms and lumbago respond in general well to decompression in contrast to neurogenic bladder that does not improve beyond infancy.

Surgery in symptomatic children stabilizes the neurological deficits in the majority and improves them in about 50 % in newer studies. Precise data are available for congenital lumbosacral lipoma and spinal congenital dermal sinuses: Out of 93 patients with the former diagnosis and a follow-up of >5 years, 42 % have been asymptomatic and 58 % symptomatic before surgery. Significant improvement was attained in 50 and 100 % of symptomatic lipomas of the conus and filum, respectively. The asymptomatic cases with lipoma of the conus were still asymptomatic in ≥50 % after >5 years, and all were asymptomatic in lipoma of the filum. Ninety-two percent of the children >1 years of age had neurological deficits in the cohort with spinal congenital sinus # versus 50 % of the children <1 year of age. Tethered cord was present at surgery in 22, inclusion tumor in 4, and arachnoiditis in 6 of the 28 children of whom 43 % were neurologically improved, 39 % intact, 7 % remained neurologically unchanged, and 11 % were worse at a mean follow-up of 2.9 years.

35.3　Sacrococcygeal Teratoma

Occurrence

Albeit rare, sacrococcygeal teratoma is the most common tumor of the newborn, and this location belongs with almost 50 % to the most frequent site of germ cell tumors. More than two thirds are girls.

Clinical Significance

- Sacrococcygeal teratoma with prenatal diagnosis must be followed in short intervals until birth because of possible shock (spontaneous bleedings and intratumoral vascular shunts), hydrops fetalis, and disproportion at birth.
- After birth, spontaneous hemorrhage may occur at any time and risk of malignant degeneration increases with time. Therefore, rapid resection is indicated in the first days after birth.
- Sacrococcygeal teratoma with exclusively presacral location (type IV) may escape early diagnosis if the possibility of presacral sacrococcygeal teratoma is not considered in the differential diagnosis of postnatal constipation or disorders of micturition.

Forms and Types

Overall, about 50 % of teratomas are mature, <25 % immature, and >25 % malignant. The following types of tumor extension are observed arranged in order of frequency: The teratoma lies visible in the region of the buttocks with possible presacral elements (type I); the external tumor is combined with a significant intrapelvic component (type II); the tumor has external, pelvic, and significant intra-abdominal extension (type III), and the tumor is exclusively presacral (type IV).

Clinical Findings

Instead of normal appearing buttocks, a large asymmetrical, solid and cystic subcutaneous mass extends from the anterior aspect of the coccyx in caudal and dorsal direction # with anterior displacement of the anus #. In types (I), II–IV, a firm mass is felt with the small finger behind the anorectum and a lower abdominal tumor in type II and III on abdominal palpation.

Usually, motor and sensorial function of the legs is intact as well as bladder and anorectal function. Type IV teratoma may be overlooked because no tumor is visible from the outside. *Neonatal constipation, disorders of micturition, and some weaknesses of the legs that are followed by rectal examination lead to its detection.*

Prenatal diagnosis by ultrasound is increasingly observed (large mass at the lower end of the spine). Polyhydramnios, fetal hydrops, or stillbirth in the last weeks of pregnancy and disproportion, heart failure (because of intratumoral shunting), intratumoral hemorrhage, and tumor rupture at delivery may endanger the fetus.

Differential Diagnosis, Work-Ups

Depending on the type of main extension, different differential diagnoses must be considered: in types I–III, meningocele, lipomyelocele, myelocystocele, vascular malformations, lipoma, or soft tissue tumor of the buttocks; and in type IV, anterior meningocele or rectal duplication; and in type II and III, lower abdominal tumor.

Clinical findings and radiological imaging (CT or MRI) permit usually typifying of the teratoma and delineation from the other differential diagnoses ([myelo] meningocele or myelocystocele has water and lipomyelomeningocele lipoma density). Markers of possible malignant components are abnormal values of α-fetoprotein and β-hCG. Plain abdominal x-rays display irregular spotted calcification in 40 % and anterior displacement of the air-filled anorectum.

Treatment, Prognosis

Every teratoma with prenatal diagnosis needs close supervision during pregnancy, at birth, and thereafter because of the inherent risks. Tumors larger than 5 cm diameter after the 32nd week of gestation need C-section and all newborns supervision on the ICU. Fetal surgery with tumor resection is rarely necessary.

Anesthesia needs special supervision of cardiovascular and respiratory system, and temperature, safe venous accesses, sufficient cross-matched blood, preoperative retrograde irrigation and package of the anorectum, and transurethral catheter.

Surgery is performed in prone position with raised lower abdomen with flexed hips and dropped feet using a lithotomy attachment of the operating table. After an inverted Y-incision of the skin, the superior margins of the incision are dissected and the tumor is completely resected close to its pseudocapsule starting with the complete removal of the coccyx. After ligature and division of the midsacral artery and/or branches of the hypogastric artery, the tumor is removed from above downward including a possible presacral extension. On the dorsal aspect of the tumor, the pseudocapsule is dissected by diathermy from the subcutaneous fat and extremely thinned muscles of the buttocks that should be carefully preserved. Dissection of the anterior aspect is more difficult because of the close proximity of the rectum that can be felt because of package. After resection of tumor including some overlying skin, the levator ani is reconstructed and reattached by sutures of its ends behind the rectum, and the skin is closed leaving some drainage of the different spaces.

Relatively small and low presacral tumor (type IV) may be resected by a PSAR approach. Large abdominal components (types II and III) need additional abdominal access.

For final diagnosis, a throughout histological examination of the whole tumor must be performed.

Mayor risks of surgery are shock due to intratumoral bleeding or shunting, and incomplete resection leaving minimal residual tumor.

Long-term follow-ups are therefore necessary. Final bladder and anorectal function are normal, although disorders of micturition (urinary retention) may be observed for a variable time.

The tumor prognosis depends on the time of surgery, completeness of resection, and final histological work-up. If the age is <2 months, the tumor is in <10 and 10 % respectively malignant and if the age is >2 months, the tumor is in about 50 % and two thirds malignant. Those with mature or immature histology have usually a permanent cure although recurrences are observed in <5 % of the mature forms and in <15 % in the immature forms within the first 2 years after surgery (immature forms may produce malignant germ cell tumors).

35.4   Dermal Sinus of the Coccyx

Occurrence, Clinical Significance

A skin pit over the coccyx between the buttocks is quite frequently observed and already in the newborn if examined carefully. Its clinical significance is as follows:

- Dermal sinus of the coccyx may be considered by mistake as a marker of spina bifida occulta.
- Dermal sinus of the coccyx can lead to recurrent infection and abscess.

Clinical Presentation

The appearance of such sinuses is quite variable extending from a superficial and shallow pit to a small opening of a deep sinus tract that leads to the periosteum of the coccyx #. Occasionally, some hair and sebum are visible at the depth of the pit corresponding to an associated dermoid cyst. *The blind end of the dermal sinus can be felt with a probe and the underlying coccyx with the fingers* on clinical examination.

Differential Diagnosis, Work-Ups

A **dermal sinus that is a part of minimal spinal dysraphism** lies *more cranially in the lumbosacral region*. Regardless of their depth, those below the top of the intergluteal crease never end intraspinally.

The so-called **pilonidal sinus** of adolescents and young adults is an acquired disorder because of inflammation of the hair follicles. The term "jeep disease" should be better named "cycle disease" because it is caused today mainly by intensive cycling, especially in sports. *Local abscess and pain with serous or bloody-purulent secretions are the symptoms, and its asymmetrical location between the buttocks is combined with multiple fistulas as the typical local findings.*

Treatment, Prognosis

Deep sinuses with small openings and pits or sinuses combined with dermoid cyst need elective complete excision including the periosteum of the coccyx after resolution of a possible infection. Recurrences are unusual in contrast to the pilonidal sinus that is best treated by secondary healing after complete excision. Histological examination of the sinus tract and especially of its base is recommended because of the possibility of dermoid cyst or tumor such as ependymoma.

Webcodes

The following webcodes can be used on www.psurg.net for further images and data.

3501 Lumbosacral myelomeningocele (MMC)	3517 Lipomyelomeningocele
3502 Thoracolumbar MMC	3518 Vascular malformation, minimal spinaldysraphism
3503 Sacral meningocele	3519 Hairy patch, minimal spinal dysraphism
3504 Lipomyelomeningocele	3520 Skin pit, minimal spinal dysraphism
3505 Medullary plate, at the level of spine	3521 Tail, minimal spinal dysraphism
3506 Medullary plate, at the level of cyst	3522 Neurogenic clubfoot, minimal spinaldysraphism
3507 High lesion with reflex activity	3523 Constipation, minimal spinal dysraphism
3508 Neurogenic club foot	3524 MRI, lipomyelomeningocele with conus involvement
3509 Stepping response	3525 Lipomyelomeningocele, intraoperative conus tethering and
3510 Rectal and vaginal prolapse, pelvic floor paresis	3526 Subcutaneous and intraspinal/intradural part resected
3511 Widened interpeduncular distances	3527 Dermal sinus at surgery
3512 Bladder in untreated neurogenic bladder	3528 Large sacrococcygeal teratoma
3513 Upper urinary tract before	3529 Perineal view of sacrococcygeal teratoma
3514 And after CIC in neurogenic bladder	3530 Dermal sinus of the coccyx
3515 Thoracic minimal spinal dysraphism, diastematomyelia	
3516 Stalk of minimal spinal dysraphism withlipoma	

Bibliography

Section 35.1

Adzick NS (2010) Fetal myelomeningocele: natural history, pathophysiology, and in-utero intervention. Semin Fetal Neonatal Med 15:9–14.

Bauer SB (2008) Neurogenic bladder: etiology and assessment. Pediatr Nephrol 23:541–551

Buyse G, Verpoorten C, Vereecken R, Casaer P (1995) Treatment of neurogenic bladder dysfunction in infants and children with neurospinal dysraphism with clean intermittent (self) catheterization and optimized intravesical oxybutynin hydrochloride therapy. Eur J Pediatr Surg 5(Suppl I):31–34

Casari EF, Fantino AG (1998) A longitudinal study of cognitive abilities and achievement status of children with myelomeningocele and their relationship with clinical types. Eur J Pediatr Surg 5(Suppl I):52–54

Cochrane DD, Irwin B, Chambers K (2001) Clinical outcomes that fetal surgery for myelomeningocele needs to achieve. Eur J Pediatr Surg 11(Suppl I):18–20

Dave S, Salle JL (2008) Current status of bladder neck reconstruction. Curr Opin Urol 18:419–424

Deshpande AV, Sampang R, Smith GH (2010) Study of botulinum toxin A in neurogenic bladder due to spina bifida in children. ANZ J Surg 80:250–253

Dillon CM, Davis BE, Duguay S, Seidel KD, Shurtleff DB (2000) Longevity of patients born with myelomeningocele. Eur J Pediatr Surg 10(Suppl I):33–34

Freeman JM (1974) Practical management of myelomeningocele. University Park Press, Baltimore

Honein MA, Paulozzi LJ, Mathews TH et al (2001) Impact of folic acid fortification of the US food supply on the occurrence of neural tube defects. JAMA 285:2981–2986

Kaiser G, Rüdeberg A (1986) Comments on the management of newborns with spina bifida cystica – active treatment or no treatment. Z Kinderchir 41:141–143

Knab K, Langhans B, Behrens R, Strehl AE (2001) The neuropathic bowel in spina bifida – a cross-sectional study in 226 patients. Eur J Pediatr Surg 11(Suppl): S41–S42

Mc Lone D et al (1985) Concepts in the management of spina bifida. In: Humphreys RP (ed) Concept pediat neurosurg. Karger, Basel

Patricolo M, Noia G, Pomini F, Perilli L, Iannace E, Catesini C, Mancuso S, Caione P (2002) Fetal surgery for spina bifida aperta: to be or not to be? J Pediatr Surg 12:S22–S24

Peacock WJ (1998) Management of spina bifida, hydrocephalus, central nervous system infections, and intractable epilepsy. In: O'Neill JA Jr et al (eds) Pediatric surgery, vol II, 5th edn. Mosby, St Louis

Schulman SL, Duckett JW (1998) Disorders of bladder function. In: O'Neill JA Jr et al (eds) Pediatric surgery, vol II, 5th edn. Mosby, St Louis

Shurtleff DB (2000) 44 years experience with management of myelomeningocele: presidential address, society of research into hydrocephalus and spina bifida. Eur J Pediatr Surg 10(Suppl I):5–8

Shurtleff DB, Duguay S, Duguay G, Moskowitz D, Weinberger E, Roberts T, Loeser J (1997) Epidemiology of tethered cord with meningomyelocele. Eur J Pediatr Surg 7(Suppl I):7–11

Sinha CK, Butler C, Haddad M (2008) Left antegrade continent enema (LACE): review of the literature. Eur J Pediatr Surg 18:215–218

Stark GD (1971) Neonatal assessment of the child with myelomeningocele. Arch Dis Child 46:539–548

Woodhouse CRJ (2008) Myelomeningocele: neglected aspects. Pediatr Nephrol 23:1223–1231

Section 35.2

Ackerman LL, Menezes AH (2003) Spinal congenital dermal sinuses: a 30-year experience. Pediatrics 112:641–647

Ackerman LL, Menezes AH, Follett KA (2002) Cervical and thoracic dermal sinus tracts. A case series and review of the literature. Pediatr Neurosurg 37: 137–147

Bruce DA, Schut L (1979) Spinal lipomas in infancy and childhood. Childs Brain 5:192–203

Cornette L, Verpoorten C, Lagae L, Plets C, Van Calenbergh F, Casaer P (1998) Closed spinal dysraphism: a review on diagnosis and treatment. Eur J Paediatr Neurol 2:179–185

Dias MS, Pang D (1995) Split cord malformations. Neurosurg Clin N Am 6:339–358

Drake JM (2007) Surgical management of the tethered spinal cord – walking the fine line. Neurosurg Focus 23:E4

Garg N, Sampath S, Yasha TC, Chandramouli BA, Devi BI, Kovoor JM (2008) Is total excision of spinal neurenteric cysts possible? Br J Neurosurg 22:241–251

Guggisgerg D, Hadj-Rabia S, Viney C, Bodemer C, Brunelle F, Zerah M, Pierre-Kahn A, de Prost Y, Hamel-Teillac D (2004) Skin markers of occult spinal dysraphism in children: a review of 54 cases. Arch Dermatol 140:1109–1115

Hertzler DA 2nd, DePowell JJ, Stevenson CB, Mangano FT (2010) Tethered cord syndrome: a review of the literature from embryology to adult presentation. Neurosurg Focus 29:E1

Hoffman HJ, Hendrick EB, Humphreys RB (1976) The tethered spinal cord: its protean manifestation, diagnosis, and surgical correction. Childs Brain 2: 145–155

Humphreys RP (1991) Current trends in spinal dysraphism. Paraplegia 29:79–83

Lapras CL, Patet JD, Huppert J, Bret P, Mottolese C (1985) The tethered cord syndrome (experience of 58 cases). J Pediatr Neurosci 1:39–50

Liptak GS (1995) Tethered spinal cord: update of an analysis of published articles. Eur J Pediatr Surg 5(Suppl II):21–23

Lowe LH, Johanek AJ, Moore CW (2007) Sonography of the neonatal spine: part 2, spinal disorders. Am J Roentgenol 188:739–744

Morandi X, Mercier P, Fournier HD, Brassier G (1999) Dermal sinus and intramedullary spinal cord abscess. Report of two cases and review of the literature. Childs Nerv Syst 15:202–206

Pierre-Kahn A, Zerah M, Renier D, Cinalli G, Sainte-Rose C, Lellouch-Tubiana A, Brunelle F, Le Merrer M, Giudicelli Y, Pichon J, Kleinknecht B, Nataf F (1997) Con-genital lumbosacral lipomas. Childs Nerv Syst 13:298–334; discussion 335

Sattar MT, Bannister CM, Turnbull IW (1996) Occult spinal dysraphism – the common combination of lesions and the clinical manifestations in 50 patients. Eur J Pediatr Surg 6(Suppl I):10–14

Savage JJ, Casey JN, McNeill IT, Sherman JH (2010) Neurenteric cysts of the spine. J Craniovertebr Junction Spine 1:58–63

Shurtleff DB, Duguay S, Duguay G, Moskowitz D, Weinberger E, Roberts T, Loeser J (1997) Epidemiology of tethered cord with meningomyelocele. Eur J Pediatr Surg 7(Suppl I):7–11

Singh DK, Kumar B, Sinha VD, Bagaria HR (2008) The human tail: rare lesion with occult spinal dysraphism – a case report. J Pediatr Surg 43:e41–e43, Comment in: J pediatr Surg (2009) 44:477–478

Steinbok P (1995) Dysraphic lesions of the cervical spinal cord. Neurosurg Clin N Am 6:367–376

Steinbok P, MacNeily AE (2007) Section of the terminal filum for occult tethered cord syndrome: toward a scientific answer. Neurosurg Focus 23:E5

Wraige E, Borzyskowski M (2002) Investigation of daytime wetting: when is spinal cord imaging indicated? Arch Dis Child 87:151–155

Section 35.2 Differential Diagnosis

Bucher HU, Boltshauser E, Friderich J, Isler W (1980) Traumatische Quer-schnittslähmung im Kindesalter. Schweiz med Wschr 110:331–337

Cirak B, Ziegfeld S, Knight VM, Chang D, Avellino AM, Paidas CN (2004) Spinal cord injuries in children. J Pediatr Surg 39:607–612

Ebisu T, Odake G, Fujimoto M, Ueda S, Tsujii H, Morimoto M, Sawada T (1990) Neurenteric cysts with meningomyelocele or meningocele. Split notochord syndrome. Childs Nerv Syst 6:465–467

Harris BH, Stylianos S (1998) Special considerations in trauma: child abuse and birth in-juries. In: O'Neill JA Jr et al (eds) Pediatric surgery, vol I, 5th edn. Mosby, St Louis

Kumar R, Jain R, Rao KM, Hussain N (2001) Intraspinal neuroenteric cysts – report of three paediatric cases. Childs Nerv syst 17:584–588

Lee JH, Sung IY, Kang JY, Park SR (2009) Characteristic of pediatric-onset spinal cord injury. Pediatr Int 51: 254–257

Luerssen TG (1998) Central nervous system injuries. In: O'Neill JA Jr et al (eds) Pediatric surgery, vol I, 5th edn. Mosby, St Louis

Sutton LN (1998) Central nervous system tumors and vascular malformations. In: O'Neill JA Jr et al (eds) Pediatric surgery, vol I, 5th edn. Mosby, St Louis

Vialle R, Piétin-Vialle C, Vinchon M, Dauger S, Ilharreborde B, Glorion C (2008) Birth-related spinal cord injuries: a multicentric review of nine cases. Childs Nerv Syst 24:79–85

Section 35.3

De Backer A, Erpicum P, Philippe P, Demarche M, Otte JB, Schwagten K, Vande-lanotte M, Docx M, Rose T, Verhelst A, De Caluwé D, Deconinck P (2001)

Sacro-coccygeal teratoma: results of a retrospective multicentric study in Belgium and Luxembourg. Eur J Pediatr Surg 11:182–185

Tapper D, Sawin R (1998) Teratomas and other germ cell tumors. In: O'Neill JA Jr et al (eds) Pediatric surgery, vol I, 5th edn. Mosby, St Louis

Section 35.4

Martinez-Lage JF, Villarejo Ortega FJ, Galarza M, Felipe-Murcia M, Almagro MJ (2010) Coccygeal dermal sinus: clinical relevance and management. An Pediatr (Barc) 73:352–356

Perruchoud C, Vuilleumier H, Givel JC (2002) Pilonidal sinus: how to choose between excision and open granulation versus excision and primary closure. Swiss Surg 8:255–258

Blended Learning and Formative Assessments for Specialist Training and Continuing Education in Pediatric Surgery

36

This chapter discusses the synergy between this book and the accompanying online resource psurg.net. It points out to the reader the possibilities and advantages of the concept of blended learning as well as the effects of formative assessments on the successful deepening of knowledge in pediatric surgery. These aspects are then connected to the theoretical basis for teaching in medical education.

36.1 Blended Learning with psurg.net

At the end of each chapter in this book, there is a reference list pointing to illustrations and secondary texts which can be accessed on the internet at psurg.net. Each reference has a number – the so-called webcode – and can be accessed by simply entering the code at psurg.net. The presented online contents relating to pediatric surgery go beyond in depth and width the limitations to which the respective topics in the book chapters are bound; also, being an online medium, their structure is different. While the book chapters initiate and maintain a linear, self-contained reading and learning process with a sharp focus and text-centered knowledge transfer complemented by illustrations, the online medium psurg.net inverts the signs, as it were in the center are pictures – photographs and illustrations – with texts and captions being their complements. On-screen reading and learning is not necessarily

linear anymore; exploration or specific research (e.g., with full-text search) comes to the fore.

This media and method mix (blending) combines the best of both worlds: the unsurpassed readability of textual information on paper with its focus- and concentration-enhancing linearity teams up with the potential of online media to provide effectively and efficiently large amounts of image material and to offer a high degree of interactivity. This is not an end in itself but should be seen as supportive to learning, for example, formative assessments with automatic analysis, or the search engine. Book and internet are an unbeatable team; none can do without the other.

According to Sauter and Bender (2004), blended learning refers to a form of learning which aims at a sensible combination of traditional lectures given to a live audience and modern forms of e-learning. Its concept combines the flexibility and effectiveness of electronic learning with the social aspects of face-to-face communication and, where appropriate, practical learning activities. In this form of learning, different teaching methods and media and different approaches in learning theory coexist. A more general use of the term "blended learning" is the educationally and economically sensible combination of various methods and media in the context of teaching and learning approaches, in which traditional lectures are not necessarily a part of it. Considering all that, the combination of book and medium "Internet" can certainly be addressed as blended learning.

G.L. Kaiser, *Symptoms and Signs in Pediatric Surgery*,
DOI 10.1007/978-3-642-31161-1_36, © Springer-Verlag Berlin Heidelberg 2012

Blended learning's added value lies not only in making use of the different advantages of various methods and media but also in taking into account the learner's preferences.

36.2   Formative Assessment at psurg.net

This book is accompanied on the Internet by formative assessments. Thirty-seven questionnaires allow the reader to test online the status quo of his or her learning process. Two different methods are used: In the differential diagnosis module, the reader has to compare image pairs or sets of image pairs and assign the correct diagnosis. There, the "drill and practice" mode is supported, in which incorrect assignments automatically prompt the repetition of the problem. The presentation that follows discusses in detail the correct solution and the learner's assessment. The second modality offers multiple-choice questions on issues discussed in the book. These questionnaires are analyzed automatically, and items answered wrong are repeated.

Formative assessment's primary objective is not assessing the learner but providing a structured confrontation with the learning contents, allowing activating energy to flow into the learning process. In other words, looking up content during a formative assessment is not forbidden, but actually encouraged!

According to current theory, formative assessment is part of good teaching, and good formative assessments require the involvement of the tutor as a consultant. In the context of advanced training and continuing education with use of electronic media, measures must be taken to ensure that a consultation loop is feasible, not only because the receiver is physically separated from the transmitter but also because of the large number of students a tutor may be faced with in virtual space. In order to meet these educational demands, the readers of this book are given the opportunity to ask questions at psurg.net. Already asked questions and their answers are available at the specific forums so that 1-on-1 tutoring may evolve to or turn into a 1:n learning process or even an n:m teaching and learning process.

36.3   Selected Content for Undergraduate Medical Students

Pediatric surgery is a specialty that is implemented differently in the curricula of undergraduate medical students. To date, there is no conclusive answer to the question of which specific aspects of pediatric surgery are to be taught in what width and depth to future doctors. Students may weigh the contents of this book for relevance to their undergraduate curriculum by checking out the "learning path for students" at psurg.net. This path guides learners through pediatric surgery as a whole but tries to indicate the desirable breadth and depth of learning. The learning path for students is completed with an online quiz encouraging them to close discovered knowledge gaps.

36.4   Certification of Advanced Training and Continuing Education with psurg.net

Medical doctors can have their advanced training and continuing education certified in eight different fields of pediatric surgery at psurg.net. To that end, they go through tutorials, in which both the book at hand and psurg.net are employed. At the end of each thematic complex, there is a multiple-choice-type summative assessment. Awarded certificates can be filed with the professional societies for the purpose of getting credits. The time required to complete a subject area is 2–5 h.

Bibliography

Bell B, Cowie B (2001) The characteristics of formative assessment in science education. Sci Educ 85(5): 536–553

Black P, Wiliam D (1998) Assessment and classroom learning. Assess Educ 5(1):7–74

Black P, William D (2009) Developing the theory of formative assessment. Educ Assess Eval Account 21(1):5–31

Buck G et al (2010) Making formative assessment discernible to pre-service teachers of science. J Res Sci Teach 47(4):402–421

Chen I et al (2010) Augmenting a web-based learning environment through blending formative assessment services. J Web Eng 9(1):48–65

Cook D et al (2008) Internet-based learning in the health professions: a meta-analysis. JAMA 300(10): 1181–1196

Costa S et al (2010) A web-based formative assessment tool for masters students: a pilot study. Comput Educ 54(4):1248–1253

Fordis M et al (2005) Comparison of the instructional efficacy of internet-based CME with live interactive CME workshops: a randomized controlled trial. J Am Med Assoc 294(9):1043–1051

Harris J et al (2002) Can internet-based education improve physician confidence in dealing with domestic violence? Fam Plann Perspect 34(4):287–292

Hitzler P, Krötzsch M, Rudolph S (2009) Foundations of semantic web technologies. CRC Press, Boca Raton

Hmelo-Silver C, Barrows H (2006) Goals and strategies of a problem-based learning facilitator. Interdiscip J Probl Based Learn 1(1):21–39

Leung C, Mohan B (2004) Teacher formative assessment and talk in classroom contexts: assessment as discourse and assessment of discourse. Lang Test 21(3): 335–359

McDonald B, Boud D (2003) The impact of self-assessment on achievement: the effects of self-assessment training on performance in external examinations. Assess Educ Princ Policy Pract 10(2):209–220

Nicol D (2010) From monologue to dialogue: improving written feedback processes in mass higher education. Assess Eval High Educ 35(5):501–517

Nicol D, Macfarlane-Dick D (2006) Formative assessment and self-regulated learning: a model and seven principles of good feedback practice. Stud High Educ 31(2):199–218

Pachler N et al (2010) Formative e-assessment: practitioner cases. Comput Educ 54(3):715–721

Pryor J, Crossouard B (2010) Challenging formative assessment: disciplinary spaces and identities. Assess Eval High Educ 35(3):265–276

Ryan G et al (2007) Online CME: an effective alternative to face-to-face delivery. Med Technol Neurosurg 29(8):e251–e257

Sauter W et al (2004) Blended Learning. Effiziente Integration von E-Learning und Präsenztraining. Luchterhand, Unterschleissheim/München

Wang J et al (2010) Distance learning success – a perspective from socio-technical systems theory. Behav Inf Technol 29(3):321–329

Index

Printed by Publishers' Graphics LLC